At a Glance

T0342555

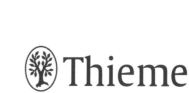

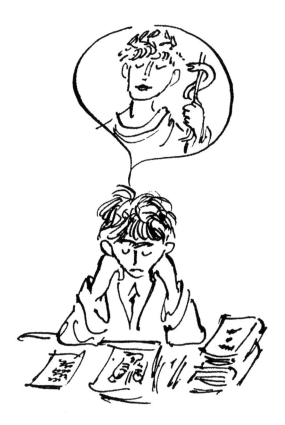

Illustration by Robert Wyss
(1925–2004)

Fundamentals of Neurology

An Illustrated Guide

2nd Revised and Updated Edition

Heinrich Mattle, MD
Professor of Neurology
Senior Consultant and formerly Vice-Chairman of the Department of Neurology
Head of the Neurological Policlinic and Stroke Center
Inselspital, University of Bern
Bern, Switzerland

Marco Mumenthaler†, MD
Professor of Neurology
Formerly Chairman of the Department of Neurology
Inselspital, University of Bern
Bern, Switzerland

With assistance from the
Institute for Diagnostic and Interventional Neuroradiology
Inselspital, University of Bern
Bern, Switzerland
Professor Jan Gralla, MD
Professor Gerhard Schroth, MD

Translated and adapted by Ethan Taub, MD

567 illustrations

Thieme
Stuttgart • New York • Delhi • Rio de Janeiro

Library of Congress Cataloging-in-Publication Data is available from the publisher.

This book is an authorized translation of the 4th German edition published and copyrighted 2015 by Georg Thieme Verlag, Stuttgart. Title of the German edition: Kurzlehrbuch Neurologie

Translator: Ethan Taub, MD, Department of Neurosurgery, University Hospital Basel, Basel, Switzerland

Illustrators: Karin Baum, Paphos, Cyprus; Malgorzata and Piotr Gusta, Paris, France; and Helmut Holtermann, Dannenberg, Germany

© 2017 by Georg Thieme Verlag KG

Thieme Publishers Stuttgart
Rüdigerstrasse 14, 70469 Stuttgart, Germany
+49 [0]711 8931 421, customerservice@thieme.de

Thieme Publishers New York
333 Seventh Avenue, New York, NY 10001 USA
+1 800 782 3488, customerservice@thieme.com

Thieme Publishers Delhi
A-12, Second Floor, Sector-2, Noida-201301
Uttar Pradesh, India
+91 120 45 566 00, customerservice@thieme.in

Thieme Publishers Rio de Janeiro, Thieme Publicações Ltda.
Edifício Rodolpho de Paoli, 25º andar
Av. Nilo Peçanha, 50 – Sala 2508
Rio de Janeiro 20020-906 Brasil
+55 21 3172 2297 / +55 21 3172 1896

Cover design: Thieme Publishing Group
Cover image: www.siemens.com/presse
Typesetting by DiTech Process Solutions, Mumbai, India

Printed in Germany by Beltz Grafische Betriebe   5 4 3 2 1

ISBN 978-3-13-136452-4

Also available as an e-book:
eISBN 978-3-13-202212-6

Important note: Medicine is an ever-changing science undergoing continual development. Research and clinical experience are continually expanding our knowledge, in particular our knowledge of proper treatment and drug therapy. Insofar as this book mentions any dosage or application, readers may rest assured that the authors, editors, and publishers have made every effort to ensure that such references are in accordance with **the state of knowledge at the time of production of the book.**

Nevertheless, this does not involve, imply, or express any guarantee or responsibility on the part of the publishers in respect to any dosage instructions and forms of applications stated in the book. **Every user is requested to examine carefully** the manufacturers' leaflets accompanying each drug and to check, if necessary in consultation with a physician or specialist, whether the dosage schedules mentioned therein or the contraindications stated by the manufacturers differ from the statements made in the present book. Such examination is particularly important with drugs that are either rarely used or have been newly released on the market. Every dosage schedule or every form of application used is entirely at the user's own risk and responsibility. The authors and publishers request every user to report to the publishers any discrepancies or inaccuracies noticed. If errors in this work are found after publication, errata will be posted at www.thieme.com on the product description page.

Some of the product names, patents, and registered designs referred to in this book are in fact registered trademarks or proprietary names even though specific reference to this fact is not always made in the text. Therefore, the appearance of a name without designation as proprietary is not to be construed as a representation by the publisher that it is in the public domain.

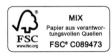

For our grandchildren Alma, Mio, and Jim, who give us a lot of joy

Heinrich Mattle, MD

For Stephi, with deep gratitude and love

Marco Mumenthaler, MD

Contents

Foreword

The second edition of *Fundamentals of Neurology* by Mattle and Mumenthaler is an excellent introductory neurology textbook that covers a broad range of topics related to how to approach patients with neurologic and muscular disorders. The initial chapters describe how to interview, examine, and order/interpret appropriate testing for such patients and then how to use the information to localize where in the nervous system the likely abnormality is. Subsequent chapters cover in detail a broad range of commonly encountered neurologic and muscular diseases. Major strengths of the book include the straightforward and easily understood presentation of the material, the excellent numerous figures and tables, and the comprehensive discussion of a wide range of neurologic and muscular disorders.

Fundamentals of Neurology is an appropriate introductory neurology textbook for medical students, trainees in a variety of medical disciplines, including neurology, and physicians in practice who need an easily accessible source of information about neurologic and muscular disorders. I highly recommend it to all of these physicians and physicians in training, and predict that it will be frequently used by them as they encounter patients with neurologic and muscular disorders.

Marc Fisher, MD
Professor, Department of Neurology
Beth Israel Deaconess Medical Center
and Harvard Medical School
Boston, Massachusetts, USA

Preface

Just a few decades ago, neurology and the neurosciences in general were contemplative disciplines oriented toward clinical phenomena and their correlation with pathoanatomic findings. Definitive diagnosis and treatment were only rarely feasible. Today, clinicians and researchers can use newly developed technologies to detect a wide variety of diseases of the central and peripheral nervous system. With the advent of improved diagnostic methods, computer technology, microtechnology, and new, highly effective drugs, neurology is no longer merely contemplative and has become a highly dynamic field. Many symptomatic and, often, causally directed treatments are now available for the treatment or even prevention of neurologic disease.

Fundamentals of Neurology provides a window onto the fascinating world of clinical neurology. Although students sometimes find neurology bewilderingly complicated, it is in fact firmly based on logic and the known correlations between clinical phenomena and the sites of the lesions that cause them. In the first few chapters of this book, the emphasis lies on fundamentals, the clinical examination, topical diagnosis, and the differential diagnosis of neurologic manifestations and syndromes. This knowledge equips the student to understand the subsequent chapters, which concern diseases of the central and peripheral nervous system. For most patients, the history and physical examination will point to the correct neurologic diagnosis. Targeted ancillary testing can be used to verify, document, and refine the presumptive diagnosis that has already been made on clinical grounds, and thus lead the way to proper treatment. Today more than ever, it bears repeating that the clinical neurologic evaluation is indispensable; the clinical findings provide a context for the proper interpretation of the ancillary test findings, so that the correct treatment can be chosen.

This second edition of *Fundamentals of Neurology* is based on the fourth edition of the German text by the same authors entitled *Kurzlehrbuch Neurologie*. The original English and German editions of this book were meant as a guide to the clinical neurologic examination and as a shorter version of our comprehensive textbook of neurology, of which the fourth and most recent English edition appeared in 2004, and the 13th German edition in 2013. A new layout, clear diagrams, and numerous tables make the material easier to understand and to learn. The text has been thoroughly updated, and many of the illustrations and diagrams have been revised or are entirely new.

Sadly, Professor Marco Mumenthaler did not live to see the publication of the second edition of *Fundamentals of Neurology*. He died in January 2016 of pneumonia, having suffered from progressively severe congestive heart failure for some time. His mind was alert and bright until the end.

Special thanks for this new English translation are due to Dr. Martina Habeck of Thieme Publishers and to the translator, Dr. Ethan Taub.

Heinrich Mattle, MD

Translator's Note

"What the heart devises belongs to man; what the tongue responds is from the Lord" (Proverbs 16:1). Language, a seemingly transcendental gift to humanity and the unique function of the human brain, has always been a source of fascination and wonderment —especially so for physicians and neurologists, for as long as these professions have existed. Translating a textbook of neurology is thus a peculiarly self-referential activity in which one mobilizes one's own (fallible) nervous system to recast a verbal description of itself, employing a different set of symbols but keeping the sense intact.

It has been my privilege to translate this thoroughly revised and updated work by Professor Mattle and our late, most honored colleague and teacher, Professor Mumenthaler. The new *Fundamentals of Neurology* incorporates classic clinical wisdom along with the most recent scientific advances. Like its predecessor, it is packed with vital information presented clearly and succinctly. The book should be a major help to its readers as they try to help those who suffer from neurologic disease.

Ethan Taub, MD

Professor Marco Mumenthaler, MD
July 23, 1925 – January 30, 2016

Marco Mumenthaler was born in Bern to Swiss parents, spent his childhood and youth in Italy and in the Swiss Canton of Ticino, studied medicine in Zurich and Basel, was trained as a neurologist in Paris and Zurich, and rounded out his training with a year of research at the National Institutes of Health in Bethesda, MD, USA. In 1962, he assumed the chairmanship of the Neurology Department at the Inselspital Bern, Switzerland, which he transformed from a small neurology service to an internationally renowned academic department and then successfully directed for nearly three decades, becoming Professor Emeritus in 1990. He served as Rector of the University of Bern from 1989 to 1991. In the years that followed, he had a private neurologic practice in Zurich and remained intensely active in continuing medical education.

Professor Mumenthaler's research interests were decidedly clinical. He published countless scientific papers, at first on muscle diseases, later on a wide variety of practically important topics in neurology. He also wrote many monographs and textbooks, which saw multiple editions, on general neurology, lesions of the peripheral nerves, and neurologic differential diagnosis. His textbook of neurology was translated into 14 languages.

Alongside his activities as a university teacher and head of a clinical department, Professor Mumenthaler was actively involved in university affairs, matters of national health policy, and humanitarian interventions. His lucid thinking and eloquence in multiple languages made him a persuasive speaker and a successful leader. From 1989 to 1993, as a member of the International Committee of the Red Cross in Geneva, he took part in many missions in war and crisis zones. His tireless and fruitful activities earned him many honors, including membership in numerous scientific societies in Switzerland

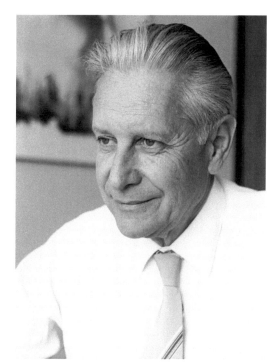

Professor Marco Mumenthaler, 1989

as well as in Europe and North America. He was Honorary President of the Swiss Neurological Society.

Professor Mumenthaler remained mentally alert and bright into old age but suffered increasingly under the physical limitations of congestive heart failure. He developed pneumonia in December 2015 and died of subsequent complications on January 30, 2016.

All of us who knew Marco Mumenthaler personally will remember him as an outstanding personality, as an exceptionally skilled physician, clinical researcher, and teacher, and as a dear friend. He made a major contribution to the development of neurology as we know it today.

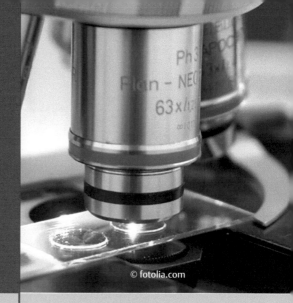

© fotolia.com

Chapter 1

Fundamentals

Introduction

Neurologic diseases can only be understood on the basis of the anatomy and physiology of the nervous system. Genetic abnormalities underlie many of them. Modern methods such as electron microscopy, electrophysiologic testing, and biochemical and molecular-biological analysis have yielded new insights into neural structure and function that are playing an increasingly important role in the classification and diagnosis of nervous diseases, as well as in their treatment.

It follows that a basic knowledge of neuroanatomy (both gross and microscopic), neurophysiology, and neurogenetics is indispensable for contemporary medical practice. In this chapter, we briefly recapitulate the essential facts in these three areas.

For the student, the important questions are:
- What are the microscopic building blocks of which the nervous system is composed?
- What are the fundamental processes in neurophysiology?
- What role do genetic factors play in the pathogenesis of disease?

The last question is becoming ever more important. Many neurologic diseases are hereditary, that is, partly or entirely due to genetic abnormalities; they will come to the reader's attention again and again in the pages of this book. At present, in the era of molecular biology, the genetic defects underlying many of them have already been identified (with still more to come). For these diseases, diagnosis by deoxyribonucleic acid (DNA) testing is now possible even before the patient develops any overt symptoms. Such testing should be done only after the patient has been thoroughly informed of the potential consequences.

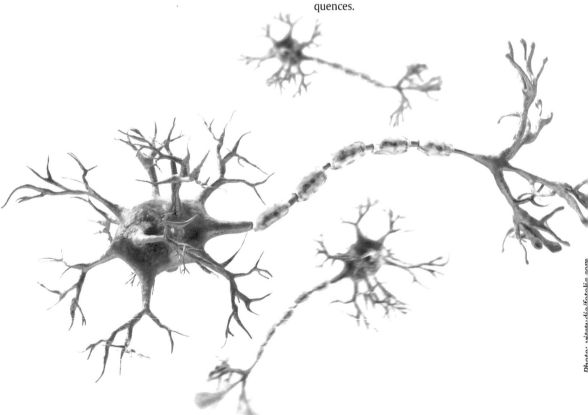

1.1 Microscopic Anatomy of the Nervous System

Key Point

Neurons are the structural and functional building blocks of the nervous system. They are specialized for the reception, integration, and transmission of electric impulses.

1.1.1 Neurons

The neuronal cell body (**soma**) is enclosed by the cell membrane and contains the cell nucleus, mitochondria, endoplasmic reticulum, neurotubules, and neurofilaments (**Fig. 1.1**). **Dendrites** are short, more or less extensively branched cellular processes that conduct *afferent* impulses toward the soma. They provide the cell with a much larger surface area than the soma alone, thereby increasing the area available for intercellular contact and for the deployment of cell membrane receptors. Each type of neuron has its own characteristic dendritic structure: the dendritic tree of a cerebellar Purkinje cell, for example, resembles a deer's antlers (**Fig. 1.2**). The **axon** is a single, elongated cell process that emerges from the soma at the axon hillock. It conducts *efferent* impulses away from the soma to another neuron or to an effector organ.

In general, every neuron has a soma, an axon, and one or more dendrites. The structure and configuration of the neuronal processes (especially the dendrites) vary depending on the function of the neuron. Thus, neurons can be classified into several morphologic subtypes (**Fig. 1.3**).

1.1.2 Neuroglia

The neurons are traditionally thought to constitute the important functional part of the nervous system; they are surrounded by *supportive cells*, which are collectively called neuroglia. **Astrocytes** are neuroglial cells with a starlike structure. They make contact with nonsynaptic sites on the neuronal surface and also have perivascular foot processes that make contact with 85% of the capillaries of the nervous system. The astrocytes supply nutrients to the neurons and are an important constituent of the blood–brain barrier. Other types of supportive cell in the central nervous system are the **oligodendrocytes**, **microglia, ependymal cells**, and choroid plexus cells.

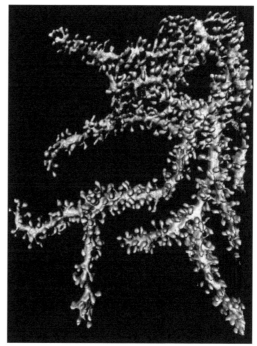

Fig. 1.2   Cerebellar Purkinje cell (microphotograph). Note the numerous synapses on the dendrites. (Image provided courtesy of Dr. Marco Vecellio, Histological Institute of the University of Fribourg, Switzerland.)

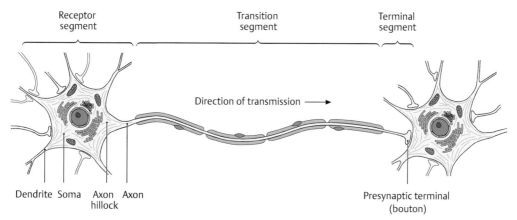

Receptor segment	Transition segment	Terminal segment

Direction of transmission ⟶

Dendrite Soma   Axon   Axon hillock

Presynaptic terminal (bouton)

Fig. 1.1   Fine structure of a neuron. (Adapted from Schuenke et al. Thieme Atlas of Anatomy. Head and Neuroanatomy. New York, NY: Thieme Medical Publishers; 2011. Illustration by Markus Voll.)

1.1.3 Myelin Sheaths

Axons less than 1 µm in diameter are usually unmyelinated; thicker ones are sheathed in myelin. The **myelin sheath** is generated when an axon "sinks" into an oligodendrocyte, giving rise to a *mesaxon*, that is, a double sheet of oligodendrocyte membrane. (In the peripheral nervous system, Schwann cells play the role of oligodendrocytes.) The mesaxon wraps around the axon multiple times to create the

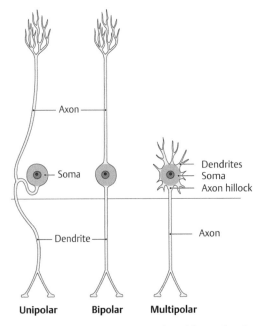

Fig. 1.3   Three types of neurons. (Adapted from Schuenke et al. Thieme Atlas of Anatomy. Head and Neuroanatomy. New York, NY: Thieme Medical Publishers; 2011. Illustration by Markus Voll.)

myelin sheath, a thick coat of electrically insulating material. Individual myelin segments (up to 1 mm long) are separated by segments of "naked" axon called **nodes of Ranvier**, which play an important role in impulse propagation (see section 1.1.4). The nodes are 1 to 4 µm wide and are only partly covered by processes of the neighboring Schwann cells. They are thus separated from the endoneural interstitium by little more than the neuronal cell membrane (called the neurilemma or axolemma). The nodal axolemma mainly contains voltage-dependent sodium channels; the axonal segments between the nodes mainly contain potassium channels.

1.1.4 Synapses

The sites at which neurons transmit impulses to each other are called synapses. The structures making up a synapse include: a bulblike expansion at the end of an axon, called an **axon terminal** (or *bouton*); the **synaptic cleft**; and the **postsynaptic membrane** of the receiving neuron or effector organ (**Fig. 1.4**). Myelinated axons lose their myelin sheath just proximal to the axon terminal. A single neuron can receive synaptic input from one or more axons, and the impulses it receives can be either excitatory or inhibitory. An axon can form a synapse onto a cell body, a dendrite, or another axon. Ongoing structural and functional changes at the synapses give the nervous system functional adaptability ("plasticity") even after the organism has reached maturity. Neural impulses are transmitted across synapses by chemical substances called **neurotransmitters**: some of the more important ones in the central nervous system are dopamine, serotonin, acetylcholine, and γ-aminobutyric acid (GABA). Specialized synapses

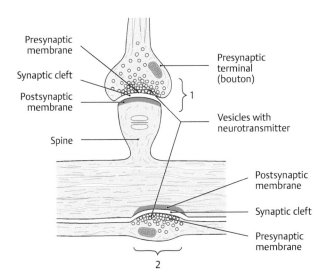

Fig. 1.4   Fine structure of a synapse. The two most common types of synapse are shown: **1** a spiny synapse and **2** a parallel contact or bouton en passage. (Reproduced from Schuenke et al. Thieme Atlas of Anatomy. Head and Neuroanatomy. New York, NY: Thieme Medical Publishers; 2011. Illustration by Markus Voll.)

connect the axons of the peripheral nervous system to effector organs such as muscle cells (motor end plates, see section 15.1.3) or secretory cells in glands.

1.2 Elements of Neurophysiology

🔱 **Key Point**

The resting membrane potential of a neuron or myocyte can undergo a rapid, transient change, called an action potential, in response to an incoming stimulus or impulse. The action potential is generated by transient changes of ion permeability across the cell membrane. Action potentials along neuronal processes and chemical impulse transmission between neurons at synapses are the mechanisms used by the nervous system for information transfer.

1.2.1 Ion Channels

Neurons are enclosed by a double-layered cell membrane with an inner phospholipid layer and an outer glycoprotein layer. Specialized protein molecules within the cell membrane form channels that are selectively permeable to sodium, potassium, or chloride ions. Some ion channels (e.g., in synapses) open only when a specific ligand binds to them, for example, a neurotransmitter molecule. These channels are called **ligand-dependent ion channels**. **Voltage-dependent ion channels**, on the other hand, are found mainly on axons. They open and close depending on the transmembrane electric potential.

1.2.2 Resting Potential

An electric potential difference arises across the neuronal membrane because of the unequal concentrations of ions in the intracellular and extracellular spaces (ICS, ECS), combined with the varying electric conductivity of the membrane to different types of ion. This resting potential is mainly determined by the **ratio of intra- to extracellular potassium concentration**. Its origin can be explained as follows. At rest, the membrane is highly permeable to potassium ions and relatively impermeable to sodium ions. The potassium concentration in the ICS is roughly 35 times higher than in the ECS. Thus, potassium ions tend to diffuse out of the cell. A buildup of negative charge on the inner surface of the membrane results; this, in turn, generates a difference of electric potential across the membrane that opposes further potassium ion outflow. An equilibrium is reached at which the potential difference exactly cancels out the force arising from the difference in potassium ion concentration. As there is no further net transfer of potassium ions across the membrane, the resting membrane potential remains stable, with a value ranging from –60 to –90 mV.

1.2.3 Action Potential

Because the sodium ion concentration is roughly 20 times higher in the ECS than in the ICS, the neurotransmitter-induced opening of ligand-sensitive postsynaptic sodium channels is followed by a **rapid influx of sodium ions** into the cell. The inner surface of the cell membrane becomes positively charged, and an action potential is generated whose amplitude and time course are independent of the nature and intensity of the depolarizing impulse (this is the **all-or-nothing law** of cellular excitation). The transmembrane potential difference reaches a peak ranging from + 20 to + 50 mV. Then, after a brief delay, the cell membrane becomes more permeable to potassium, and a net outflow of potassium ions results. This compensates for the preceding sodium influx and causes membrane repolarization. An active sodium pump also participates in this process. Until repolarization is complete, the membrane cannot conduct any further impulses; there is an initial *absolute* **refractory period**, followed by a *relative* refractory period.

1.2.4 Impulse Conduction

The axon potential begins at the axon hillock and is conducted along the axonal membrane by the successive opening of voltage-dependent sodium channels. This wave of excitation (local depolarization) travels down the axon at a speed depending on the thickness of the axon and the thickness of its myelin sheath. The nodes of Ranvier play a major role in this process: the myelin sheaths lower the capacitance of the axonal membrane and raise its electric resistance. The action potentials are therefore initiated only at the nodes of Ranvier, "jumping over" the internodal segments (so-called **saltatory conduction**). This mechanism enables myelinated nerve fibers to conduct action potentials much more rapidly than unmyelinated fibers. The normal motor and sensory conduction velocity of peripheral nerves is 50 to 60 m/s.

1.3 Elements of Neurogenetics

 Key Point

Many neurologic diseases are caused by a genetic defect or favored by a genetic predisposition. In this section, we present the basics of both "classic" (mendelian) inheritance and molecular genetics, which are prerequisites for the understanding of these diseases and the counseling of affected patients and their families.

1.3.1 General Genetics

> **NOTE**
>
> The physical characteristics of an organism in health and in disease, its phenotype, are determined by its genetic makeup, or genotype, along with environmental factors. DNA is the carrier of genetic information.

DNA molecules are located in the cell nucleus and mitochondria. A segment of DNA containing the information needed for the synthesis of a protein molecule is called a gene, and the totality of the organism's genes is called the genome. Human nuclear genes are contained in 23 pairs of chromosomes: 22 pairs of autosomes and 1 pair of sex chromosomes (gonosomes), which are either XX (in females) or XY (in males).

Genetic Recombination

Growth requires many cell divisions (**mitoses**). In each mitosis, the nuclear genetic material doubles in amount (replicates) and is distributed to the two daughter cells, so that each one, like the original cell, contains a complete (diploid) set of chromosomes. For sexual reproduction, a reductive cell division (**meiosis**) occurs, producing germ cells with a haploid set of chromosomes—that is, only one of each chromosome. The union of an egg cell and a sperm cell yields a zygote with a full (diploid) complement of chromosomes, half derived from the maternal genome and half from the paternal genome.

By the rules of mendelian inheritance, maternally derived and paternally derived properties (genes) are assorted randomly and independently to the germ cells, and thereby to the offspring. Yet, the independence of gene transmission is not total, because genes that lie on the same chromosome are usually transmitted together to the daughter cells. There is a phase of meiosis in which corresponding DNA segments on homologous chromatids can be exchanged with each other to produce a new arrangement of genetic material; this is called **crossing-over** or genetic recombination. The further apart two genes are on a chromosome, the more often recombination will occur between them.

Alongside these physiologic mechanisms of genetic change and reassortment (random mixing of maternal and paternal chromosomes in meiosis and fertilization, recombination of genes on homologous chromosomes), genes can also undergo spontaneous change, that is, **mutation**. Mutations in the germ line are passed on to the offspring (see later).

Unlike nuclear DNA, mitochondrial DNA is passed on only from the mother to her offspring, by way of the egg cell.

Autosomal Dominant Inheritance

An allele (version of a gene) that markedly influences or completely determines the phenotype of the individual in the heterozygous state (i.e., even if it is present in only one copy) is called dominant. If either parent is heterozygous for a dominant allele, then the child has a 50% chance of being affected in both genotype and phenotype.

Autosomal Recessive Inheritance

An allele of an autosomal gene that has an overt effect only in the heterozygous state (i.e., only if present in two copies) is called recessive. If *both* parents are heterozygous for such an allele, then 50% of their children will be asymptomatic heterozygotes (carriers) and 25% will be symptomatic homozygotes, and 25% will not inherit the recessive allele from either parent and will thus be both genetically and phenotypically normal.

X-chromosomal Inheritance

Sons receive an X-chromosome from their mother and a Y-chromosome from their father; daughters receive X-chromosomes from both parents. A mother who is heterozygous for an abnormal X-chromosomal allele will pass it on to half of her children (of either sex), while a father bearing such an allele will pass it on to all of his daughters, but none of his sons. Dominantly inherited X-chromosomal diseases affect both sexes; recessively inherited X-chromosomal diseases mainly affect males, with females affected only if they have received the abnormal allele from both parents. Any affected male must have received the allele from his mother; as long as his mate is not a carrier, all of his daughters will be carriers. Female carriers with unaffected mates will pass on the disease to 50% of their sons; all of their daughters will be phenotypically normal, but half will be carriers.

Maternal Inheritance of the Mitochondrial Genome

Mitochondrial DNA is inherited exclusively in the maternal line. Thus, mitochondrial genetic diseases are passed on only by mothers to their children (both male and female), but never by fathers. Mitochondria with mutated DNA can coexist in the same cell with other mitochondria whose DNA is normal. This phenomenon, called **heteroplasmy**, has no counterpart in the nuclear genome, which is the same in all cells of the body. In mitochondrial genetic diseases, the extent of abnormality of the cells and tissues (the phenotype) depends on the number of mutated mitochondria and on the ratio of mutated to normal mitochondrial DNA.

Mutations

Mutations are necessary for evolution; without them, no species (including man) could exist. Unfortunately, adverse mutations can also cause deformity and disease. Mutations are classified as either *genomic* or *intragenic*.

Genomic Mutations

These are of two types, called **numerical** and **structural chromosomal aberrations**. In the former, the number of chromosomes is abnormal (e.g., monosomy, trisomy). In the latter, a chromosome has an abnormal structure—caused by a deletion, translocation, or inversion of a chromosomal segment.

Intragenic Mutations

Intragenic mutations involve alterations of the DNA. Within each chromosome, DNA is arranged linearly. The DNA segments (genes) that code for amino acid sequences (proteins), which are called *exons*, alternate with noncoding sequences called *introns*. Exons make up only ~5% of human chromosomal DNA. When the DNA is transcribed into RNA, the primary RNA transcript still contains a copy of the introns, which are then removed by "splicing" to yield the mature transcript, *messenger RNA* (mRNA).

Each trinucleotide sequence in the mRNA molecule (called a *triplet* or *codon*) encodes an amino acid in the protein being synthesized. "Stop codons" between exons signal the beginning and end of the gene and thereby determine the length of the protein. The replacement of a DNA nucleotide by a different one can alter the sense of the codon to which it belongs (**missense** mutations), causing the "wrong" amino acid to be inserted into the gene product. This can affect its function in a variety of ways. If a nucleotide replacement happens to generate or destroy a stop codon, then either a truncated protein or an excessively long one will be produced (**nonsense** mutations). Mutations involving either the *insertion* of an extra nucleotide into the DNA or the *deletion* of a nucleotide will alter the rhythm of nucleotide triplets and are therefore called **frameshift** mutations: these tend to cause marked abnormalities of protein structure and function (e.g., Duchenne muscular dystrophy; see section 15.3.1).

Expanded Repetitive DNA Sequences

Another type of mutation of special importance in neurology changes the number of trinucleotides (triplets) in a gene. Normal human DNA contains many repetitive trinucleotide sequences that affect gene function and expression. An important group of neurodegenerative diseases is caused by mutations involving abnormally long (expanded) triplet repeat sequences; these are called **trinucleotide** or **triplet repeat** diseases. A normal repeat sequence might contain only a few triplets; diseased sequences contain dozens or even hundreds. The longer the expansion, the earlier the age of onset of disease and the more severe its manifestations. The abnormal repeat sequences tend to lengthen from one generation to the next, so that the disease tends to appear ever earlier ("anticipation"), and in ever greater severity, as it is passed down through the generations.

Mutations of Mitochondrial DNA

These impair oxidative metabolism in the mitochondria, causing various kinds of disease, including **mitochondrial encephalomyopathies** (see section 15.5.2).

1.3.2 Neurogenetics

> **NOTE**
>
> The triplet diseases are of special relevance in neurology.

Triplet repeat diseases. The neurodegenerative diseases caused by expanded triplet repeats are listed in **Tab. 1.1**; their common features are as follows:

- Autosomal dominant or X-chromosomal inheritance.
- Onset usually between the ages of 25 and 45 years.
- Gradual progression of disease.
- Symmetric neuronal loss and gliosis in the brain.
- Anticipation (earlier disease onset in successive generations).
- The diagnosis can be established by DNA analysis.
- The number of triplet repeats is correlated with the age of onset and the severity of the disease.

Most common inherited mitochondrial diseases.
- Progressive external ophthalmopathy.
- Kearns–Sayre syndrome.
- Leber's hereditary optic neuropathy.
- Mitochondrial encephalomyopathy with lactic acidosis and stroke.
- Leigh disease.
- Neuropathy, ataxia, and retinitis pigmentosa syndrome.
- Myoclonus epilepsy with ragged red fibers.
-

Myoneurogastrointestinal encephalopathy.

> **Practical Tip**
>
> Ever more genetic defects are being identified. Rapid access to current knowledge is best obtained via the Internet. Two useful sites are Online Mendelian Inheritance in Man (OMIM) and Medline/Pubmed.

1

Tab. 1.1

Some neurodegenerative diseases caused by triplet repeat expansions

Disease	Major clinical manifestations	Triplet	Chromosomal localization
Fragile X-chromosome	Diminished intelligence, sometimes facial dysmorphism, connective tissue dysplasia	CGG	Xq27.3
Fragile X tremor/ataxia syndrome (FXTAS)	Progressive intention tremor, extrapyramidal hypokinesia, impotence, and cognitive impairment in old age	CGG	Xq27.3
Myotonic dystrophy of Steinert (DM1)	Progressive, mainly distal muscular dystrophy and myotonia	CTG	19q13.3
Myotonic dystrophy type 2 (proximal myotonic myopathy, PROMM, DM2)	Mainly proximal muscular dystrophy and myotonia	CCTG	3q13.3-q24
Friedreich ataxia	Ataxia, areflexia, pyramidal tract signs, dysarthria	GAA	9q13-q21.1
Spinobulbar muscle atrophy (Kennedy syndrome)	Muscle atrophy, dysarthria, fasciculations, gynecomastia	CAG	Xq13-q21
Huntington disease	Chorea, rarely spasticity or rigidity, cognitive and behavioral disturbances	CAG	4p16.3
Dentate-rubro-pallido-Luysian atrophy (DRPLA)	Ataxia, myoclonus, epilepsy, choreoathetosis, dementia	CAG	12p13.31
Spinocerebellar ataxia type 1 (SCA1)	cerebellar ataxia, sometimes chorea or dystonia, polyneuropathy, often pyramidal tract signs, sometimes dementia	CAG	6p22.3
Spinocerebellar ataxia type 2 (SCA2)	Cerebellar ataxia, sometimes chorea or dystonia, myoclonus, polyneuropathy, sometimes pyramidal tract signs and dementia	CAG	12q24.12
Spinocerebellar ataxia type 3 (SCA3); Machado–Joseph disease	Cerebellar ataxia, sometimes chorea or dystonia, polyneuropathy, sometimes pyramidal tract signs and dementia	CAG	14q32.12
Spinocerebellar ataxia type 6 (SCA6)	Cerebellar ataxia, sometimes polyneuropathy and pyramidal tract signs	CAG	19p13.2
Spinocerebellar ataxia type 7 (SCA7)	Cerebellar ataxia, sometimes chorea or dystonia, retinal degeneration, polyneuropathy, sometimes pyramidal tract signs	CAG	3p14.1
Spinocerebellar ataxia type 8 (SCA8)	cerebellar ataxia, spasticity, impaired vibration sense	CTG	13q21.33
Spinocerebellar ataxia type 10 (SCA10)	cerebellar ataxia, epileptic seizures, sometimes polyneuropathy	ATTCT	22q13.31
Spinocerebellar ataxia type 12 (SCA12)	Cerebellar ataxia, extrapyramidal hypokinesia, later dementia	CAG	5q32
Spinocerebellar ataxia type 17 (SCA17)	Cerebellar ataxia, spasticity, cognitive impairment, psychosis, epileptic seizures	CAG	6q27

1.3.3 Genetic Counseling

Many genetic mutations can be detected directly by DNA analysis. The results are highly specific. Thus, many diseases can be diagnosed even before they become symptomatic. Sadly, these diseases are generally untreatable and inexorably progressive.

NOTE

The findings of DNA analysis can be emotionally devastating for the patient. Before DNA analysis, the patient must be thoroughly informed and counseled by a physician.

Before obtaining a DNA analysis, the treating physician should:
- Perform a meticulous clinical examination.
- Obtain a detailed family history and personally examine the patient's relatives, if possible.
- Inform the patient and his or her relatives in detail about the suspected disease.
- Explain the consequences of the proposed DNA analysis to them in a readily understandable manner.

A negative DNA analysis can provide relief and freedom from anxiety. A positive result, on the other hand, can propel the patient into a severe depression, as he or she will then face the certainty of developing a hereditary disease, often with a grim prognosis, and may not be able to cope with this knowledge. A known genetic defect can also severely strain a marriage or other relationship. Social problems of other kinds can arise as well, because, unfortunately, persons with inherited diseases can easily become pariahs in our postindustrial society. They may have difficulties finding or keeping a job, not least because they may become uninsurable. For all these reasons, genetic testing generally causes fewer problems if it is performed *after* the disease has become symptomatic. Asymptomatic children should not have their DNA tested even if their parents ask for it. They should decide for themselves whether to be tested once they are mature enough to do so and have attained legal majority.

Many patients and their relatives decide not to be tested after being fully informed about their potential genetic disease and the consequences of DNA analysis. In particular, pre- and asymptomatic persons often prefer not to know whether they are going to develop the disease in the future. A positive test result would destroy their hopes for good health in later life.

If the patient does decide to undergo DNA analysis and then tests positive, the physician should inform the patient and his or her relatives in a personal discussion, with ample time to address all of the implications. Test results should never be imparted over the telephone or in writing. Patients who have tested positive often need long-term psychotherapy. Nor does the physician–patient relationship end when the test results are given: many persons with hereditary diseases are greatly helped by ongoing psychological support and symptomatic treatment.

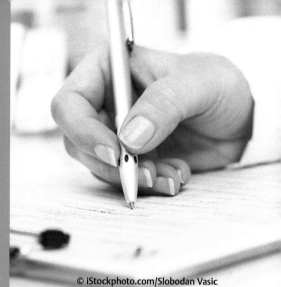

© iStockphoto.com/Slobodan Vasic

Chapter 2

The Clinical Interview in Neurology

Is It in My Head?

A 47-year-old elementary-school teacher consults a neurologist after being referred by her family physician.

"Good morning. What seems to be the trouble?"

"Doctor, I've been having headaches for a while now. I've never had headaches before, and I've always been healthy, but now I'm getting a little worried."

"How long have the headaches been bothering you?"

"About six months, I'd say. I've been having a lot of stress at work lately, and my mother died six months ago. I had to clear out her old apartment. Could that have something to do with it?"

"Perhaps, but let's concentrate on the headaches for a moment. How would you describe them?"

"It's as if my head's going to explode. Everything feels so tight!"

"As if you were wearing a tight ring around your head, is that it?"

"Well, the pressure actually seems to be coming from the inside, but it's sort of like a tight ring, too. Anyway, it's a feeling of pressure. That's the best way to describe it."

"Do you have a headache all the time?"

"Not always. Some days are better, and I sometimes forget about the headaches entirely, but they always come back—sometimes for a couple of hours, but sometimes for a whole day or even two."

"Are the headaches located anywhere in particular, such as only in the front of your head, behind your eyes, or on the right or left side?"

"No, they're all over my head."

"Do they keep you from doing things you want to do?"

"Well, of course."

"I mean, can you go to work even when you have a headache?"

"Oh. Yes, I've been going to work anyway, and then I had all that stress with my mother's apartment. No matter what, I still have to take care of my family and do my job, don't I? I can't take a holiday from life just because I have headaches."

"Have you been having any other problems aside from headaches? Nausea or vomiting? Ringing in the ears? Oversensitivity to noise or bright light? Dizziness?"

"No, basically I just have headaches. That's already bad enough, I think."

"Have you taken anything for them?"

"No, I'm not a big fan of taking medicines. Thank God I never needed any regularly."

"Are there situations in which the headaches are more likely to arise?"

"Well, yes, I think the stress of the last couple of weeks has had a lot to do with it, and then all that running around because of the apartment. My mother lived far away from here, I forgot to tell you, in the south of France."

"Yes, I can imagine that gave you quite a lot of trouble. So, you think the headaches have to do with your mother's death?"

"I suppose they do, somehow. By the way, my mother died of a brain tumor. Tell me, doctor … do you think I might have one, too?"

This dialogue exemplifies a typical headache history. Precise history-taking usually lets the physician formulate a tentative diagnosis that can serve as a basis for the physical examination and further testing (if indicated). To fulfill this purpose, history-taking should follow a few basic rules, particularly regarding the physician's demeanor and a systematic approach to questioning. The emotional aspects and the patient's own interpretation of the symptoms must never be ignored. The general aspects of history-taking are discussed in this chapter.

This patient's history suggests she is most likely suffering from tension-type headaches, which may or may not be related to her mother's death and the stressful situations she describes. The physician must nonetheless respect her interpretation and address the matter again once the diagnostic evaluation is complete. It was not till the very end of the interview that she revealed her likely motivation for the consultation—fear of a brain tumor, that is, fear of having (and perhaps dying from) the same disease her mother had. The physician should do his or her best to assuage this fear, even while the diagnostic evaluation is still in progress.

2.1 General Principles of History-Taking

 Key Point

The clinical history is of paramount importance in neurology, perhaps more so than in any other medical specialty. It is indispensable as a diagnostic instrument, it helps establish a doctor–patient relationship built on trust, and it is a prerequisite for the success of any subsequent treatment. The history should always be taken with utmost care.

The general type of neurologic disturbance from which the patient is suffering can usually be determined from a carefully obtained clinical history even before the physical examination or any further tests are performed. Often, the physician can pinpoint the diagnosis from the history alone—but only after attentive listening and an adequate investment of time.

> **NOTE**
> "A blind neurologist is better than a deaf neurologist."

2.1.1 General Prerequisites for Good History-Taking

In any branch of clinical medicine, not just in neurology, a good history can be taken only if the patient has full confidence in the physician. Introduce yourself to the patient and take the history in a place that offers the necessary privacy and discretion. The patient should be comfortably seated and emotionally at ease, as far as the circumstances allow, and must not feel rushed. If anyone else is present during the interview, for example, a medical student, introduce this person and make sure the patient has no objection to his or her presence. Persons other than the physician who is taking the history should behave unobtrusively. The history should be detailed and complete.

2.1.2 General Principles of the Clinical Interview

While interviewing the patient, observe these principles:
- At first, the patient should be doing most of the talking, and you should say as little as possible.
- You do indeed have to elicit all of the important historic data by specific inquiry, but only after the patient has finished describing the problem in his or her own words.
- Even if the patient's story is rambling or vague, you should take care not to betray any impatience or irritation.

- Once your turn comes, you must amplify and refine this initial information by persistent or even stubborn questioning, until at last you have a clear picture of the present illness.
- Never reject the patient's own interpretation of his or her symptoms, even if it seems implausible or absurd. You will then come across as a scoffing know-it-all and will have broken your line of communication with the patient.

2.1.3 Your Demeanor toward the Patient

Every patient has the right to be treated courteously and tactfully and to have the physician's full attention for an adequate period of time. You should perform a meticulous physical examination only after listening carefully to the patient's story and rounding it out with further, detailed questioning. The patient has the right to be told what your findings are and what they imply about his or her illness. Explain these matters truthfully, in language that the patient can understand, and with due respect for his or her feelings. You will often find yourself having to steer a difficult course between bluntness and reassurance.

If the patient is accompanied by another person, such as a spouse, parent, other relative, or friend, the patient should remain the focus of your attention, even if he or she is a child or adolescent or is cognitively impaired. Communicate mainly with the patient. You may have to ask accompanying persons to leave the room for part of the clinical interview or physical examination, but do not neglect their needs, either; the persons closest to the patient, after all, may have an important role to play later on, during treatment. Courtesy and consideration for the patient as a fellow human being, palpable respect for his or her dignity, and genuine understanding and sympathy are the foundations of a trusting relationship between the patient and the physician and are therefore essential preconditions for successful treatment.

2.1.4 The History and Physical Examination

The patient history and the physical examination are independent and equally important components of the clinical diagnostic evaluation. They must complement each other and should, to some extent, be performed in parallel. An experienced clinician, while listening to the patient's history, will already be thinking of specific abnormalities to look for on physical examination. If the examination reveals other, perhaps unexpected findings, the clinician can amplify the history with specific questions. Ideally, the clinician will be able to make the diagnosis from the history and physical examination alone.

2.2 Special Aspects of History-Taking

Key Point

The "classic" history has certain standard components (Table 2.1) and is meant to provide a complete picture of the patient, including his or her present complaints, past medical history, personality, and life situation.

2.2.1 The Present Illness

When taking a clinical history, always first give the patient a chance to state his or her **current complaints** and the **reason for the consultation**. Only afterward should you begin interrogating the patient systematically to make the history complete. Systematic history-taking is performed in standard fashion in all branches of clinical medicine; a basic outline is provided in **Table 2.1**. In each specialty, however, there are further important issues that tend to arise regularly, and these should be asked about

Table 2.1

Outline of the general clinical history

Element of the clinical history	Details
Current complaints	— Information spontaneously provided by the patient — Direct questioning to obtain more precise information — Systematic analysis of the current complaints (see **Table 2.2**)
Past medical and surgical history	— Information spontaneously provided by the patient — Specific questioning by the physician, particularly about earlier conditions that may be relevant to the current complaints — Gestational history, birth history, and childhood developmental history, if indicated
Life habits	— Alcohol and tobacco — Medications — Illicit drugs — Potentially toxic environmental influences
Neurovegetative functions	— Sleep — Digestion — Micturition — Sexual function
Personality and social situation	— The patient's personal and social setting (education, occupation, familial/social/financial position, and any current problems or conflicts in these areas); such information lets the physician assess the factors that might help or hinder the patient in coping with medical problems — The patient's behavior, manner of speaking, gestures, facial expressions, emotional responses, reactions to questions, etc., give the examiner an overall impression of the patient's personality

Table 2.2

History of the present illness

Symptoms	Details
Major symptom(s)	— The patient's **spontaneous description**, refined by **specific questioning** — **How long** have the symptoms been present? **Where** are they located? — **How did they begin** (suddenly, gradually, or after a specific inducing event)? — **How have they developed** over time (constant, increasing, decreasing, fluctuating)? — **What influences the symptoms** (ameliorating/aggravating influences, medications)? — **Effects—how severe** are the symptoms? How do they affect everyday life, at home and at work, and the patient's emotional well-being? Is treatment needed?
Current accompanying symptoms	— Here it is particularly important to supplement the patient's spontaneous complaints with specific questioning. An experienced clinician knows what questions to ask even if the patient has provided very little information.
Relevant past medical history	— Did the patient already have **earlier symptoms** that might be relevant to the current complaints (e.g., earlier transient ischemic attacks in a patient suffering from acute stroke)? — Does the patient have any **predisposing factors** for conditions that might account for the current complaints (e.g., cigarette smoking leading to a Pancoast tumor of the apex of the lung)?
Relevant family history	— This may lend support to a conjectural diagnosis: for example, similar symptoms in blood relatives of the patient's parents if a recessively inherited condition is suspected, or hemicranial headaches in the mother of a patient with suspected migraine

specifically. The important questions to ask in the neurologic history are summarized in **Table 2.2**.

2.2.2 Past Medical History, Family History, and Social History

Once you have a clear and complete picture of the patient's current complaints, you can begin to ask about **earlier symptoms and illnesses**, proceeding from the general to the specific. Always ask about problems that might bear a relation to the present illness: a patient suffering from ischemic stroke, for instance, should be asked about hypertension, heart disease, and smoking. Ask about the health of the patient's blood relatives, particularly with regard to neurologic and other hereditary diseases. Finally, ask about the patient's **familial and social setting**: marriage or other partnership, children, occupation, and any potential problems or conflicts in these areas. Ascertain how the patient's current (or earlier)

medical problems affect him or her in everyday life, both at home and in the workplace. Broach these matters as discreetly as possible, as needlessly aggressive questioning may give the impression that you have already written off the patient's problems as psychogenic. Of course, if your thorough evaluation reveals that a psychogenic mechanism is indeed the most likely cause, then this, too, should be discussed openly with the patient.

A carefully elicited clinical history enables an experienced clinician to formulate a **tentative diagnosis** even before proceeding to the physical examination. With the tentative diagnosis in mind, you can focus your attention on certain aspects of the examination. Of course, you must not allow your findings to be so heavily influenced by your expectations that they are no longer reliable. The tentative diagnosis should inform the physical examination, not convert it into a pointless exercise.

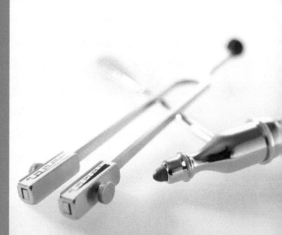

Chapter 3

The Neurologic Examination

A Fateful Diagnosis

A 62-year-old woman is referred by her family physician to a neurologist. She has been feeling exhausted for several months. Recently, she has also been suffering from muscle cramps, and she has noticed that food occasionally "goes down the wrong pipe." The neurologist's examination reveals the following:

Head and cranial nerves: Gag reflex not clearly elicitable, all findings otherwise normal.

Speech: Mildly slurred.

Upper and lower limbs: Asymmetric, marked atrophy of various muscles, no clear abnormality of muscle tone, surprisingly brisk reflexes even in the muscles that are markedly weak and atrophic, visible fasciculations.

Babinski reflex weakly elicitable bilaterally. Coordination normal. Sensation intact in all modalities.

Stance and gait: Marked difficulty standing on the toes and heels due to weakness.

Psychopathologic state: Patient worried and anxious, otherwise normal.

Neuropsychological state: No evident deficits.

General physical examination: Impaired nutritional state and mildly impaired general state of health, blood pressure mildly elevated, cardiovascular examination otherwise normal. Chest clear, abdomen soft, all peripheral pulses palpable.

Assessment: The patient is a 62-year-old woman with muscle atrophy and weakness but no accompanying sensory disturbance. This constellation of findings is present only in myopathy or a disease of the ventral horns of the spinal cord. The fasciculations point toward ventral horn dysfunction rather than myopathy. A disease affecting the nerve roots or peripheral nerves might cause muscle atrophy and weakness, but would also be expected to cause sensory deficits and hypo- or areflexia. This patient'sreflexes are brisker than normal, indicating that her condition affects the pyramidal tracts as well—an inference solidly confirmed by the Babinski sign. Combined dysfunction of the ventral horns and pyramidal tracts is the clinical hallmark of amyotrophic lateral sclerosis, and this diagnosis appears highly likely from the physical findings. The patient's mildly slurred speech indicates bulbar involvement.

Although many highly informative ancillary tests are available, it would be an error to work up neurologically abnormal patients with only neuroimaging and other high-technology diagnostic procedures. Rather, the neurologist must take a thorough history, perform a full, meticulous clinical neurologic examination, and then document all findings in full. On the basis of these findings, the neurologist can decide what additional tests to order next, in case any are needed.

In this chapter, the components of a systematic neurologic examination (including a neuropsychological examination, if indicated) are described in detail, along with the main abnormal findings. The information provided here should enable the examining physician to localize the underlying lesion in the nervous system anatomically on the basis of the findings. Anatomic localization does not, in itself, reveal the etiology of the problem; further information from the history and additional tests will be needed for this.

3.1 Basic Principles of the Neurologic Examination

Key Point

Neurologic diseases can often be diagnosed on the basis of a carefully elicited history in combination with the physical examination. To ensure completeness, the examining physician should examine all patients according to the same general scheme.

One may either examine the individual components of the nervous system in a particular sequence (cranial nerves, reflexes, and motor, sensory, and autonomic function) or conduct the examination along topographic lines (head, upper limbs, trunk, lower limbs). The presentation in this chapter is **topographically organized**.

Neurology stands by itself as an independent medical specialty and field of research. Most neurologic illnesses affect only the nervous system. Nonetheless, general medical illnesses often manifest themselves with neurologic symptoms and signs (cf. section 6.8). The clinical neurologic examination must therefore always include a **general physical examination**.

The practicing neurologist should emphasize the neurologic aspects of the physical examination without neglecting its general aspects.

Here are some **basic principles** of physical examination:

The examiner must **talk to the patient**, briefly explaining the purpose of individual steps in the examination where appropriate. This affords the examiner the opportunity to obtain more information on certain aspects of the clinical history, if necessary.

In principle, the neurologic examination should always be **complete** and should always be performed in the same sequence, though the examiner is free to use whatever sequence he or she prefers. The individual components of the examination are listed in **Table 3.1**. In certain exceptional situations, or on repeated follow-up, a highly experienced clinician may choose to perform only a partial examination. This is generally to be avoided, however, as even the best neurologist can miss something important in this way. A thorough, methodical examination also helps reassure the patient that the physician is competent and attentive.

Patients should be examined **unclothed**, after being given clear instructions about which clothes to remove, usually everything but their underwear. The spine cannot be examined if the upper body is covered; if the patient is wearing socks, sensation

cannot be tested in the feet, and the Babinski reflex cannot be elicited.

Although the examination should always be **systematic and complete**, the tentative diagnosis (or diagnoses) suggested by the history will direct the clinician to **pay particular attention to certain aspects of the examination**. There is no sense in the mechanical, unthinking performance of a rigidly identical examination on every patient.

Deviating from the usual order of examination may be advisable for psychological reasons. For example, if the patient mainly has symptoms in the lower limbs or the back, one can begin the examination with the spine.

As soon as possible after the examination is completed, the examiner should **document the findings in writing**. Global statements such as "Neuro OK" are worthless. The findings can be summarized in an outline such as the one provided in **Table 3.1**. The main purpose of precise documentation is to let the clinician follow the development of a disease process from one examination to the next. It is also obviously indispensable for medicolegal reasons.

Moreover, certain findings should be **quantified or numerically graded**, particularly muscle strength (see **Table 3.5**). Sensory disturbances should be documented precisely in terms of their topography and extent.

3.2 Stance and Gait

Key Point

Stance and gait should be tested systematically with the patient unclothed and barefoot. Inspection of the standing patient at rest may already reveal signs of disease. Next, the patient's gait is examined, usually with special tests of walking and balance.

3.2.1 General Remarks

Though stance and gait are listed at the bottom of **Table 3.1**, we in fact recommend testing these functions as the first step in the examination of the unclothed patient.

Inspection of the standing patient can already reveal evidence of a disease process, for example, muscle atrophy, spinal deformities, and winging of the scapula. The patient's **posture at rest** may be abnormal, for example, the exaggerated lumbar lordosis of muscular dystrophy (cf. **Fig. 15.3**) or the stooped, rigid posture of the patient with Parkinson disease (cf. **Fig. 6.55**, **Fig. 6.56**). The testing of **stance and gait** often yields important clues to the disease process. The sequence of tests is shown in **Fig. 3.1a–h**.

Table 3.1

The neurologic examination

Region	Findings
General	— *Blood pressure, pulse*
	— Weight, height
	— Temperature
	— Heart
	— Lungs
	— Lymph nodes (enlarged?)
	— Peripheral pulses (palpable?)
Cognition and behavior	— *Handedness* (right or left)
	— *Level of consciousness* (awake, somnolent, stuporous, comatose)
	— Behavior (normal, abnormal)
	— Mood (normal, depressed, euphoric)
	— Orientation (day, month, year, location)
	— *Language*
	• Production (normal, aphasic, dysarthric, hoarse)
	• Comprehension
	• Repetition
	• Naming, word-finding
	— *Memory*
	• History (clear, vague, unobtainable)
	• Short-term memory (number sequence forward and backward; words)
	— Apraxia? (use of toothbrush, comb, and hammer)
	— Neglect? (none, visual, somatosensory, motor)
Head and cranial nerves	— Head freely mobile, no meningismus
	— Skull not tender to percussion
	— No supra- or infraorbital point tenderness
	— Carotid pulsations strong bilaterally, without bruits
	— Temporal artery pulsations strong bilaterally, without tenderness
	— No meningismus
	— No bruits
	— No occipital point tenderness
	— Perioral reflexes not exaggerated
	Olfactory nerve (CN I)
	— Coffee correctly identified by smell in both nostrils (spontaneously named/chosen from list)
	Optic nerve (CN II)
	— Corrected visual acuity (*distance*): R/L
	— *Visual fields* full to confrontation
	— Optic discs normal bilaterally
	Oculomotor, trochlear, and abducens nerves (CN III, IV, and VI)
	— Eye movements full and coordinated
	— *Eye position* parallel, cover test normal
	— *No pathologic nystagmus*
	— *Pupils* equal, round, midsized, and symmetric, with prompt reaction to light and convergence
	Trigeminal nerve (CN V)
	— *Sensation* in the face intact
	— Corneal reflex symmetrically elicitable
	— Masseter strong bilaterally
	Facial nerve (CN VII)
	— Spontaneous *mimesis* normal
	— Voluntary *movement of facial muscles* normal
	Vestibulocochlear nerve (CN VIII)
	— *Hearing* subjectively normal
	— Finger-rubbing heard in both ears
	— Weber test: not lateralized
	— Head-impulse test: normal bilaterally
	— VOR suppression test normal
	Glossopharyngeal and vagus nerves (CN IX and X)
	— *Palatal veil* symmetric at rest, elevates symmetrically
	— Gag reflex intact
	— Swallowing subjectively unimpaired

| Table 3.1 |

The neurologic examination *(continued)*

Region	Findings
	Accessory nerve (CN XI)
	— *Sternocleidomastoid* strength and bulk full and symmetric
	— Trapezius strength and bulk full and symmetric
	Hypoglossal nerve (CN XII)
	— *Tongue* symmetric, protrudes in the midline, freely mobile
Upper limbs	— *Bulk* normal bilaterally
	— *Tone* normal bilaterally
	— Full mobility throughout
	— *Raw strength* normal in all muscle groups (weakness should be graded on scale of **Table 3.5**)
	— *Postural testing* normal bilaterally, without sinking or pronator drift
	— *Rapid alternating movements* performed well bilaterally
	— No rebound phenomenon
	— Finger-tapping
	— Finger–nose test accurate bilaterally, no intention tremor
	— No hand or finger tremor
	— Reflexes:
	• Biceps, triceps, and brachioradialis reflexes symmetric, of medium strength
	• Mayer reflex elicitable bilaterally
	• Hoffmann sign, Trömner reflex not exaggerated bilaterally
	— Sensation bilaterally intact to *touch*
	— Pain sensation bilaterally intact
	— *Temperature sensation* bilaterally intact
	— Two-point discrimination < 5 mm bilaterally
	— Position sense in the fingers bilaterally intact
	— Vibration sense bilaterally intact
	— Stereognosis bilaterally intact, prompt
	— Coin recognition bilaterally intact
Trunk	— Spine unremarkable, no tenderness to percussion
	— Sensation on trunk intact; "saddle" sensation intact
	— Reflexes:
	• Abdominal skin reflex symmetrically intact
	• Cremaster reflex bilaterally present (males only)
	— Small Schober index: .../... cm
	— Finger-to-floor distance: .../... cm
Lower limbs	— *Bulk* normal bilaterally
	— *Tone* normal bilaterally
	— Full mobility throughout
	— *Raw strength* normal in all muscle groups (weakness should be graded on scale of **Table 3.5**)
	— Lasègue sign negative bilaterally
	— No nerve trunk tenderness
	— Postural testing (supine position) normal bilaterally, without sinking
	— Heel–knee–shin test accurate bilaterally
	— Reflexes:
	• *Quadriceps* reflex and *Achilles* reflex symmetric, of medium strength
	• *Babinski* response absent bilaterally
	• Gordon reflex negative bilaterally
	• Oppenheim reflex negative bilaterally
	— Sensation bilaterally intact to *touch*
	— Pain sensation bilaterally intact
	— *Temperature sensation* bilaterally intact
	— *Vibration sense* bilaterally intact
	— Position sense in the toes bilaterally intact
	— Graphesthesia (number recognition) good on both legs
Stance and gait	— Patient can stand up normally from a sitting position
	— Upright stance
	— Romberg test negative (with various positions of the head)
	— Can stand on either leg for 5 seconds
	— Normal *gait* with normal accessory movements
	— Normal *length of steps*
	— Number of steps needed to turn 180 degrees
	— Walks well on heels bilaterally
	— Walks well on tiptoes bilaterally
	— Steady tandem gait
	— Can hop on either leg
	— Postural stability intact
	— No gait deviation with eyes closed

Abbreviations: CN, cranial nerve; VOR, vestibulo-ocular reflex.
Note: If this table, or one like it, is used in practice to document the findings of the clinical neurological examination, the examiner should note all abnormal findings in the appropriate place and place a check (✓) or plus sign (+) next to all examined items that are normal. The record will then show which (if any) elements of the examination have been omitted.
Items in italics should, in principle, be examined in every patient. Only experienced examiners should perform a restricted neurologic examination.

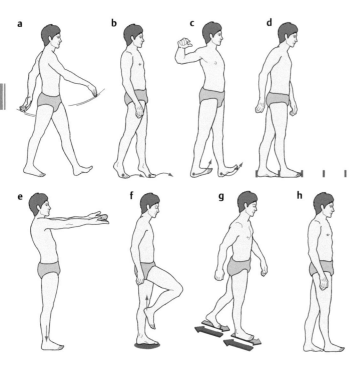

Fig. 3.1   Tests of stance and gait. a Normal gait. Note normal step length and arm swing. **b** Walking on tiptoes. **c** Walking on heels. **d** Heel-to-toe (tandem) walking. One foot is placed precisely in front of the other. **e** Romberg test with eyes closed, combined with postural test of the upper limbs. **f** Unterberger step test: walking in place with eyes closed. **g** Babinski–Weil test with "star gait" (*marche en étoile*): the patient is asked to take two steps forward and two steps back, repeatedly, with eyes closed. **h** Tandem stance: standing with one foot precisely in front of the other. For interpretation, see text.

| NOTE |

In the assessment of stance and gait, attention should be paid to the following:
- Does the patient walk fluidly, symmetrically, and without a limp? If the patient has a limp, then the side that bears weight for the *shorter* time is the abnormal side.
- How long are the patient's steps, and how are the feet placed on the ground and rolled off it?
- How do the arms move while the patient walks?

Some characteristic disturbances of gait are described in **Table 3.2**.

3.2.2 Special Stance and Gait Tests

The clinician can judge the strength of the calf muscles and the foot and toe extensors by making the patient **walk on tiptoe and on the heels** (**Fig. 3.1b,c**). If the plantar flexors are only mildly weak, the patient will still be able to walk on tiptoe, but will not be able to raise himself or herself on tiptoe while standing on one leg, or hop repeatedly on one foot (10 times in succession) (see **Fig. 13.66**).

The "**tightrope walk**" (heel-to-toe walk, tandem walk) (**Fig. 3.1d**) is a very sensitive test of equilibrium and gait stability. The patient is instructed to place one foot firmly and directly in front of the other, at first while looking at the floor, then while looking straight ahead, and finally while looking at the ceiling. Heel-to-toe walking should be possible under all of these conditions. Heel-to-toe walking with the eyes closed is a more difficult task that many normal persons cannot perform.

The **Romberg test** (**Fig. 3.1e**) is a further test of equilibrium. The patient is asked to stand with the feet together and parallel and with eyes closed, for at least 20 seconds. This should be accomplished calmly and easily, without any appreciable swaying. The test can be made more difficult by having the patient turn or incline the head to one side. It can also be performed in combination with postural testing of the arms (see later). Other demanding tests of equilibrium include standing with one foot precisely in front of the other (**tandem stance, Fig. 3.1h**) and standing on one foot. Normal persons can stand on one foot for at least 5 seconds and, for example, put their trousers on or take them off while standing freely; persons older than 70 years cannot always do this.

The functions of the vestibular system (section 12.6.2) and cerebellum (section 5.5.6) can be tested in several ways:
- In the **Unterberger step test** (**Fig. 3.1f**), the patient is made to walk with the eyes closed, raising the knee to (or above) the horizontal with each step. After 50 steps, the patient should have rotated no more than 45 degrees from his or her original position. Larger rotations suggest dysfunction of the vestibular apparatus on the side

Table 3.2

Characteristic disturbances of gait

Designation	Abnormalities of gait	Causes/remarks
Spastic gait (Fig. 3.2)	Slow, stiff, with audible dragging of the soles of the feet across the ground	Bilateral pyramidal tract lesion
Ataxic gait (Fig. 3.2)	Uncoordinated, stamping, unsteady, deviating irregularly from a straight line; heel-to-toe walking impossible	Cerebellar dysfunction, posterior column dysfunction, polyneuropathy
Spastic–ataxic gait (Fig. 3.2)	Combination of the two disturbances described above; jerky, stiff, inharmonious gait	Most commonly seen in multiple sclerosis
Dystonic gait	Irregular additional movements interfering with the normal course of gait	Basal ganglionic disease causing choreoathetosis or dystonia
Hypokinetic gait (Fig. 3.2 and Fig. 6.56)	Slow gait, stiff, bent posture, small steps, lack of accessory arm movements; turning requires multiple small steps	Most commonly seen in Parkinson disease; similar picture in the lacunar state (cerebral microangiopathy, cf. section 6.5.6)
Small-stepped gait ("marche à petits pas")	Small steps, unsteady, resembles hypokinetic gait but with more normal accessory arm movements	"Old person's gait" most commonly seen in the lacunar state, i.e., multiple small infarcts in the basal ganglia and along the corticospinal tracts; distinguishable from parkinsonian gait mainly by the different accompanying signs
Circumduction (Fig. 3.2)	Increased tone in the extensors of the paretic leg, which comes forward in a gentle outward arc, with a strongly plantar-flexed foot; hardly any accompanying movement of the flexed and adducted ipsilateral arm	Central (spastic) hemiparesis
Steppage gait	The advancing leg is raised high and then placed on the ground toe first, often with an audible slap	Unilateral: foot drop, e.g., in peroneal nerve palsy; bilateral: e.g., polyneuropathy or Steinert myotonic dystrophy
Hyperextended knee (Fig. 3.2)	With each step, the knee of the stationary leg is hyperextended	Prevents buckling of the knee when the knee extensors are weak—unilaterally, e.g., in quadriceps weakness due to a lesion of the femoral nerve; bilaterally, e.g., in muscular dystrophy
Hyperlordotic gait (Fig. 15.3a)	Exaggerated lumbar lordosis	For example, in muscular dystrophy affecting the pelvic girdle, in boys with Duchenne muscular dystrophy
Trendelenburg gait (Fig. 3.2)	With each step, the pelvis tilts downward on the side of the swinging leg	Severe hip abductor weakness—unilaterally, e.g., in lesions of the superior gluteal nerve; bilaterally, e.g., in muscular dystrophy affecting the pelvic girdle and in bilateral hip dislocation
Duchenne gait (Fig. 3.2)	With each step, the upper body tilts to the side of the stationary leg	Mild or moderate weakness of the hip abductors (as in Trendelenburg gait, but less severe), or as an antalgic maneuver in disorders of the hip joint

to which the patient has turned or of the cerebellar hemisphere on that side.

— In the "**star gait**" test of Babinski and Weil (**Fig. 3.1g**), the patient keeps the eyes closed and walks two steps forward and two steps back, repeatedly. Dysfunction of the vestibular system manifests itself as involuntary turning to the side of the lesion.

— In **blind walking**, the patient first looks at the examiner, who is standing some distance away, then closes the eyes, and walks toward him or her. Vestibular lesions usually cause a deviation to the side of the lesion.

Several common gait abnormalities are illustrated in **Fig. 3.2**.

3.3 Head and Cranial Nerves

 Key Point
One should note the shape of the head and face, the range of motion of the cervical spine, and the intrinsic reflexes of the facial muscles. The skull and the neck vessels are auscultated, and the functions of the cranial nerves are tested.

3.3.1 Head and Cervical Spine

The examiner should first note the **general appearance** of the head and cervical spine (e.g., sunken temples in Steinert myotonic dystrophy) and the patient's **facial expressions** (e.g., paucity of facial expression in Parkinson disease). Next, the **range of**

3

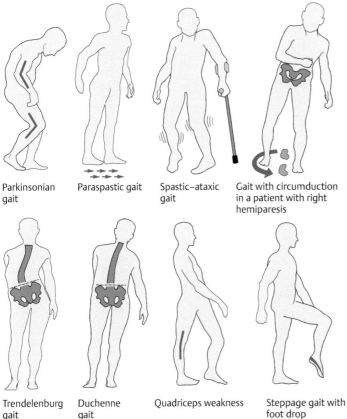

Parkinsonian gait

Paraspastic gait

Spastic–ataxic gait

Gait with circumduction in a patient with right hemiparesis

Trendelenburg gait

Duchenne gait

Quadriceps weakness

Steppage gait with foot drop

Fig. 3.2   Common gait disturbances.

motion of the cervical spine is tested: young, healthy persons should be able to turn the neck and head almost 90 degrees in either direction, so that the eye that is farther from the examiner disappears behind the root of the patient's nose. Further, the patient should be able to incline the head laterally 45 degrees in either direction and to rotate it 60 degrees to the right or left when the neck is maximally flexed (this rotation occurs only at the atlantoaxial and atlanto-occipital joints).

Testing for **meningismus** is performed with the patient supine. This finding, if present, usually indicates meningeal irritation due to meningitis or subarachnoid hemorrhage, but is sometimes a reflex response to a mass lesion in the posterior fossa. Meningismus consists of isolated opposition to neck flexion, while the head can still be rotated. To test for meningismus, the examiner flexes the neck of the supine patient by passively bending the head forward. In genuine meningismus, the **Lasègue sign** (see section 13.1.2, Radicular Syndromes due to Intervertebral Disk Herniation) is usually positive, often with a positive Bragard sign as well. If attempted passive flexion of the neck also induces flexion of the lower limbs at the knee or hip joint, this is called a positive

cervical **Brudzinski sign**. This sign is often accompanied by a **positive Kernig sign**: when the patient is in the sitting position, the knee cannot be passively extended, and when the patient is supine, passive straight leg raising induces reflex knee flexion.

Auscultation of the skull may reveal a pulse-synchronous bruit over an arteriovenous fistula or malformation. A carotid bruit may be due to stenosis.

The intrinsic reflexes of the facial musculature should always be examined. Tapping a finger placed over the lateral canthus of the patient's eye normally induces contraction of the ipsilateral orbicularis oculi muscle. This reflex normally weakens (habituates) on repeated tapping; if it does not, or if there is excessively intense, bilateral contraction of the orbicularis oculi when the examiner taps on the patient's glabella (the **glabellar or nasopalpebral reflex**), then Parkinson disease or another type of bilateral lesion of the corticobulbar pathways is probably present. Tapping on a tongue depressor held loosely on the patient's lips may induce lip protrusion (positive **snout reflex**). The **masseter reflex** (jaw jerk reflex) is elicited by gently tapping the patient's jaw from above when the patient's mouth is half open. Another way to elicit this reflex is to tap on a tongue depressor laid on the patient's mandibular teeth. Very intense contraction of the perioral musculature indicates bilateral involvement of the corticobulbar pathways; the most common cause is a microangiopathic lacunar state. The **corneomandibular reflex** ("winking jaw phenomenon") consists of deviation of the slightly opened jaw when the cornea is touched. Its presence on only one side, or any marked asymmetry, implies an interruption of the ascending and descending brainstem pathways terminating in the pontomesencephalic reticular formation.

3.3.2 Cranial Nerves

Next, the cranial nerves are examined individually. **Fig. 3.3** and **Table 3.3** provide an overview of the anatomy and function of the 12 cranial nerves. The clinical syndromes associated with lesions of individual cranial nerves are presented systematically in Chapter 12. In the current chapter, we will describe the main examining techniques and a selection of the important abnormal findings that can be elicited with each technique.

> **NOTE**
>
> The first two cranial nerves (the olfactory and optic nerves) are actually not peripheral nerves at all, but rather are portions of the brain that happen to be situated in the periphery. The remaining 10 structurally and functionally resemble the other peripheral nerves of the body. They have motor, somatosensory, special sensory, and autonomic functions.

Cranial Nerve I: Olfactory Nerve

> **NOTE**
>
> For the nuclei and functions of this nerve, see **Table 3.3**. For a detailed discussion of olfactory disturbances, see section 12.1.

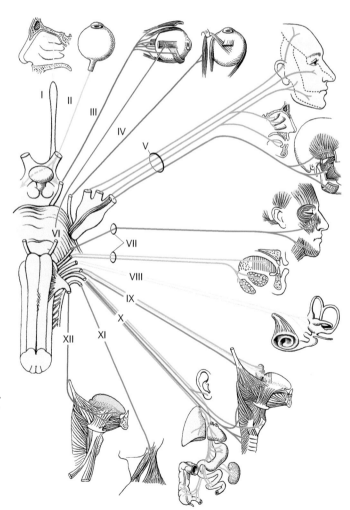

Fig. 3.3   The cranial nerves: overview of their sites of exit from the brainstem, components, and areas of innervation. I = olfactory nerve, **II** = optic nerve, **III** = oculomotor nerve, **IV** = trochlear nerve, **V** = trigeminal nerve, **VI** = abducens nerve, **VII** = facial nerve, **VIII** = vestibulocochlear nerve, **IX** = glossopharyngeal nerve, **X** = vagus nerve, **XI** = accessory nerve, **XII** = hypoglossal nerve. (Reproduced from Bähr M., Frotscher M. Neurologisch-topische Diagnostik. 9th ed. Stuttgart: Thieme; 2009.)

Table 3.3

The 12 cranial nerves, their brainstem nuclei, and their functions

Cranial nerve	Anatomic substrates (peripheral and central); *innervated structures*	Function
I Olfactory nerve	— Sensory neurons of the nasal mucosa (olfactory zone) — Olfactory fila — Olfactory bulb and tract — Olfactory striae — Amygdala	— Perception of odors (only substances dissolved in the fluid of the nasal mucosa can be perceived)
II Optic nerve	— Retina — Optic nerve — Optic chiasm — Optic tract — Lateral geniculate body — Optic radiation — Primary visual cortex on the banks of the calcarine fissure	— Visual perception
III Oculomotor nerve	— Nucleus of the oculomotor nerve and Edinger–Westphal nucleus (both are in the midbrain) — Peripheral nerve — *Levator palpebrae muscle; superior, inferior, and medial rectus muslces; and inferior oblique muscle, as well as the constrictor pupillae muscle*	— Elevation of the upper lid — Most of the movements of the globe (eyeball) — Constriction of the pupil
IV Trochlear nerve	— Nucleus of the trochlear nerve (midbrain at its junction with the pons) — Peripheral nerve — *Superior oblique muscle*	— Depression of the adducted globe — Internal rotation of the abducted globe
V Trigeminal nerve	— Pontine and spinal nuclei of the trigeminal nerve (sensory root) — Motor nucleus of the trigeminal nerve (motor root) — Gasserian ganglion — Three peripheral nerve branches (the ophthalmic, maxillary, and mandibular nerves) — *Skin and mucosa of the head and face; muscles of mastication (temporalis, masseter, and medial and lateral pterygoid muscles)*	— Sensation on the face and external ear — Sensation on mucosal surfaces of the head — Innervation of the muscles of mastication
VI Abducens nerve	— Nucleus of the abducens nerve (pons), intramedullary fascicle nerve — *Lateral rectus muscle*	— Lateral gaze (nucleus) — Abduction of the globe (fascicle or peripheral nerve)
VII Facial nerve	— Nucleus of the facial nerve (pons, motor fibers for the *muscles of facial expression*) — Superior salivatory nucleus (secretory fibers for the *lacrimal, nasal, and palatal glands*) — Nucleus of the tractus solitarius (gustatory fibers for the *anterior two-thirds of the tongue*) — Peripheral nerve	— Innervation of the muscles of facial expression and the stapedius muscle — Lacrimation and salivation — Taste on the anterior two-thirds of the tongue
VIII Vestibulocochlear nerve (statoacoustic nerve, auditory nerve)	— Sensory neurons in the cochlea (cochlear root) and in the semicircular canals — Utricle and saccule (vestibular root) — Peripheral afferent nerve trunk — Brainstem nuclei and projecting fibers to higher regions of the CNS	— Perception of sound and of bodily position, movement, and acceleration — Regulation of balance
IX Glossopharyngeal nerve	— Nucleus ambiguus (medulla, motor fibers for the *muscles of the soft palate and pharynx*) — Nucleus of the tractus solitarius (gustatory fibers from the *posterior third of the tongue, somatosensory fibers from the palatal and pharyngeal mucosa*) — Inferior salivatory nucleus, otic ganglion (secretory fibers for the *parotid gland*) — Peripheral nerve	— Motor innervation of the palatal and pharyngeal muscles — Somatosensory innervation of the palatal and pharyngeal mucosa — Taste on the posterior third of the tongue — Control of swallowing
X Vagus nerve	— Nucleus ambiguus (medulla, motor fibers for the muscles of the soft palate and pharynx) — Dorsal nucleus of the vagus nerve, nucleus of the tractus solitarius (visceromotor and viscerosensory fibers for the thoracic and abdominal viscera) — Spinal nucleus of the trigeminal nerve (sensory fibers from the pharynx, larynx, and external auditory canal) — Nerve trunk	— Innervation of the laryngeal musculature (speech) — Sensation in the external ear canal and the posterior cranial fossa — Autonomic fibers to the thoracic and abdominal viscera
XI Accessory nerve	— Nucleus ambiguus (medulla, cranial root) — Spinal nucleus of the accessory nerve (C1–C5, spinal root) — Nerve trunk — *Sternocleidomastoid muscle and upper portion of the trapezius muscle*	— Turning the head to the opposite side — Shrugging the shoulders

Table 3.3

The 12 cranial nerves, their brainstem nuclei, and their functions *(continued)*

Cranial nerve	Anatomic substrates (peripheral and central); *innervated structures*	Function
XII Hypoglossal nerve	— Nucleus of the hypoglossal nerve (medulla) — Nerve trunk — *Muscles of the tongue*	— Movement of the tongue

Abbreviation: CNS, central nervous system.

The sense of smell is tested individually in each nostril. The patient is asked to close his or her eyes and then to identify (or at least perceive) **aromatic substances** such as coffee, peppermint, cinnamon, or vanilla that are held under the open nostril. Three-quarters of normal individuals can correctly identify coffee grounds. If there is doubt about the patient's ability to smell, asafetida (onion extract), a substance with an unpleasant odor, is used. Only a complete loss of the sense of smell (anosmia; see section 12.1), not a mere diminution of it, is neurologically relevant. Anosmia is most commonly a sequel of severe traumatic brain injury but may also be due to frontal tumors, particularly olfactory groove meningioma, or postinfectious abnormalities of the nasal mucosa, for example, after an upper respiratory "cold," or in ozena.

NOTE

If it is unclear whether anosmia is of neurologic origin, the patient is given a dilute ammonia solution to smell. The unpleasant irritation that this produces is mediated, not by the olfactory nerve, but by the trigeminal nerve. If the patient fails to react, then he or she is probably suffering either from an acute process affecting the nasal mucosa (e.g., acute rhinitis) or from a psychogenic disturbance. The anosmia is not neurogenic in either case.

Cranial Nerve II: Optic Nerve

NOTE

For the nuclei and functions of this nerve, see **Table 3.3**. For a detailed discussion of optic nerve disturbances, see section 12.2.

Ophthalmoscopy

Inspection of the optic nerve papillae (optic discs) with the ophthalmoscope is an important technique for assessment of the optic nerve. Abnormal pallor indicates an optic nerve lesion (**Fig. 3.4b**). In addition, **inspection of the fundus** can provide evidence of subacutely or chronically elevated intracranial pressure: in **papilledema**, the papillae are raised and hyperemic, and their margins are blurred. Enlarged

retinal veins indicate impaired venous drainage due to intracranial hypertension (cf. **Fig. 12.3**). A raised papilla with blurred margins can also be a sign of an inflammatory process affecting the optic nerve (see section 12.2.2, Progressive Impairment of Visual Acuity in One or Both Eyes).

NOTE

Intracranial hypertension causes papilledema, which can be seen by ophthalmoscopy. Papilledema may, however, be absent if the intracranial hypertension is acute.

Visual Acuity

For neurologic purposes, visual acuity is usually tested with a **wallchart** seen from a distance. Patients who wear eyeglasses should wear them for this test.

Perimetry

Visual field testing is of special importance in neurology. The visual fields can be roughly assessed in the neurologist's office or at the bedside with so-called **finger perimetry** (or digital confrontation; **Fig. 3.5**). The examiner sits directly in front of the patient and the patient fixes one eye on the examiner's nose. The examiner then moves a finger in each of the four quadrants of the visual field, testing first the right eye, then the left. The patient is asked whether he or she can see the finger. This method can reveal a major visual field defect, for example, **bitemporal hemianopsia** or **quadrantanopsia** (see section 12.2.1). If the visual acuity is impaired, the visual fields of the two eyes should be tested separately; if the visual acuity is normal, the visual fields can be tested with both eyes open, because the lesion, if any, lies behind the optic chiasm and any visual field defect will therefore be homonymous.

If **visual neglect** (see section 12.2.1, Etiologic Classification of Visual Field Defects) is suspected, the examiner should next perform double simultaneous stimulation of the visual field by moving the two index fingers at the same time in corresponding quadrants in the two halves of the field (left and right hemifields). The patient should report seeing both fingers. If both fingers are perceived on

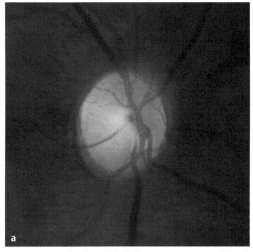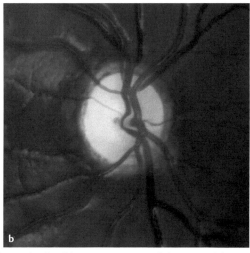

Fig. 3.4 Optic disc (papilla) of the right eye. a Normal disc. **b** Pale, atrophic disc. (These images are provided courtesy of the Department of Ophthalmology, University of Bern.)

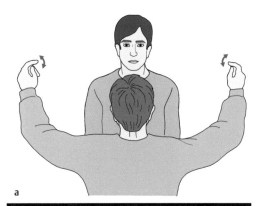

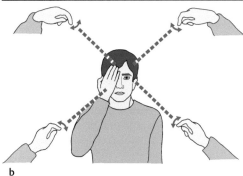

Fig. 3.5   Testing the visual fields by digital confrontation. a Double simultaneous testing for the detection of visual

Smaller (monocular or binocular) visual field defects can sometimes be detected by confrontational perimetry with a red object, but are usually revealed only by formal testing with equipment such as the Goldmann perimeter or octopus (see section 4.5.3).

Cranial Nerves III, IV, and VI: Oculomotor, Trochlear, and Abducens Nerves

> **NOTE**
>
> For the nuclei and functions of these nerves, see **Table 3.3**. For a detailed discussion of oculomotor and pupillary disturbances, see section 12.3.

Inspection

The examiner should first note the **position of the eyes at rest**, paying particular attention to the following: parallel position of the eyes, possible prominence of one eye, and symmetry of the palpebral fissures and of the pupils. The parallel position of the eyes is best assessed by observation of the small reflected images of light sources in the examining room in the patient's eyes, which should be at an analogous position on the two corneas (**Fig. 3.6**). A prominent globe (exophthalmos) can sometimes be appreciated by viewing the eyes tangentially from above (**Fig. 3.7**).

Ocular Motility

The function of the extraocular muscles is summarized in **Table 3.3** and **Fig. 3.8**. **Eye movements** are tested by having the patient keep the head stationary and follow the examiner's finger with his or her eyes. The motility of the globes is assessed along the vertical and horizontal axes. If abnormalities of eye

individual testing, but only one is seen on double simultaneous stimulation, this may be due to visual neglect. **Monocular visual field defects** are revealed by separate testing of the four quadrants of the visual field in each eye, with a finger starting in the periphery and moving gradually toward the center.

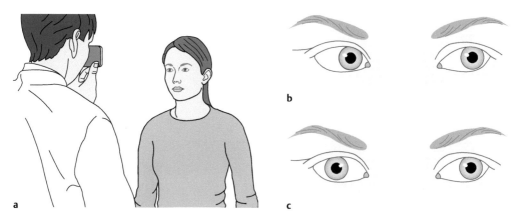

Fig. 3.6   Light reflected from the cornea (i.e., the Purkinje–Sanson reflex image) as used to assess the positions of the eyes.
a The examiner holds the flashlight near his or her own eyes and shines it into the eyes of the patient, who looks at the light.
b If the axes of the globes are parallel, the reflex images are on the same position of the cornea in the two eyes. **c** Dissimilar images indicate that the patient has a squint (strabismus).

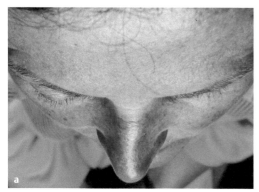
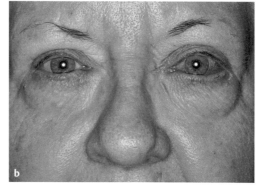

Fig. 3.7   Exophthalmos due to a fistula between the internal carotid artery and the cavernous sinus. a Fistula on the right side: the tangential view from above reveals exophthalmos. **b** Fistula on the left side: the elevated venous pressure has also caused conjunctival injection.

movement can be seen directly by the examiner, or if the patient reports double vision (**diplopia**), then the manner in which eye movement is restricted (including any abnormality of the resting position of the eyes) and the type of double vision enable the examiner to determine which muscle(s) is (are) paretic and, therefore, which cranial nerve is dysfunctional (**paralytic strabismus**). The eye muscles may, however, be weakened by intrinsic muscle lesions, rather than by cranial nerve palsies. A general principle for the interpretation of findings is that the positions of the eyes are farthest apart, and diplopia is therefore worst, when the patient looks in the direction of function of the paretic muscle (see section 12.3.4, Oculomotor Nerve Palsy).

NOTE

In diplopia, the farther image is always the one seen by the abnormal eye.

A **conjugate gaze palsy** (see section 12.3.3, Horizontal Gaze Palsy) is the inability to perform a conjugate eye movement to direct the gaze in a particular direction. In such patients, the lesion is not in the peripheral portion of a cranial nerve; it is located centrally, within the brain (a supranuclear lesion, i.e., one that lies above the nuclei of the cranial nerves that innervate the extraocular muscles). In contrast to peripheral lesions, the eyes remain parallel and there is no double vision. A gaze palsy can be either horizontal or vertical.

NOTE

When testing eye movements, the examiner should deliberately look for nystagmus (see section 12.3.2). Diplopia arises when the visual axes of the two eyes are not parallel. This can be detected objectively by the examiner from the nonidentically positioned reflected images on the patient's corneas.

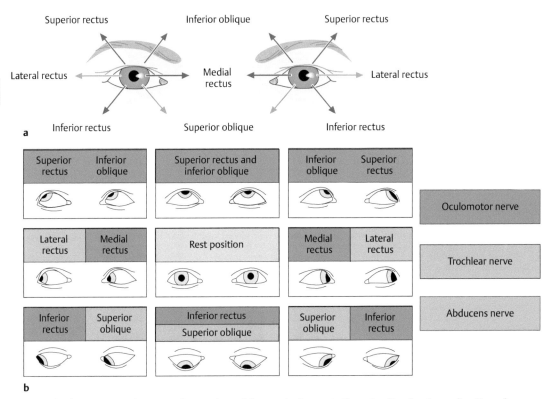

Fig. 3.8 **The three nerves to the extraocular muscles and the muscles innervated by each. a** The **six primary directions of gaze** are clinically tested (see arrows). The medial and lateral rectus muscles deviate the globe medially and laterally, respectively. The oblique muscles elevate and depress the adducted globe, while the superior and inferior rectus muscles elevate and depress the abducted globe. **b Scheme of Hering** indicating the direction of gaze in which the main function of each eye muscle is most strongly in evidence.

A nonparallel (skewed) position of the two eyes without diplopia implies that the patient has **concomitant strabismus**, a result of longstanding impaired vision in one eye (usually from birth or early childhood). No cranial nerve palsy is present. Concomitant strabismus can be demonstrated with the aid of a **cover test** (**Fig. 3.9**). The patient keeps both eyes open while the examiner covers one eye and asks the patient to fix his or her gaze on a particular object in the room. The cover is then rapidly switched to the other eye, so that the previously covered eye must jump into position to keep the gaze fixed on the same object. The initially uncovered eye, now covered, deviates to one side, as can be shown by switching the cover back again (alternating concomitant strabismus; usually divergent, but sometimes convergent).

Pupils

The examiner should note the **appearance**, **shape** (round or oblong), and **size** (narrow, normal, wide) of the pupils. Normal pupils are generally of equal size and react equally to light. Inequality of the pupils is called **anisocoria**. When the examiner illuminates the pupil of one eye, there should be reflex constriction of that pupil (the **direct light response**), accompanied by an equal reflex constriction of the other pupil (the **consensual light response**). To ensure that only one pupil is illuminated, the examiner shines a flashlight on one eye while blocking the light from the other eye with his or her own hand, held in the midline over the root of the patient's nose. The direct and consensual light responses should be tested in both eyes. **Convergence** is tested by having the patient fix his or her gaze on a distant object and then look at the examiner's finger, which is held close to the patient's face. The normal reaction is adduction of both eyes (convergence) accompanied by simultaneous reflex constriction of the pupils (the **near response**).

Pathologic abnormalities of the pupillary reflexes and their significance with regard to localization are presented in **Fig. 12.16**.

3

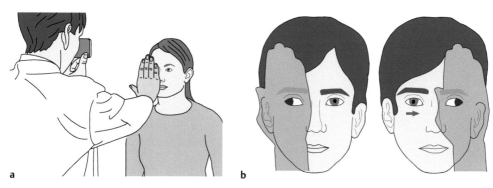

a   b

Fig. 3.9   Cover test. In concomitant, alternating, divergent strabismus, the covered eye, i.e., the one that is not fixating, deviates outward. **a** The examiner covers one of the patient's eyes while observing the position of the uncovered, freely fixating eye, as well as the corneal light reflex. The light source is held in front of the examiner's eyes. **b** When the cover is rapidly switched to the other eye, the newly uncovered eye moves to the fixating position, while the other eye deviates outward with a positioning saccade (→), indicating strabismus. The absence of a saccade implies that the axes of the two eyes were parallel.

Cranial Nerve V: Trigeminal Nerve

> **NOTE**
>
> For the nuclei and functions of this nerve, see **Table 3.3**. For a detailed discussion of trigeminal nerve disturbances, see section 12.4.

Testing Sensation in the Face

The somatosensory portion of this mixed cranial nerve originates in the ganglion cells of the gasserian ganglion. The cutaneous and mucosal zones innervated by the trigeminal nerve are shown in **Fig. 3.10**. **Sensation** should be tested with a cotton swab or a piece of tissue paper. The latter can also be used to test the **corneal reflex**: the patient is asked to look upward and the tactile stimulus is delivered to the lower edge of the cornea to avoid engendering a visually induced fright reaction. The reflex response consists of immediate closure of both eyes.

Examination of the Muscles of Mastication

The motor portion of the trigeminal nerve runs in its third branch (the mandibular nerve) to supply the muscles of mastication, that is, the masseter and temporalis muscles and the medial and lateral pterygoid muscles. The examiner tests the **function of the muscles of mastication** by placing his or her fingers in front of the angle of the jaw bilaterally and asking the patient to clamp the jaw tightly (press the teeth together). In unilateral (motor) trigeminal nerve paresis, the contraction of the masseter muscle on the affected side is palpably weaker and the **masseter reflex** may be weaker as well. When the patient opens the jaw, the mandible deviates to the side of the lesion because of the dominant effect of the pterygoid muscles on the healthy side. An excessively brisk masseter reflex (the intrinsic reflex of the muscles of mastication) indicates an upper-motor-

neuron lesion, that is, a supranuclear brainstem lesion or a lesion of the corticobulbar pathways.

Cranial Nerve VII: Facial Nerve

> **NOTE**
>
> For the nuclei and functions of this nerve, see **Table 3.3**. For a detailed discussion of facial nerve disturbances, see section 12.5.

Muscles of Facial Expression

The anatomy of the seventh cranial nerve is shown in **Fig. 12.19**. In assessing its function, the examiner should note any **asymmetry of the face**, spontaneous **facial expression** (mimesis), and contractions of the facial muscles during **movement**: the patient should be systematically asked to furrow the brow, close the eyes tightly, show his or her teeth, and whistle. In lesions of the facial nerve, the **corneal reflex** is weak because the efferent arm of the reflex arc is interrupted (rather than the afferent arm, as in trigeminal lesions). The clinical findings in facial nerve palsy, and the differentiation of peripheral and central facial weakness, are presented in **Fig. 12.21** and **Fig. 12.23**. The elicitation of the perioral reflexes is described in **Table 3.8**; markedly increased contraction of the perioral muscles is a sign of corticobulbar, extrapyramidal, or diffuse cerebral dysfunction.

Taste, Lacrimation, and Salivation

The facial nerve also contains gustatory fibers supplying **taste** to the anterior two-thirds of the tongue. When a facial nerve lesion is suspected, taste in this region can be tested by the application of substances with the four basic modalities of taste—sweet, salty, sour, and bitter—to the corresponding half of the tongue. Appropriate solutions to use are, for example, 20% glucose, 10% sodium chloride, 5% citric acid,

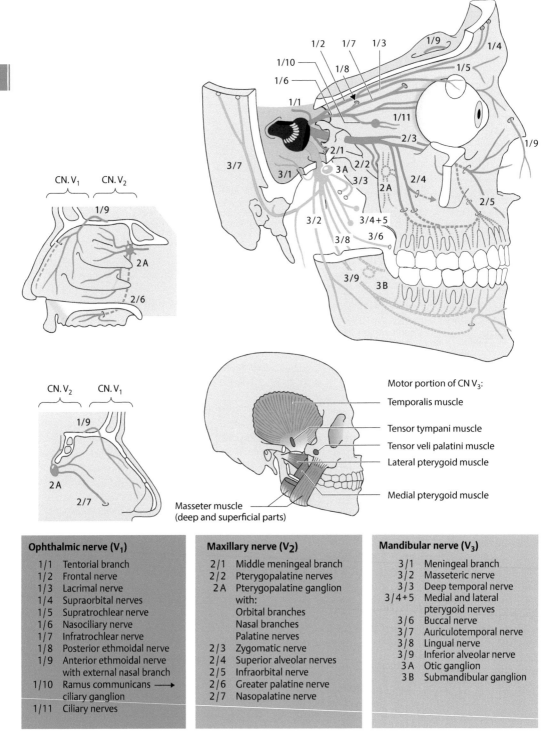

Ophthalmic nerve (V₁)

1/1	Tentorial branch
1/2	Frontal nerve
1/3	Lacrimal nerve
1/4	Supraorbital nerves
1/5	Supratrochlear nerve
1/6	Nasociliary nerve
1/7	Infratrochlear nerve
1/8	Posterior ethmoidal nerve
1/9	Anterior ethmoidal nerve with external nasal branch
1/10	Ramus communicans ⟶ ciliary ganglion
1/11	Ciliary nerves

Maxillary nerve (V₂)

2/1	Middle meningeal branch
2/2	Pterygopalatine nerves
2A	Pterygopalatine ganglion with:
	Orbital branches
	Nasal branches
	Palatine nerves
2/3	Zygomatic nerve
2/4	Superior alveolar nerves
2/5	Infraorbital nerve
2/6	Greater palatine nerve
2/7	Nasopalatine nerve

Mandibular nerve (V₃)

3/1	Meningeal branch
3/2	Masseteric nerve
3/3	Deep temporal nerve
3/4+5	Medial and lateral pterygoid nerves
3/6	Buccal nerve
3/7	Auriculotemporal nerve
3/8	Lingual nerve
3/9	Inferior alveolar nerve
3A	Otic ganglion
3B	Submandibular ganglion

Fig. 3.10   Anatomy of the somatosensory and motor portions of the trigeminal nerve.

and 1% quinine. (Note: "bitter" is perceived in the mucosa of the posterior third of the tongue; this sensation is thus mediated by the glossopharyngeal nerve, not the facial nerve.) Peripheral lesions of the facial nerve also cause diminished **lacrimation and salivation**, which are usually not noticed by the patient and require special tests to demonstrate. There may also be hypersensitivity to sound (**hyperacusis**).

Cranial Nerve VIII: Vestibulocochlear Nerve

> **NOTE**
>
> For the nuclei and functions of this nerve, see **Table 3.3**. For a detailed discussion of vestibulocochlear nerve disturbances, see section 12.6.

Hearing

The anatomy of the vestibulocochlear nerve is depicted in **Fig. 3.11** and **Table 3.3**. The neurologist's assessment of the patient's hearing is generally limited to determining whether (uni- or bilateral) **hearing loss** is present and, if so, whether it is due to **impaired conduction of sound** (middle ear process, obstruction of the external auditory canal) or a **sensorineural deficit** (process affecting the inner ear or the cochlear portion of the eighth cranial nerve). The examiner tests hearing separately in each ear, rubbing two fingers together in front of the right ear, then the left, and asking whether the patient hears this equally on the two sides (or at all); a more precise test is to speak or whisper words from a distances of ~5 m and ask the patient to repeat them. The patient must inactivate hearing in the ear not being tested by vigorously rubbing a finger back and forth in the ear canal. Total deafness, that is, deafness even for very loud sounds, is never due to a conductive deficit alone.

Differentiation of Conductive and Sensorineural Hearing Loss

These two types of hearing loss can be distinguished by the Rinne and Weber tests (**Fig. 3.12**).

— **Rinne test**: Air conduction of sound is normally better than bone conduction, as can be demonstrated as follows: first, a vibrating tuning fork is placed on the mastoid process. As soon as the subject can no longer hear the tone, the tuning fork is removed from the mastoid process and placed next to the ear. The tone should then be heard again, and should take approximately twice as long to disappear as it did on the mastoid process. This is called a "positive," that is, normal, Rinne test. If the air-conduction tone disappears sooner than this or is not heard at all, then the Rinne test is negative, indicating conductive

hearing loss (due either to a middle ear process or to obstruction of the external auditory canal). In patients with sensorineural hearing loss, the Rinne test is positive (normal).

— **Weber test**: The vibrating tuning fork is placed in the center of the forehead or on the vertex. Normally, the tone is heard equally loudly in both ears and is localized to the midline. It is lateralized to the affected ear in conductive hearing loss and to the normal ear in sensorineural hearing loss (caused by a process affecting the cochlea or the cochlear portion of the eighth cranial nerve). When unilateral hearing loss has been present for many years, the Weber test no longer lateralizes.

> **NOTE**
>
> — **Conductive hearing loss:**
>   • Rinne test: negative = bone conduction better than air conduction.
>   • Weber test: lateralization to the side of the hearing loss.
> — **Sensorineural hearing loss:**
>   • Rinne test: positive = air conduction better than bone conduction.
>   • Weber test: lateralization to the normal side.

Vestibular Function

The most common symptom of a lesion affecting the labyrinth or the vestibular portion of the vestibulocochlear nerve is **vertigo**. Patients usually describe a directional or systematic type of vertigo, for example, rotational vertigo ("like on a merry-go-round"), a feeling of being tilted to one side, or an "elevator" feeling. They can often say in which direction they seem to be rotating. In contrast, dizziness of nonvestibular origin—for example, due to a brainstem lesion—is often less well defined; patients may complain of giddiness, swaying, or seeing black before their eyes (see also section 12.6.2).

The objective sign of a lesion of the vestibular portion of the vestibulocochlear nerve is **nystagmus**—a rapid, rhythmic jerking movement of both eyes in the same direction (also called "jerk nystagmus"). There is a slow conjugate deviation in one direction, followed by a rapid conjugate movement returning the eyes to the original position, and then the cycle starts again. The slow deviation is the pathologic component of nystagmus; the rapid component is a reflex correction to preserve fixation. By convention, however, the direction of nystagmus is stated as the direction of the rapid phase. Nystagmus may be **horizontal** (toward the right or the left), **vertical** (upbeat or downbeat), or **rotatory** (clockwise or counterclockwise). Nystagmus of vestibular origin can sometimes be seen even when the patient looks straight

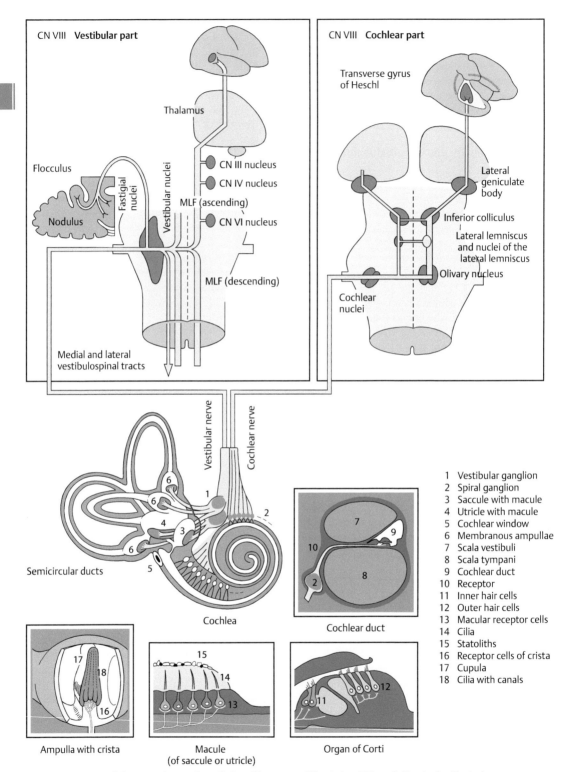

CN VIII   Vestibular part

Thalamus

Flocculus

Fastigial nuclei

Vestibular nuclei

Nodulus

CN III nucleus
CN IV nucleus
MLF (ascending)
CN VI nucleus

MLF (descending)

Medial and lateral vestibulospinal tracts

CN VIII   Cochlear part

Transverse gyrus of Heschl

Lateral geniculate body

Inferior colliculus

Lateral lemniscus and nuclei of the lateral lemniscus

Olivary nucleus

Cochlear nuclei

Vestibular nerve

Cochlear nerve

Semicircular ducts

Cochlea

Cochlear duct

Ampulla with crista

Macule (of saccule or utricle)

Organ of Corti

1 Vestibular ganglion
2 Spiral ganglion
3 Saccule with macule
4 Utricle with macule
5 Cochlear window
6 Membranous ampullae
7 Scala vestibuli
8 Scala tympani
9 Cochlear duct
10 Receptor
11 Inner hair cells
12 Outer hair cells
13 Macular receptor cells
14 Cilia
15 Statoliths
16 Receptor cells of crista
17 Cupula
18 Cilia with canals

Fig. 3.11   Anatomy of the internal ear and vestibulocochlear nerve. Abbreviation: MLF, medial longitudinal fasciculus.

3

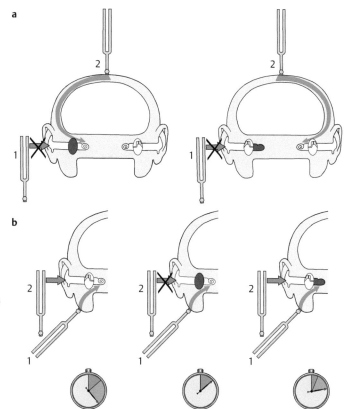

Fig. 3.12   Weber and Rinne hearing tests.
a Weber test: in a patient with right-sided conductive hearing loss (picture at left), the tuning fork cannot be heard when held next to the ear (1). If it is placed on the forehead (2), the vibratory tone is heard and localized to the side of the hearing loss, i.e., to the right ear. In contrast, in a patient with right-sided sensorineural hearing loss (picture at right), the tone is localized to the normal (left) ear. **b Rinne test:** the tuning fork is first placed on the mastoid process (1). As soon as the tone disappears, the tuning fork is held next to the ear. The tone will now be heard again if hearing is normal (2), but will not be heard at all if there is right-sided conductive hearing loss (middle picture; negative Rinne test). In right-sided sensorineural hearing loss, the tone will be heard, but for a shorter time than normal, both by bone conduction and with the tuning fork held next to the ear (positive, i.e., normal Rinne test).

ahead (nystagmus that beats spontaneously in this way is called **spontaneous nystagmus**); in other cases, it appears only when the examiner asks the patient to look to one side. Nystagmus of vestibular origin always beats away from the side of the lesion, regardless of whether it appears when the patient looks straight ahead, to the right, and/or to the left. Spontaneous nystagmus of vestibular origin is to be distinguished from **physiologic end-gaze nystagmus** and from **gaze-evoked nystagmus**. End-gaze nystagmus arises when the patient looks all the way to one side or the other (into the monocular visual field); its rapid phase beats in the direction of gaze, it is seen in both eyes to the same extent, and it disappears spontaneously after several beats. It is found symmetrically in normal individuals. If end-gaze nystagmus is seen on examination, the examiner should bring the test object ~10 degrees back into the binocular visual field. The nystagmus is clinically significant only if it is still present after this maneuver (gaze-evoked nystagmus). Some common pathologic types of nystagmus are listed and described in **Table 12.2**.
Further evidence for a vestibular disturbance can be obtained from the **head-thrust test** (Halmagyi test)

for the function of the horizontal semicircular canals (**Fig. 3.13**). The patient looks at the nose of the examiner, sitting opposite. The examiner (or a third person) rapidly rotates the patient's head at least 45 degrees to one side. Normally, the patient's gaze remains fixed on the examiner's nose because of the rapid function of the vestibulo-ocular reflex. If one horizontal semicircular canal is defective, however, the eyes turn along with the head toward the side of the lesion and then make a rapid corrective saccade back to the original fixation point.
Certain **abnormalities of stance and gait** also indicate vestibular dysfunction (the Unterberger step test, the star gait test, and blind walking, described in section 3.2.2), as does the **Bárány pointing test**: the patient stretches one arm out forward, then lowers it to point to a previously indicated target, for example, the examiner's index finger. Next, the patient repeats this maneuver with his or her eyes closed, trying to hit the target as precisely as possible. A unilateral vestibular lesion (or a lesion in the ipsilateral cerebellar hemisphere) causes the arm to deviate to the side of the lesion during its downward course.

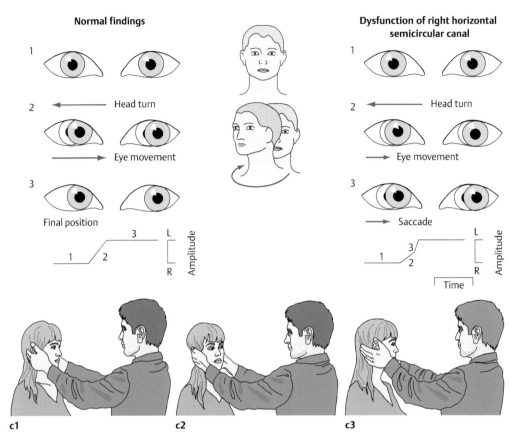

Fig. 3.13   Head-impulse test for the function of the horizontal semicircular canal (as described by Huber). a Normal finding.
b Finding with functional loss of the right horizontal semicircular canal. **c** Performance of the head-impulse test. **c1**: The examiner gently moves the patient's head back and forth, so that the patient relaxes the nuchal muscles while keeping the eyes fixated on the examiner's nose. **c2**: The examiner turns the patient's head to the right with a quick jerk. If the semicircular canal is functioning normally, the vestibulo-ocular reflex causes the eyes to move promptly leftward, so that they remain fixated on the examiner's nose; no corrective positioning saccade is necessary. A saccade thus indicates dysfunction of the semicircular canal. **c3**: Rapid turning of the head to the left.

Various **instruments** are available for examining vestibular function.

— **Frenzel goggles** make nystagmus easier to observe. They contain strong magnifying lenses that make the patient unable to fixate, as well as a lamp to illuminate the globes. Vestibular nystagmus, which can often be suppressed by fixation, may only be visible when the patient wears Frenzel goggles. Head-shaking is a further provocative maneuver. The magnification provided by the Frenzel lenses also makes it easier for the examiner to see fine movements.

— Vestibular lesions can be examined objectively by testing of the **rotational** and **caloric excitability** of the corresponding labyrinth. In the normal case, irrigation of the external auditory canal with warm water induces nystagmus with the rapid phase toward the irrigated ear (with cold-water irrigation, the rapid phase is toward the opposite ear). If a vestibular lesion is present, the induced nystagmus is diminished or absent.

Cranial Nerves IX and X: Glossopharyngeal and Vagus Nerves

| NOTE

For the nuclei and functions of these nerves, see **Table 3.3**. For a detailed discussion of disturbances of the glossopharyngeal and vagus nerves, see section 12.7.

The efferent fibers from the nucleus ambiguus to the muscles of the palate, larynx, and pharynx reach these structures through the glossopharyngeal and vagus nerves. The larynx is innervated by two vagal branches, the superior laryngeal nerve and the recurrent laryngeal nerve. The glossopharyngeal nerve carries somatosensory fibers from the soft palate, the posterior pharyngeal wall, the tonsillar fossa, and the middle ear, as well as gustatory fibers from the posterior third of the tongue. Somatosensory fibers from the external auditory canal, part of the external ear, and the meninges of the posterior fossa travel along the vagus nerve into the brainstem. The vagus nerve also carries efferent parasympathetic fibers to the thoracic and abdominal viscera (cf. **Table 3.3**).

The motor function of the 9th and 10th cranial nerves is assessed by **inspection of the palate and throat** and, more importantly, by observation of the movements of these structures during **phonation** ("aaah ...") and after induction of the **gag reflex** by touching the posterior pharyngeal wall with, for example, a cotton swab. Unilateral weakness of the palatal veil and the pharyngeal muscles makes these structures deviate laterally away from the side of the lesion, as shown in **Fig. 3.14**. Hoarseness due to a unilateral recurrent laryngeal nerve palsy can sometimes be heard only when the patient sings. Unilateral absence of the gag reflex also indicates dysfunction of the glossopharyngeal and vagus nerves.

Cranial Nerve XI: Accessory Nerve

> **NOTE**
>
> For the nuclei and functions of this nerve, see **Table 3.3**. For a detailed discussion of accessory nerve disturbances, see section 12.8.

The external (final) branch of the accessory nerve, which is a purely motor nerve, innervates the sternocleidomastoid muscle and the upper portion of the trapezius muscle. To test the **sternocleidomastoid muscle** on one side, the examiner instructs the patient to turn the head to the opposite side against resistance and then observes and palpates the muscular contraction at the anterior edge of the lateral triangle of the neck (**Fig. 3.15**).

The **upper portion of the trapezius muscle** is examined as follows: the examiner stands in front of the patient, puts both hands on the patient's shoulders, grasps the upper edge of the trapezius muscle on either side between the thumb and index finger, and asks the patient to shrug the shoulders against resistance. In unilateral accessory nerve palsy, the shrug is less powerful on the affected side, and the trapezius muscle is palpably thinner and weaker (**Fig. 3.16**).

Cranial Nerve XII: Hypoglossal Nerve

> **NOTE**
>
> For the nuclei and functions of this nerve, see **Table 3.3**. For a detailed discussion of hypoglossal nerve disturbances, see section 12.9.

The 12th cranial nerve is a purely motor nerve to the muscles of the tongue. Hypoglossal nerve dysfunction is evident on **inspection of the tongue**;

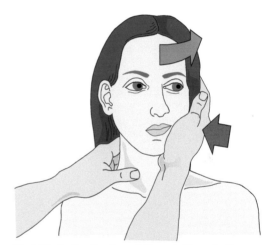

Fig. 3.15 Testing the sternocleidomastoid muscle. The patient tries to turn the head to the left against the examiner's resistance. The right sternocleidomastoid muscle contracts.

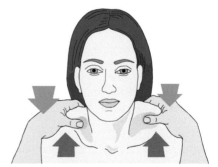

Fig. 3.16 Testing the upper portion of the trapezius muscle. The examiner places his or her hands on the patient's shoulders, grasps the upper edge of the trapezius muscle on each side between his or her thumb and index finger, and asks the patient to shrug the shoulders. Unilateral weakness, reduced contraction, or diminished volume of the trapezius muscle can be palpated.

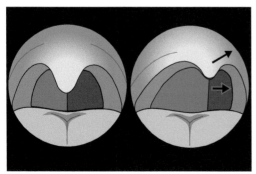

Fig. 3.14 Palatal deviation. In right glossopharyngeal nerve palsy, the palate and posterior pharyngeal wall deviate to the normal left side when the patient gags.

3

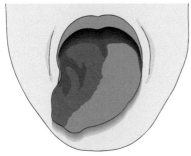

Fig. 3.17 Atrophy and weakness of the right half of the tongue in a lesion of the right hypoglossal nerve.

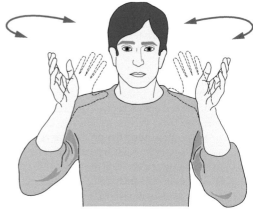

Fig. 3.18 Testing of diadochokinesis by rapid pronation and supination of the forearms.

lesions of this nerve produce tongue atrophy and weakness. A unilateral lesion usually produces a longitudinal furrow; when protruded, the tongue deviates to the weaker side because of the predominant force of the intact contralateral genioglossus muscle, which "pushes" the tongue forward (**Fig. 3.17**).

Phonation, Articulation, and Speech

Assessment of the patient's **voice** and **speech** is an obligatory part of the neurologic examination. The examiner should pay attention to hoarseness, to the volume of speech (e.g., hypophonia in Parkinson disease; see section 6.9.2), and to disturbances of articulation (dysarthria), of the tempo of speech, and of its linguistic form and content (aphasia; see section 3.9.2).

3.4 Upper Limbs

 Key Point

The upper limb examination begins with inspection: the examiner should assess the spontaneous movements and any postural abnormalities of the arms, hands, and fingers, as well as muscle bulk and skin consistency. Any involuntary movements, such as tremor or fasciculations, should be noted. Next, the range of motion of the larger joints is tested, and the pulses are palpated. The neurologic examination (in the narrow sense) can now be performed, with assessment of strength, reflexes, coordination, and sensation.

3.4.1 General Aspects

The examiner should ask the patient **which hand he or she mostly uses**, right or left. Only persons who use a pair of scissors, a knife, or a sewing needle with their left hand, or write with the left hand, are true left-handers. Any abnormalities of **muscle bulk** should be noted, in particular isolated atrophy of muscle groups. **Fasciculations** must be deliberately

sought: in our experience, these involuntary contractions of groups of muscle fibers, which induce no movement, can be seen under the skin only by careful observation of the unclothed patient from an adequate distance and for a sufficient length of time. The **trophic state of the skin**, the papillary pattern of the fingertips, and the configuration of the nails should also be assessed. Important positive findings include **abnormalities of finger posture, tremor**, and other **involuntary movements**. The **range of motion of the larger joints** should be tested individually and the **pulses** in the limbs should be felt. Vascular bruits should be sought in the supraclavicular fossa when indicated.

3.4.2 Motor Function and Coordination

Several standard tests are used to assess motor function and coordination.

— **Diadochokinesis** is the ability to carry out rapid alternating movements, for example, pronation and supination of the forearm (**Fig. 3.18**). Such movements will be abnormally slow (bradydiadochokinesis) or irregular (dysdiadochokinesia) on one side or both in the presence of paresis, extrapyramidal processes, and cerebellar diseases.

— Movements of the hands and fingers are tested with **finger-tapping**, which is performed with rapidly alternating flexion and extension of the thumb and the four other fingers at their metacarpophalangeal joints. Paresis or hypokinesia of extrapyramidal origin reduces the spread between the thumb and the other fingers, which becomes even smaller on repeated tapping (**Fig. 3.19**).

— In the **postural test**, the patient extends both arms horizontally in front, in supination, with eyes closed (**Fig. 3.20**). An involuntary sinking or pronation of one arm ("pronator drift"), or involuntary flexion at the elbow or wrist, indicates hemiparesis of central origin; conjugate deviation of both arms to one side implies an ipsilateral lesion of the labyrinth or cerebellum.

- In the **arm-rolling test**, the patient rapidly rotates the forearms around each other in front of the trunk (**Fig. 3.21**). Mild hemiparesis manifests itself as markedly diminished movement of the affected limb.
- In the **finger–nose test**, the patient keeps his or her eyes closed and brings the index finger slowly to the tip of the nose, in a wide arc. This can normally be done smoothly and confidently (**Fig. 3.22a**). Fluctuating deviation of the finger from the ideal arc is a manifestation of ataxia (**Fig. 3.22b**), indicating either a proprioceptive disturbance or a lesion in the ipsilateral cerebellar hemisphere. On the other hand, a deviation that first appears when the finger is near its target and then worsens as it approaches is called intention tremor (**Fig. 3.22c**) and is caused by lesions of the dentate nucleus of the cerebellum or its efferent projections.
- A positive **rebound phenomenon** consists of inadequate braking of the normal, small rebound movement that occurs when the patient isometrically contracts a muscle against the examiner's resistance and the resistance is suddenly removed (**Fig. 3.23**). If the patient is sitting, the examiner can test for rebound of the biceps brachii muscle (while taking care lest the patient hit himself or herself in the face). A patient lying on the examining table can be asked to extend one arm and raise it a little, then press strongly downward against the examiner's resistance. If the examiner suddenly lets go, a healthy subject will brake the ensuing downward movement of the arm in time, but a patient with hemiparesis or cerebellar dysfunction will hit the examining table with it.

3.4.3 Muscle Tone and Strength

Muscle Tone

Muscle tone in the upper limbs can be tested with wide-amplitude passive movement of the radiocarpal joint or the elbow joint. The movement should be rapid, but not rhythmic (so that the patient cannot predict its course).

- Diminished muscle tone (**hypotonia**) is a characteristic sign of intrinsic muscle lesions, peripheral nerve lesions, ipsilateral cerebellar dysfunction, and hyperkinetic extrapyramidal diseases.
- **Spasticity** is a type of increased muscle tone due to lesions of the pyramidal pathway (**Fig. 3.24a**). The resistance of a spastic upper limb to passive movement is usually strong at first, but may then suddenly give way ("clasp-knife phenomenon"); alternatively, it may increase on continued passive movement.

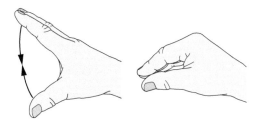

Fig. 3.19   Finger-tapping. The test involves rapid alternating flexion and extension of the thumb and the other four fingers at their metacarpophalangeal joints.

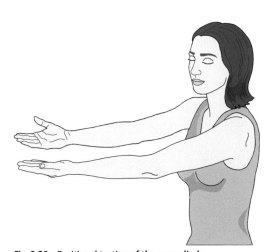

Fig. 3.20   Positional testing of the upper limbs.

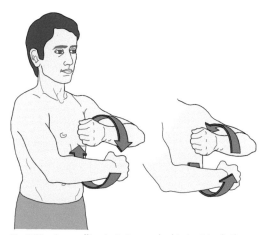

Fig. 3.21   Arm-rolling test. A normal subject rotates both arms to a roughly equal extent, while a patient with central hemiparesis (even if mild) moves the nonparetic limb much more than the paretic one.

3

- **Rigidity** is a viscous or waxy resistance to passive movement that can be felt to an equal extent throughout the entire movement. Mild rigidity may only be detectable on coactivation of the opposite limb; thus, for example, the examiner can bring out rigidity of the right wrist joint by asking the patient to move the left hand. Rigidity is most commonly found in Parkinson disease (**Fig. 3.24b**). The accompanying parkinsonian **cogwheel phenomenon** (**Fig. 3.24c**) is best appreciated at the radiocarpal joint. The examiner should fix the patient's forearm with one hand, grasp the patient's fingertips with the other, and alternately flex and extend the radiocarpal joint, slowly and with a wide excursion, but not in perfect rhythm (**Fig. 3.25**). The examiner will then feel multiple, brief impulses of resistance at irregular intervals, giving the overall impression of a saccadic movement.
- Increased muscle tone may also result from **active opposition** to passive movement, with the patient seemingly unable to relax the muscular contraction. This phenomenon, known by the German term *Gegenhalten* ("opposition"), is a sign of a frontal lobe lesion.

Strength

Strength is tested in muscle groups that carry out a single movement or, if necessary, in individual muscles. The patient is asked to **contract the corresponding muscle(s) actively against the examiner's resistance**. The strength of contraction is judged at the endpoint of the related movement: thus, the examiner tests biceps strength by trying to extend the patient's flexed elbow against resistance, and triceps strength by trying to flex the extended elbow against resistance. The evaluation of potential lesions of individual nerve roots or peripheral nerves requires specific testing of the particular muscles or muscle groups innervated by these nerves (see section 13.1). A decrease in strength is called weakness. **Table 3.4** gives an overview of terms that are used to describe it. For the purpose of documentation, muscle strength can be graded semiquantitatively with the Medical Research Council (MRC) scale shown in **Table 3.5**.

3.4.4 Reflexes

Types of Reflexes

Reflexes are processes that are induced by a specific stimulus, always take the same course, and cannot be voluntarily influenced by either the patient or the examiner.

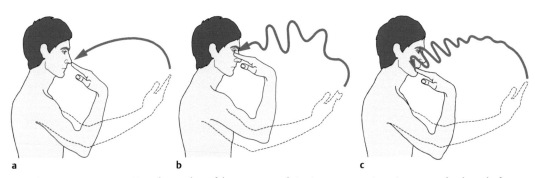

Fig. 3.22 Finger–nose test. a Normal, smooth, confident movement. **b** Ataxic movement. **c** Intention tremor: the closer the finger comes to its target (nose), the more it deviates from the ideal line of approach.

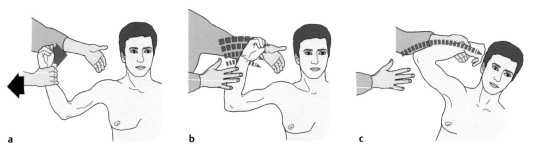

Fig. 3.23 Rebound phenomenon due to a cerebellar lesion. a Method of testing: the examiner's other hand protects the patient's face. **b** When the examiner suddenly releases the patient's actively flexed arm, the ensuing involuntary flexion is promptly braked in the normal case. **c** Braking is inadequate (the rebound phenomenon is positive) if there is an ipsilateral cerebellar lesion.

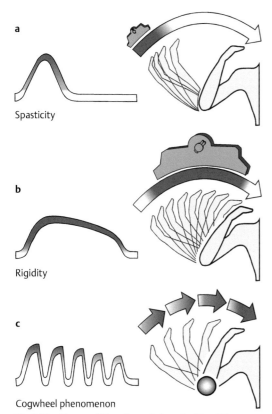

a

Spasticity

b

Rigidity

c

Cogwheel phenomenon

Fig. 3.24 Abnormalities of muscle tone (a, b) and the cogwheel phenomenon (c).

- For the **intrinsic** muscle reflexes (also called proprioceptive muscle reflexes), the site (muscle) of the eliciting stimulus is the same as that of the reflex contraction.
- For the **extrinsic** (exteroceptive) reflexes, the stimulus and the response are at different sites, and the afferent and efferent arms of the reflex loop, therefore, belong to different peripheral nerves or segmental nerve roots. Extrinsic reflexes become less intense ("habituate") on repeated stimulation.
- **Pathologic** reflexes may be present in normal children but are seldom seen in normal adults;

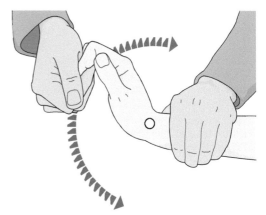

Fig. 3.25 Testing for the cogwheel phenomenon in the radiocarpal joint. The examiner fixes the patient's forearm with one hand, grasps the patient's fingers with the other, and moves them slowly (but not rhythmically) back and forth.

Table 3.4

Terms used to describe weakness

Term	Meaning
Paresis	Weakness but not paralysis
Plegia	(Total) paralysis
Hemiparesis/hemiplegia	Weakness or paralysis of one side of the body
Monoparesis/monoplegia	Weakness or paralysis of one limb
Paraparesis/paraplegia	Weakness or paralysis of both lower limbs
Brachial diplegia	Weakness or paralysis of both upper limbs
Quadriparesis/quadriplegia	Weakness or paralysis of all four limbs

Table 3.5

Grading of muscle strength (0 to 5 scale of the British Medical Research Council)

M0 = no muscle contraction
M1 = visible contraction not resulting in movement
M2 = movement of the body part only when the effect of gravity is eliminated
M3 = movement against gravity
M4 = movement against moderate resistance
M5 = full strength

Note: Grades M3 and M4 can be optionally subdivided by adding plus or minus signs.

they can be due to various central nervous diseases. Some pathologic reflexes are of the extrinsic type.

The more important reflexes and the segmental nerve roots and peripheral nerves mediating them are listed in **Table 3.6**, **Table 3.7**, and **Table 3.8**.

Intrinsic Muscle Reflexes of the Upper Limb

The intrinsic muscle reflexes are elicited by a rapid, forceful blow on the tendon of a muscle or on the bone to which the tendon is attached. The resulting, transient stretching of the muscle excites receptors in the muscle spindles, so that afferent impulses are generated. These travel to the spinal cord and excite the α-motor neurons innervating the stimulated muscle (usually by way of interneurons at the same segmental level). The upper limb reflexes that are usually tested are the **triceps**, **biceps**, and **radial periosteal reflexes** (**Table 3.6**). The radial periosteal reflex is elicited by a tap on the styloid process of the radius; this is followed by contraction, not only of the brachioradialis muscle, but also of the biceps and brachialis muscles. The elicitation of these reflexes is illustrated in **Fig. 3.26**.

The two important finger flexor reflexes are essentially variations of the same reflex. The **Trömner reflex** is elicited by a rapid tap on the pads of the patient's lightly flexed fingers (**Fig. 3.27**). The response consists of flexion of the distal interphalangeal joints of the fingers and thumb (only in the hand that was stimulated, not in the other hand). To elicit the **Hoffmann sign**, the examiner gently grasps the distal phalanx of one of the patient's fingers (usually the middle finger) between his or her own thumb and index finger, and then lets it snap back as the thumb slides off the patient's fingernail. The response is the same as in the Trömner reflex (**Fig. 3.27**).

The more common abnormalities of the intrinsic muscle reflexes and their significance are presented in **Table 3.9**.

Facilitating Maneuvers

Initially faint or not clearly elicitable intrinsic muscle reflexes can be enhanced with various maneuvers, which are based on the principle that preloading of the intrafusal muscle spindle fibers makes them more sensitive to stretch. Forceful contraction of practically any muscle group in the body results in a generalized sensitization of all muscle spindle fibers. Thus, all of the intrinsic muscle reflexes can be made stronger by having the patient forcefully lift his or her head from the headrest (in the supine position), clench the teeth, make fists, strongly plantar-flex the feet, or interlock the hands and pull hard (this is called the **Jendrassik handgrip**). These maneuvers are illustrated in **Fig. 3.28**.

Pyramidal Tract Signs in the Upper Limb

Lesions in the pyramidal pathway cause characteristic changes in the pattern of the reflexes that are normally present and bring out pathologic reflexes

Table 3.6

The most important normal intrinsic muscle reflexes

Reflex	Stimulus	Response	Muscle(s)	Peripheral nerve	Segment
Masseter reflex	Tap on the chin or a tongue depressor laid on the lower teeth, with slightly opened mouth	Brief mouth closure	Masseter muscle	Trigeminal nerve	CN V
Trapezius reflex	Tap on the lateral attachment of the trapezius to the coracoid process	Shoulder elevation	Trapezius muscle	Accessory nerve	CN XI C3–C4
Scapulohumeral reflex	Tap on the medial edge of the lower half of the scapula	Adduction and external rotation of the dependent arm	Infraspinatus and teres minor muscles	Suprascapular and axillary nerve	C4–C6
Biceps reflex	Tap on the biceps tendon with flexed elbow	Elbow flexion	Biceps brachii muscle	Musculocutaneous nerve	C5–C6
Brachioradialis reflex ("radial periosteal reflex")	Tap on the distal end of the radius with lightly flexed elbow and pronated forearm	Elbow flexion	Brachioradialis muscle (biceps brachii and brachialis muscles)	Radial and musculo-cutaneous nerves	C5–C6
Pectoralis reflex	Tap on the scapulohumeral joint from anteriorly	Forward movement of the shoulder	Pectoralis major and minor muscles	Medial and lateral pectoral	C5–T4

Table 3.6

The most important normal intrinsic muscle reflexes *(continued)*

Reflex	Stimulus	Response	Muscle(s)	Peripheral nerve	Segment
Triceps reflex	Tap on the triceps tendon with bent elbow	Elbow extension	Triceps brachii muscle	Radial nerve	C7–C8
Thumb reflex	Tap on the flexor pollicis longus tendon in the distal third of the forearm	Flexion of the thumb at the interphalangeal joint	Flexor pollicis longus muscle	Median nerve	C6–C8
Wrist reflex	Tap on the dorsum of the wrist, proximal to the radiocarpal joint	Extension of the wrist and fingers (inconstant)	Wrist extensors and long extensors of the fingers	Radial nerve	C6–C8
Finger flexor reflex	Tap on the examiner's thumb, which is laid in the palm of the patient's hand; or, tap on the flexor tendons on the volar surface of the wrist	Flexion of the fingers (and of the wrist)	Flexor digitorum superficialis muscle (flexor carpi muscles)	Median (ulnar) nerve	C7–C8
Trömner reflex	Patient's hand held at the middle finger; tap on the volar side of the distal phalanx of the middle finger	Flexion of the distal phalanges of the fingers (including the thumb)	flexor digitorum profundus muscle	Median (ulnar) nerve	C7–C8 (T1)
Adductor reflex	Tap on the medial condyle of the femur	Leg adduction	Adductors	Obturator nerve	L2–L4
Quadriceps femoris reflex ("patellar tendon reflex," "knee-jerk reflex")	Tap on the quadriceps tendon below the patella with the knee lightly flexed	Knee extension	Quadriceps femoris muscle	Femoral nerve	(L2) L3–L4
Tibialis posterior reflex	Tap on the tibialis posterior tendon behind the medial malleolus	Supination of the foot (inconstant)	Tibialis posterior muscle	Tibial nerve	L5
Peroneus muscle reflex (foot extensor reflex)	Foot lightly flexed and supinated; examiner's finger placed over the distal end of the metatarsal bones; tap on the finger, especially over the first and second metatarsal bones	Dorsiflexion and pronation of the foot	Long extensors of the foot and toes, peronei	Peroneal nerve	L5–S1
Semimembranosus and semitendinosus reflex	Tap on the tendon of the medial knee flexors (patient prone, knee lightly flexed and relaxed)	Palpable muscle contraction	Semimembranosus and semitendinosus muscles	Sciatic nerve	S1
Biceps femoris reflex	Tap on the tendon of the lateral knee flexors (patient prone, knee lightly flexed and relaxed)	Muscle contraction	Biceps femoris muscle	Sciatic nerve	S1–S2
Triceps surae reflex ("Achilles reflex," "ankle-jerk reflex")	Tap on the Achilles tendon (knee lightly flexed, foot in right-angle posture)	Plantar flexion of the foot	Triceps surae muscle (and other plantar flexors)	Tibial nerve	S1–S2
Toe flexor reflex (Rossolimo sign)	Tap on the pads of the toes	Flexion of the toes	Flexor digitorum and flexor hallucis longus muscles	Tibial nerve	S1–S2

Abbreviation: CN, cranial nerve.

Table 3.7

The most important normal extrinsic muscle reflexes

Reflex	Stimulus	Response	Muscle(s)	Peripheral nerve	Segment
Pupillary reflex	Incident light, convergence	Constriction	Constrictor pupillae muscle	Optic and oculomotor nerves	Diencephalon, midbrain, pons
Corneal reflex	Gently touching the cornea from the side, e.g., with a wisp of cotton or piece of tissue paper, while the eye looks medially	Eye closure (and simultaneous upward movement of the globes = Bell phenomenon)	Orbicularis oculi muscle	Trigeminal and facial nerves	Midpons
Bell phenomenon (palpebro-oculogyric reflex)	Attempted active eye closure while the examiner holds the upper lids open	The globes normally turn upward	Superior rectus and inferior oblique muscles	Trigeminal and oculomotor nerves	Pons
Auriculopalpebral reflex	Sudden noise from a source that the patient cannot see	Blink	Orbicularis oculi muscle	Vestibulocochlear and facial nerves	Caudal pons
Palatal reflex and pharyngeal (gag) reflex	Touching the soft palate or the posterior pharyngeal wall with a tongue depressor	Elevation of the palatal veil and symmetric contraction of the posterior pharyngeal wall	Palatal and pharyngeal musculature	Glossopharyngeal and vagus nerves	Medulla
Mayer reflex of the proximal interphalangeal joint	Forced passive flexion of the proximal interphalangeal joints of the third and fourth fingers	Adduction and opposition of the first metacarpal bone	Adductor pollicis muscle, opponens pollicis muscle	Ulnar and median nerves	C6–T1
Abdominal skin reflex	Rapidly and lightly stroking the abdominal skin from lateral to medial	Movement of the abdominal skin, including the umbilicus, toward the side of the stimulus	Abdominal musculature	Intercostal nerves, hypogastric nerves, and ilioinguinal nerve	T6–T12
Cremaster reflex (in males)	Stroking the skin on the upper medial surface of the thigh (or pinching the proximal adductor muscles)	Retraction of the testes	Cremaster muscle	Genital branch of the genitofemoral nerve	L1–L2
Gluteal reflex	Stroking the skin over the gluteus maximus muscle	Contraction of the gluteus maximus muscle (inconstant)	Gluteus medius muscle, gluteus maximus muscle	Superior and inferior gluteal nerves	L4–S1
Bulbocavernosus reflex (in males)	Gently pinching the glans penis; pinprick on the skin of the dorsum of the penis	Contraction of the bulbocavernosus muscle (visible at the root of the penis in the perineum, or palpable by rectal examination)	Bulbocavernosus muscle	Pudendal nerve	S3–S4
Anal wink reflex	Pinprick on the skin of the perianal region or perineum, with patient in lateral decubitus position, hips and knees flexed	Visible contraction of the anus	External anal sphincter	Pudendal nerve	S3–S5

Table 3.8

The most important pathologic reflexes

Reflex	Stimulus	Response	Significance
Orbicularis oculi reflex (glabellar reflex, nasopalpebral reflex)	Tap on the glabella or on a finger, applied to the lateral edge of the orbit while the orbicularis oculi muscle is contracted	Narrowing of the palpebral fissure by contraction of the orbicularis oculi muscle (possibly bilaterally)	Exaggerated in supranuclear lesions of the corticopontine pathway and in extrapyramidal diseases
Corneomandibular reflex (winking jaw)	Like the corneal reflex; mouth slightly open	The jaw deviates to the side opposite the stimulus	Release of an older functional synergy between the orbicularis oculi muscle and the lateral pterygoid muscle; due to an ipsilateral lesion of the corticobulbar pathway, lacunar state, or bulbar palsy
Marcus Gunn phenomenon (winking jaw)	Opening the mouth and moving the jaw	A previously ptotic eyelid is very strongly elevated	Proof that ptosis is not due to peripheral paresis or myasthenia
Bulldog reflex	Placing a tongue depressor between the patient's teeth	The patient bites down so hard that the head can be lifted by the tongue depressor	Release phenomenon (disinhibition) due to diffuse cortical injury, e.g., postanoxic
Orbicularis oris reflex (snout reflex, nasomental reflex)	Gentle tap on a finger or tongue depressor placed on the lateral corner of the mouth or on the lips (can sometimes also be elicited from the glabella)	Contraction of the orbicularis oris muscle with pursing of the lips	Absent or only faintly present in normal individuals; exaggerated as a result of lesions affecting the supranuclear corticopontine pathways (status lacunaris, multi-infarct dementia, extrapyramidal diseases such as Parkinson disease)
Suck reflex	Slowly, gently stroking the lips	Sucking and, possibly, swallowing movements; occasionally, biting; mouth opening and turning of the head toward the stimulus (termed a magnet reaction if present as soon as an object is brought near the mouth)	Severe, diffuse brain injury, decorticate state; e.g., in apallic syndrome after anoxia or severe traumatic brain injury (normal in infants; pathologic release phenomenon in later life)
Wartenberg reflex ("thumb sign")	Forceful passive flexion of the second through fifth fingers	Flexion of the thumb	Indicates a pyramidal tract lesion
Palmomental reflex (exaggerated or asymmetric)	Intensely stroking the ball of the thumb or the palm of the hand with a fingernail or wooden stick	Contraction of the ipsilateral chin muscles	In diffuse cerebral injury (multi-infarct syndrome, brain atrophy, postanoxic); if unilateral, indicates contralateral brain lesion
Grasp reflex	Stroking the palm	Finger flexion, possibly grasping of the stimulating object	Normal in infants; later a sign of diffuse brain injury (mainly in the frontal lobes); seen contralateral to a frontal lobe lesion or ipsilateral to a lesion in the basal ganglia
Grasping and groping (magnet phenomenon)	Object brought near the palm of the (conscious) patient	The hand follows the presented object like a magnet, making grasping movements	
Gegenhalten	Attempted passive stretching of a muscle (e.g., pushing down on the lower jaw, or forcibly extending the flexed fingers)	The patient actively and intensely contracts the muscle in question, preventing passive stretch (in the absence of generalized negativism)	In diffuse frontal lobe disease and lesions of the basal ganglia
Mass reflexes of the lower limbs in paraplegia	For example, forceful passive flexion of the toes and forefoot (Marie–Foix handgrip)	Retraction of the (otherwise plegic) lower limb by flexion at the knee and hip	Reveals the intactness of the spinal reflex arc and therefore of the peripheral nervous system (useful as a "trick" facilitating the nursing care of patients with spastic rigidity)
Babinski reflex (Fig. 3.34a)	Stroking the lateral edge of the foot from the heel to the little toe (or else transversely across the plantar arch)	Tonic (slow) extension of the big toe, while the other toes remain in their original position or are splayed (like a fan)	Indicates a lesion of the corticospinal (pyramidal) pathway on the corresponding side
Oppenheim reflex (Fig. 3.34b)	Forcefully stroking the anterior margin of the tibia from proximal to distal (painful)		
Gordon reflex (Fig. 3.34c)	Forcefully stroking or squeezing the calf muscles		

3

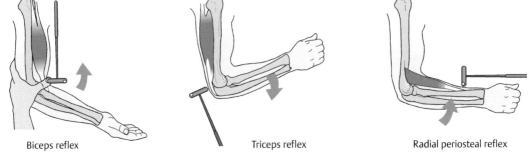

Biceps reflex   Triceps reflex   Radial periosteal reflex

Fig. 3.26   Elicitation of the intrinsic muscle reflexes of the upper limb.

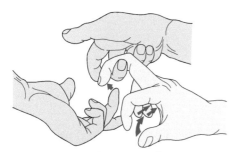

Fig. 3.27   Elicitation of the Trömner reflex.

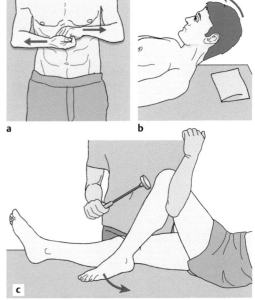

a   b

c

Fig. 3.28   Facilitation maneuvers make the intrinsic muscle reflexes more intense and easier to elicit. **a** Jendrassik handgrip. **b** Same effect with active, strong raising of the head off the headrest. **c** Active plantar flexion of the foot.

that are normally absent. The evidence for a pyramidal lesion is generally less obvious in the upper limbs than in the lower, as there are no "classic pyramidal tract signs" for the lower limbs (cf. see also section 3.6.3, Pathologic Reflexes). One important clue is **exaggeration of the physiologic intrinsic muscle reflexes**, especially if asymmetric. There may also be **spreading of the reflex zones** and **ease of elicitation** of certain intrinsic reflexes that, under normal circumstances, are only barely elicitable or not at all, for example, the trapezius and pectoralis reflexes (cf. **Table 3.6**). The Trömner reflex and Hoffmann sign can also be of pathologic significance if abnormally brisk or unilaterally exaggerated. **Absence of the Mayer reflex of the metacarpophalangeal joint** is also considered a pyramidal tract sign: forceful passive flexion of the middle finger at the metacarpophalangeal joint is normally followed by reflex adduction of the metacarpal bone of the thumb (**Fig. 3.29**), but not if there is a lesion in the pyramidal pathway. Another pyramidal tract sign is flexion and opposition of the thumb when the examiner forcefully pulls on an actively flexed finger.

3.4.5 Sensation

Sensory testing takes time, patience, and cooperation from the patient. Its goal is to identify sensory deficits, delimit their site and extent, and determine which sensory modalities are affected. The pattern of findings obtained in this way usually permits classification of the causative lesion as central, radicular, or peripheral. Before examining the patient, the clinician should have a clear idea of what he or she is

Table 3.9

3

Significance of the more common abnormalities of the intrinsic muscle reflexes

Abnormality	Significance	Remarks
Apparent absence of all reflexes	Very weak reflexes, or inadequate examining technique	Facilitation maneuvers, e.g., Jendrassik handgrip (**Fig. 3.28a**)
True generalized areflexia	Polyneuropathy, polyradiculopathy	Sensory deficit, perhaps paresis
	Anterior horn cell disease	Muscle atrophy without sensory deficit
	Lambert–Eaton syndrome	
	Myopathy	
	Adie syndrome	Inspect pupils
	Congenital areflexia	Often familial
Absence of an individual reflex or reflexes	Nerve root lesion	For example, triceps reflex (C7), Achilles reflex (S1)
	Peripheral nerve lesion	For example, biceps reflex (musculocutaneous nerve), knee-jerk reflex (femoral nerve)
Very weak reflexes	Usually without pathologic significance	Often seen in older patients
Very brisk reflexes	If generalized, often without pathologic significance	Often seen in younger patients
Pathologically exaggerated reflexes	"Pyramidal tract signs," spasticity	Compare sides (hemiparesis?) and compare upper with lower limbs (paraparesis?)
Positive Hoffmann sign and Trömner reflex	Normal if symmetric and without any accompanying "pyramidal tract signs"	

looking for, where in the body to look for it, and what examining techniques are to be used.

The Sense of Touch

The sense of touch (**esthesia**) is tested with the patient's eyes closed. The examiner lightly touches various sites on the patient's body with a finger, a feather, a piece of tissue paper, or the like. Precise quantitative testing can be performed with graded instruments, such as von Frey's hairs or an adjustable Wartenberg pinwheel, but is not necessary in routine practice. (Sharp instruments for multiple use, e.g., pinwheels, can transmit infectious diseases such as hepatitis and AIDS and should be avoided. If they are nonetheless used in exceptional cases, sterilization before each use is mandatory.) It usually suffices to describe a deficit as either a deficient sense of touch (**hypesthesia**) or an absent sense of touch (**anesthesia**). Depending on the clinical situation, the examiner may want to measure sensation quantitatively in a particular dermatome or in the distribution of a particular peripheral nerve, or to compare sensation on mirror-image sites on the body. Sensory dysfunction can also involve an excess of sensation. **Paresthesia** is an abnormal, positive sensation of some kind, whether spontaneous or evoked, for example, the pins-and-needles sensation of polyneuropathy. An abnormal, positive sensation that is unpleasant or painful is called **dysesthesia** (e.g., a burning sensation due to a peripheral nerve injury). The elicitation of pain by a stimulus that is not normally painful (such as lightly stroking the skin) is called **allodynia**.

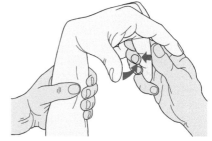

Fig. 3.29 The Mayer reflex of the metacarpophalangeal joint is elicited by forceful passive flexion of the middle finger. Involuntary adduction of the thumb normally follows; absence of the reflex suggests a lesion of the pyramidal pathway.

Two-Point Discrimination, Stereognosis

The **epicritic** component of the sense of touch (derived from Greek *krites*, "judge") is tested on the pads of the fingers, for example, by determining the patient's ability to discriminate two simultaneous stimuli located close together. This can be done with a pair of calipers or simply with the two points of an unfolded paper clip. The two ends are placed on the skin simultaneously, initially very close together, and then at increasing distances until the patient reports feeling two separate stimuli. The threshold distance is usually larger when the stimuli are simultaneous than when they are successively applied; on the fingertips, it should be no more than 5 mm. Epicritic sensation can also be tested by having the patient identify a coin by touch or "read" a number written on the patient's fingertip. Normal performance on these tests also requires intact **stereognosis**.

3

Vibration and Position Sense

Vibration sense (**pallesthesia**) is tested with a vibrating 64- or 124-Hz tuning fork solidly placed on various bony prominences of the body, that is, sites where the bone is covered only by skin. The intensity of vibration can be graduated, if desired, with the aid of special adjustable tuning forks, such as the Rydel–Seiffer model, which allows grading in eighths. This is mostly unnecessary, as there is an easier method: as soon as the patient reports that the vibration is no longer felt, the examiner tests his or her own vibration sense with the same tuning fork at an analogous position. If the examiner still clearly feels the vibration, then the patient unquestionably has a deficit of vibration sense (the rarely used scholarly terms are **pallhypesthesia** for a partial deficit and **pallanesthesia** for a total deficit). Milder deficits are usually detectable only in the periphery (e.g., at the ankles), while more severe ones are evident further up the trunk.

| NOTE |

Vibration sense usually declines by one- or two-eighths over the course of normal aging.

The examiner tests **position sense** by passively moving some part of the patient's body (in the hands, usually the middle finger) and asking the patient in which direction it is being moved. The patient should look away or keep the eyes closed in order not to see the movement. The body part in question should be held from the sides to eliminate surface pressure as a cue.

Temperature Sense

Temperature sense (**thermesthesia**) should be tested when a central lesion is suspected, because the pain and temperature pathways run separately from those of the other sensory modalities in the spinal cord and brainstem, joining them only in the thalamus (see **Fig. 5.2**).

A lesion affecting the spinothalamic tract in the spinal cord or brainstem but sparing the other sensory pathways produces a **dissociated sensory deficit**: pain and temperature sensation are impaired in the affected area of the body, but the sense of touch is preserved. A partial deficit of temperature sense is called **thermhypesthesia** and a total one **thermanesthesia**.

To test the sense of temperature, the examiner fills two test tubes or special-purpose metal containers with cold and warm water and applies them to various sites on the skin. Thermal stimuli can be delivered in graded fashion, if desired, by varying their temperature, area, and duration.

Pain

The ability to feel pain (**algesia**) should be tested by pinching a fold of skin, never by pinprick. A partial deficit is called **hypalgesia** and a total one **analgesia**.

Other Sensory Qualities

Allesthesia or **allocheiria** is the perception of a tactile stimulus somewhere other than the site at which it was delivered. This phenomenon can occur in normal individuals and is of uncertain significance.

3.5 Trunk

 Key Point

The shape and range of motion of the spine are evaluated with the patient standing. Sensation is tested with the patient lying down; particular attention should be paid to a sensory level or to a deficit in a saddle or genital distribution. The motor innervation of the trunk is assessed with the intrinsic abdominal muscle reflexes and the extrinsic reflexes (abdominal skin reflex, cremasteric reflex).

3.5.1 Back and Spine

The back and spine are examined with the patient standing. **Inspection** may reveal scoliosis or a deviation from the normal lordosis or kyphosis of particular segments of the vertebral column. Protruding ribs on one side (often visible only when the patient bends forward) are a sign of torsional scoliosis. As one looks at the patient from behind, there is a triangular gap to either side of the patient's waist, formed by the dependent arm, the rib cage, and the upper border of the pelvis; asymmetry of this gap is a further sign of scoliosis. A plumb line from the spinous process of C7 should overlie the natal cleft; deviations should be measured and documented (preferably in centimeters, rather than fingerbreadths). One should also look for stepping of the lumbosacral vertebrae (e.g., in spondylolisthesis, described in section 14.5.2) or tenderness of the spinous processes to pressure or percussion. Techniques for testing the **mobility of the cervical spine** were described in section 3.3.1. The mobility of the thoracolumbar spine is tested by having the patient bend the trunk forward, backward, and to either side, and then rotate it to either side. On forward bending with extended knees, young patients should be able to touch the ground (**finger-to-ground distance**: 0 cm). Spinal mobility can be quantified with the two **Schober tests**: the small Schober index pertains to the lumbosacral spine and the large Schober index to the thoracic spine.

- To measure the small Schober index, place a mark on the patient's skin 10 cm above the spinous process of L5, have the patient bend forward as far as possible, and measure the distance again; it should now be at least 15 cm.
- The large Schober index is measured similarly, starting from a point 30 cm below the spinous process of C7, which on maximal forward bending should move to at least 32 cm below it.

Any diminution of the normal cervical lordosis is best seen when the patient stands with shoulders and heels to the wall and bends the head as far back as possible. The back of the patient's head normally touches the wall; if not, the distance from the occipital protuberance to the wall should be measured in centimeters. An abnormality of this type is found, for example, in ankylosing spondylitis.

3.5.2 Reflexes

The **abdominal skin reflexes** are extrinsic muscle reflexes. They are tested by rapid stroking of the abdominal skin (e.g., with a wooden stick) from lateral to medial, at three different segmental levels, on either side (**Fig. 3.30a**). They can be enhanced, if necessary, by having the patient lift his or her head off the headrest (**Fig. 3.28b**). Diminution of the abdominal skin reflexes indicates a lesion of the pyramidal pathway. A diminished or absent reflex at only one level on one side suggests a segmental peripheral lesion. Total bilateral absence is usually an artifact of deficient examining technique, but may also be caused by an obese or flaccid abdominal wall (e.g., after pregnancy). "True" bilateral absence of all abdominal skin reflexes is seen in bilateral lesions of the pyramidal pathway; an accompanying sign in such patients is unusual briskness of the **intrinsic reflexes of the abdominal musculature**. These are tested by tapping at the sites of muscle attachment, for example, at the costal margin or the symphysis pubis (**Fig. 3.30b**). Alternatively, the examiner can place his or her own hand on the abdomen and tap on it.

The **cremaster reflex** is tested (in males) by stroking the medial surface of the thigh or by forceful pressure with a finger near the origin of the adductor muscles. The **anal reflex** is tested by lightly scratching the perianal skin with, for example, a pointed wooden stick. This induces reflex contraction of the anal sphincter. The anal reflex is sometimes easier to appreciate on rectal examination with a gloved finger (with which the examiner can also assess sphincter tone); it is abolished by lesions of the cauda equina and conus medullaris (described in section 7.1.2).

3.5.3 Sensation

Sensation on the trunk is tested to localize a possible **sensory level** (segmentally delimited sensory deficit)

due to a spinal cord lesion. A sensory level caused by a bilateral lesion of one or more spinal nerve roots is limited to one or a few dermatomes; one caused by spinal cord transection covers the entire region of the body from the toes up to the rostral border of the injured spinal segment. A sensory level should be localized to a particular numbered segment as precisely as possible by testing both from above and from below. If a lesion of the cauda equina is suspected, sensation should be meticulously tested in the sacral dermatomes, the so-called **saddle area**.

3.6 Lower Limbs

Key Point

The examination of the lower limbs, too, begins with inspection: the examiner assesses the posture and spontaneous movements of the legs and feet, muscle bulk, skin condition, and any abnormal movements that may be present. Next, the mobility of the major joints is tested, and the pulses are palpated. The neurologic examination per se then follows, with testing of strength, reflexes, coordination, and sensation.

3.6.1 General Aspects

The procedure here is the same as in the upper limbs (cf. section 3.4). The muscles are inspected and palpated for **tone and bulk**. Atrophy of individual muscle groups should be looked for (especially the tibialis anterior muscle); any **fasciculations** (definition: **Table 5.3**) should be noted. **Involuntary movements** should be observed, if present. The **mobility of the larger joints**, particularly the hip joints, should be tested individually. The **Lasègue sign** (see section 13.1.2, Radicular Syndromes due to Intervertebral Disk Herniation) should be tested, and the examiner should check for tenderness of the peripheral nerve trunks. The **trophic state of the skin** and the **peripheral pulses** should be assessed as well. The pedal and popliteal pulses should be palpated; the pulses in the abdominal vessels should be examined by auscultation, as should those of the femoral artery, both in the groin and in the proximal adductor canal. The **Ratschow test** is a provocative test of the blood supply to the leg: the examiner holds up both legs of the supine patient and the patient rotates the feet back and forth. A normal individual can do this for several minutes without difficulty, but, if arterial insufficiency is present, pain soon arises. In addition, when the legs are brought back to the horizontal position, the skin takes a longer time than normal to regain its usual pink color (in patients of light complexion) and venous refilling is likewise delayed.

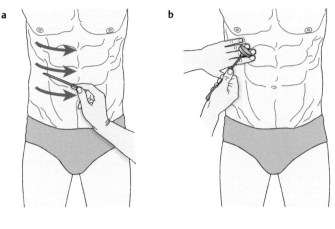

Fig. 3.30 The abdominal skin reflexes.
a Elicitation of the extrinsic reflexes by stroking the abdominal skin from lateral to medial.
b The intrinsic reflexes are elicited by striking the sites of muscle attachment.

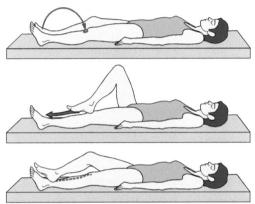

Fig. 3.31 The heel–knee–shin test. With eyes closed, the patient touches one heel to the opposite knee and then slides it down the shin.

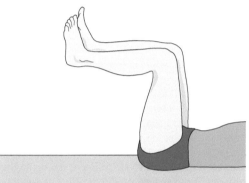

Fig. 3.32 Postural test of the legs in the supine position.

3.6.2 Coordination and Strength

The following motor tests should be performed:

- In the **heel–knee–shin** test, the patient closes the eyes, brings the heel of one leg through the air in a wide arc to place it on the opposite knee, then slides the heel down the shin to the front of the ankle, and finally back up to the knee (**Fig. 3.31**). Unsteadiness indicates ataxia.
- In the **postural test**, the patient lies supine, raises the lower limbs so that the hips and knees are at right angles, and holds them in this position (**Fig. 3.32**). The examiner looks for possible sinking of a leg, indicating (mild) paresis.
- **Strength**, too, should be tested in the supine patient. Additional special tests are used for individual muscle groups. For example, a patient with quadriceps weakness has trouble stepping up onto a stool or chair, or standing up from a sitting position (if the weakness is bilateral). The dorsiflexors of the feet and toes should always be tested, because these distal muscles are frequently weakened early in the course of many

different neurologic disorders. Dorsiflexion of the big toe, for example, is weak in L5 radiculopathy. In suspected polyneuropathy, it may be useful to palpate the contractions of the muscles of the dorsum of the foot and to compare the patient's ability to spread the toes on the two sides. Mild weakness of the calf muscles (i.e., of dorsiflexion of the foot) is best tested by having the patient hop on one foot or stand repeatedly on the tip of one foot (see **Fig. 13.66**).

3.6.3 Reflexes

Intrinsic Muscle Reflexes

The **quadriceps reflex** (patellar tendon reflex) and **Achilles reflex** are the most important intrinsic muscle reflexes of the lower limb. They should be tested in every patient (**Fig. 3.33**, **Table 3.6**). In some situations, it may also be advisable to test the adductor reflex or the knee flexor reflexes. The latter are elicited by tapping the biceps femoris tendon (lateral border of the popliteal fossa) and the semimembranosus and semitendinosus tendons (medial border of the popliteal fossa). The inconstantly present tibialis posterior reflex is elicited by a tap on the tendon of this muscle behind the medial malleolus while the foot is held in mild pronation. The response consists of supination.

Pathologic Reflexes

There are several important pathologic reflexes in the lower limbs that signify a lesion of the pyramidal pathway. Chief among these is the **Babinski reflex** or "Babinski sign" (**Fig. 3.34a, Table 3.8**). To elicit it, the examiner forcefully strokes the lateral plantar surface of the patient's foot, proceeding from the heel toward the toes. The pathologic response is a slow, tonic dorsiflexion of the big toe, usually accompanied by fanning of the other toes. (Babinski himself called these phenomena *signe de l'orteil*—the big toe sign—and *signe de l'éventail*—the fan sign.) The same response can sometimes be elicited by stroking other parts of the foot, particularly the anterior ball of the foot from lateral to medial. The **Oppenheim sign** is the Babinski phenomenon evoked by a painfully intense stroke along the edge of the tibia, from the knee downward (**Fig. 3.34b**); the **Gordon sign** is the same phenomenon evoked by pressing or forcefully squeezing the calf muscles (**Fig. 3.34c**). The **Rossolimo sign** (toe flexor reflex) consists of flexion of the second through fifth toes in response to a tap from the plantar side on their distal phalanges, produced with a reflex hammer or the examiner's fingers. It is a somewhat unreliable indicator of a pyramidal tract lesion.

> **NOTE**
>
> If the "classic" Babinski sign is present, there is no need to look for additional pyramidal tract signs. These should be sought only if the Babinski sign is absent or unclear in a clinical situation where a pyramidal tract lesion is suspected.

A "mute sole," that is, the lack of any toe movement at all when the Babinski reflex is tested, is a preliminary stage of the Babinski reflex in some patients and clinically meaningless in others. Mute soles in deeply comatose patients are associated with a poorer prognosis.

Further signs of a pyramidal tract lesion include brisk or asymmetric intrinsic muscle reflexes and clonus on elicitation of the quadriceps or Achilles reflex. The main intrinsic muscle reflexes of the lower limbs are summarized in **Table 3.6**, the extrinsic reflexes in **Table 3.7**, and the pathologic reflexes in **Table 3.8**.

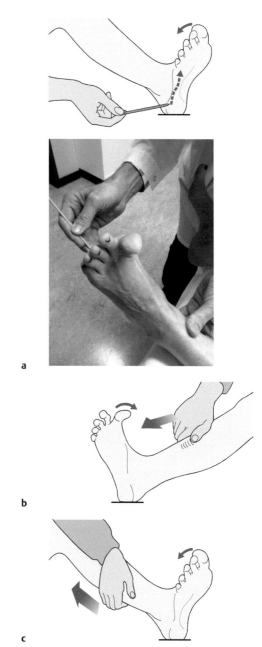

a

b

c

Fig. 3.34   Pyramidal tract signs in the lower limbs. **a** Babinski sign. **b** Oppenheim reflex. **c** Gordon reflex.

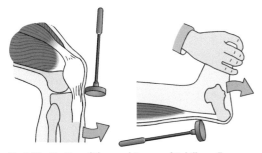

Fig. 3.33   Testing of the quadriceps and Achilles reflexes.

3.6.4 Sensation

The earliest and most sensitive evidence of a mainly distal sensory deficit in the lower limbs, for example, in polyneuropathy, is an impairment of **vibration sense**. Normal persons can feel vibration in all joints down to the distal interphalangeal joints of the toes (**Fig. 3.35a**); this can be tested and quantified with a graded tuning fork (see section 3.4.5, Vibration and Position Sense). They can also recognize numbers drawn on the skin of the leg (**Fig. 3.35b**) and usually on the pad of the big toe as well (**stereognosis**). **Position sense** in the big toe is tested by holding it on both sides and alternately dorsiflexing and plantar-flexing it (**Fig. 3.35b**); the patient should be able to state in which direction the toe was moved. Position sense is impaired, for example, by posterior column lesions.

3.7 Autonomic Nervous System

Key Point

The autonomic nervous system is affected in many neurologic and general medical conditions. The examiner should look for disturbances of postural blood-pressure regulation, sweating, trophic state of the skin and nails, micturition, and sexual function.

For the anatomy of the autonomic nervous system, see **Fig. 16.1**, **Fig. 16.2**, and **Fig. 16.3**. Many clinical tests of the autonomic nervous system have been devised; a few are rather cumbersome. We will merely mention some of them here: testing of pupillary reactivity by the local application of various substances, measurement of the rise in blood pressure after the administration of ephedrine, observation of changes in blood pressure with orthostasis or on a tilt table, observation and measurement of sweating after warming of the body or observation of local sweating with pilocarpine iontophoresis, measurement of the pulse on inspiration and expiration or after the administration of 1 mg of atropine, assessment of voiding and erectile function (in males), etc. Such tests are generally used only in selected patients to answer specific questions. All patients, however, should be asked about possible disturbances of autonomic function when the history is taken (urination, defecation, sexual function, sweating).

3.8 Neurologically Relevant Aspects of the General Physical Examination

Key Point

Many general medical and rheumatologic illnesses have neurologic symptoms and signs, sometimes as the main or sole manifestation of

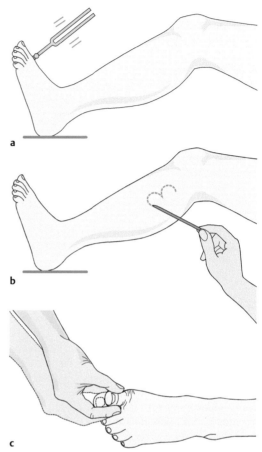

Fig. 3.35 Sensory testing in the lower limbs. a Vibration sense, **b** stereognosis, **c** position sense (the examiner grasps the patient's big toe from the sides).

disease. The clinician performing a neurologic examination should pay special attention to any symptoms or signs indicating a condition that is not limited to the nervous system.

The patient's **general appearance** may suggest a wasting illness, such as a malignant neoplasm, or an endocrinopathy. Organomegaly or lymphadenopathy should be noted. Abnormal skin pallor may be a sign of anemia and a straw-yellow coloration may indicate pernicious anemia due to vitamin B_{12} deficiency. The **skin** should also be carefully inspected for evidence of neurocutaneous diseases, vasculitic processes, or collagen vascular disease, which, taken together, are not at all rare. Findings to look for include the cafe-au-lait spots of neurofibromatosis (von Recklinghausen disease; see **Fig. 6.5**), abnormal shape and consistency of the nails, herpetic vesicles, etc. The **cardiovascular examination** is very important: the blood pressure must be measured, pulses felt in the upper and lower limbs, and vascular bruits listened for, particularly in the neck, the supraclavicular fossae, the abdomen, and the groin bilaterally.

3.9 Neuropsychological and Psychiatric Examination

 Key Point
Many neurologic illnesses are associated with more or less severe disturbances of cognitive and emotional function. The organic neurologic clinical picture is only complete when any psychopathologic abnormalities that may be present have been thoroughly assessed and documented. The goal of the neuropsychological examination is to reveal cognitive deficits (especially aphasia, agnosia, and apraxia) and processing disturbances that imply the presence of a focal brain lesion.

3.9.1 Psychopathologic Findings
The examiner should first determine whether the patient is awake and alert. If not, he or she will be unable to receive and process incoming stimuli in the normal way. The patient may have an **impairment of consciousness** ranging in severity from drowsiness to coma, as described in **Table 3.10**.

In addition to the patient's level of consciousness and attention, the examiner should assess his or her **orientation**, **concentration**, **memory**, **drive**, **affective state**, and **cognitive ability**. The overall psychopathologic picture is composed of these elements. If mental functioning is disturbed by an underlying neurologic illness (so-called *psycho-organic syndrome* or *organic brain syndrome*), the manifestations often progress in a characteristic sequence, regardless of the etiology. At first, short- and long-term memory, concentration,

and attention are impaired; the patient is easily fatigued and has difficulty processing new information or performing complex tasks. Later, the patient becomes progressively disoriented, first to time, then to place, and then to person (self). Reactive depression is common at this stage. Ultimately, all spontaneous activity ceases; the patient loses interest, lacks drive, and becomes permanently confused. Disturbances of this type can often be discerned in the patient's behavior before the formal examination begins, growing increasingly evident to the examiner during history-taking and physical examination. Further details of the patient's history from the family can often help. The **Mini-Mental State Examination** (**Table 3.11**, **Fig. 3.36**) and the **clock test** (**Table 3.12**) are widely used to assess cognitive function; the MOCA test is a well-validated alternative (see www.mocatest.org). For acquired dementia, see section 6.12.

3.9.2 Neuropsychological Examination
The localizing significance of various neuropsychological deficits is shown in **Fig. 3.37**. An overview of important neuropsychological terms and syndromes is provided in **Table 3.13**.

Aphasia
Language is a complex process encompassing numerous individual functions (**Table 3.14**).
Cortical disturbances of language are called **aphasia** and are due to a lesion in the language-dominant hemisphere. The left hemisphere is dominant for language in nearly all right-handers and in most left-handers as well. The clinical varieties of aphasia are:
- Disturbances of language production (**motor aphasia** or Broca aphasia; **Fig. 3.38** and **Fig. 4.12**):

Table 3.10	

Degrees of impairment of consciousness, and other abnormal states of consciousness

Designation	Features
Normal consciousness	Oriented to place, time, and person (self), answers questions promptly and appropriately, follows commands correctly
Drowsiness	Mostly awake, responds to questions and commands slowly but usually correctly (after repetition if necessary), moves in response to a sufficiently intense stimulus, usually oriented and coherent
Somnolence	Mostly asleep, arousable with a moderately intense stimulus, generally requires repetition of questions or commands but then responds correctly, reacts slowly and after a delay but usually correctly
Stupor	Asleep unless awakened, can only be awakened with a strong (auditory) stimulus or perhaps only with a mechanical stimulus, cannot answer questions or follow commands or does so only after intense repetition, and then only incompletely
Coma	Unconscious, cannot be awakened, does not respond to a verbal or auditory stimulus, may respond to painful stimuli of graded intensities with specific (localizing) self-defense, nonlocalizing withdrawal of a limb, or abnormal flexion or extension responses
Confusion	Inappropriate spontaneous behavior and responses to questions and commands, deficient orientation to place, time, and/or person (self); the confused patient may be fully conscious, less than fully conscious, or agitated (see below)
Agitation	Motor unrest, inappropriate spontaneous behavior, cannot be calmed by verbal persuasion, more or less disoriented, does not follow commands appropriately

| Table 3.11 |

Mini-Mental State Examination

Parameter	Questions
Name of patient: Date of birth: Date of examination: 1 point for each correct answer	
Orientation in time	
1.	— "What day of the week is it?"
2.	— "What is today's date?"
3.	— "What is the current month?"
4.	— "What is the current season?"
5.	— "What year is it?"
Orientation to place	
6.	— "Where are we (hospital, old age home, etc.)?"
7.	— "On what floor?"
8.	— "In what city?"
9.	— "In what state (canton, province, etc.)?"
10.	— "In what country?"
Retentiveness	
	"Please repeat the following words" (to be spoken at one word per second; to be performed only once)
11.	— "Lemon"
12.	— "Key"
13.	— "Ball"
Attention and calculations	
14.	"Please count from 100 backward by sevens" (serial-7 test). One point for each correct subtraction, maximum five points
Recent memory	
15.	"Which three words did you repeat earlier?" One point for each word correctly recalled
Language, naming	
16.	— "What is this?" (show a pencil)
17.	— "What is this?" (show a watch)
18.	— "Please say after me: 'No ifs, ands, or buts'"
Language comprehension, motor execution	
19.	— "Take this piece of paper in your hand"
20.	— "Fold it down the middle"
21.	— "Put it on the ground" (each command to be given only once)
Reading	
22.	"Please do what it says on this card" (show card: "Close your eyes") (**Fig. 3.36a**)
Writing	
23.	"Write any sentence" (the patient is given a piece of paper and something to write with)
Drawing	
24.	"Please copy this drawing" (overlapping pentagons, **Fig. 3.36b**; all 10 edges of the two pentagons must be drawn, and the pentagons must overlap, for the patient to receive one point for this task)
Level of wakefulness:	
Total points achieved:	

Source: Adapted from Folstein MF, Folstein SE, McHugh PR. "Mini-mental state". A practical method for grading the cognitive state of patients for the clinician. J Psychiatr Res 1975;12(3):189–198.

the patient's spontaneous speech is not fluent, even though the "organic prerequisites" for speech production (phonation, breathing, orofacial musculature) are all apparently unimpaired.
— Disturbances of language comprehension (**sensory aphasia** or Wernicke aphasia; **Fig. 3.38** and **Fig. 4.12**): the patient has trouble understanding speech despite intact hearing and auditory processing. The patient's spontaneous speech is fluent.
— Disturbances of speech repetition. The patient cannot correctly repeat words or sentences spoken by the examiner.
— Nearly all patients with aphasia have difficulty with naming and word-finding.

The examiner begins to assess the patient's sponta-neous speech while taking the history; if necessary, the patient can be given specific language tasks, for example, "Describe this picture." Various kinds of

abnormality may be noted. The patient's utterances may be found to be unusually poor in meaning-bearing words and overloaded with connectives and "function words." Sentences may be faultily con-structed (**paragrammatism**). The flow of speech may be either considerably greater than normal or slow and hesitant (**telegraphic speech**). Individual words may be deformed in certain characteristic ways (e.g., sound substitutions or **phonemic paraphasias**, such as "cog" for "dog"), or words may be used in place of other words from the same semantic category (**semantic paraphasias**, e.g., "table" for "chair"). Some words may be replaced by invented pseudowords (**neologisms**). Impaired language comprehension may be manifested by the patient's inability to point out various objects in the room, including parts of his or her own body, when these are named by the examiner. Complex commands are an even more sensitive functional test. The patient can be asked, for example, to place a certain named object in between two other named objects, or to interpret a complicated sentence, such as the following: "Not in the closet, but on top of it, was where he had put his hat. Where was the hat?" Aphasic patients often make mistakes when they repeat spoken sentences or name objects (including parts of the body) that

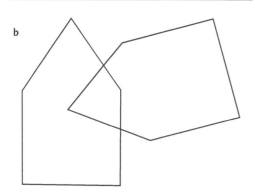

a Close your eyes

b

Fig. 3.36 Forms for the Mini-Mental State Examination. **a** A written command for the patient to follow (Task 22 in **Table 3.11**). **b** Pentagons to be copied (Task 24 in **Table 3.11**). (Reproduced from Mattle H, Mumenthaler M. Neurologie. 13th ed. Stuttgart: Thieme; 2013.)

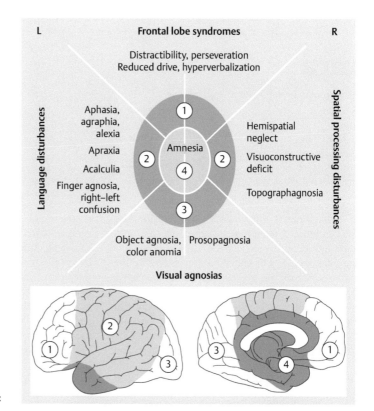

Fig. 3.37 Cognitive deficits that typi-cally result from various focal brain lesions. (Adapted from Schnider A. Verhaltensneurologie. 2nd ed. Stuttgart: Thieme; 2004.)

3

Table 3.12

The clock test

Task

The patient is given a piece of paper with an empty circle drawn on it and is asked to complete the drawing of a clock, including numbers and hands. The time shown should be 10 minutes past 11 o'clock.

Interpretation	Points if correct
Are all 12 numbers present?	1
Is the number "12" at the top?	2
Are two hands of different lengths present?	2
Is the indicated time correct?	2

Note: A score of 5 or below raises the suspicion of dementia.

Table 3.13

Important neuropsychological terms and syndromes

Aphasia	Cortical disturbance of language, usually due to a left-hemispheric lesion
Spatial processing disturbance	Difficulty drawing or copying three-dimensional figures (cube, house, five-pointed star); neglect of the left side of space or the left side of the body (so-called hemispatial neglect); usually due to a right-hemispheric lesion
Apraxia	Disturbance of the goal-directed execution of complex behaviors or behavioral sequences, or of the use of tools: — **Ideomotor apraxia**: individual components of a single action are not put together correctly. — **Ideational apraxia**: individual actions cannot be combined in complex action sequences. More common with left-hemispheric than with right-hemispheric lesions
Agnosia	Disturbance of the ability to recognize and correctly interpret various kinds of sensory stimuli, despite intact sensory function. — **Visual agnosia**: inability to recognize objects visually despite intact vision. Special types: color agnosia, prosopagnosia (inability to recognize faces). The responsible lesion is located in the occipital or occipitotemporal visual cortex — **Tactile agnosia**: objects cannot be recognized by touch with the eyes closed — **Anosognosia**: deficit of self-awareness, i.e., denial or trivialization of one's own pathologic deficits

Table 3.14

Functions that are needed for normal language

Function	Disturbance
Hearing	Hearing impairment, deafness (section 12.6.1)
Comprehension	Sensory aphasia
Construction of words and thoughts	
Construction of speech	Motor aphasia
Phonation and articulation	Hoarseness (section 12.7), dysarthria (see sections 3.9.1, 5.5.5, and 12.9)

are pointed out to them. Reading and writing may also be impaired, often to a greater extent than spoken language.

The different types of aphasia are classified by the characteristics of the patient's spontaneous speech, comprehension and repetition of speech, word-finding, and naming (**Table 3.15**). An aphasic patient whose spontaneous speech lacks fluency speaks slowly, with effort, in short sentences containing many meaning-bearing words, with paraphasias and altered melody of speech (dysprosody). An aphasic patient with fluent spontaneous speech speaks at normal speed, effortlessly, and with the normal melody of speech (prosody), but the sentences are of normal length but contain relatively few meaning-bearing words in relation to meaningless filler words and literal and semantic paraphasias.

Dysarthria is not a disturbance of language, but of the mechanical process of speech production (articulation); the content of speech is normal. When the motor apparatus of speech is affected by a central paresis or a muscular coordination disorder, the patient's speech becomes unclear or slurred, perhaps even unintelligible.

Disturbances of Spatial Processing

Disturbances of spatial processing are usually caused by right-hemispheric lesions. They are manifested,

| Table 3.15 |

The classification and differential diagnosis of aphasia

Type of aphasia	Spontaneous speech	Comprehension	Repetition	Naming, word-finding
Motor aphasia (Broca)	Nonfluent	Normal	Impaired	Impaired
Sensory aphasia (Wernicke)	Fluent	Impaired	Impaired	Impaired
Conduction aphasia	Fluent	Normal	Impaired	Impaired
Global aphasia	Nonfluent	Impaired	Impaired	Impaired
Transcortical motor aphasia	Nonfluent	Normal	Normal	Impaired
Transcortical sensory aphasia	Fluent	Impaired	Normal	Impaired
Anomic aphasia	Fluent	Normal	Normal	Impaired

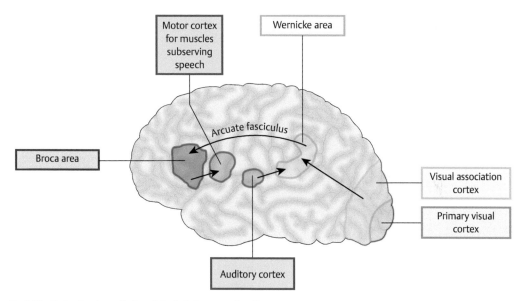

Fig. 3.38   Brain structures that participate in language function.

for example, by unusual difficulty in spontaneously drawing or copying three-dimensional figures (cube, house, etc.) (**Fig. 3.39a**). Deficits of this kind are often accompanied by neglect of the left side of space and the left half of the patient's own body (**hemispatial neglect**; **Fig. 3.39b,c**).

Memory and Amnesia

| NOTE |

Memory enables us to store and recall information; it makes learning possible. There is a somewhat arbitrary distinction between **short- and long-term memory**; the latter, in turn, is divided into **recent and old memory**.

Short-term memory, also called **working memory**, is that which we are able to keep in mind at any one moment. Its content is rapidly lost unless it is kept active by repetition and transferred to long-term memory.

The examiner gains a first impression of the patient's short- and long-term memory while taking the history. To test **short-term memory**, one can ask the patient to repeat sequences of numbers forward and backward or to take mental note of a sequence of 3 to 10 words and repeat them, immediately and a few minutes later.

Old memory can be tested by asking the patient to state autobiographic data that can be checked against other sources, facts about his or her own

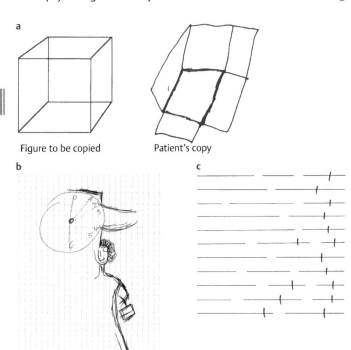

a

Figure to be copied   Patient's copy

b   c

**Fig. 3.39 Spatial processing and neglect.
a Cube-drawing as a test of spatial processing.** This drawing is by a patient with a
right parietal lesion. **b Drawings of a clock
and a woman.** The left half of each is missing, indicating severe left hemineglect. The
patient had sustained an acute hemorrhage
in the right parietal lobe. **c Line-dividing
test.** The patient was a university professor
with left-sided neglect due to a tumor (astrocytoma) in the right hemisphere. (Reproduced from Mattle H, Mumenthaler M.
Neurologie. 13th ed. Stuttgart: Thieme;
2013.)

family, or information about historical dates, political
events, or public figures. The findings should be
interpreted in the light of the patient's premorbid
level of intelligence and education.

Short-term memory and verbal memory are
mainly subserved by the limbic system (section
5.5.4) and hippocampus. Memory disturbances are
called **amnesia**.

> **NOTE**
>
> **Amnesia** is the inability to store or recall conscious
> memories. **Anterograde** amnesia is the inability to lay
> down new memories from the moment of a brain
> injury onward. **Retrograde** amnesia is the inability to
> recall information that was acquired before the brain
> injury. Persistent amnesia is the main clinical manifes-
> tation of dementia (section 6.12).

Apraxia

Disturbances in the goal-directed execution of
complex actions or sequences of actions, or in the
use of objects, are known as **apraxia**. If the individual components of a *single* action cannot be
put together correctly, the patient is suffering
from **ideomotor apraxia**. Different parts of the
body can be affected individually. In facial apraxia,
for example, the patient may be unable to follow
commands to execute certain motor tasks with
the face, e.g., drinking through a straw or clicking the
tongue. A patient with ideomotor apraxia of the
upper limbs may be unable to salute or to mime the
action of slapping someone in the face; a patient with
ideomotor apraxia of the lower limbs may be unable
to kick an imaginary football. In **ideational apraxia**,
individual actions can be performed, but cannot be
combined into more complex sequences. A patient
might thus be unable to ready a letter for mailing, as
this requires several steps: folding the letter, putting
it in the envelope, sealing the envelope, and putting a
stamp on it. Cortical lesions causing apraxia are usually on the left side.

Agnosia

Agnosia is an inability to recognize and correctly
interpret incoming stimuli in a particular sensory
modality, even though sensation as such is intact.
A patient with **visual agnosia**, for example, has no
visual impairment but cannot recognize objects on
sight; the patient can name an object only after
feeling or hearing it (e.g., the jangling of a bunch
of keys). Special types of visual agnosia include an
inability to recognize colors (color agnosia) or
faces (prosopagnosia). The responsible lesion is in
the visual association cortex, that is, in the occipital or occipitotemporal region, in one or both
hemispheres.

Stereognosis is tested by putting a familiar object (key, pair of scissors) in the patient's hand and asking him or her to palpate and name it (with eyes closed). An inability to do this despite intact sensation is called **tactile agnosia**. Further special types of agnosia are finger agnosia and autotopagnosia (difficulty recognizing parts of one's own body).

Anosognosia is the denial or trivialization of one's own neurologic deficits, for example, hemiplegia or even blindness.

Higher Cognitive Functions

For an individual to thrive in his or her social environment and cope adequately with the demands of everyday life, more is needed than just a properly functioning interaction of the basic neuropsychological functions described earlier. A person's fund of knowledge, memory, intelligence (i.e., the capacity for abstract thought and problem-solving), personality, and social behavior are all of vital importance, as are his or her mood and motivation. The assessment of these higher cognitive functions requires careful weighing of biographic historical information (particularly useful when derived from persons in the patient's social environment: family, friends, colleagues), as well as standardized neuropsychological testing. For example, there are specific tests for the patient's fund of knowledge, logical thinking, and cognitive skills such as difference recognition, category formation, and the interpretation of symbolic information, for example, proverbs. These higher integrative functions are performed by the cerebral cortex in collaboration with other, deeper regions of the brain.

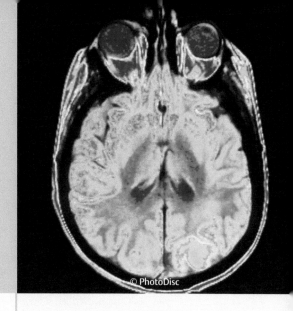
© PhotoDisc

Chapter 4

Ancillary Tests in Neurology

Stay Alert!

The patient, a 72-year-old woman who worked at the checkout counter in a family-owned grocery store, consulted her family physician in January 2001 because of a reduction of sensation in her left thumb, index finger, and middle finger. The doctor suspected carpal tunnel syndrome and prescribed a volar hand splint to be worn at night.

The splint did not help much, and the patient wore it only irregularly. Electroneurography (ENG) 2 years later revealed normal sensory nerve conduction velocities and a normal distal motor latency in the median nerve. By this time, the sensory disturbance had spread to include the fourth and fifth fingers of the left hand as well. The left biceps reflex was weak, but all other proprioceptive reflexes in the upper limb were normal. The family physician recommended that she try wearing the splint more consistently. As time went on, the patient noticed weakness of the left hand. She began dropping things involuntarily out of the left hand and, a few months later, she consulted a neurologist. She now had paresthesiae in the first through third digits of the right hand as well.

The most common cause of a sensory disturbance in the hands is carpal tunnel syndrome, a compressive neuropathy of the median nerve under the transverse carpal ligament. The clinical diagnosis is confirmed by ENG: typically, the sensory nerve conduction velocity across the carpal canal is low, or the distal motor latency of the median nerve is prolonged. The normal ENG findings in this patient should have led her doctor to suspect a C6 radiculopathy, particularly in view of the weak biceps reflex. Nothing more was done, however, and she only presented to a neurologist when the strength of the hand was affected.

The neurologist's examination revealed spastic quadriparesis, more pronounced in the upper limbs, particularly the left hand. The biceps and triceps reflexes were not elicitable on the left, but all other reflexes in the upper and lower limbs were very brisk. Babinski signs were present bilaterally. Pain and temperature sensation were markedly diminished from C6 downward, with a lesser diminution of touch and position sense. There was no sensation whatever in the C7 and C8 segments. These findings pointed to a central spinal cord lesion; the slow progression of symptoms (years) suggested syringomyelia or a spinal cord tumor as the most likely elements in the differential diagnosis. Cervical spinal magnetic resonance imaging (MRI) revealed an intramedullary tumor at the C5 and C6 levels, with a tumor-associated cyst above it and spinal cord edema below it. A neurosurgical procedure was performed, and the diagnosis of ependymoma was histologically confirmed.

This case illustrates the importance of ancillary tests, which are often indispensable for determining the etiology of a medical problem but should only be used in targeted fashion and always in correlation with the clinical findings. No imaging study is needed in a classic case of carpal tunnel syndrome; an imaging study should have been performed much earlier in the present case, however, as a weak biceps reflex is incompatible with the diagnosis of carpal tunnel syndrome. Failure to pursue the implications of this finding greatly delayed the diagnosis and treatment of this patient's tumor.

4.1 Fundamentals

 Key Point
Neurologic conditions can often be correctly diagnosed from the history and physical examination alone, but ancillary tests of various kinds are nonetheless vitally important, in many patients, to confirm the diagnosis and identify the etiology precisely. In this section, we will discuss imaging studies (primarily computed tomography [CT] and MRI), electrophysiologic studies (including electroencephalography [EEG], electromyography [EMG], ENG, and evoked potentials), and ultrasonography, as well as the laboratory testing of bodily fluids (blood, cerebrospinal fluid [CSF]) and the histopathologic and cytologic study of biopsy specimens.

Whenever an ancillary diagnostic test is proposed, the **specific indication for the test** should be considered carefully and critically:
— The test should be done only after:
  • Thorough and meticulous clinical history-taking and neurologic examination.
  • The formulation of a clinical differential diagnosis, in which all of the competing diagnoses are ranked by probability.
— The test to be done is the one whose result is most likely to affect the further diagnostic and therapeutic management:
  • But only if this will be of clear benefit to the patient.
  • Only if the risks of performing it do not outweigh any potential benefit that its findings might bring.
— Multiple tests that yield the same diagnostic information should not be done merely for repeated confirmation of the findings.
— A test should not be done if, regardless of its result, another study will have to be performed that will probably yield at least as much information.
— Only very rarely should tests be done to confirm a diagnosis that is already practically certain.
— The costs must be kept in mind in view of the wide variety of tests that can be performed, some of which are very expensive.

| NOTE
The potential consequences of any ancillary test should be discussed thoroughly with the patient and his or her family before it is performed

4.2 Imaging Studies

 Key Point
Imaging studies, particularly CT and MRI, are a very important means of determining the etiology of neurologic diseases. They are applied in targeted fashion, after history-taking and physical examination, to obtain an image of the pathologic process at the site of the functional disturbance.

4.2.1 Conventional Skeletal Radiographs

| NOTE
Conventional radiography can reveal fractures, osteolysis, degenerative changes, and postural abnormalities of the bony structures. It is now only rarely indicated, as it has largely been supplanted by tomographic imaging.

Even though newer techniques are available, plain X-rays of the skull and spine can still occasionally be of diagnostic use.
Skull X-rays are performed for very few purposes nowadays and are hardly ever indicated. (They cannot be used as a substitute for CT in head trauma; if a CT is indicated, but unavailable for some reason, then the patient should be transported to a center where a CT can be performed.) Plain films of the skull enable visualization of the following:
— Fractures (though much less well than on CT; see **Fig. 4.1**).
— Congenital malformations of the skull.
— Various developmental disorders.
Skull radiographs are useless in the diagnostic evaluation of headache or intracranial processes.
Spinal X-rays are sometimes useful for the demonstration of the following:
— Fractures.
— Bony tumors (which, however, are more easily seen by CT or MRI—see **Fig. 4.2**).

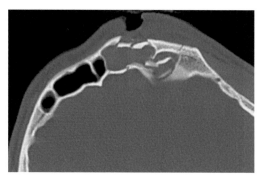
Fig. 4.1   Head CT: fracture of the frontal sinus on the left side. The anterior wall of the sinus is shattered, and the sinus cells on the left are filled with blood.

4

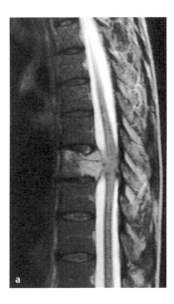

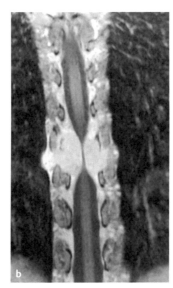

Fig. 4.2   Chordoma of the T7 vertebral body in a 48-year-old woman. **a** Sagittal MR image: the spinal cord is posteriorly displaced and compressed. **b** Frontal MR image: after contrast medium has been administered, a tumor is seen that envelops the spinal cord.

- Degenerative diseases and slippage (olisthesis) of the spine.
- Bone infections.
- Axial skeletal deformities.
- Dynamic abnormalities (abnormal mobility or instability of individual spinal segments).

CT and MRI are more sensitive than plain X-rays for the demonstration of pathologic abnormalities and are generally a better aid to diagnosis.

4.2.2 Computed Tomography

> **NOTE**
>
> CT is a tomographic imaging method that employs X-rays to visualize soft tissue and bone. It is particularly suitable for the visualization of the skeleton and for emergency diagnosis. CT angiography and CT perfusion studies reveal vascular abnormalities and perfusion deficits.

Technique. CT yields horizontal (axial) sectional images in which the bone and soft tissues are well seen. The images can also be digitally reconstructed in other planes, if desired. In CT, one or more rotating X-ray sources emit a beam that penetrates the tissue from many different directions, either in a single plane of section or in a spiral. The beam is attenuated to different degrees by tissues of different radiodensities, and its amplitude after attenuation is measured by a circular array of up to 320 detectors and amplifiers. From the resulting pattern of attenuation, the radiodensity at each location (voxel) in the interior of the brain is calculated by specialized computer software. There may be, for example, 512 × 512 voxels in each axial section. A visual image is then created in which the

radiodensity at each voxel is depicted on an analogue grayscale; anatomic structures can be visualized because of the differences in radiodensity between adjacent tissues (**Fig. 4.3**). Bony structures are well seen in CT images, especially in three-dimensional CT reconstructions (**Fig. 4.4**). Blood vessels, too, can be visualized.

Currently, **spiral CT scanners** are in widespread use: these contain multiple X-ray sources and detectors that rotate in a spiral, that is, the X-ray tube(s) swivels around the patient's head while the table on which the patient is lying is slowly advanced, at constant velocity, along the long axis of the body. The resulting spiral dataset is numerically converted into axial sections. This technique shortens the time required for a complete scan.

The **radiation load** associated with a CT scan of the head is roughly that of a chest X-ray. CT is somewhat less expensive than MRI.

Indications. The indications for, and diagnostic utility of, CT versus MRI are shown in **Table 4.1**.

Special CT Techniques

The administration of **intravenous contrast medium** increases the sensitivity and specificity of CT scanning.

- **Blood–tissue (or blood–CSF) barrier**: the penetration of contrast medium into brain tissue or tumor tissue (contrast enhancement) indicates disruption of the blood–tissue barrier or the blood–CSF barrier.
- **Blood vessels** can also be selectively imaged with the injection of contrast medium (**CT angiography**). This technique reveals vascular lesions such as aneurysms, intra-arterial plaques, stenosis, and occlusion.

4

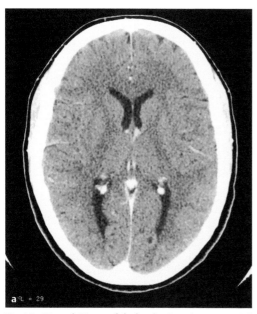
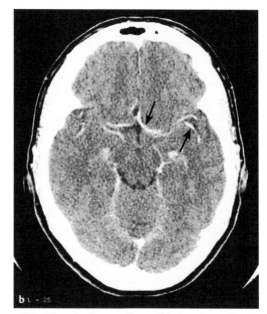

Fig. 4.3   Normal CT scan of the head. a Note the symmetrical, normal-sized frontal and occipital horns of the lateral ventricles. The cerebral cortex and deep white matter are clearly demarcated from each other, and the falx cerebri is seen in both the frontal and occipital regions. Several blood vessels can be seen. Also, note the bilateral calcifications of the choroid plexus of the lateral ventricles. **b** Some of the blood vessels around the base of the brain (arrows) are well seen after the administration of contrast medium.

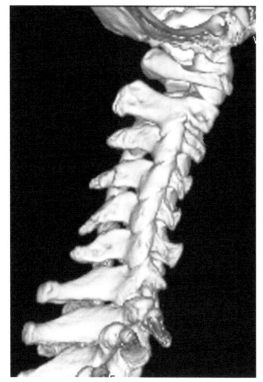

Fig. 4.4   Three-dimensional CT reconstruction of the cervical spine.

— **Perfusion CT** (**Fig. 4.5**) employs short image-acquisition times with the simultaneous injection of contrast medium to enable the visualization of brain perfusion.

4.2.3 Magnetic Resonance Imaging

| NOTE

MRI employs magnetic fields and radio waves to induce hydrogen atoms in the body's tissues to emit signals that can be displayed on sectional images. MRI is particularly suitable for the visualization of soft-tissue lesions but can also be used for vascular imaging and for functional diagnostic studies.

MRI is a sectional imaging technique that does not rely on the use of ionizing radiation.

Technical description. The underlying physical principles of MRI are as follows: the most common atomic nuclei in all tissues of the body are hydrogen nuclei (protons). They are positively charged and possess an intrinsic magnetic property known as "**spin**," which can be imagined as a rotation of the proton around its own axis. Each proton thus has its own small magnetic field. A proton to which an external magnetic field is applied orients itself in the field like a compass needle (**Fig. 4.6**). When the protons in a particularly bodily tissue are aligned in this way, and then stimulated with a radiofrequency pulse at a particular frequency (the resonance or Larmor frequency), they will take on energy and reorient themselves opposite the field. Once the

Table 4.1

Comparative indications of CT and MRI of the head

Location and type of pathology	CT	MRI
Brain atrophy	+++	+++
Acute infarct	++	+++
Older infarct	++	+++
Lacunar state	+++	+++
Acute intraparenchymal hemorrhage	++	+++
Subarachnoid hemorrhage	+++	+
Aneurysm	+	++
Venous thrombosis	+	+++
Brain tumor (cerebral hemispheres)	++	+++
Pituitary tumor	+	+++
Brain metastases	+++	+++
Carcinomatous meningitis	–	++
Hydrocephalus	+++	+++
Head trauma: skull injury	+++	+
Head trauma: brain injury	++	+++
Head trauma: acute sub- or epidural hematoma	+++	+++
Meningoencephalitis	++	+++
Abscess	++	+++
Parasitic cyst(s)	+	+++
Arachnoid cyst	++	+++
Posterior fossa	+	+++
Pathology of the white matter	+	+++
Multiple sclerosis	–	+++
Atlanto-occipital joint	+	+++
Lesions of the skull	+++	+
Lesions of the spine (bone)	++	++
Lesions of the spinal cord and nerve roots	+	+++

Note: +++ = most suitable study, usually adequate for diagnosis; ++ = study generally useful; + = study occasionally necessary or indicated in addition to other tests; – study not useful.

stimulating pulse is switched off, the protons release the energy that they previously absorbed as they return to their original orientation. The released energy can be detected with a radio antenna or coil and is called the **magnetic resonance signal**. The signals from different points in a slab of tissue are distinguished from one another with gradient fields, that is, smaller magnetic fields overlying the main field. The MR image is a gray-scale map of the different intensities of MR signal coming from the tissue (**Fig. 4.7**) and can be computed in any desired plane of section. Gadolinium–DTPA can be given intravenously as a **contrast medium** for MRI. Caution is advised in patients with renal dysfunction, in whom gadolinium may lead to nephrogenic systemic fibrosis.

The MR signal intensity of tissue is a function of its local physical and chemical properties, which determine, for example, the length of time that the hydrogen nuclei need to return to their initial orientation (T_1 and T_2 relaxation times). The signal intensity is further influenced by the technical parameters of the scanner (e.g., the strength of the applied magnetic field and the frequency of the stimulating impulses).

Indications. The MRI signal characteristics of various normal and pathologic tissues in the brain are listed in **Table 4.1**. The main types of signal abnormality that are important for neurologic diagnosis are indicated in **Table 4.2**.

MR Angiography

When the spin-echo technique is used in MRI scanning, flowing blood gives rise to a signal only if it is excited by two radio wave pulses that arrive one after the other at the same location. If the blood passes rapidly through the imaging plane, the bit of blood that received the first excitatory pulse has already flowed away by the time the second pulse arrives, and no signal is generated—the vessel appears dark (there is a "flow void"). However, if the blood flows slowly enough to receive both pulses in the imaging plane, the vessel appears bright. When gradient-echo sequences are used, flowing blood always appears bright, while stationary tissue appears dark.

Computer algorithms can combine the individual sectional images, processing them to generate a projectional image resembling a conventional angiogram;

| Table 4.2 |

MRI signal intensities of normal and abnormal structures

Tissue	T1-weighted image	T2-weighted image
Cerebrospinal fluid	Dark	Very bright
Brain		
White matter	Bright	Slightly dark
Gray matter	Slightly dark	Slightly bright
MS plaque	Intermediate to dark	Bright
Bland infarct	Dark	Bright
Tumor/metastasis	Dark	Bright
Meningioma	Intermediate	Intermediate
Abscess	Dark	Bright
Edema	Dark	Bright
Calcification	Intermediate or bright	Intermediate or dark
Fat	Very bright	Intermediate to dark
Cyst		
Containing mostly water	Dark	Very bright
Containing proteinaceous fluid	Intermediate to bright	Very bright
Containing lipids	Very bright	Intermediate to dark
Bone		
Cortical bone	Very dark	Very dark
Yellow bone marrow	Very bright	Intermediate to dark
Red bone marrow	Intermediate	Slightly dark
Bone metastasis		
Lytic	Dark	Intermediate to bright
Sclerotic	Dark	Dark
Cartilage		
Fibrous	Very dark	Very dark
Hyaline	Intermediate	Intermediate
Intervertebral disk		
Normal	Intermediate	Bright
Degenerated	Intermediate to dark	Dark
Muscle	Dark	Dark
Tendons and ligaments		
Normal	Very dark	Very dark
Inflamed	Intermediate	Intermediate
Torn	Intermediate	Bright
Contrast enhancement with gadolinium–DTPA		
Low concentration	Very bright	Bright
High concentration	Intermediate to dark	Very dark
Hematoma		
Hyperacute	Intermediate	Intermediate to bright
Acute	Intermediate to dark	Dark to very dark
Subacute	Bright rim, intermediate	Bright rim, dark center, later all bright
Chronic	Dark rim, bright center, later all dark	Dark rim, bright center, later all dark

Abbreviations: DTPA, diethylenetriaminepentaacetic acid; MS, multiple sclerosis.
Source: Adapted from Edelman RR, Warach S. Magnetic resonance imaging (1). N Engl J Med 1993;328(10):708–716.
Note: Bright = hyperintense; dark = hypointense; intermediate = isointense in comparison to brain tissue.

this is called a **magnetic resonance angiogram** (**Fig. 4.8**). The technique that exploits signal timing and flow voids is called time-of-flight magnetic resonance angiography, or TOF-MRA. It can be used for the noninvasive diagnosis of, for example, a carotid artery occlusion.

Contrast-enhanced MR angiography is now being performed increasingly often. In this technique, the signal is produced not by the flowing of the blood per se, but by the contrast medium in the bloodstream (**Fig. 4.9**).

Susceptibility-weighted MR sequences have also entered into widespread clinical use. They permit

4

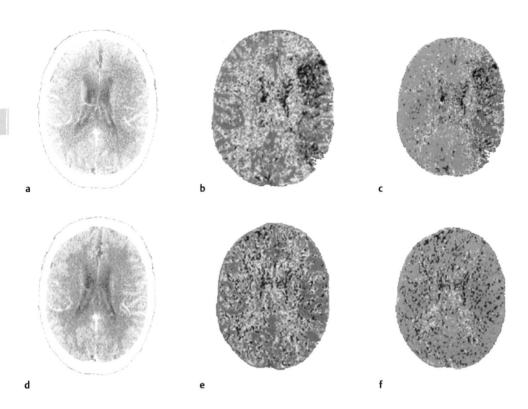

a   b   c

d   e   f

Fig. 4.5   Perfusion CT in acute occlusion of the left middle cerebral artery (MCA; upper row of images, a–c) and after reperfusion (lower row, d–f). a CT without contrast medium reveals no abnormality. **b** Visualization of regional cerebral blood flow (rCBF), as calculated from the regional blood volume and the mean contrast-medium transit time (MTT), reveals hypoperfusion of the entire left MCA territory. **c** MTT is prolonged in the MCA distribution. **d** After successful reperfusion by thrombolysis, there is no infarct; **e** the blood flow and **f** transit time are normal again.

the demonstration of acute embolic or thrombotic vascular occlusion (**Fig. 4.10**).

Further MR Techniques

The passage of contrast medium through the organs can be detected with rapid imaging sequences, so that organ perfusion can be measured (**perfusion MRI**). The technique of perfusion MRI is based on the loss of signal caused by contrast media such as gadolinium on gradient-echo images.

The diffusive movement of hydrogen nuclei (protons) can also be visualized with special diffusion-weighted sequences (**diffusion MRI**). This technique enables the detection of acute ischemia, because protons in ischemic tissue diffuse much less readily in the initial hours and days after the event. The use of diffusion gradients in all three spatial dimensions (**diffusion tensor imaging**) enables detection of the preferential direction of diffusion in each voxel of tissue. This technique is used to depict fiber tracts and display their course between different regions of the brain (**Fig. 4.11**).

Functional MRI enables the visualization of regional blood-flow changes that correspond to increases or decreases in regional neuronal activity. Changes in blood flow are reflected in an altered ratio of oxy- to deoxyhemoglobin, which can be detected with gradient-echo imaging and an averaging technique. This method is used, for example, to demonstrate the activation of language areas in the brain when the patient speaks (**Fig. 4.12**).

4.2.4 Angiography with Radiologic Contrast Media (Digital Subtraction Angiography)

> **NOTE**
>
> Digital subtraction angiography (DSA) enables the precise diagnostic visualization of vascular abnormalities such as stenosis, acute occlusion, aneurysms, fistulae, and arteriovenous malformations. Because of its risks, DSA should only be performed when strictly indicated. DSA is particularly useful for treatment planning and is indispensable for the endovascular treatment of the above-mentioned vascular abnormalities.

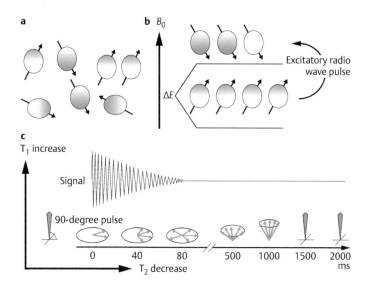

Fig. 4.6   Physical principles of magnetic resonance imaging. Adapted from Edelman RR, Warach S. Magnetic resonance imaging (1). N Engl J Med 1993;328(10):708–716. **a** The magnetic axes of the protons are randomly distributed over space. **b** When a magnetic field B_0 is applied to the protons, they align themselves either parallel or antiparallel to the field. A proton aligned parallel to B_0 has a lower energy than one aligned antiparallel to it; therefore, most protons have a parallel alignment at first. If radio waves of a specific frequency (the Larmor frequency) are now applied, protons can absorb the energy they need to "flip" from the lower-energy to the higher-energy state, thereby becoming antiparallel to the field B_0. The flipped protons then gradually return to the parallel, lower-energy state (relaxation). The speed of relaxation is determined by two tissue-specific constants called T_1 and T_2. **c** After the 90-degree excitatory pulse is delivered, the protons precess in the transverse plane. They are in phase at first, and therefore give off a maximally intense signal. Very small inhomogeneities of the magnetic field make the protons precess at slightly different speeds, resulting in "dephasing" and loss of signal intensity. This process, which takes only a few milliseconds, is called T_2 relaxation. The MR signal is usually measured during T_2 relaxation. The restoration of magnetization parallel to B_0 is a somewhat slower process, called T_1 relaxation. Several techniques (e.g., gradient echo, spin echo) are used to generate the largest possible MR signal.

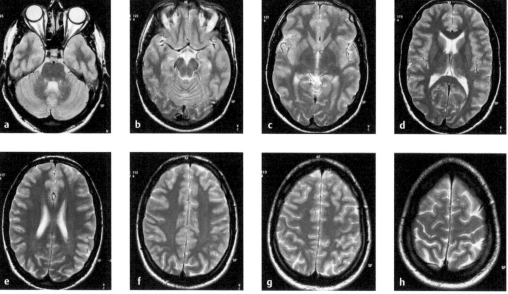

Fig. 4.7   a–h Normal MRI of the brain in 5-mm sections from base to vertex.

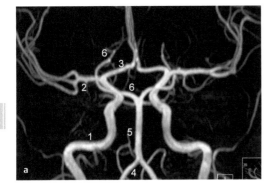

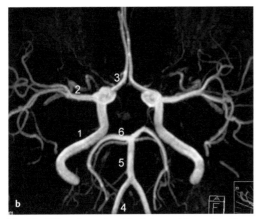

Fig. 4.8 MR angiography of the intracranial vessels. a Coronal and **b** axial projections of the circle of Willis, revealing the internal carotid artery (**1**), the middle cerebral artery(**2**), the anterior cerebral artery (**3**), the vertebral artery (**4**), the basilar artery (**5**), and the posterior cerebral artery (**6**).

Methods and risks. Conventional biplanar arteriography, also known as **angiography with radiologic contrast media**, is indicated for certain special purposes, for example, the preoperative visualization of intracranial aneurysms or arteriovenous malformations. This type of study involves the introduction of an intra-arterial catheter by way of the femoral artery along a guidewire all the way up to the great vessels that supply the brain. Contrast medium is injected into these vessels while fluoroscopic images are simultaneously obtained. The image changes from one second to the next, as the contrast medium distributes itself in the cerebral vasculature. All of the images are digitized, and an image obtained before contrast medium was injected is subtracted from each of the images obtained with contrast medium to generate a **digital subtraction angiogram**, which displays nothing but the blood vessels supplying the head and brain (both extra- and intracranial). Contrast medium can be injected into the carotid artery to display the anterior circulation (**Fig. 4.13**), or into the vertebral artery to display

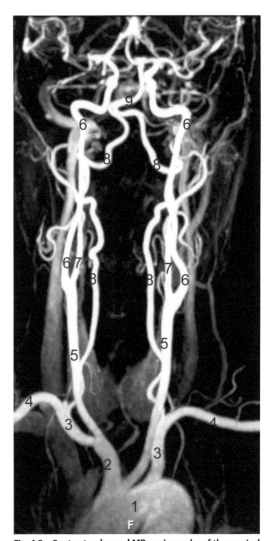

Fig. 4.9 Contrast-enhanced MR angiography of the cervical vessels. Coronal image. The visualized structures include the aortic arch (**1**) and the cervical and brachial arteries that emerge from it: the brachiocephalic trunk (**2**), the subclavian artery (**3**), the axillary artery (**4**), the common carotid artery (**5**), the internal carotid artery (**6**), the external carotid artery (**7**), the vertebral artery (**8**), and the basilar artery (**9**). The only abnormality here is an unusual elongation of the basilar artery.

the posterior circulation (**Fig. 4.14**). The **blood vessels of the spinal cord** can also be studied angiographically, for example, for the diagnosis and treatment of spinal arteriovenous malformations or dural fistulae.

Rotational angiography (**rotational DSA**) is a further development of the technique, which, like CT, enables the generation and display of three-dimensional reconstructed images (e.g., syngo DynaCT (Siemens Healthineers); **Fig. 4.15**).

The **risks** of angiography include hemorrhage or dissection at the femoral puncture site, the detachment of atherosclerotic plaques from arterial walls by the

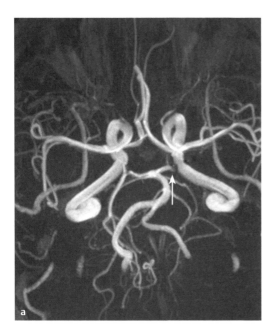

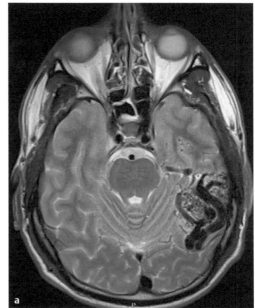

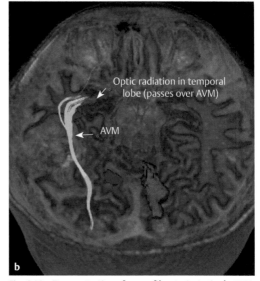

Fig. 4.11   Demonstration of nerve fiber trajectories by MRI with diffusion tensor imaging (DTI). **a** T2-weighted MRI reveals an arteriovenous malformation (AVM) in the posterior portion of the left temporal lobe. **b** DTI reveals that the visual pathway (green) lies superior to the AVM as it courses toward the occipital lobe. (This view is from above, and the AVM is therefore on the left side of the image.)

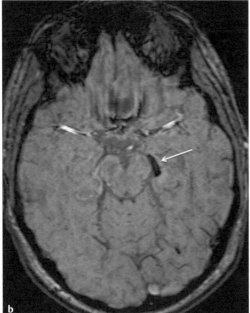

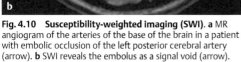

Fig. 4.10   Susceptibility-weighted imaging (SWI). a MR angiogram of the arteries of the base of the brain in a patient with embolic occlusion of the left posterior cerebral artery (arrow). **b** SWI reveals the embolus as a signal void (arrow).

tip of the catheter, and the induction of vasospasm leading to cerebral ischemia and stroke. Angiographic contrast media can also have side effects.

The general rule, when a diagnostic study of the blood vessels is desired, is to choose a study that is likely to

yield sufficient information for effective diagnosis and treatment without putting the patient at excessive risk. MR angiography, conventional MRI (see **Fig. 4.16**), CT angiography, or Doppler ultrasonography (Section 4.4) will suffice for most purposes.

Indications. Angiography is used not just for diagnostic purposes, but also increasingly often for

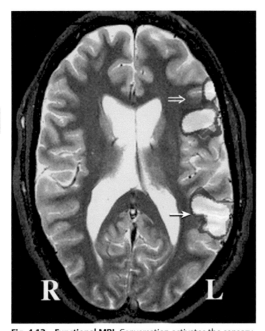

Fig. 4.12 Functional MRI. Conversation activates the sensory (Wernicke) language area at the junction of the temporal and parietal lobes (thin arrow), as well as the motor (Broca) language area in the left inferior frontal gyrus (thick arrow).

treatment, for example, for the obliteration of aneurysms and fistulae, the opening of stenoses of the intra- or extracranial vessels, or the mechanical or pharmacologic recanalization of occluded brain arteries in acute stroke. The particular indications for cerebral angiography can be listed as follows:

− Visualization of saccular aneurysms.
− Visualization of arteriovenous malformations and fistulae.
− Detailed visualization of saccular aneurysms (after diagnosis by MRI or CT as an aid to treatment by neurosurgical or interventional neuroradiologic methods).
− Detailed visualization of arteriovenous malformations (after diagnosis by MRI or CT as an aid to treatment by neurosurgical or interventional neuroradiologic methods).
− Visualization of other vascular anomalies:
  • Moyamoya.
  • Agenesis of vessels and other developmental anomalies.
  • Vascular stenosis or occlusion.
  • Arterial dissection.
− Treatment:
  • Extra- and intracranial arterial stenoses, arterial occlusion in acute stroke (recanalization).

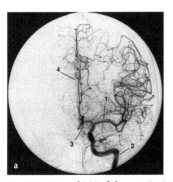
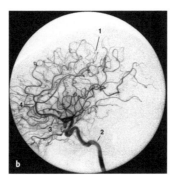
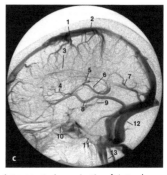

Fig. 4.13 Normal DSA of the anterior intracranial circulation (carotid distribution). a Anteroposterior projection. **b** Lateral projection. **c** Venous phase, lateral projection. **a and b: 1** MCA = middle cerebral artery; **2** ICA = internal carotid artery; **3** ACA = anterior cerebral artery; **4** pericallosal artery. **c: 1** Superior cerebral veins (rolandic and Trolard); **2** superior sagittal sinus; **3** inferior sagittal sinus; **4** septal vein; **5** thalamostriate vein; **6** internal cerebral vein; **7** straight sinus; **8** vein of Labbé = inferior anastomotic vein; **9** basal vein of Rosenthal; **10** cavernous sinus; **11** inferior petrosal sinus; **12** lateral sinus; **13** jugular vein.

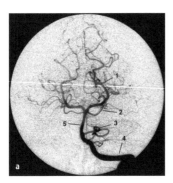
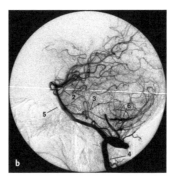

Fig. 4.14 Selective angiography of the left vertebral artery. a Arterial phase, anteroposterior projection. **b** Arterial phase, lateral projection. **1** posterior cerebral artery; **2** superior cerebellar artery; **3** anterior inferior cerebellar artery (AICA); **4** left vertebral artery; **5** basilar artery; **6** posterior inferior cerebellar artery (PICA).

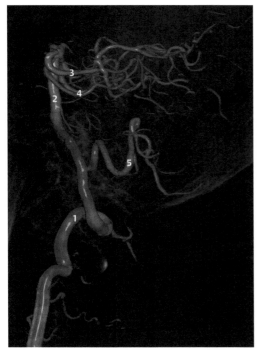

Fig. 4.15 Three-dimensional image of the posterior circulation reconstructed from a dataset obtained by rotational DSA (syngo DynaCT). The arteries visualized include the left vertebral artery (**1**) and the basilar artery (**2**), together with their main branches. The posterior cerebral artery is uppermost (**3**), with the superior cerebellar artery immediately inferior to it (**4**). The inferior cerebellar artery originates from the vertebral artery above its C1 loop (**5**).

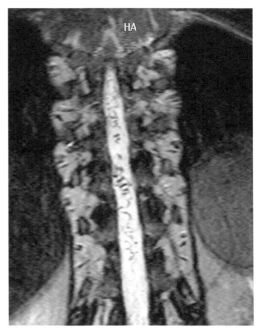

Fig. 4.16 Arteriovenous malformation on the surface of the cervical spinal cord ("varicosis spinalis" in earlier terminology). The T2-weighted MR image reveals the vessels of the malformation as voids within the bright-appearing CSF.

- Vasospasm, for example, after subarachnoid hemorrhage.
- Endovascular occlusion of aneurysms, arteriovenous malformations, and fistulae with spiral coils, or redirection of blood flow with flow diverters.

4.2.5 Myelography and Radiculography

> **NOTE**
>
> Myelography and radiculography (together usually called "myelography" in short) display the intraspinal structures and spinal nerve roots with the aid of contrast medium injected into the subarachnoid space. This technique is generally used when CT or MRI alone cannot reveal whether the spinal cord or nerve roots are compressed by structural changes of the vertebral column or by a mass lesion.

Technical description. Myelography generally involves the injection of 10 to 15 mL of water-soluble contrast medium into the subarachnoid space via lumbar puncture (LP)—or, rarely, suboccipital puncture. The passage of contrast medium through the subarachnoid space, including the nerve root sleeves, can then be followed on the radiologic image, and any obstructions to the flow of contrast medium can be identified (e.g., spinal tumors). The nerve roots appear as filling voids within the nerve root sleeves. The vertebral column is seen on the myelographic images as well and can be evaluated at the same time.

Indications. The indications for myelography are listed in **Table 4.3**, together with those of other competing types of study. CT and MRI have now replaced myelography for most indications. Postmyelographic CT is a useful adjunct to myelography (**Fig. 4.17**).

Typical findings. Some of the more common myelographic findings are shown schematically in **Fig. 4.18**. Further myelographic images can be found elsewhere in this book: lumbar intervertebral disk herniation, **Fig. 13.9**; cervical myelopathy, **Fig. 7.10**; spinal cord tumors, **Fig. 7.6**, **Fig. 7.7**, **Fig. 7.8**, and **Fig. 7.9**.

4.2.6 Diagnostic Techniques of Nuclear Medicine

CSF Scintigraphy/Isotope Cisternography

Technique. The subarachnoid space is entered with a fine needle in the suboccipital or lumbar region and a radiolabeled substance, for example, human albumin labeled with ^{131}I, is injected into the CSF. The

Table 4.3

Indications for contrast myelography as compared with other imaging techniques

Condition/suspected pathology	Plain X-ray	CT	MRI	Contrast myelography, radiculography, myelo-CT
Pain without neurologic deficit	+ +			
Clinically localizable radiculopathy		+ +	+ + +	
Clinically evident lumbar radiculopathy with unclear CT or MRI findings	E.g., in vertebral body tumors			+ +
Suspected radiculopathy, but no clear segmental localization		+	+ + +	
Suspected spinal cord compression		+ +	+ + +	
Suspected spinal stenosis	+ +	+ +	+ + +	+
Clinically evident spinal stenosis			+ + +	+ +
Suspected myelopathy due to cervical spondylosis		+	+ + +	+
Suspected myelitis or demyelination			+ + +	

Abbreviations: CT, computed tomography; MRI, magnetic resonance imaging.
Note: + + + = most suitable study, usually adequate for diagnosis; + + = study generally useful; + = study occasionally necessary or indicated in addition to other tests.

radioactive contrast medium should be detectable 1 to 2 hours later in the basal cisterns, 4 to 6 hours later over the cerebral convexity, and 24 hours later in the superior sagittal sinus. In normal individuals, it is never detected in the lateral ventricles.

Indications. This type of study is used, for example, to localize a fistula through which CSF is leaking from the subarachnoid space into the nasal cavity (where it can be detected on a nasal tampon), or to demonstrate malresorptive hydrocephalus, in which contrast medium enters the lateral ventricles. Scintigraphy is now only rarely indicated, as CT and MRI yield more useful information in most cases.

SPECT

Technique. Single-photon emission computed tomography (SPECT) employs either a 99^m-technetium compound or 133^I-amphetamine as a tracer. The purpose of this type of study is to measure regional cerebral blood flow (rCBF).

Indications. See the following section, "PET."

PET

Technique. Positron emission tomography (PET) uses the short-lived positron-emitting radionuclides ^{11}C, ^{14}O, or ^{18}F and can therefore only be performed near a cyclotron in which these isotopes are produced. It yields quantitative tomographic images of rCBF, cerebral blood volume, oxygen consumption (the cerebral metabolic rate for oxygen, CMR-O_2), and glucose consumption (CMR-Gluc).

Indications for PET and SPECT. PET and SPECT are indicated for the demonstration of hypoperfusion, for example, in stroke, or of reduced metabolic activity in the brain, for example, reduced activity in the

temporal and parietal lobes in Alzheimer disease (**Fig. 4.19b**). They can also be used to detect focal pathologic processes of other types, such as epileptogenic foci (**Fig. 4.19c**). With PET, physicians can perform biochemical studies in vivo. The radioactive labeling of substances that are metabolized in the brain makes it possible to measure their concentration and kinetics in specific brain areas. Thus, for example, the localization and concentration of injected DOPA can be studied in patients with suspected Parkinson disease (see **Fig. 6.57**).

Optical Coherence Tomography

Optical coherence tomography employs low-coherence interferometry to produce images of optically scattering tissue. It is mainly used for diagnostic evaluation of the retina, including the macula and the optic disc. It can resolve lesions of the order of magnitude of a micron (**Fig. 4.20**).

4.3 Electrophysiologic Studies

Key Point
The investigation of electrophysiologic processes in muscle and nerve cells with suitable techniques can shed light both on the normal functioning of these processes in normal individuals and on disturbances caused by neurologic disease.

4.3.1 Fundamentals

Electrophysiologic processes are an intrinsic part of all cellular activity (Section 1.2). Differences in electrical potential and changes in these differences over time can be amplified, displayed on an oscilloscope, and recorded on paper or in digitized form. **EEG** records the activity of cortical neurons and neuronal populations; **EMG** records that of muscle cells. The

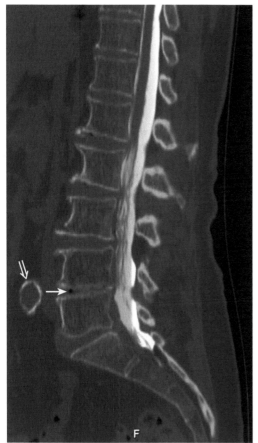

Fig. 4.17 Postmyelographic CT of a 79-year-old woman with an ischemic lesion of the conus medullaris. A sagittal reconstruction of the lumbar spine after the injection of contrast medium into the lumbar theca reveals the thoracic spinal cord and conus medullaris as a solid, dark void within the bright CSF. The nerve roots are seen as dark strands. Note the spinal degenerative changes (with prominent ventral spondylophytes) and the loss of disk height at L4–L5, indicating osteochondrosis (thin arrow). The aorta is calcified (thick arrow). The spinal canal is not narrowed to any significant extent by the degenerative changes.

conduction of spontaneous or evoked impulses in peripheral nerves is assessed by **ENG**. Repeated stimulation of the receptors of a particular sensory system (e.g., the retina, by visual stimuli) and simultaneous measurement of the ensuing cortical activity enable determination of the conduction velocity within the sensory system in question (**evoked potential studies**). The complex electrophysiologic phenomena of sleep are studied with **somnography** (sleep studies). These electrophysiologic diagnostic techniques offer a practically risk-free means of assessing the functional state of the nervous system, although some of them are rather unpleasant for the patient. Despite the absence of risk, they should only be performed for strict indications, in accordance with the general principles outlined in Section 4.1.

4.3.2 Electroencephalography

> **NOTE**
>
> The surface EEG registers fluctuations in electrical potential that are generated by the cerebral cortex. These represent the sum of the excitatory and inhibitory synaptic potentials. EEG is mainly used to characterize epilepsy and disturbances of consciousness.

Technique. Electrodes are placed on the scalp according to the internationally standardized **ten–twenty system** (**Fig. 4.21**). The fluctuations of electrical potential at each electrode are recorded, either in bipolar mode (i.e., differences between adjacent electrodes) or in unipolar mode (i.e., differences between each electrode and a reference electrode). Their magnitude at the scalp is 10 to 100 μV. They are amplified and recorded on paper in 12 parallel channels. Fluctuations in electrical potential are classified by frequency. Certain maneuvers, for example, opening and closing the eyes, hyperventilation, and rhythmic photic stimulation, affect the EEG tracing in characteristic ways and may induce pathologic waves in patients with epilepsy. A standard EEG recording takes approximately 20 minutes. Long-term recording

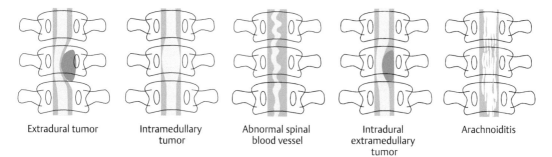

| Extradural tumor | Intramedullary tumor | Abnormal spinal blood vessel | Intradural extramedullary tumor | Arachnoiditis |

Fig. 4.18 Typical findings in contrast myelography.

4

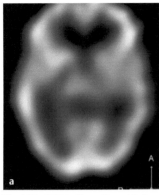 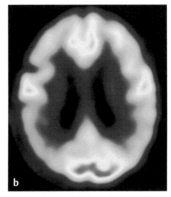 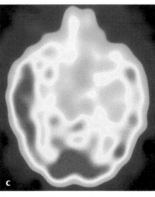

Fig. 4.19   PET studies. a Normal findings. **b** In a patient with Alzheimer disease, PET reveals bilateral parietotemporal hypometabolism. **c** In a patient with complex-partial epilepsy, ictal PET reveals increased neuronal activity in the right temporal lobe.

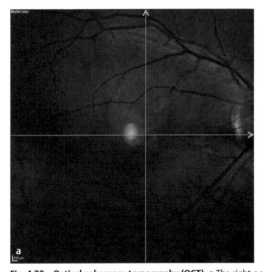 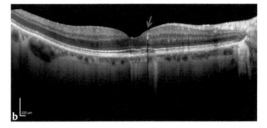 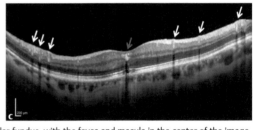

Fig. 4.20   Optical coherence tomography (OCT). a The right ocular fundus, with the fovea and macula in the center of the image. A small, nonspecific retinal scar is seen at the nasal edge of the fovea. **b** Horizontal OCT and **c** vertical OCT along the green arrows of part **a** enable visualization of the intraretinal structures and layers, the retinal scar (red arrow), and multiple vascular "shadows" (white arrows).

or an EEG after sleep deprivation may be necessary for the study of certain types of epilepsy.

Evaluation. A normal EEG tracing is shown in **Fig. 4.22**, and the main physiologic and pathologic graphic elements of the EEG are shown schematically in **Fig. 4.23**. A predominantly occipital α rhythm is the main component of the EEG tracing in a normal, awake, relaxed individual. There is a progressive slowing of frequencies during sleep, depending on the sleep stage (depth of sleep). The following EEG changes indicate a pathologic process in the brain:

- **General changes. Slowing** of the background rhythm in an awake patient is abnormal, as is **acceleration** of background activity (e.g., a β rhythm). The latter is often due to medication use.

- **Focal findings.** Slowing of background activity (e.g., in the form of theta or delta waves) limited to a circumscribed area of the brain reflects focal cortical dysfunction. Findings of this type are often due to structural lesions (e.g., tumors; see **Fig. 4.24**).

- **Sharp waves and spikes.** These characteristically shaped abnormal potentials are seen in persons with epilepsy. During a seizure, typical seizure-related potentials appear (spikes followed by a prolonged wave— the "spike-and-wave" pattern). They are visible in all leads in generalized seizures; in focal seizures, or before the secondary generalization of an initially focal seizure, rhythmic steep potentials are generally seen only over a few leads. Pathologic EEG changes are not necessarily present between seizures, and a normal interictal EEG does not rule out epilepsy.

a

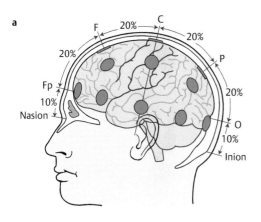

b

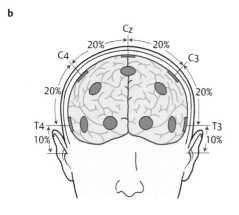

c

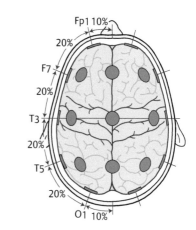

d

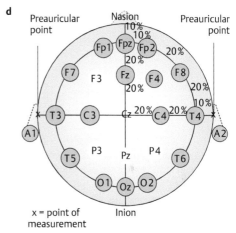

x = point of measurement

Fig. 4.21   Placement of EEG electrodes according to the ten–twenty system. a Lateral view. The electrodes are placed at fixed percentage intervals between the nasion and the inion. **b** Frontal view. The preauricular points serve as reference points for the placement of the central transverse row of electrodes. C_z is the intersection of the central transverse and longitudinal rows. **c** Superior view. **d** Names of electrodes in the ten–twenty system. (Adapted from Masuhr KF, Neumann M. Duale Reihe Neurologie. Stuttgart: Thieme; 2013.)

EEG changes are also seen in many other disease processes affecting the brain.

The main indications for EEG.

— Confirmation of the diagnosis of epilepsy.
— Determination of the type of epilepsy that is present.
— Brief, episodic impairment of consciousness of unknown etiology.
— Longer-lasting disturbances of consciousness, delirium.
— Metabolic disturbances.
— Creutzfeldt–Jakob disease.
— Sleep studies (e.g., in suspected narcolepsy).

Polysomnography

Technique. Polysomnography is a special application of EEG in which the EEG is recorded simultaneously with several other electrophysiologic parameters. It is used to assess sleep and disturbances of sleep. The EEG changes normally occurring during sleep reflect the progression of the individual through various sleep stages, including deep or REM sleep (REM = " rapid eye movement"). The recorded parameters include eye movements (by electro-oculography), respiratory excursion, airflow in the nostrils, muscle activity (by surface EMG), cardiac activity (by ECG), and the partial pressure of oxygen (by transcutaneous pulse oximetry) (**Fig. 4.25**). These are displayed together with the EEG in a polygraph recording (**polysomnogram**).

Indications. The most common indication for a sleep study is a clinical suspicion of sleep apnea syndrome (Section 10.3.1 and **Fig. 10.1**) based on a characteristic history obtained from the patient or bed partner, together with related physical findings and a low partial pressure of oxygen measured during sleep by

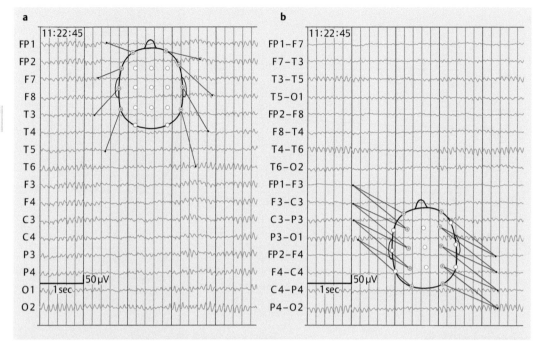

Fig. 4.22   Normal EEG. a Monopolar recording. **b** Bipolar recording.

pulse oximetry. Polysomnography is also indicated for the diagnosis of narcolepsy, as well as for the assessment of excessive fatigue and daytime somnolence.

4.3.3 Evoked Potentials

NOTE

Evoked potentials are electrical signals generated by the nervous system in response to repetitive stimuli. They reflect the electrical conducting activity of functional systems.

General principles. Evoked potentials are used to assess the integrity of individual functional systems (visual, auditory, somatosensory, or motor). The system under study is activated with a repeatedly delivered stimulus. The resulting fluctuations of electrical potential in the brain can be detected by summation of the potentials that are recorded when the excitatory stimulus has been delivered a large number of times. Evoked potentials provide evidence of whether impulse conduction in the system in question is intact from the site of stimulation all the way to the cerebral cortex. Sometimes a partial or total conduction block can be localized precisely between two of the relay stations for neural transmission along a particular functional pathway. Evoked potentials can also reveal subclinical lesions. The most

important types of evoked potential for clinical practice are outlined in the following paragraphs.

Visual Evoked Potentials

The patient fixates on a video screen displaying a checkerboard pattern that is regularly and periodically inverted, while electrical potentials are recorded through a needle electrode in the scalp at the occiput. Evoked potentials are obtained by summation; the largest fluctuation is a positive wave that appears 100 milliseconds after the stimulus. Delay of this wave is found early in the course of optic neuritis and persists thereafter (**Fig. 4.26**).

Auditory Evoked Potentials

A click stimulus delivered periodically to one ear induces the generation of neural impulses that travel along the auditory nerve to the brainstem, the thalamus, and finally the cerebral cortex. The electrophysiologic response is measured from the vertex of the head in relation to a reference electrode on the earlobe or mastoid process. The normal auditory evoked potential contains five different waves, each of which is generated by a different structure along the chain of impulse transmission.

Somatosensory Evoked Potentials

When a repetitive electrical stimulus is applied to the skin, impulses are generated at the terminal

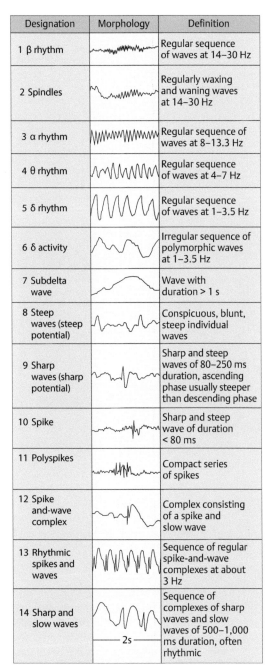

Designation	Morphology	Definition
1 β rhythm		Regular sequence of waves at 14–30 Hz
2 Spindles		Regularly waxing and waning waves at 14–30 Hz
3 α rhythm		Regular sequence of waves at 8–13.3 Hz
4 θ rhythm		Regular sequence of waves at 4–7 Hz
5 δ rhythm		Regular sequence of waves at 1–3.5 Hz
6 δ activity		Irregular sequence of polymorphic waves at 1–3.5 Hz
7 Subdelta wave		Wave with duration > 1 s
8 Steep waves (steep potential)		Conspicuous, blunt, steep individual waves
9 Sharp waves (sharp potential)		Sharp and steep waves of 80–250 ms duration, ascending phase usually steeper than descending phase
10 Spike		Sharp and steep wave of duration < 80 ms
11 Polyspikes		Compact series of spikes
12 Spike and-wave complex		Complex consisting of a spike and slow wave
13 Rhythmic spikes and waves		Sequence of regular spike-and-wave complexes at about 3 Hz
14 Sharp and slow waves		Sequence of complexes of sharp waves and slow waves of 500–1,000 ms duration, often rhythmic

Fig. 4.23 The most important graphoelements in EEG: designations, morphology, and definitions. (Adapted from Schliack H, Hopf HC. Diagnostik in der Neurologie. Stuttgart: Thieme; 1988.)

sensory branch of a peripheral nerve and conducted centrally via the peripheral nerve, nerve root, posterior columns/spinothalamic tract, medial lemniscus, and thalamocortical connections. A lesion at any point along this pathway can alter the evoked potentials, which are recorded first over Erb's point (for the median nerve) or the lumbar spine (for the tibial

nerve), and then through a scalp electrode in the parietal region on the side opposite the stimulus. An example of delayed conduction in the central somatosensory pathway is shown in **Fig. 4.27**.

4.3.4 Electromyography

NOTE

EMG measures the electrical activity of muscle in the resting state and during voluntary contraction. In combination with the clinical findings, EMG can reveal whether weakness is due to myopathy, a peripheral nerve lesion, a lesion of the anterior horn of the spinal cord, or a more centrally located disturbance.

Principle. The electrical activity of a muscle is recorded through bipolar needle electrodes, first with the muscle at rest and then with light and maximal voluntary contraction. The recorded potentials are displayed visually on an oscilloscope and also converted into an audio signal. With light contraction of the muscle, potentials arising from individual motor units can be observed. (A motor unit is the set of muscle fibers innervated by a single motor anterior horn cell, by way of its multiple axon collaterals.) With stronger or maximal contraction, a large number of motor unit potentials come together to form an interference pattern.

— **Insertional activity and spontaneous activity.** At rest, muscles are normally electrically silent; when the needle is inserted, there are normally only a few positive sharp waves or fibrillations. **Pathologic spontaneous activity** of a muscle manifests itself as prolonged insertional activity as well as pathologic fibrillation potentials and positive sharp waves (**Fig. 4.29**). This spontaneous activity reflects denervation of the muscle. Fasciculations and complex repetitive discharges are further forms of pathologic spontaneous activity, as are myotonic repetitive discharges.

— **Electrical activity on voluntary contraction.** Muscle action potentials are observed when the muscle is voluntarily contracted. The amplitude and duration of individual motor unit potentials are proportional to the size of the motor unit, that is, the number of muscle fibers it contains. The more strongly a muscle is contracted, the more motor units will be recruited. When a large number of motor units are active, their potentials can no longer be seen individually. Instead, they summate to form a (complete) interference pattern (**Fig. 4.30a**). The size and shape of electromyographic potentials are altered by many different types of neuromuscular disease.

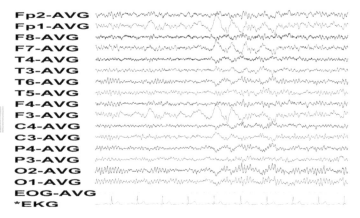

```
Fp2-AVG
Fp1-AVG
F8-AVG
F7-AVG
T4-AVG
T3-AVG
T6-AVG
T5-AVG
F4-AVG
F3-AVG
C4-AVG
C3-AVG
P4-AVG
P3-AVG
O2-AVG
O1-AVG
EOG-AVG
*EKG
```

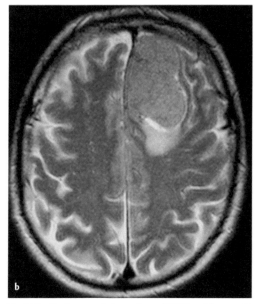

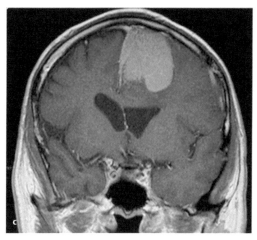

Fig. 4.24 **Electroencephalography and MRI in a 65-year-old man who presented with a single nocturnal seizure and was found to have a left frontal convexity meningioma.** **a** The EEG reveals a left frontal focus of delta-wave activity corresponding to the site of the tumor on MRI; **b** axial T2-weighted image; **c** contrast-enhanced coronal T1-weighted image. Note the homogeneous uptake of contrast medium that is typical of meningioma.

- **Myopathy** is characterized by a diffuse loss of individual muscle fibers in all motor units of the affected muscle(s). Each motor unit potential is therefore of lower amplitude and shorter duration (**Fig. 4.30d**). In principle, all of the motor units are still present but contain fewer muscle fibers than before; thus, on maximal voluntary contraction of the muscle, the interference pattern is full, but of lower than normal amplitude.
- In contrast, in a **neuropathic process** (chronic denervation of a muscle), the motor units are larger than normal because of repeated denervation and reinnervation. When the nerve fiber innervating a particular motor unit degenerates, axon collaterals sprouting

from the nerves of adjacent motor units take over the muscle fibers of the denervated unit, so that the surviving motor units actually contain more muscle fibers than before. Their motor unit potentials are usually polyphasic and of increased amplitude and duration (**Fig. 4.30b**). Because there are fewer motor units, maximal voluntary contraction of a denervated muscle yields a markedly attenuated interference pattern, in which the individual action potentials of the remaining motor units appear as large oscillations.

- **Electrical activity at the motor end plate.** EMG can also reveal dysfunction of the motor end plate affecting neuromuscular transmission. On repetitive electrical stimulation of a peripheral motor

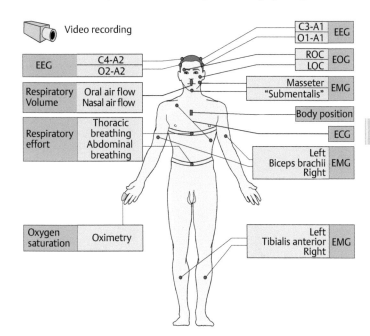

Fig. 4.25   Recording scheme for polysomnography.

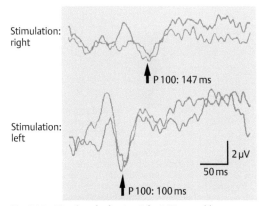

Fig. 4.26   Visual evoked potentials. A 38-year-old woman with multiple sclerosis and right optic neuritis. The cortical response on the right side is significantly delayed compared with the normal left side.

nerve, the muscle action potential becomes smaller with each stimulus (decrement phenomenon; see **Fig. 15.17**).

Indications. In disorders affecting muscle, EMG can be used to determine whether the underlying pathologic process is located in the muscle itself (a myopathic process), in the nerve innervating it (a neuropathic process), or at the neuromuscular junction. EMG can also be used to grade the severity of muscle denervation and the extent of reinnervation, if any. In combination with ENG (see later), EMG is a very important ancillary test for the evaluation of neuromuscular diseases. The indications for these two methods are listed side by side in **Table 4.4**.

4.3.5 Electroneurography

> **NOTE**
>
> ENG records the action potentials that are generated after the electrical stimulation of a nerve and measures the conduction velocity of the most rapidly conducting nerve fibers. Slowed conduction, low-amplitude action potentials, or conduction blocks are evidence of a mono- or polyneuropathy. ENG helps localize such disturbances and determine their etiology.

Principle. ENG is a method of measuring the **motor and sensory conduction velocities** of a peripheral nerve. The result of measurement is always the conduction velocity of the most rapidly conducting fibers. The technique involves the placement of stimulating and recording electrodes at some distance from each other along the course of the nerve. The measured conduction velocity is then the time elapsed between the stimulus and the beginning of the response, divided by the distance between the electrodes. Normal values in the upper limbs are 50 to 70 m/s and in the lower limbs 40 to 60 m/s. The amplitude and duration of the response depend on the number of functioning axons and the degree of dispersion of their conduction velocities. The case presented in **Fig. 4.31** (localized compression of the common peroneal nerve at the head of the fibula) illustrates the clinical utility of ENG.

4

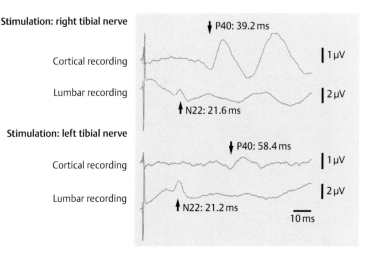

Stimulation: right tibial nerve

Cortical recording

Lumbar recording

Stimulation: left tibial nerve

Cortical recording

Lumbar recording

Fig. 4.27 Somatosensory evoked potentials of the tibial nerve in a 44-year-old woman with multiple sclerosis. There is a normal lumbar N22 potential on both sides. The cortical P40 potential appears at a normal latency of 39.2 milliseconds on the right, but is significantly delayed on the left, with a latency of 58.4 milliseconds, and also abnormally small. These findings indicate impaired conduction in the spinothalamic pathways.

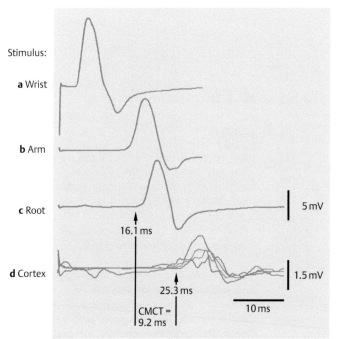

Stimulus:

a Wrist

b Arm

c Root

d Cortex

Fig. 4.28 Motor evoked potentials in a 61-year-old man with cervical syringomyelia. Recording of motor potentials from the abductor digiti minimi muscle after electrical stimulation of the ulnar nerve at the wrist, the forearm, and the C8 root (tracings **a–c**). After cortical stimulation (**d**), the recorded motor evoked potential is reduced in amplitude and somewhat delayed. The calculated central motor conduction time (CMCT) of 9.2 milliseconds is prolonged in comparison to the normal value of 8.7 milliseconds. These findings suggest impaired conduction in the pyramidal tract in the cervical spinal cord.

F wave

When a peripheral motor nerve is stimulated, impulses travel not only orthodromically (in the normal direction of transmission, i.e., distally, toward the muscle), but also antidromically (toward the spinal cord). The antidromic impulse reaches the ganglion cells of the anterior horn and is then reflected back to the periphery; this echo is the F wave. Thus, *two* orthodromic impulse waves travel down the peripheral nerve—the original one, produced by the stimulus, and the F wave. The F wave is later and of lower amplitude. Sometimes it is not seen at all. If the F wave is delayed longer than usual, this may indicate slowed conduction in the plexus or nerve roots.

4.3.6 Other Electrophysiologic Studies

Other types of electrophysiologic study are used less commonly in neurologic diagnosis. We will only briefly mention a few of them here. **Oculography** is a study of the electrical potentials accompanying eye movements. It can be used for objective documentation of gaze saccades and pathologic eye movements. When oculography is used to study vestibular disturbances, it is called **electronystagmography**. **Retinography** is mainly used to determine whether the lesion causing a visual disturbance is in the retina or the optic nerve.

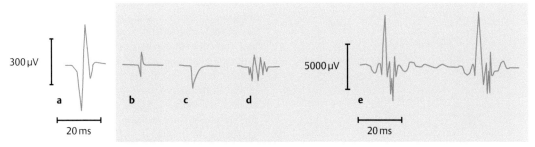

Fig. 4.29 Different types of potentials in an electromyogram. a Normal motor unit potential. **b** Fibrillation potentials in denervation. **c** Positive sharp waves in denervation. **d** Fragmented polyphasic low-amplitude potential, as seen in reinnervation. **e** Abnormally prolonged and high-amplitude motor unit potential ("giant potential") in chronic anterior horn cell disease.

| Table 4.4 |

Indications for EMG and ENG

Condition/suspected pathology	EMG (needle myography)	ENG (electro-neurography)	Remarks
Suspected anterior horn cell disease	+ +	+	ENG reveals normal conduction velocities and sometimes low amplitude of the summed muscle potential
Suspected nerve root lesion	+	+ + (F wave)	Imaging studies may be more important
Suspected plexus lesion (differentiation from peripheral nerve lesion)	+	+ + (F wave)	
Focal peripheral nerve lesion	+ +	+ +	Severity of injury, evidence of regeneration, localization of injury
Polyneuropathy	+	+ +	
Myopathy	+ +	Normal	
Ischemic muscle damage	+ +		
Myasthenia gravis	+ +		Repetitive stimulation, jitter phenomenon

Abbreviations: EMG, electromyography; ENG, electroneurography.
Note: + + = indicated test; + = may be additionally useful.

4.4 Ultrasonography (Neurosonography)

 Key Point

Neurovascular ultrasound studies (Doppler and duplex sonography) are used for the noninvasive diagnostic evaluation of the vessels that bring blood to the brain. They reveal stenoses and occlusions of the extracranial arteries due to arteriosclerosis and other causes, as well as stenoses, occlusions, or spasm of the intracranial arteries. They can also reveal collateral vessels and fistulae.

Principle. The 19th-century Austrian physicist Christian Doppler discovered that the frequency of a wave changes when its source and receiver are in relative motion. Thus, when ultrasound pulses are directed at erythrocytes in flowing blood, the ultrasound waves reflected back from the erythrocytes are altered in frequency to a degree that depends on the flow velocity. In fact, the Doppler shift is directly proportional to the flow velocity.

Technique. The ultrasound probe contains both a transmitter and a receiver of ultrasonic waves. The angle of insonation should be as steep as possible to minimize angle-dependent variations in the measured values, so that the results will be consistent from study to study. There are two types of Doppler system: **continuous-wave (CW)** systems detect all moving wave reflectors within the cone of insonation, while **pulsed-wave** systems detect only those at a particular depth, which can be chosen by the examiner. In CW Doppler studies, the signals of different vessels may overlie one another.

The Doppler signal is visually displayed as a frequency spectrum that varies over time (**Fig. 4.32b–d**). It is also transduced into an audio signal. Ultrasound waves are reflected to varying extents depending on the acoustic resistance of tissue; thus, the profile of reflected echo intensities can be used to construct a two-dimensional sectional image of

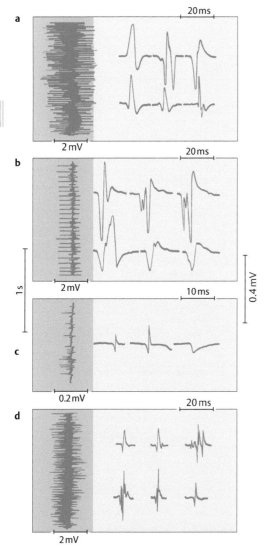

Fig. 4.30 Various EMG findings. a Normal electromyogram with full interference pattern. **b** Individual oscillations in the reinnervation stage after a peripheral nerve injury. **c** Total denervation. Fibrillation potentials and positive sharp waves are seen. **d** Myopathy. Despite muscle weakness, there is a complete interference pattern. The individual potentials making up the interference pattern are of low amplitude; some of them are polyphasic and fragmented.

the insonated tissue. The so-called B image ("brightness mode") or **echotomogram** is a grayscale representation of tissue echo density. The combination of Doppler flow measurement with B imaging is called **duplex ultrasonography**. The velocity of blood flow can be color-coded and displayed as an overlay on the B image; this is called **color duplex ultrasonography** (**Fig. 4.32a**, **Fig. 4.33**, and **Fig. 4.34**).

Indications. The velocity and flow profile (laminar vs. turbulent) of the blood flowing within a particular vessel depend, among other things, on the

vessel's caliber and the nature of its wall. Ultrasound studies can detect vascular stenosis and occlusion, vessel wall irregularities, abnormalities of the speed and direction of blood flow, and turbulent flow. Insonation of the extra- and intracranial vessels (e.g., of the middle cerebral artery through the thin bone of the "temporal window," or of the basilar artery through the foramen magnum) yields an informative picture of the state of blood flow in the brain. This diagnostic technique is inexpensive, noninvasive, and entirely safe.

4.5 Other Ancillary Studies

 Key Point
CSF studies, histopathologic studies of biopsy specimens, and the precise localization of visual field defects are further types of ancillary test that yield important diagnostic information in a variety of neurologic diseases.

4.5.1 Cerebrospinal Fluid Studies

| **NOTE** |

Infectious and inflammatory diseases of the nervous system call forth reactive changes in the CSF. CSF studies are mainly used to detect or rule out the presence of infection and inflammation in the central nervous system, the nerve roots, and the meninges.

Technique. CSF is usually obtained by **LP** below the level of the conus medullaris, most often at L4–L5 (occasionally at L3–L4 or L5–S1). Suboccipital puncture is fraught with a much higher rate of complications and is performed only when meningitis is suspected and no fluid can be obtained by LP ("dry tap"), or when LP is contraindicated because of a known purulent process in the lumbar region. LP is performed with sterile technique on a patient in the lateral decubitus position (or, occasionally, sitting up). The recommended positioning is shown in **Fig. 4.35**; the proper level for puncture is generally located on the line between the iliac crests. The physician performing the puncture measures the CSF pressure with a manometer and visually assesses the color of the fluid. The laboratory tests to be performed include cell count, glucose and protein content, and others (especially cultures) depending on the clinical situation. The most important CSF tests are listed in **Table 4.5**. **Normal CSF values** are listed in **Table 4.6** together with the corresponding serum values.

Indications. LP is an aid to the diagnosis of all diseases affecting the meninges, brain, spinal cord, and nerve roots that can alter the biochemical or cellular

Motor neurography of the common peroneal nerve

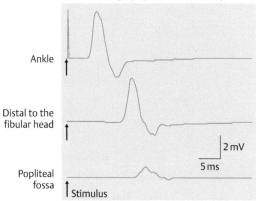

Ankle

Distal to the
fibular head

2 mV

5 ms

Popliteal
fossa

Stimulus

Fig. 4.31 Electroneurography of the right common peroneal nerve in pressure palsy at the fibular head. The farther the stimulating electrode is from the recording electrode (in the peroneal muscles), the longer the latency until the summed muscle potential appears. When the stimulus is delivered in the popliteal fossa, the amplitude of the summed potential collapses. This implies that conduction in all axons is blocked at a site that must lie between the popliteal fossa and the stimulation site distal to the fibular head. This finding is typical of pressure palsy.

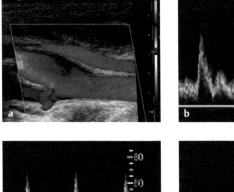

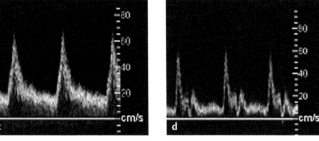

Fig. 4.32 Doppler study of a normal carotid bifurcation. a Two-dimensional sectional image (blue) of the carotid bifurcation. Right side, common carotid artery; left side, internal carotid artery above external carotid artery. The origin of the superior thyroid artery (red) is just distal to that of the external carotid artery. **b–d Doppler frequency-time spectra** in the common carotid **(b)**, internal carotid **(c)**, and external carotid arteries **(d)**. The end-diastolic velocity is higher in the internal than in the external carotid artery because of the lower resistance of the cerebral vasculature.

properties of the CSF. The most important abnormal CSF findings are listed in **Table 4.7**.

The **Reiber diagram** is a tool for comparing the immunoglobulin content of CSF and serum. The CSF/serum quotient of the immunoglobulin concentration is plotted on the y-axis and that of albumin concentration on the x-axis. A data point lying above the normal range indicates intrathecal immunoglobulin synthesis and is thus evidence of inflammation or infection within the central nervous system. On the other hand, a data point to the right of the normal range indicates elevated permeability of the blood–brain barrier and is thus evidence of inflammation or infection outside the central nervous system.

Contraindications. Intracranial hypertension is the most important contraindication to LP. Before any LP is performed, the patient's optic discs should be inspected with an ophthalmoscope to rule out papilledema. **An LP should never be performed if the platelet count is below 5,000/μL.** It should only rarely be performed, for strict indications and with utmost caution, in anticoagulated patients or when the platelet count is below 20,000/μL.

Complications. Complications of LP are rare overall. If the patient harbors an intracranial mass causing elevated intracranial pressure, CSF removal may be followed by herniation of parts of the brain into the tentorial notch or the foramen magnum, potentially resulting in death. If an intraspinal mass is present, preexisting paraparesis may worsen after LP. Persistent leakage of CSF out of the subarachnoid space through the puncture hole(s) in the dura mater may cause symptomatic **intracranial hypotension** with orthostatic headache (see Section 14.2.4). Other very rare complications include iatrogenic infection and spinal epidural hematoma, potentially causing cauda equina syndrome.

4

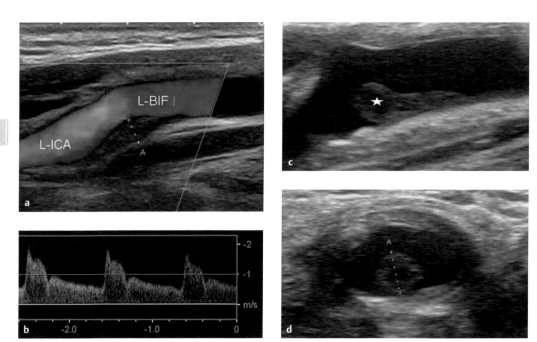

Fig. 4.33   Color-coded duplex sonography of carotid stenosis. a Color duplex sonography of a soft plaque at the carotid bifurcation (L-ICA = left internal carotid artery, L-BIF = carotid bifurcation). **b** The Doppler frequency-time spectrum reveals mildly elevated flow velocities, indicating mild stenosis. **c** Sagittal B image of a thrombus (asterisk) in a carotid bifurcation. **d** Axial image of the carotid bifurcation with the thrombus

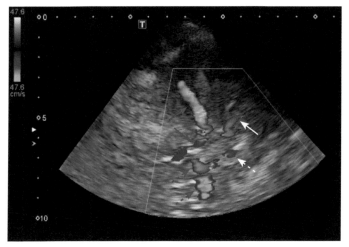

Fig. 4.34   Transcranial color duplex sonography of the basal intracranial arteries. The probe is over the right temple. Right middle cerebral artery (red arrow), right anterior cerebral artery (blue arrow), and right posterior cerebral artery (white arrow). The dashed arrows indicate the corresponding contralateral arteries.

4.5.2 Tissue Biopsies

| NOTE |

Tissue biopsy is needed to diagnose diseases of the brain, nerves, and muscles if no noninvasive or minimally invasive test can definitively establish the diagnosis. Biopsy findings often determine the further course of treatment.

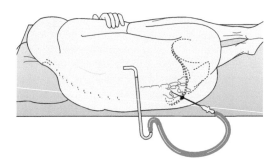

Fig. 4.35   Patient positioning for lumbar puncture.

Table 4.5

Clinically relevant CSF studies

Parameter	
Routinely performed tests	— Pressure
	— Color (turbidity, xanthochromia, bloody tinge?)
	— Cell count and differential
	— Protein
	— Glucose
Tests to be performed under special circumstances	— Immunoglobulins
	— IgG-albumin index
	— Oligoclonal bands
	— Measurement of specific IgG, IgA, and IgM against *Borrelia*, parasites, and viruses
	— Cultures: bacterial, fungal, viral, mycobacterial
	— Gram and Ziehl–Neelsen staining, touch prep
	— VDRL and FTA tests for syphilis
	— Cytologic examination for malignant cells
	— DNA amplification (polymerase chain reaction) in suspected tuberculosis or viral diseases
	— Cystatin C in amyloid angiopathy
	— Antineuronal antibodies in suspected paraneoplastic syndromes
	— Protein 14-3-3 in suspected prion disease

Abbreviations: FTA, fluorescent treponemal antibody; Ig, immunoglobulin; VDLR, Venereal Disease Research Laboratory.

Table 4.6

Normal CSF values and corresponding serum values in adults

	CSF	Serum
Pressure	5–18 cm H_2O	
Volume	100–160 mL	
Osmolarity	292–297 mOsm/L	285–295 mOsm/L
Electrolytes		
— Na	137–145 mmol/L	136–145 mmol/L
— K	2.7–3.9 mmol/L	3.5–5.0 mmol/L
— Ca	1.0–1.5 mmol/L	2.2–2.6 mmol/L
— Cl	116–122 mmol/L	98–106 mmol/L
pH	7.31–7.34	7.38–7.44
Glucose	2.2–3.9 mmol/L	4.2–6.4 mmol/L
— CSF/serum glucose ratio[a]	>0.5–0.6	
Lactate	1–2 mmol/L	0.6–1.7 mmol/L
Total protein	0.2–0.5 g/L	55–80 g/L
— Albumin	56–75%	50–60%
— IgG	0.010–0.014 g/L	8–15 g/L
— IgG index[b]	<0.65	
Leukocytes	<4/µL	
Lymphocytes	60–70%	

Abbreviations: CSF, cerebrospinal fluid; IgG, immunoglobulin G.
[a]Because there is normally an equilibrium between CSF and serum, it is advisable to measure CSF and serum values at the same time.
[b]IgG index = [CSF IgG (mg/L) × serum albumin (g/L)]/[serum IgG (mg/L) × CSF albumin (mg/L)]

Muscle Biopsy

Muscle biopsy is justified in patients with neuromuscular disease when the clinical history, MRI, physical examination, and electromyographic, chemical, and/or genetic studies fail to yield a sufficiently precise diagnosis. It should be performed under local anesthesia in a muscle that is known to be affected by the disease process but is not so atrophic as to lessen the chance of a diagnosis. In many cases, a needle biopsy alone suffices. Depending on the clinical situation, histochemical and/or electron-microscopic study of the tissue specimen may be indicated, in addition to conventional histologic staining.

Table 4.7

CSF analysis: main indications and findings

Condition/suspected pathology	Appearance	Cell count and type	Protein	Pressure	Special remarks
Bacterial meningitis	Turbid	↑↑ Mostly granulo-cytes	↑	Possibly ↑	
Viral meningitis	Usually clear	↑ Mostly lympho-cytes	Possibly ↑	Normal	
Chronic meningitis	Usually clear	Mildly ↑ Mostly lympho-cytes	↑↑	Normal	Low glucose
Encephalitis	Clear	↑ Mostly lympho-cytes	Possibly ↑	Possibly ↑	
Subarachnoid hemorrhage	Bloody–xanthochro-mic	↑ Erythrocytes	Possibly ↑	Possibly ↑	Xanthochromia arises in 6 h to 6 d
Intracerebral hemorrhage	Xanthochromic	Possibly ↑ Erythrocytes	Normal	↑	LP not indicated
Subdural hematoma	Xanthochromic	Usually normal	↑	Normal, ↑, ↓	LP not indicated
Low CSF pressure syndrome	Clear	Normal	↑ to ↑↑	↓↓↓	Aspirate if no spon-taneous CSF flow

Abbreviations: CSF, cerebrospinal fluid; LP, lumbar puncture.

Nerve Biopsy

Nerve biopsy is performed under local anesthesia. A relatively unimportant sensory nerve is chosen for biopsy, usually the sural nerve. The ensuing sensory deficit on the lateral edge of the foot is generally an acceptable price to pay for a firm diagnosis, but the patient must be informed of it before granting his or her consent to the procedure. Part of the specimen is used to make a teased preparation in which nerve fibers and their myelin sheaths can be seen over a certain length of nerve. More importantly, very thin cross-sections of the nerve are prepared that can be microscopically examined for various abnormalities, including disordered myelination and inflammatory changes of the vasa nervorum.

Brain Biopsy

Brain biopsy is performed by a neurosurgeon, usually with stereotactic technique, for very strict indications. Its purpose is the histologic diagnosis of (potentially treatable) structural changes of the brain that have been revealed by imaging studies but whose precise nature remains unclear, for example, a brain tumor or an infectious or inflammatory process.

4.5.3 Perimetry

NOTE

Perimetry is used to detect and quantify visual field defects (Section 12.2.1).

Goldmann Perimetry

Goldmann perimetry is a dynamic method in which moving spots of light of variable size and intensity are presented in the patient's visual field, starting in the periphery and moving toward the center. Typical findings associated with different types of visual field defect are illustrated in **Fig. 12.1**.

Static Computed Perimetry

Static computed perimetry is performed with the Octopus apparatus (Haag-Streit). The brightness of a stationary light source is increased until the patient can see it. The measured brightness thresholds at all tested points in the visual field can be displayed visually as raw numbers, on a grayscale, or as a pseudo-three-dimensional visual field "landscape."

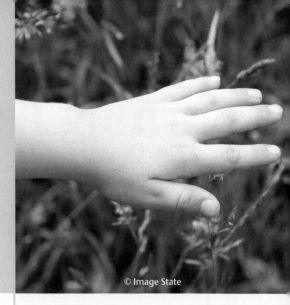
© Image State

Chapter 5

Topical Diagnosis and Differential Diagnosis of Neurologic Syndromes

Burning Feet

The patient, a 52-year-old baker, had received the diagnosis of diabetes mellitus 5 years before his presentation to the neurologist and had been taking insulin for 2 years, with regular blood-sugar checks, under his family physician's supervision. Despite good drug compliance and strict adherence to a low-sugar diet, he had had repeated episodes of hyperglycemia.

He presented complaining of burning pain in the toes of both feet, of 1 year's duration, which had become progressively worse and then nearly intolerable. The neurologist found markedly diminished vibration sense in both feet and absent Achilles reflexes bilaterally. The patient could not spread his toes; when he dorsiflexed them, there was no palpable contraction of the muscles on the dorsum of the foot. The rest of the neurologic examination was normal.

The first step in neurologic diagnosis is always to pinpoint the site of the lesion in the nervous system with the aid of the detailed history and the neurologic examination. The findings generally reveal where the lesion is, as different parts of the nervous system serve different functions, and a loss of function in any particular part calls forth a characteristic collection of neurologic deficits, that is, a characteristic syndrome, as will be discussed in detail in this chapter.

This patient's lesion must be situated in the peripheral nervous system, as can be seen from a combination of findings: the absent Achilles reflexes signify an interruption of the peripheral reflex arc, that is, damage to either its afferent (sensory) or its efferent (motor) component. The marked deficit of vibration sense and the spontaneous dysesthesia are evidence of an impairment of afferent fibers from the feet. The patient's inability to spread his toes indicates weakness of the interosseous muscles of the feet, supplied by the tibial nerve on each side; weakness of the dorsal pedal muscles implies dysfunction of the motor fibers of the fibular nerve. All these findings taken together indicate a more or less symmetric impairment of motor and sensory fibers in multiple peripheral nerves—in particular, the longest nerves of the human body, those supplying the feet. This type of disturbance is called polyneuropathy. The cause here is diabetes mellitus, which impairs nerve function both directly (by hypoglycemia itself) and indirectly by way of diabetic microangiopathy and nerve ischemia. The longest nerve fibers are the most vulnerable ones to this type of disturbance, and thus diabetic polyneuropathy tends to begin in the feet.

The diagnosis of diabetic polyneuropathy motivated an attempt to optimize this patient's glycemic control. To treat the pain, he was initially given lipoic acid for a few weeks, with indifferent results. A switch to carbamazepine led at first to transient and mild side effects, and thereafter to highly satisfactory, albeit subtotal, pain relief.

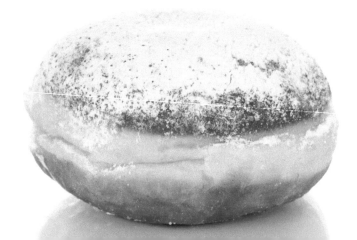

5.1 Fundamentals

Key Point

The clinical manifestations of neurologic disease are determined above all by the site of the lesion. Thus, the first step in neurologic diagnosis is always the *localization* of the disease process in the nervous system. This can usually be done very precisely on the basis of the patient's symptoms and the findings of the neurologic examination. The *etiology* is sought in a second (or parallel) step with the aid of further information: the course of the disease over time, any accompanying nonneurologic manifestations, and ancillary test results.

In this chapter, we will show how the clinical manifestations of neurologic disease can be used to make inferences about the site of the lesion and its possible etiologies. We will first describe the typical findings of lesions affecting individual functional systems (the motor and somatosensory systems) and then those of lesions in particular areas of the brain. The manifestations of diseases affecting the spinal cord and peripheral nerves will be discussed later on in the relevant chapters.

5.2 Muscle Weakness and Other Motor Disturbances

Key Point

Weakness can result from a disturbance at the level of the first motor neuron (cerebral cortex and pyramidal tract) or of the second motor neuron (anterior horn cells of the spinal cord, anterior root, peripheral nerve), or else from impaired conduction at the neuromuscular junction or from a disease of muscle. Disturbances of extrapyramidal structures cause complex movement disorders and abnormalities of muscle tone.

5.2.1 Anatomic Substrate of Motor Function

It is a useful simplification to consider the motor system as consisting of the first and second motor neurons, the neuromuscular junction, and the musculature (**Fig. 5.1**).

First (Central) Motor Neuron. The first motor neuron is located in the precentral gyrus. The axons travel in the corticobulbar and corticospinal tracts through the internal capsule and cerebral peduncle and terminate either in the cranial nerve nuclei of the pons and medulla (corticobulbar tract) or on the anterior horn cells of the spinal cord (pyramidal tract). Lesions of the first motor neuron in the precentral gyrus, or at any other site, produce the following deficits:

— **Spastic weakness** (elevated muscle tone, diminished raw strength, and impaired fine motor control).
— **Increased intrinsic muscle reflexes, spreading of reflex zones, and pathologic reflexes** (Babinski, Oppenheim, and Gordon reflexes, pathologically brisk Hoffmann sign, and Trömner reflex, inextinguishable or asymmetrically persistent clonus).
— Diminished or absent extrinsic muscle reflexes (e.g., abdominal skin reflex).
— No muscle atrophy (though there may be mild atrophy of disuse in the later course of disease).
— Reflex asymmetry if the lesion is unilateral.

Second (Peripheral) Motor Neuron. The second motor neuron originates in one of the motor relay stations mentioned earlier (the motor cranial nerve nuclei or the anterior horn cells of the spinal cord). It consists of a cell body (ganglion cell) and an axon that travels by way of a spinal nerve root, plexus, and peripheral nerve to the skeletal muscle. Each ganglion cell, together with its axon and the muscle fibers that it innervates (there may be many or only a few), comprises a single motor unit. The following deficits are associated with a **lesion of the second motor neuron:**

— **Flaccid weakness** (diminished muscle tone and raw strength).
— **Diminished** or **absent intrinsic muscle reflexes**.
— **Muscle atrophy** becoming evident about 3 weeks after injury and progressing thereafter.

Motor End Plate and Muscle. Normal motor function requires effective impulse transmission from the peripheral nerve to the muscle fiber, followed by fiber contraction. A lesion or functional disturbance of either or both of these elements causes **flaccid weakness**, usually accompanied by **atrophy** and **diminished reflexes** (see **Table 15.1**).

Coordination of Anatomic Structures. Because every movement, as we have seen, is the product of a complex interaction of many different anatomic structures, motor processes are subject to a wide range of pathologic disturbances.

— Typical findings of lesions of individual components of the motor system are listed in **Table 5.1**.
— Some typical constellations of motor deficits, the likely site(s) of the lesion producing each, and some of the possible etiologies are listed in **Table 5.2**. This table reflects the classic threefold paradigm of clinical inference, from the findings to the site of the lesion to the diagnosis.

5.2.2 Motor Regulatory Systems

The smooth, precise, and economic execution of a movement requires a properly functioning regulatory system, in addition to the effector components

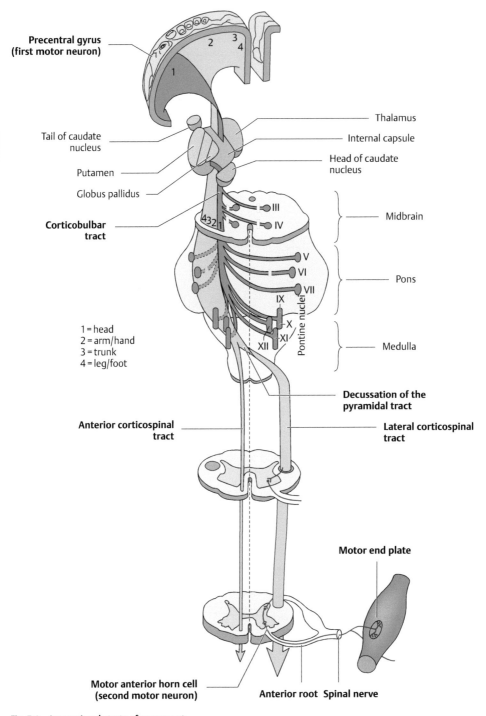

**Precentral gyrus
(first motor neuron)**

2 3
4

1

Thalamus

Internal capsule

Tail of caudate
nucleus

Head of caudate
nucleus

Putamen

Globus pallidus

III

**Corticobulbar
tract**

432 1

IV

Midbrain

V

VI

VII

IX

Pons

X
XI

1 = head
2 = arm/hand
3 = trunk
4 = leg/foot

XII

Pontine nuclei

Medulla

**Decussation of the
pyramidal tract**

**Anterior corticospinal
tract**

**Lateral corticospinal
tract**

Motor end plate

**Motor anterior horn cell
(second motor neuron)**

Anterior root Spinal nerve

Fig. 5.1   Anatomic substrate of movement.

discussed earlier. The regulatory system must do the
following:

− **Integrate proprioceptive input** from the peripheral nerves, posterior columns (fasciculus gracilis and fasciculus cuneatus), thalamus, and

thalamocortical pathways, along with further
input from the vestibular apparatus and the
visual system, and use these "feedback" data to
optimize each phase of the movement at every
moment.

Table 5.1

Aspects of motor function and their localizing significance

Criterion	Motor neuron in anterior horn	Spinal nerve root or peripheral nerve	Central motor pathway (corticobulbar and corticospinal)	Extrapyramidal system	Cerebellum
Raw strength	↓	↓	↓	Normal	Normal
Tone	↓	↓	↑	Possibly rigid, possibly ↑	↓
Muscle atrophy	+ +	+ +	Ø (except for possible atrophy of disuse)	Ø	Ø
Intrinsic muscle reflexes	↓ or absent	↓ or absent	↑	Normal	Normal
Extrinsic muscle reflexes	↓ or absent	↓ or absent	↓	Normal	↓
Pyramidal tract signs	Ø	Ø	+	Ø	Ø
Coordination	↓	↓	↓	Normal or ↓	↓ ↓
Distribution of weakness	No rule	Corresponding to the affected root or nerve	Hemi-, para-, or quadriparesis, depending on site of lesion	No weakness	No weakness
Fasciculations	+ +	Rare	Ø	Ø	Ø

- Plan the force and amplitude of the movement (extrapyramidal system and cerebellum).
- Coordinate the activity of all of the muscles taking part in the movement and, in particular, ensure the effective complementary functioning of agonist and antagonist muscles (extrapyramidal system, cerebellum, and spinal cord).

Loss of function of one or more components of this regulatory system impairs the execution and coordination of movement. Such disturbances typically manifest themselves as **ataxia, hypokinesia,** and **involuntary movements.**

Ataxia

Ataxia is an impairment of the smooth performance of goal-directed movement, with **repeated deviation from the ideal line of a movement**. The different types of ataxia have specific clinical features, depending on the nature and location of the underlying lesion.

Cerebellar Ataxia. This form of ataxia is characterized by irregularity of the entire course of a movement. A lesion in a **cerebellar hemisphere** produces ataxia in the ipsilateral limbs, while a **vermian** lesion mainly produces truncal ataxia (ataxia of stance and/or gait; see **Fig. 3.2**). On the other hand, involvement of the **dentate nucleus** or **its efferent fibers** causes intention tremor: in targeted movements, such as pointing movements, the deviation from the ideal line of approach increases as the limb nears the target (see **Fig. 3.22**).

Central sensory ataxia. This form of ataxia reflects impaired position sense due to lesions of the somatosensory cortex, the **thalamus,** or the **thalamo-cortical pathways** to the parietal lobe.

Posterior column ataxia (spinal ataxia). Spinal ataxia is produced by lesions of the afferent somatosensory pathways in the dorsal portion of the spinal cord (**fasciculus gracilis** and **fasciculus cuneatus**—also known as the columns of Goll and Burdach). It is most apparent when the patient walks; it is regularly accompanied by impaired proprioception and position sense. Patients can compensate for posterior column ataxia to some extent with visual cues; the ataxia is thus appreciably worse in the dark, or when the patient's eyes are closed, than in a well-lit room with the patient's eyes open.

Practical Tip

The distinguishing characteristic of spinal, as opposed to cerebellar, ataxia is that it is mainly evident when visual input is removed.

Peripheral sensory ataxia. This form of ataxia is caused by **diseases affecting the peripheral sensory nerves,** for example, polyneuropathy, and is associated with loss of reflexes and impaired epicritic sensation.

Other types of ataxia. Frontal lobe lesions sometimes cause contralateral ataxia; **motor weakness** can also impair motor coordination, causing ataxia. **Psychogenic ataxia** is typified by its irregularity and by the lack of constant, objectifiable neurologic deficits. Patients with psychogenic ataxia do not fall.

Table 5.2

Patterns of distribution of weakness and their localizing significance

Pattern of distribution of weakness	Type of paralysis	Anatomic substrate	Causative illnesses; remarks
Focal, isolated, usually asymmetric weakness of individual muscles or muscle groups	Flaccid	Peripheral nerve lesion	When a purely motor nerve is involved, usually high-grade paresis of the muscle(s) that it innervates; when a mixed nerve is involved, there are additional sensory and/or autonomic deficits
	Flaccid	Nerve root lesion	Paresis and reflex deficits (if any) in the segmentally innervated muscle(s), usually accompanied by a sensory deficit in the dermatome of the affected nerve root
	Flaccid	Loss of anterior horn ganglion cells	Initial stage of spinal muscular atrophy; fasciculations are usually seen in the muscles innervated by the lost anterior horn cells
	Flaccid	Muscle ischemia	Compartment syndromes, e.g., tibialis anterior syndrome; sensation intact, muscle shortened (contracture)
Symmetric, mainly proximal weakness	Flaccid	Myopathy	Initial stage of limb girdle muscular dystrophies; also seen in polymyositis
	Flaccid	Loss of anterior horn ganglion cells	Initial stage of certain types of spinal muscular atrophy
Symmetric, mainly distal weakness	Flaccid	Myopathy	Initial stage of certain types of muscular dystrophy or myotonia, e.g., Steinert myotonic dystrophy (in such cases usually beginning distally, and involving mainly extensor muscles)
	Flaccid	Lesion of distal portion of multiple peripheral nerves	Polyneuropathy; often accompanied by paresthesiae and sensory deficits
Hemiparesis			
Hemiparesis including the face	Spastic	Lesion of the contralateral motor cortex or corticobulbar and corticospinal pathways as they pass through the corona radiata and internal capsule, down to the level of the cerebral peduncle	Ischemic stroke, intracerebral hemorrhage, tumor, trauma, infection, or inflammation; the weakness is usually mainly distal (the ends of the limbs, especially the hands, have a larger cortical representation) and accompanied by impairment of fine motor control and sensation
Hemiparesis sparing the face (no weakness of the muscles of facial expression)	Spastic	Lesion of the contralateral caudal portion of the brainstem	Focal lesion, usually microinfarct (contralateral hemiparesis usually accompanied by sensory deficits and caudal cranial nerve deficits, see below)
	Spastic	Hemisection of the spinal cord at a high cervical level, on the side of the paretic limbs	For example, trauma or compression by a tumor; may be accompanied by ipsilateral hypesthesia and contralateral (dissociated) deficit of pain and temperature sensation below the level of the lesion, as well as segmentally delimited flaccid paresis at the level of the lesion (because of anterior horn cell involvement)
Special form: crossed unilateral weakness (face on one side, body on other side)	Spastic	Brainstem lesion (medulla, pons, or midbrain)	Combination of ipsilateral cranial nerve deficit and contralateral hemiparesis; if a motor cranial nerve nucleus is involved, there may be flaccid weakness in the muscles it innervates

Table 5.2

Patterns of distribution of weakness and their localizing significance *(continued)*

Pattern of distribution of weakness	Type of paralysis	Anatomic substrate	Causative illnesses; remarks
Quadriparesis/ global weakness	Spastic	Lesion of the cerebral cortex of both hemispheres	For example, hypoxic brain injury after cardiorespiratory arrest
	Spastic	Lesion of the deep cerebral white matter of both hemispheres	For example, multiple sclerosis
	Spastic	(Partial) transverse lesion of the brainstem interrupting all corticospinal projections	For example, locked-in syndrome
	Spastic	High cervical spinal cord transection	For example, trauma or compression by tumor; accompanied by sensory deficit in all modalities below the level of the lesion (sensory level) and segmentally delimited flaccid weakness at the level of the lesion
	Mixed spastic/flaccid	Loss of central motor neurons and anterior horn ganglion cells	Amyotrophic lateral sclerosis
	Flaccid	Loss of anterior horn ganglion cells at many different spinal cord levels	Acute anterior poliomyelitis, advanced stage of spinal muscular atrophy
	Flaccid	Lesion of multiple nerve roots at multiple segmental levels	For example, advanced stage of Guillain–Barré syndrome (acute or chronic recurrent)
	Flaccid	Impaired neuromuscular transmission	Generalized form of myasthenia gravis; Lambert–Eaton myasthenic syndrome
	Flaccid	Myopathy	Advanced stage of various types of muscular dystrophy, generalized form of myasthenia; myositis
	Usually no objective evidence of weakness	Disease of an internal organ	For example, thyroid dysfunction
		Psychogenic	Depression
Paraparesis	Spastic	Bilateral parasagittal lesion (cortical representation of the lower limbs in the precentral gyri)	Often in falx meningioma; sometimes accompanied by sensory deficits in the lower limbs due to simultaneous involvement of the postcentral gyri; there may also be neuropsychological abnormalities and urinary dysfunction
	Spastic	Thoracic spinal cord transection	For example, trauma or compression by tumor; sensory level, possible segmentally delimited weakness at the level of the lesion
	Spastic	Disease process affecting the corticospinal tracts bilaterally	Spastic spinal paralysis; purely motor deficit (no sensory deficit)
	Flaccid	Acute lesion of multiple lumbar nerve roots	Initial stage of Guillain–Barré syndrome (often with ascending weakness); cauda equina syndrome due to massive lumbar intervertebral disc herniation
	Flaccid	Lesion of multiple peripheral nerves of the lower limbs	Polyneuropathy; usually in combination with sensory deficits and reflex deficits (e.g., Achilles reflex)
	Flaccid	Myopathy	For example, initial stage of myotonic dystrophy

Hypokinesia

Hypokinesia is defined as **generalized slowing** of all types of movement.

It is typically found in (hypokinetic) **Parkinson disease** (section 6.9). Spontaneous movements are sparse or absent, automatic accessory movements cease (e.g., arm movements during walking), and all voluntary movements are slowed. The muscles are rigid, and the cogwheel phenomenon (see section 3.4.3 and **Fig. 3.24c**) is usually present. Hypokinesia is also found in **depression** as a sign of generally diminished drive; in such cases, it is not accompanied by any other neurologic deficit.

Involuntary Movements

Involuntary movements come in many varieties, of which the main ones are listed in **Table 5.3**. The phenomenology and localizing significance of each type of involuntary movement are described.

5.3 Sensory Disturbances

Key Point

Sensory disturbances of peripheral origin are due to lesions of the peripheral nerves or nerve roots, while those of central origin are due to lesions of the spinal cord, brainstem, thalamus, thalamocortical projection to the parietal lobe, or parietal cortex. The nature of the sensory disturbance and its extent and distribution on the skin often enable the physician to infer the site of the lesion. Because different sensory modalities are subserved by different afferent pathways in the spinal cord, a lesion in the spinal cord can also cause a dissociated sensory disturbance.

5.3.1 Anatomic Substrate of Sensation

It is another useful simplification to consider the somatosensory system as consisting of the following components (**Fig. 5.2**, **Table 5.4**).

Table 5.3

Involuntary movements and movement disorders

Designation	Manifestations	Localization; remarks
Spontaneous muscle activity not producing movement		
– **Fibrillations**	Phasic contractions of individual muscle fibers, not visible to the naked eye, only demonstrable by EMG	Due to contractions of individual muscle fibers; pathologic at rest or as prolonged insertional activity in the EMG (section 4.3.4)
– **Fasciculations**	Brief, irregular contractions of individual groups of muscle fibers, visible to the naked eye	Due to contractions of individual motor units; in the presence of muscle weakness and atrophy, fasciculations indicate an anterior horn lesion; in the absence of weakness and atrophy, fasciculations (e.g., of the calves) may be benign
– **Myokymia**	Visible waves of contraction passing across many different fiber bundles in a muscle or group of muscles	Unknown
Hyperkinetic phenomena		
– **Myorhythmia**	Rhythmic twitching in a muscle group (always the same one) producing movement; frequency usually 1 to 3 Hz	Central nervous system
– **Myoclonus**	Nonrhythmic, rapid, large-amplitude, sometimes very intense twitching of one or more muscles, producing visible movement	Cerebral cortex, cerebellum; seen physiologically in persons who are falling asleep (hypnagogic myoclonus)
– **Tremor**	Rhythmic oscillation at a frequency that remains roughly constant for the affected individual, of more or less constant localization; may be observed at rest (rest tremor) or with action (action tremor; e.g., postural tremor, kinetic tremor, intention tremor)	Central nervous system (mainly cerebellum, extrapyramidal system)
– **Chorea**	Brief and relatively rapid, shooting muscle contractions, mainly distal, nonrhythmic, irregular, of varying localization, sometimes putting the joints into extreme positions for a brief period of time	Basal ganglia/striatum
– **Athetosis**	Like chorea, but slower, writhing movements with longer-lasting hyperflexion or hyperextension of the joints	Basal ganglia

Table 5.3

Involuntary movements and movement disorders *(continued)*

Designation	Manifestations	Localization; remarks
— **Ballism**	Brief, shooting muscle contractions, mainly proximal and therefore causing pronounced movement (flinging movements of the limbs, jactation)	Subthalamic nucleus
— **Dystonia**	Involuntary, longer-lasting muscle contraction that slowly overcomes the resistance of the antagonist muscles, usually leading to rotatory movements and bizarre postures of individual parts of the body (trunk, limbs, head)	Basal ganglia
— **Tics and tic-like movements**	Irregular muscle contraction limited to certain parts of the body; rapid, but not lightning-like	Psychogenic or tic disorder (e.g., Gilles de la Tourette syndrome)
Other		
— **Spasms**	Muscle contractions of variable frequency and intensity, occurring at irregular intervals, occasionally painful; two examples are hemifacial spasm (**Fig. 12.24**) and blepharospasm	Facial nerve lesion, extrapyramidal dystonic movement disorder; very rarely psychogenic
— **Cramps**	Long-lasting, tonic contractions of individual muscles or muscle groups, fixed	Of muscular origin

5.3.2 The Peripheral Part of the Somatosensory System

The peripheral part of the somatosensory system contains **sensory (afferent) nerves** and **receptors** that are specialized for the perception of the individual modalities of somatic sensation.

Sensory receptors in the periphery. These receptors are classified into three principal types:

- **Exteroceptive receptors** (exteroceptors) transduce physical stimuli from the external environment (e.g., mechanoreceptors, thermoreceptors).
- **Proprioceptive receptors** (proprioceptors) inform the nervous system about head and body posture, the positions of the joints, and tension in muscles and tendons (muscle spindles and Golgi tendon organs).
- **Nociceptors,** which subserve pain, occupy an intermediate position between the extero- and proprioceptors.

The density of somatosensory receptors is greatest in the skin, but they are also found in most other tissues of the body, including the viscera (but not the brain or spinal cord).

In small-fiber neuropathies, the peripheral receptors and their nerve fibers are dysfunctional. This manifests itself clinically as an impairment of pain and temperature sensation (see section 11.3.1, Small-Fiber Neuropathy).

Afferent sensory nerve fibers. Afferent sensory nerve fibers run in the **peripheral nerves, plexuses,** and **posterior spinal nerve roots**. These are the axons of the first somatosensory neurons, whose cell bodies lie outside the spinal cord in the dorsal root ganglia.

All other sensory neurons have their cell bodies within the central nervous system.

5.3.3 The Central Part of the Somatosensory System

The central part of the somatosensory system comprises all of the somatosensory pathways and nuclei of the **spinal cord, brainstem,** and **cerebral hemispheres**. These can be classified, according to their function, as follows.

Posterior column system. The centripetal processes of the pseudo-unipolar spinal ganglion cells (first sensory neuron) that subserve **epicritic sensation** carry information both from **exteroceptors** (tactile sense, stereognosis, and vibration) and from **proprioceptors** (position sense). They travel via the posterior columns to terminate in the nucleus gracilis and nucleus cuneatus of the medulla, without any intervening relay in the spinal cord. These two medullary nuclei contain the second sensory neurons, whose axons, in turn, form the medial lemniscus, which travels onward to the thalamus.

Lesions affecting the posterior column system impair all of the "high-resolution" somatosensory modalities:

- **Astereognosia** (inability to recognize objects by touch) and **impaired two-point discrimination**.
- **Impaired vibration sense** (pallhypesthesia or pallanesthesia).
- **Impaired position sense and kinesthesia**.
- **Spinal ataxia** (unsteady stance and gait, see section 5.2.2) due to the lack of proprioceptive feedback concerning the posture and movements of the head, trunk, and limbs.

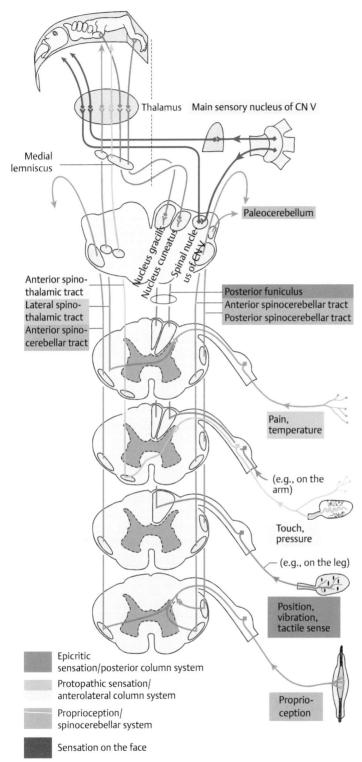

Fig. 5.2 Anatomic substrate of somatic sensation.

Anterolateral column system. The centripetal processes of the first sensory neuron that subserve **protopathic sensation** (pain, temperature sensation, coarse touch, and pressure) form synapses onto second sensory neurons in the posterior horn of the spinal cord. The axons of these cells cross the midline in

Table 5.4

The somatosensory system

Structures	Components
Peripheral portion	
Receptors	— Exteroceptors (mechano- and thermo-receptors) — Proprioceptors (body posture, joint position, tension in muscles and tendons) — Nociceptors
Nerve fibers	— Peripheral nerves — Plexuses — Posterior roots
Central portion	
Spinal cord	— Posterior columns — Anterolateral columns — Spinocerebellar tracts
Brainstem	— Posterior column fibers terminate in synaptic relay stations in the medulla (nucleus gracilis, nucleus cuneatus); the efferent fibers of these nuclei ascend in the brainstem as the medial lemniscus and terminate in the thalamus — The spinothalamic tracts ascend the spinal cord in the anterolateral columns and terminate in the thalamus — The spinocerebellar tracts terminate in the cerebellum
Cerebral hemispheres	— Thalamus — Thalamocortical tracts — Somatosensory cortex

the anterior spinal commissure and then ascend in the spinal cord and through the brainstem to terminate in the thalamus. Fibers subserving pain and temperature sensation travel in the **lateral spinothalamic tract**, and those subserving coarse touch and pressure travel in the **anterior spinothalamic tract**.

Lesions affecting the lateral spinothalamic tract in the spinal cord or brainstem, or the corresponding thalamic nuclei, produce a **dissociated sensory deficit**: pain and temperature sensation are impaired below the level of the lesion, while touch remains intact. The deficit is contralateral to the lesion, because the lateral spinothalamic tract is crossed.

Thalamocortical system. The axons of the second neurons of both the posterior column system and the anterolateral column system terminate in the thalamic nuclei that contain the third neurons of the somatosensory system. These neurons, in turn, send their axons by way of the posterior limb of the internal capsule to the primary somatosensory cortex (postcentral gyrus) and the neighboring association areas. The third neurons thus belong to the so-called thalamocortical system.

Lesions of the third sensory neuron produce a contralateral hemisensory deficit, which usually affects all of the somatosensory modalities, though sometimes to varying extents.

Spinocerebellar system. The spinocerebellar system conveys information regarding **tension and stretch of muscles and tendons** from the muscle spindles and Golgi tendon organs to the paleocerebellum. The main spinal pathways used by this system are the **posterior spinocerebellar tract** (which exclusively carries information from the ipsilateral half of the body) and the **anterior spinocerebellar tract** (which carries information from both sides of the body). The paleocerebellum, in turn, is the origin of multiple efferent pathways, which influence muscle tone to ensure the smooth cooperative functioning of agonist and antagonist muscle groups in standing and walking. The paleocerebellum thus plays an important role in the regulation of balance, though its activity is wholly unconscious.

Lesions of the spinocerebellar pathways and paleocerebellum cause ataxia of stance and gait (see earlier).

Overview.

— **Table 5.5** contains an overview of the typical constellations of somatosensory deficits and their pathoanatomic basis. For the sake of clarity, we have not mentioned any specific diagnoses in this table.

Some of the typical clinical findings are illustrated in **Fig. 5.3**.

5.4 Disturbances of Consciousness

 Key Point

Intact consciousness requires the normal functioning of the cortex of both cerebral hemispheres. The "driving force" of cortical activity, however, is located in a lower center—a group of neurons in the brainstem called the reticular formation, which sends impulses toward the cerebral cortex by way of the intralaminar thalamic nuclei. The reticular formation and its ascending projections are collectively termed the ascending reticular activating system (ARAS). Disturbances of consciousness can be due either to dysfunction of the ARAS or to the simultaneous dysfunction of both cerebral hemispheres.

5.4.1 Somnolence, Stupor, and Coma: Severity and Causes

Depending on their severity, impairments of consciousness are termed **somnolence, stupor, or coma** (see **Table 3.10**). Coma, the most severe impairment of consciousness, can be more finely graded with a widely used semiquantitative scheme called the **Glasgow Coma Scale (GCS)** (see **Table 6.5**).

Table 5.5

Patterns of distribution of somatosensory deficits

Pattern of distribution of deficit	Sensory qualities affected	Anatomic substrate; remarks
Asymmetric		
— Sharply delimited, unilateral, focal	All	Lesion of the **peripheral (sensory) nerve trunks**; maximal sensory deficit in the autonomous zone of the affected nerve; hypesthesia generally more pronounced than hypalgesia; concomitant impairment of sweating in the area of the deficit (cf. **Fig. 5.3a**)
— Less sharply delimited, unilateral, segmental	All	Lesion of the spinal nerve roots; hypalgesia more pronounced than hypesthesia in monoradicular lesions (cf. **Fig. 5.3b**)
Bilaterally symmetric		
— **Gradually increasing from proximal to distal** (stocking-and-glove distribution)	Diminished vibration and position sense at first; the remaining sensory qualities may be lost as the deficit progresses	**Polyneuropathy**; sometimes also seen in polyradiculopathy (cf. **Fig. 5.3c**)
— **Segmental**	Pain and temperature sense	Lesion of the **anterior commissure** of the spinal cord, which contains the decussating fibers of the **lateral spinothalamic tract**; exclusively at a particular segmental level, without damage to ascending pathways
— **Below a given spinal cord level**	All modalities	**Complete spinal cord transection**; regularly accompanied by spastic paraparesis below the level of the lesion and bilateral flaccid paresis at the level of the lesion. The sensory deficits are found below the highest segmental level that is involved by the lesion (the same holds for spinal cord hemisection). Bladder and bowel function are impaired as well
Unilateral		
— **Below a given spinal cord level**	Pain and temperature sense	Lesion of the **contralateral lateral spinothalamic tract**
	Vibration and position sense	Lesion of the **ipsilateral posterior columns**
	All qualities other than pain and temperature on the side of the lesion; pain and temperature contralaterally	Lesion of **one-half of the spinal cord**, regularly producing ipsilateral spastic paresis below the level of the lesion, as well as ipsilateral segmental flaccid paresis at the level of the lesion
— **Including the face**	All	Lesion of the **contralateral thalamus**, or of the **ascending thalamocortical projection** as it passes through the **internal capsule**; contralateral parietal cortex (rare)
	Pain and temperature sense	**Thalamic lesion** on the side opposite the sensory deficit; may be accompanied by spontaneous pain on the affected side of the body, as well as abnormally prolonged pain in response to a stimulus that usually produces only brief pain (= hyperpathia); very rarely due to a cortical lesion
— **Sparing the face**	All	Circumscribed lesion of the **contralateral dorsal internal capsule**, or unilateral high cervical cord lesion (see above)

Consciousness can be impaired either by a structural lesion of brain tissue or else indirectly by a systemic disturbance of some kind (metabolic, toxic, or anoxic coma; see later).

 Practical Tip

If a structural lesion is the cause, there are often accompanying focal neurologic deficits that enable the clinician to infer the site of the lesion. Focal neurologic signs are usually absent in purely metabolic, toxic, or anoxic coma.

When a structural lesion is present, the direct cause of the impairment of consciousness is often not the lesion itself, but rather the **cerebral edema** surrounding it (cf. **Table 5.6**).

Bilateral cortical dysfunction can also be the result of an **epileptic seizure** or an **infectious/inflammatory process** such as meningitis or encephalitis (in which case meningismus is usually present). Finally, there are also purely psychogenic states (**psychogenic stupor**) that can superficially resemble an organic impairment of consciousness.

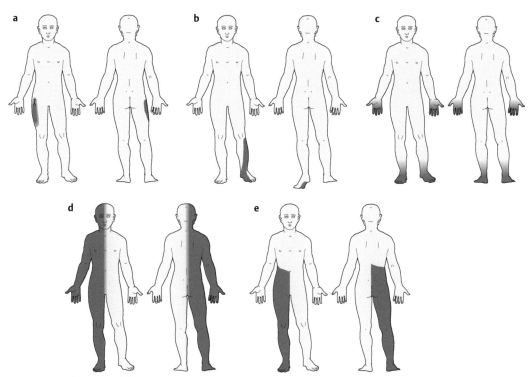

Fig. 5.3   Typical patterns of distribution of somatosensory deficits. (a) Peripheral nerve lesion: meralgia paresthetica due to a lesion of the lateral femoral cutaneous nerve. **(b) Radicular lesion:** typical sensory deficit in L5 radiculopathy. **(c) Polyneuropathy:** distal, stocking-and-glove sensory deficit. **(d) Central lesion:** contralateral hemisensory deficit. **(e) Spinal cord lesion** at the T6 level: hemihypesthesia below the level of the lesion.

Table 5.6

Causes of impaired consciousness

Clinical situation	Possible causes
Impaired consciousness or coma without focal signs or meningismus (purely toxic/metabolic or anoxic coma)	**Metabolic:** various metabolic disorders — Hypo- or hyperglycemia — Uremia — Liver failure — Endocrine dysfunction — Electrolyte disturbances — Metabolic acidosis or alkalosis
	Toxic: intoxications (e.g., alcohol, medications, carbon monoxide)
	Cardiac/anoxic: acute heart failure hypovolemia (anoxic encephalopathy) — Myocardial infarction — Atrial fibrillation — Cardiac tamponade — Hypovolemic shock — Cardiorespiratory arrest, etc. Focal neurologic signs are absent only if cerebral ischemia and hypoxia have not yet caused irreversible structural damage to the CNS
Impaired consciousness or coma without focal signs, with meningismus	**Meningitis**
	Subarachnoid hemorrhage
Impaired consciousness or coma with focal signs (structural lesion)	**Supratentorial lesions** — **Acute:** infarct, trauma, intracranial hemorrhage, subdural/epidural hematoma — **Subacute/chronically progressive:** infections, tumors Impairment of consciousness is often due to edema in the brain tissue around the lesion and the resulting intracranial hypertension and capillary hypoxia, sometimes accompanied by midline shift and herniation, with secondary brainstem damage
	Infratentorial lesions — Acute: infarct, trauma, hemorrhage — Subacute/chronically progressive: infections, tumors
Transient impairment of consciousness, possibly accompanied by involuntary movements	**Generalized epileptic seizure**

The main causes of impaired consciousness are listed in **Table 5.6**. Here we have classified all impairments of consciousness into four basic clinical situations and listed the common etiologies of each.

5.4.2 The Differential Diagnosis of Coma

We will now briefly describe different types of coma and other disturbances of consciousness that must be distinguished from coma.

Coma due to a brainstem lesion. Bilateral brainstem lesions (section 5.5.5), such as those produced by basilar artery thrombosis (described in section 6.5.7), can damage the reticular formation, cranial nerve nuclei, and long tracts on both sides. Comatose patients with such lesions often have asymmetric pupillary responses, impaired corneal reflexes, and absent vestibulo-ocular reflexes, as well as long tract dysfunction that manifests itself as (for example) asymmetric withdrawal of the limbs from painful stimulation.

Apallic syndrome/coma vigile. The apallic syndrome, also called "coma vigile" and "persistent vegetative state," is usually due to severe and extensive brain damage. It is characterized by a complete uncoupling of midbrain and diencephalic activity from cortical activity and thus by a complete dissociation of wakefulness and consciousness. (The term "apallic" signifies "without cortex.") The vegetative functions (breathing, cardiovascular regulation, sleep–wake cycle) are preserved, though possibly abnormal to some extent. Cognitive or goal-directed motor activity is entirely lacking. Unlike the comatose patient, the apallic patient lies in bed with eyes open, staring blankly into the distance, not fixating the gaze on anything, and not responding to verbal or noxious stimuli. At other times, the patient is in a sleeplike state, with eyes closed. Muscle tone is elevated, and automatisms and primitive reflexes are sometimes observed about the mouth. Common types of autonomic dysfunction seen in apallic patients include tachycardia, excessive sweating, and rapid breathing.

Akinetic mutism. This is often due to extensive, bilateral frontal lobe damage or to a lesion affecting the projections of the ARAS to the frontal lobes, for example, a bilateral thalamic or midbrain lesion. Swallowing and the extrinsic muscle reflexes are intact, and the patient's eye movements are usually normal, yet spontaneous verbal or motor activity is absent. The patient nonetheless looks "awake."

NOTE

Locked-in syndrome (described in section 5.5.5) is **not** a disturbance of consciousness, though it can be mistaken for one. The patient is **awake and alert**, but can express him- or herself only through vertical eye

---

movements and eyelid movements, because all four limbs are paralyzed, as well as all of the muscles innervated by the lower cranial nerves. The unwary clinician may gain the false impression of a comatose, unresponsive patient.

5.5 Dysfunction of Specific Areas of the Brain

 Key Point

Up to this point, we have described the characteristic neurologic deficits produced by lesions of individual functional components of the nervous system. Usually, however, more than one functional component is affected. There is often simultaneous impairment of motor function, coordination, sensation, and possibly consciousness. The individual clinical signs and symptoms described earlier often appear together in particular constellations (syndromes) that are characteristically associated with the site of the lesion and are largely independent of its nature.

We will now describe the major syndromes of individual regions of the brain.

5.5.1 Syndromes of the Individual Lobes of the Cerebral Hemispheres

Frontal Lobe Syndrome

Frontal lobe syndrome is characterized by the following manifestations, in variable severity, depending on the extent and precise location of the causative lesion:

— **Abnormalities of personality and behavior**: loss of drive and initiative, apathy, indifference; if only the orbitofrontal cortex is affected, there may be disinhibition, absentmindedness, and socially inappropriate behavior.

— **Primitive reflexes**, for example, grasp reflex and brisk palmomental reflex.

— **Motor phenomena**, for example, spontaneous, compulsive grasping of objects, copying of other people's gestures (echopraxia), and motor perseveration. The last-named phenomenon can be demonstrated with the clapping test: the examiner claps three times and asks the patient to do the same; the patient then claps four or more times. There may also be a contralateral gaze paresis.

— **Lateralizing deficits**: motor aphasia in lesions of the language-dominant hemisphere, anosognosia (nonrecognition of one's own manifestations of illness, e.g., hemiparesis), and contralateral apraxia (see section 3.9.2, Apraxia) in lesions of the nondominant hemisphere.

- **Akinetic mutism**, usually caused by extensive bilateral lesions (the patient is awake, but does not speak or respond to stimuli).
- In lesions affecting the frontal eye fields: **déviation conjuguée** to the side of the lesion, because voluntary gaze to the opposite side is not possible (cf. **Fig. 12.7**).
- **Irritative signs:** adversive seizures (epileptic seizures in which the head and trunk are involuntarily turned to the side opposite the lesion; the contralateral arm is sometimes raised as well).

Syndromes of Lesions of the Pre- and Postcentral Gyri

Each of these gyri contains a somatotopic cortical representation of the entire body, as described in detail 50 years ago by the neurosurgeon Wilder Penfield (the classic "**Penfield homunculus**" is shown in **Fig. 5.4**). Lesions involving these paracentral gyri thus impair the function of specific parts of the body, with the specific site and extent of bodily dysfunction depending on the site and extent of the brain lesion. This can be most impressively observed in **lesions of the precentral gyrus**:

- There are **focal motor deficits**, for example, monoplegia of a limb; if the lesion is restricted to the precentral gyrus itself, the weakness may be flaccid, but this is rarely the case. Simultaneous dysfunction of the premotor cortex usually causes spastic weakness.
- **Sensory deficits** are less commonly observed in such patients and cannot be clinically distinguished from those caused by thalamic lesions.
- The contralateral **intrinsic muscle reflexes** are generally increased and there are accompanying **pyramidal tract signs**.
- **Irritative phenomena** may appear, for example, in the form of jacksonian epilepsy of focal onset (motor and/or somatosensory) or Kozhevnikov epilepsia partialis continua (section 9.3.1).

Temporal Lobe Syndrome

Temporal lobe syndrome takes different forms, depending on the precise location of the lesion:

- **Impairment of memory** (e.g., in lesions affecting the hippocampus on both sides).
- **Sensory aphasia** (Wernicke aphasia, section 3.9.2) in lesions involving the language-dominant (usually left) hemisphere.

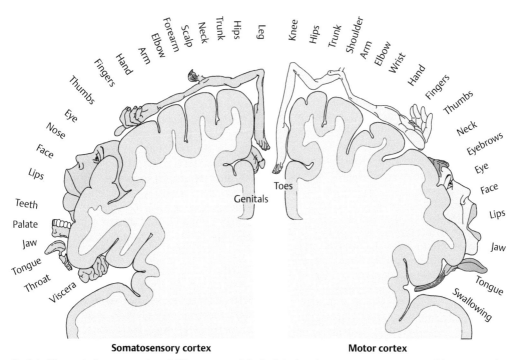

Somatosensory cortex   **Motor cortex**

Fig. 5.4   The cortical representation of different parts of the body in the primary somatosensory cortex of the postcentral gyrus (left) and the primary motor cortex of the precentral gyrus (right) in the human being. (Adapted from Penfield W, Jasper H. Epilepsy and the Functional Anatomy of the Human Brain. Boston, MA: Little Brown; 1954.)

- Possible **disturbance of spatial orientation** in lesions involving the nonlanguage-dominant (usually right) hemisphere.
- In deep-seated lesions, a **visual disturbance** in the form of contralateral homonymous upper quadrantanopsia.
- **Irritative phenomena**: complex partial seizures (temporal lobe seizures, section 9.3.2), sometimes with ictal olfactory or gustatory hallucinations (uncinate fits)—these are usually reported as unpleasant.
- **Mental abnormalities**: irritability, cantankerousness, depression.

Parietal Lobe Syndrome

Parietal lobe syndrome manifests itself in somatosensory deficits and a variety of neuropsychological abnormalities:

- The most prominent sign is usually a **hemisensory deficit**.
- **Sensory neglect** of the contralateral half of the body may arise, manifesting itself as the **extinction** phenomenon: despite intact sensation, double simultaneous stimulation on mirror-image sites on the two sides of the body is only felt on one side.
- Lesions of the language-dominant (usually left) hemisphere can cause left/right confusion, finger agnosia, acalculia (inability to do arithmetic), and agraphia (inability to write letters or words correctly; the combination of these four elements is called **Gerstmann syndrome**), and/or **astereognosia** (inability to recognize objects by touch).
- Lesions of the nondominant (usually right) hemisphere can cause **anosognosia** (inability to perceive one's own condition as pathologic).
- With regard to motor function, there are often poorly coordinated, **ataxic hand and foot movements** on the side opposite the lesion.
- Deep-seated lesions may produce **contralateral homonymous lower quadrantanopsia** or **hemianopsia**, or else only **visual neglect** for the contralateral hemifield.

Occipital Lobe Syndrome

Occipital lobe syndrome is mainly characterized by:

- A contralateral, homonymous visual field defect (usually **homonymous hemianopsia**; cf. **Fig. 12.1**).
- Possible **cortical blindness** (in the case of bilateral occipital lobe lesions), in which elementary or formed visual hallucinations, or seeing gray, may be present; patients often deny being blind (anosognosia).
- **Visual agnosia**, that is, the inability to recognize (for example) colors or shapes, despite normal visual acuity.

- **Irritative phenomena**: visual hallucinations, perhaps as the initial manifestation of an epileptic seizure.

5.5.2 Syndromes of the Extrapyramidal Motor System

Structures and Functions

NOTE

Recent research findings in neurophysiology have made it more difficult to sustain a functional distinction between the **extrapyramidal and pyramidal motor systems**. Rather, the structures making up these two "systems" are best thought of as constituting a **common motor system**. There is no objection to the continued use of the traditional terms "extrapyramidal" and "pyramidal" as long as one keeps this fact in mind.

The main nuclei of the extrapyramidal motor system are the **basal ganglia (caudate nucleus, putamen, and globus pallidus)**. These structures (strictly speaking, these structures in combination with the cerebellum and its brainstem nuclei) are traditionally held to constitute a functional system that ensures the **smooth and purposeful execution of all motor processes**, both voluntary and involuntary. The basal ganglia exert their effects almost exclusively by way of the cerebral cortex. One of their functions is to **efficiently combine individual motor components into complex patterns of movement** and to enable their **automatic execution**. Further ones are to give the signals for the **initiation and termination of movement** and to **regulate muscle tone**.

Further components of the extrapyramidal motor system are the **subthalamic nucleus** (in the diencephalon) and the **substantia nigra** and **red nucleus** (both in the midbrain), along with the **cerebellum and its brainstem nuclei**. Extensive fiber connections link these structures to each other and to higher motor cortical areas (by way of the thalamus). They influence the activity of spinal motor neurons through a multiplicity of afferent and efferent spinal pathways.

Deficits

Lesions of individual components of the extrapyramidal motor system produce **various disturbances of motor function**, depending on their location. Since the functions of the extrapyramidal system are as described earlier, these disturbances generally manifest themselves as an excess or deficiency of movement-initiating impulses, automatic movements, and/or muscle tone:

- There may be diminished spontaneity of movement, that is, **hypokinesia** (e.g., in Parkinson disease), usually combined with elevated muscle tone, that is, **rigidity**; this combination is called a **hypertonic–hyperkinetic syndrome** (cf. section 6.9).
- On the other hand, there may be **hyperkinesia** of a wide variety of types, which may be thought of as the uncontrolled expression of complex motor programs resulting from the removal of their normal inhibition by the extrapyramidal motor system. These involuntary, repetitive movements include chorea, athetosis, ballism, and dystonia, all of which are described in detail in section 6.10. Choreatic syndromes are often associated with **diminished muscle tone** and are thus called **hypotonic–hyperkinetic syndromes**.
- Acute basal ganglionic lesions can also cause transient **hemiparesis**.

5.5.3 Thalamic Syndromes

Structure and Function
The thalamus is the **synaptic relay station** for many **somatosensory and special sensory pathways**; it transmits afferent impulses from peripheral extero- and proprioceptors, as well as from the higher sensory organs (eye, ear), to higher centers. In the thalamus, impulses pertaining to the body's various senses are **integrated, affectively colored**, and then **passed on to the cortex** (conscious perception appears to be possible only if the impulses reach the cortex). The thalamus also receives neural input from the extrapyramidal motor system and participates in the **regulation of attention and drive** as a component of the ARAS (see later). Finally, certain components of the thalamus play a role in **memory**.

Deficits
Because the functions of the thalamus are as described earlier, lesions affecting it can produce the following deficits:
- **Somatosensory deficits**: these mainly consist of impaired proprioception on the side opposite the lesion. There may also be painful, burning sensations that either arise spontaneously (**dysesthesia**) or are induced by, and outlast, a tactile stimulus delivered to the skin (**hyperpathia**).
- **Deficits of movement and coordination**: there may be contralateral hemiparesis (which is usually transient) or hemiataxia.
- **Contralateral hemianopsia** may be present.

- Severe **impairment of memory** arises mainly with bilateral lesions of the thalamic nuclei. There may also be **affective disturbances** (in particular, affect lability).
- **Abnormal posture**, particularly of the hands, may be present. In the "**thalamic hand**," the metacarpophalangeal joints are flexed, while the interphalangeal joints are hyperextended (cf. **Fig. 6.59**).

5.5.4 The Limbic System

Structures and Function
The limbic system comprises a group of subcortical nuclei and neo-, archi-, and paleocortical areas that are linked together both anatomically and functionally (**Fig. 5.5**). Its main components are the parahippocampal gyrus, cingulate gyrus, subcallosal area, indusium griseum, hippocampus, fornix, amygdala, mammillary body, hypothalamus, and anterior thalamic nuclei. The limbic system plays a major role in the following:
- Regulation of the autonomic nervous system and of endocrine function.
- Regulation of emotion and control of drive and affective behavior.
- Learning and memory.

Deficits
- Lesions of the **hippocampus** mainly impair learning and short-term memory. A well-known example is Alzheimer disease, which is pathoanatomically characterized by bilateral mesiotemporal atrophy.
- Lesions of the **hypothalamus** mainly cause hormonal disturbances.
- Lesions of the **right insular region** cause sympathetic functional disturbances, while lesions of the **left insular region** cause parasympathetic functional disturbances.
- **Bilateral limbic lesions**, particularly when they affect the anterior components of the limbic system, can produce blunted emotions, depression, abnormal behavior in everyday life, disinhibition of instinctual drives, sexual promiscuity, and/or addictive behavior.
- **Bilateral temporal lesions** lead, in extreme cases, to Klüver–Bucy syndrome, which is characterized by hyperphagia, hypersexuality, affective indifference, inhibited drive, visual agnosia, and the inability to acquire and store new memories, as well as a tendency to explore objects orally and to ingest them.

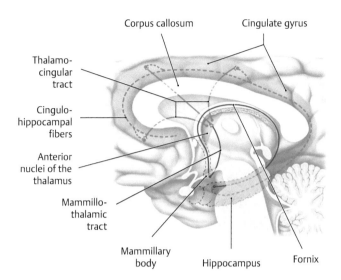

Corpus callosum

Cingulate gyrus

Thalamo-cingular tract

Cingulo-hippocampal fibers

Anterior nuclei of the thalamus

Mammillo-thalamic tract

Mammillary body

Hippocampus

Fornix

Fig. 5.5 The limbic system. The figure shows the so-called "Papez circuit" of neural connections, running from the hippocampus by way of the fornix to the mammillary body, then by way of the mammillothalamic tract to the anterior thalamic nuclei, and onward via the thalamocingular tract to the cingulate gyrus and via the cingulo-hippocampal fibers back to the hippocampus. (Reproduced from Schuenke et al. Thieme Atlas of Anatomy. Head and Neuroanatomy. New York, NY: Thieme Medical Publishers; 2011. Illustration by Markus Voll.)

Limbic encephalitis (section 6.8.8) is a disease process that specifically affects the limbic system.

5.5.5 Brainstem Syndromes

Structure and Function
The brainstem is a **"throughway" for many fiber pathways of the nervous system**, which lie adjacent to one another here in a tightly confined space. All of the motor and somatosensory projections to and from the periphery pass through the brainstem; some of them cross (decussate) here to the other side, and some undergo a synaptic relay. In addition, the brainstem contains **many nuclei**: all of the somatic and visceral motor and sensory nuclei of **cranial nerves III through XII** are contained within it. Two brainstem nuclei, the red nucleus and the substantia nigra, belong to the extrapyramidal motor system. Finally, the nuclei of the reticular formation also include the **vital autonomic regulatory centers** that control cardiovascular and respiratory function, as well as nuclei of the **ARAS** that send activating impulses to the cerebral cortex and are essential for the maintenance of consciousness.

Deficits
As one would expect from the very large number of important neural structures located in the brainstem and the fiber tracts passing through it, a correspondingly wide variety of deficits can be produced by brainstem lesions of different sizes and locations. The pattern of clinical manifestations usually enables the clinician to localize the **level of the lesion** to one of the three brainstem segments (midbrain, pons, or medulla). One can also clinically distinguish **focal**

lesions from partial or complete **cross-sectional lesions** of the brainstem:

Unilateral focal lesions. These are usually of vascular origin (lacunar infarct). The typical clinical picture is the so-called **alternating hemiplegia syndrome**, in which a cranial nerve deficit on the side of the lesion appears together with a motor and/or sensory deficit on the contralateral half of the body. There are different alternating hemiplegia syndromes depending on the level of the lesion; some of these are described further in **Table 6.17**. Focal **diencephalic lesions** can produce diabetes insipidus as well as disturbances of thermoregulation, the sleep–wake cycle, eating behavior, and other instinctual behaviors.

Bilateral partial cross-sectional lesions of the brainstem. The classic example of a disturbance produced by this type of lesion is the **locked-in syndrome**, which is due to an **extensive lesion of the ventral portion of the pons** (e.g., an infarct secondary to thrombosis of the basilar artery). **The corticobulbar and corticospinal pathways of the basis pontis are totally interrupted**, and part of the pontine reticular formation may be as well. All four limbs are paralyzed (quadriplegia), and the caudal cranial nerves are dysfunctional: the patient cannot swallow, speak, or (in most cases) produce facial expressions. Vertical eye movements and lid closure, both of which are midbrain functions, are preserved, but horizontal eye movements, which are a function of the pons, are abolished. Consciousness remains intact, because the reticular formation is largely spared. The patient can communicate only through vertical eye movements and lid closure.

Bulbar palsy and **pseudobulbar palsy** are two further syndromes caused by bilateral partial cross-sectional lesions of the brainstem. Bulbar palsy is due to system atrophy of the motor cranial nerve nuclei of the medulla and therefore manifests itself as bulbar dysarthria, dysphagia, and tongue atrophy, with fasciculations. In pseudo-bulbar palsy, the causative lesion does not involve the cranial nerve nuclei themselves, but rather their innervating corticonuclear pathways bilaterally, or else the cortical areas from which these pathways arise. The clinical picture resembles that of bulbar palsy, but tongue atrophy and fasciculations are absent, because the peripheral motor neuron is intact.

Complete cross-sectional lesions of the brainstem. Brainstem transection can be due to a pathologic process either in the posterior fossa or in the brainstem itself (**infratentorial lesion**), or else to acute **intracranial hypertension in the supratentorial compartment**, with secondary herniation and brainstem compression. Systemic processes (e.g., prolonged hypoxia or cardiorespiratory arrest) can also cause extensive damage to the brainstem, as well as to the cerebral hemispheres. Midbrain lesions cause severe **impairment of consciousness**, ranging to deep coma, and characteristic **motor and oculomotor signs**. The same is true of pontine transecting lesions. The most prominent sign of medullary transection is **loss of all autonomic function**. The level of brainstem injury can almost always be correctly deduced from the pattern of clinical deficits and the findings of a few special tests (particularly of the brainstem reflexes), as described in **Table 5.7**. A patient who survives acute, extensive damage to the midbrain will probably be quadriplegic and suffer from akinetic mutism (see earlier).

5.5.6 Cerebellar Syndromes

Structure and Function

The cerebellum carries out its two main tasks in parallel:
- Optimization of the amplitude, speed, and precision of voluntary movement.
- Preservation of equilibrium through the appropriate regulation of supportive movements and muscle tone.

The cerebellum also plays a role in the regulation of gaze-related eye movements and in ensuring the smooth complementary functioning of agonist and antagonist muscle groups.

To carry out these coordinating tasks, the cerebellum needs information from various different parts of the nervous system. Different types of incoming information are processed separately in three parts of the cerebellum that are distinct from one another both functionally and phylogenetically:
- **Impulses from the cerebral cortex** for the initiation and planning of voluntary movement travel via the corticopontocerebellar pathway, by way of the brachium pontis (middle cerebellar peduncle), to the **neocerebellum** (cerebellar hemispheres). This phylogenetically youngest part of the cerebellum is mainly responsible for the fine control of very precise movements, particularly of the limbs (especially the hands and fingers) and the motor apparatus of speech.
- **Impulses carrying information about joint position and muscle tone** from peripheral proprioceptors (muscle spindles and Golgi tendon organs) travel centrally, by way of the anterior and posterior spinocerebellar tracts and through the restiform body and brachium conjunctivum (inferior

| Table 5.7 |

Findings in deep brainstem lesions

Site of lesion or functional disturbance	Pupils: appearance and reactivity to light	Corneal reflexes	Vertical VOR (see section 12.3.2)	Horizontal VOR	Respiration
Cerebral hemispheres (bilateral)	Equal, reactive	Bilaterally present	Present	Present (elicitable in both directions)	Cheyne–Stokes respiration, continuous hyperventilation
Midbrain	Unilaterally or bilaterally fixed and dilated	Present	Absent	Present	May be irregular, with pauses
Pons	Small, equal, fixed	Unilaterally or bilaterally absent	May be absent	Absent	May be irregular, with pauses
Medulla	Equal, reactive	Present	May be absent	May be absent	Irregular, apneustic
Extensive brainstem lesion	Unilaterally or bilaterally fixed and dilated	Unilaterally or bilaterally absent	Absent	Absent	Irregular, apneustic

Abbreviation: VOR, vestibulo-ocular reflex.

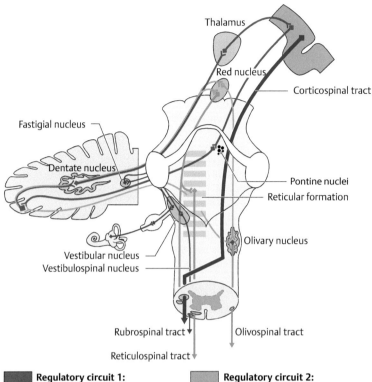

Thalamus

Red nucleus

Corticospinal tract

Fastigial nucleus

Dentate nucleus

Pontine nuclei

Reticular formation

Olivary nucleus

Vestibular nucleus
Vestibulospinal nucleus

Rubrospinal tract   Olivospinal tract

Reticulospinal tract

Regulatory circuit 1:
cortex–pontine nuclei–
cerebellar cortex–dentate
nucleus–thalamus–cortex

Regulatory circuit 2:
red nucleus–olivary nucleus–
cerebellar cortex–dentate
nucleus–red nucleus

Efferent pathways to spinal cord

Fig. 5.6   Anatomic connections of the cerebellum. The connections to the cerebral cortex, brainstem, vestibular system, and spinal cord are illustrated.

and superior cerebellar peduncles), to the **paleo-cerebellum** (located in part of the vermis and the paraflocculus). This part of the cerebellum is mainly responsible for the smooth, synergistic functioning of the muscles of stance and gait.
- **Impulses from the vestibular system** travel via the restiform body (inferior cerebellar peduncle) to the **archicerebellum** (nodulus and flocculus). This phylogenetically oldest part of the cerebellum mainly serves to keep the upright body in balance when the individual stands or walks.

The cerebellum integrates the various types of afferent impulses it receives and then influences the motor regulatory functions of the brain and spinal cord in the manner of a **feedback system**. Efferent impulses travel from the cerebellar cortex to the dentate nucleus, where further processing takes place, and then through the superior cerebellar peduncle to the lateral nucleus of the thalamus, and onward to the **cerebral cortex** (**Fig. 5.6**). Other efferent impulses travel from the dentate nucleus via the red nucleus to the thalamus, or via the red nucleus to the olive, and then back to the cerebellum. These

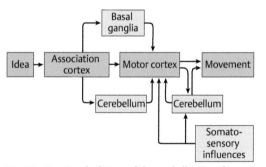

Fig. 5.7   Functional relations of the cerebellum to other motor centers. To keep the diagram simple, the sensory feedback to the cerebellum and basal ganglia is not shown. (Adapted from Allen GI, Tsukahara N. Cerebrocerebellar communication systems. Physiol Rev 1974;54(4):957–1006.

two neuronal loops give off descending fibers to the rubrospinal and reticulospinal tracts, which terminate in the **motor nuclei of the spinal cord** (**Fig. 5.6**). The integration of the cerebellum in the complex functional system controlling voluntary movement is shown in **Fig. 5.7**.

Deficits

In accordance with the functions of the cerebellum described earlier, cerebellar lesions produce **disturbances of muscle tone and movement**:

- Lesions of the cerebellar hemispheres (mainly affecting the neocerebellum) produce **impaired coordination of (fine) movements of the limbs on the side of the lesion.**
- Lesions of rostral midline portions of the cerebellum (mainly affecting the paleocerebellum) produce **impaired coordination of stance and gait.**
- Lesions of basal midline portions of the cerebellum (mainly affecting the archicerebellum) produce **disturbances of truncal posture and the maintenance of balance**, which are particularly evident when the patient tries to sit.

A detailed list of the clinical manifestations of cerebellar disease is provided in **Table 5.8**.

Table 5.8

Clinical manifestations of cerebellar disease

Clinical manifestation	Definition/description	Remarks
Diminished muscle tone	Can be felt by the examiner during repeated passive movement, e.g., pronation and supination of the forearm	
Dyssynergia	Lack of coordination of the various muscle groups participating in a single movement	For example, when walking on all fours, lack of precise alternation of limbs (each arm with opposite leg)
Dysmetria	Poor control of the force, speed, and amplitude of voluntary movement	For example, opening fingers too wide when trying to grasp a small object
Intention tremor	Alternating, progressively severe deviation from the ideal course of a directed movement as the limb approaches the target	See **Fig. 3.22**
Pathologic rebound phenomenon	When a muscle is actively contracted against resistance and the resistance is suddenly released, the antagonist muscles fail to contract within a normally brief interval after the release	See **Fig. 3.23**
Dysdiadochokinesia	The alternating contraction of agonists and antagonists cannot be performed as rapidly and smoothly as normal	See **Fig. 3.18**
Sinking of a limb in postural testing	The tonic muscle contraction needed to keep the limb in a particular antigravity posture cannot be maintained for a normal length of time on the affected side	The sinking limb is ipsilateral to the cerebellar lesion; cf. **Fig. 3.18**
Truncal ataxia	Evident when the patient tries to sit	Indicates a vermian lesion
Unsteady stance	Observable in the Romberg test	See **Fig. 3.1e**
Cerebellar gait	Wide-based, unsteady, ataxic gait	Indicates involvement of the vermis
Past-pointing in the Bárány pointing test	Slowly lowering the extended arm onto a previously demonstrated target, with eyes closed; deviation to the side of the affected cerebellar hemisphere	Also positive in ipsilateral vestibular lesions (see section 3.3.2, Cranial Nerve VIII: Vestibulocochlear Nerve)
Nystagmus	Coarse nystagmus toward the side of the lesion, increasing with gaze toward the side of the lesion, decreasing on eye closure	See **Table 12.1**
Pathologic nystagmus suppression test	The patient stands up, extends his or her arms forward, stares at his or her own extended thumbs, and keeps on doing so while the examiner rapidly rotates the patient around the bodily axis; staring at the thumbs completely suppresses the induced vestibular nystagmus in normal persons, but not in persons with cerebellar disease	See **Fig. 12.6**
Cerebellar dysarthria	Choppy, explosive speech ("scanning dysarthria")	Patients with degenerative cerebellar diseases are said to develop a "lion's voice"

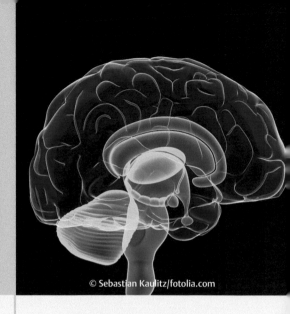

© Sebastian Kaulitz/fotolia.com

Chapter 6

Diseases of the Brain and Meninges

Suddenly Speechless

A 59-year-old manager of an information technology firm, previously in good health, suddenly felt unwell late one afternoon at work, with a warm feeling in his head that was hard to describe. He slowly cleared his desk and drove home. On arrival, he could not carry on a conversation with his wife: he understood her easily but found no words to answer her. He went to bed and slept for 2 hours, but still could not speak properly on awakening. He went to the emergency room of the nearest hospital. The neurologic examination there, 4 hours after the onset of symptoms, revealed aphasia with word-finding difficulty and paraphasic errors, as well as a mild right central facial palsy. His blood pressure was 165/95 mm Hg.

The mainly motor aphasia and the right facial palsy implied a left frontal disturbance, and the acute onset was consistent with cerebral ischemia or hemorrhage as the most likely cause. To pin down the diagnosis, a computed tomography (CT) scan was performed immediately after the examination. It showed hypodensity in the left insular cortex, most likely representing an ischemic stroke. Occlusion of a major cerebral vessel was ruled out by duplex ultrasonography. As the patient had not presented to the emergency room until 4 hours after the onset of symptoms, and the clinical and neuroradiologic workup had taken an additional 35 minutes, the temporal window for intravenous thrombolysis was already over. A magnetic resonance imaging (MRI) scan confirmed the diagnosis of a territorial ischemic stroke: the lesion was hyperintense on both the diffusion-weighted image and the T2-weighted spin-echo image. Given that occlusion of a major cerebral vessel had been ruled out, endovascular recanalization was not indicated. The need remained to find the cause of the stroke to protect the patient from further such events.

His family physician had measured mildly elevated blood pressure values at various times in the past, and he had been mildly overweight for several years, with a high cholesterol level. He had also complained of bothersome palpitations on multiple occasions over the past few months. A 24-hour electrocardiogram (ECG) showed intermittent atrial fibrillation; echocardiography revealed no other cardiac abnormality.

The most likely cause of the stroke was atrial fibrillation leading to clot formation in the left atrium and then embolism of a blood clot into the brain (cardioembolic stroke). Oral anticoagulation was begun to prevent further clot formation in the left atrium. This measure lowers the risk of a second stroke by two-thirds. An antihypertensive drug and a statin were also prescribed, and the patient was encouraged to lose weight by means of a healthier diet and regular physical exercise. His aphasia improved markedly during his hospital stay; only mild word-finding difficulty remained when he was discharged.

6.1 Congenital and Perinatally Acquired Diseases of the Brain

Key Point

The main types of brain disease that are congenitally present or acquired at the time of birth are the following: cerebral movement disorders of perinatal origin (infantile cerebral palsy), developmental disorders of the neural tube (dysrhaphias), childhood hydrocephalus, heterotopias (islands of gray matter in the brain at abnormal locations outside the cerebral cortex), combined disease of the brain and skin (phakomatoses), malformations of the skull, and infections that are acquired in utero.

6.1.1 Fundamentals

Table 6.1 contains an overview of the major types of brain damage that are present at birth, or acquired in early childhood, and their causes. The most common ones are:

— Genetic disorders.
— Disorders acquired during intrauterine life: infections (rubella embryopathy, toxoplasmosis, cytomegalovirus [CMV], syphilis, human immunodeficiency virus [HIV]) and chronic intoxications (alcohol embryopathy).

Table 6.1

Important causes of congenital and perinatally acquired brain damage

Cause	Examples
Perinatal asphyxia	
Structural anomalies of the brain	— Microcephaly — Meningoencephalocele (cf. **Fig. 6.3a**) — Meningomyelocele — Micropolygyria — Arnold–Chiari malformation (cf. **Fig. 6.3b**) — Dandy–Walker syndrome with or without hydrocephalus
Phakomatoses	— Tuberous sclerosis (Bourneville disease) — Encephalofacial angiomatosis (Sturge–Weber disease) — Neurofibromatosis, type 1 (von Recklinghausen disease) and type 2 — von Hippel–Lindau disease — Ataxia telangiectasia (Louis–Bar syndrome)
Brain damage acquired in utero	— Rubella embryopathy — Congenital toxoplasmosis — Congenital cytomegaly — Congenital syphilis — Congenital HIV infection — Alcohol embryopathy
Rh incompatibility	— Severe neonatal jaundice
Synostosis and craniostenosis (see **Fig. 6.6**)	
Traumatic intracranial hemorrhage during delivery	— Subdural hematoma — Intracerebral hemorrhage — Intraventricular hemorrhage

— Complications of delivery (cerebral hypoxia during birth, birth trauma).

Prematurity and difficult delivery are the most important risk factors.

6.1.2 Cerebral Movement Disorders

Multiple mechanisms of injury to the developing brain (cf. **Table 6.1**) can cause movement disorders of varying degrees of severity; these are known collectively as **cerebral movement disorders** or **infantile cerebral palsy**.

Clinical features. The manifestations of cerebral movement disorder include:

— **Disturbances of movement** of many different kinds; the more common ones are summarized in **Table 6.2**. These are usually accompanied by a variably severe delay of motor development.
— **Intellectual disability** (sometimes designated "childhood psycho-organic syndrome" or "attention deficit–hyperactivity syndrome") is common and is characterized by the delayed acquisition of mental abilities, impaired attention, and often also hyperactivity and inability to concentrate.
— **Epileptic seizures** often arise later on.

Practical Tip

The term psychomotor retardation refers to a combination of movement disturbances and intellectual disability.

NOTE

Possible signs of brain damage in young children include: at birth—cyanosis, a weak cry, hypotonia; in the early postnatal period—further abnormalities of muscle tone, pathologic reflexes; later on in childhood —strabismus or hip dysplasia.

Treatment. The goal of treatment is maximal independence. Physical therapy (e.g., of the Bobath or Vojta type) should be initiated as early as possible, incorporating the child's reflex behavior as well as special education, rehabilitation, ergotherapy, and speech therapy.

Prognosis. Although the neurologic deficits of cerebral palsy do not progress over time, certain manifestations may not appear until later in life (e.g., epileptic seizures), and certain symptoms may worsen over the course of the individual's life.

6.1.3 Hydrocephalus

Hydrocephalus is a pathologic **dilatation of the inner (and sometimes also the outer) cerebrospinal fluid (CSF) spaces**. Various types of hydrocephalus are listed in **Table 6.3** (see also section 6.12.6).

Table 6.2

The most important cerebral movement disorders

Disorder	Clinical features	Pathoanatomic substrate	Causes
Infantile spastic diplegia (Little disease)	Spasticity, predominantly in the legs; pes equinus, scissor gait, mentally often normal	Pachymicrogyria (abnormally hard, small gyri)	Perinatal injury (disturbance of cerebral development, embryopathy, severe neonatal jaundice)
Congenital cerebral monoparesis	Usually paresis of arm and face	Porencephaly (cavities in the brain parenchyma), localized atrophy	Birth trauma (asphyxia, hemorrhage)
Congenital hemiparesis	Arms more severely affected than legs, seizures in ~50%, usually mentally impaired	Porencephaly	Birth trauma (asphyxia, hemorrhage)
Congenital quadriparesis (bilateral hemiparesis)	Arms more severely affected than legs, occasionally bulbar signs, seizures; severe mental impairment	Porencephaly, bilateral; often hydrocephalus	Birth trauma (asphyxia, hemorrhage), also prenatal injury
Congenital pseudobulbar palsy	Dysphagia to liquids, dysarthria, usually not mentally impaired	Bilateral lesions of the corticobulbar pathways	Prenatal injury or birth trauma, congenital malformation (syringobulbia)
Bilateral athetosis (athétose double) **and congenital chorea (choreoathetosis)**	Athetotic or other involuntary movements, often combined with spastic paresis	Basal ganglionic defects, status marmoratus (multiple confluent gliotic areas in the basal ganglia); status dysmyelinisatus (Vogt) in cases of later onset	Disturbances of cerebral development, perinatal injury, especially severe neonatal jaundice
Congenital rigor	Rigor without involuntary movements, postural abnormalities, no pyramidal tract signs, severe mental impairment, seizures	Status marmoratus	Disturbances of cerebral development, perinatal injury, especially severe neonatal jaundice
Congenital cerebellar ataxia	Gait ataxia, intention tremor and impaired coordination, motor developmental retardation, dysarthria, sometimes in combination with other motor syndromes	Cerebellar developmental anomalies	Disturbances of cerebellar development

Table 6.3

Types and terminology of hydrocephalus

Internal hydrocephalus	Enlargement of the ventricles:
– Obstructive	Due to obstruction of CSF flow within the ventricular system (e.g., aqueductal stenosis) or at its exits (e.g., compression of the fourth ventricle by a mass in the posterior fossa)
– Malresorptive	Due to impaired CSF resorption (e.g., cisternal adhesions or dysfunction of the pacchionian granulations)
External hydrocephalus	Enlargement of the subarachnoid space over the cerebral convexities and/or in the cisterns
External and internal hydrocephalus	Combination of the above
Hydrocephalus ex vacuo	External and internal hydrocephalus due to brain atrophy

Pathogenesis. Hydrocephalus is due to impaired circulation or resorption of CSF (**Fig. 6.1**, **Fig. 6.2**). The most common type of hydrocephalus in childhood is **occlusive hydrocephalus**, reflecting impaired CSF outflow and generally due to one of the following:

– Gliosis, stenosis, or malformation of the cerebral aqueduct.

– Brain tumor (**Fig. 6.2b**).
– Obstruction of the foramina of Luschka and Magendie.
– Arnold–Chiari malformation (**Fig. 6.3b**).

In the **Arnold–Chiari malformation**, part of the medulla and the cerebellar tonsils are displaced below the foramen magnum into the cervical spinal

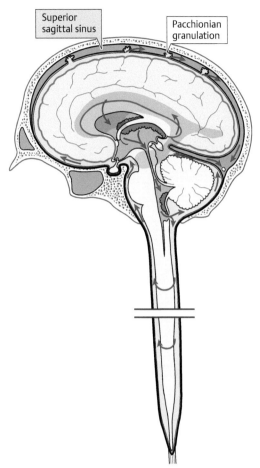

Fig. 6.1   Circulation of the cerebrospinal fluid.

canal. This anomaly may be combined with internal hydrocephalus and syringomyelia.

Malresorptive hydrocephalus is caused by an impairment of CSF resorption in the pacchionian granulations and nerve root sleeves, for example, in the aftermath of meningitis or subarachnoid hemorrhage (**Fig. 6.2c**). This form of hydrocephalus is particularly common in adults (see section 6.12.6).

Clinical features. Children with hydrocephalus have an **abnormally large head**, which may already be noted in a prenatal ultrasound study or at birth, and which progresses over time. Protrusion of the frontal bone and depression of the orbital plate make the upper part of the sclera visible and cause the lower part of the iris to sink below the lower lid, in the so-called "**setting-sun sign.**" Severe hydrocephalus causes psychomotor retardation.

Diagnostic evaluation. The essential diagnostic tests are **CT** and **MRI**.

Treatment. Surgery is necessary to prevent motor and intellectual disability. In most cases, a ventriculoperitoneal **shunt** is implanted.

Prognosis. The prognosis of isolated hydrocephalus, in the absence of other neurologic abnormalities, is good: once the hydrocephalus is treated, two-thirds of children go on to have a normal physical and mental development.

6.1.4 Microcephaly

Microcephaly is usually due to prenatal **toxic influences** (e.g., alcohol), **infections** (e.g., CMV), or **genetic factors**. Affected persons are generally of low intelligence.

6.1.5 Dysraphic Malformations

The most common type is **spina bifida with meningomyelocele**: in this disorder, there is a closure defect of the posterior arches of multiple vertebrae, usually in the lumbosacral region, accompanied by a prolapse of the meninges and spinal cord through the defect. The level and extent of spinal cord involvement determine whether paralysis of the lower limbs will be manifest at birth. Even if the defect is surgically repaired in the first few hours after birth, major sensorimotor impairment and urinary disturbances generally persist. This type of malformation may be accompanied by internal hydrocephalus and by anomalies of the craniocervical junction, which often require treatment. Prenatal intrauterine surgery for this condition is now possible.

Further dysrhaphic syndromes include the following:

— **Acrania** (partial or total absence of the skull).
— **Anencephaly** (absence or degeneration of most of the brain, with acrania—practically always a fatal condition).
— **Encephalocele** (prolapse of the meninges and brain tissue through a defect in the skull; see **Fig. 6.3a**).

6.1.6 Heterotopia

Areas of neuronal heterotopia (i.e., **islands of gray matter anomalously lying outside the cerebral cortex**) arise from a neuronal migration disturbance in early brain development. They may be found in the periventricular zones or in a subcortical layer (lamina) that creates the appearance of a "**double cortex**" on MRI. Heterotopias are genetically heterogeneous and sometimes combined with lissencephaly ("smooth brain," i.e., absence of the cerebral gyri and sulci). Heterotopia is commonly seen in patients with epilepsy and psychomotor retardation.

6.1.7 Ulegyria

Ulegyria is a type of early childhood hypoxic brain damage, anatomically characterized by **scarring** and abnormally small gyri (**microgyria**). These structural abnormalities can be seen on MRI (**Fig. 6.4**).

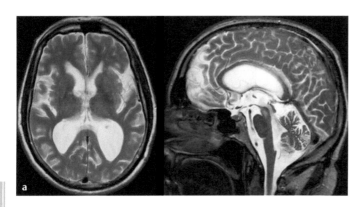

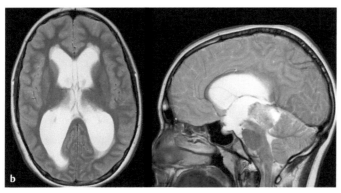

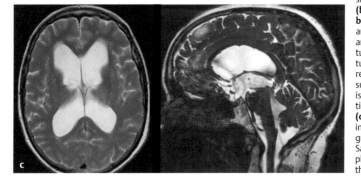

Fig. 6.2   Types of hydrocephalus.
(a) Hydrocephalus ex vacuo in degenerative brain atrophy. Axial image (left): the inner and outer CSF spaces are widened because of atrophy. Sagittal image (right): the suprahypophyseal and supraoptic recesses are acute (sharply pointed), because the third ventricle is not under pressure. The fourth ventricle is also widened. **(b) Occlusive hydrocephalus due to pineoblastoma.** Axial image (left): the ventricles are enlarged, while the external CSF spaces are barely visible. Sagittal image (right): a tumor is seen overlying the midbrain tectum. The suprahypophyseal and supraoptic recesses are wider than normal. Unlike the supratentorial ventricles, the fourth ventricle is of normal width; this implies an obstruction to CSF flow at the level of the aqueduct. **(c) Malresorptive hydrocephalus.** Axial image (left): the ventricles are enlarged to a greater extent than the external CSF spaces. Sagittal image (right): The suprahypophyseal and supraoptic recesses are wider than normal.

6.1.8 Phakomatoses

The phakomatoses are a group of genetic disorders that cause complex malformations and tumors mainly affecting ectodermally derived structures, that is, the **brain, peripheral nervous system, and skin**. They are also called **neurocutaneous disorders**. The internal organs may also be affected. An overview is provided in **Table 6.4**.

6.1.9 Brain Infections Acquired in Utero

The main types of brain infection acquired in utero are the following:

Rubella embryopathy. This syndrome is seen in 10% of infants who have been exposed to maternal rubella infection in the first trimester of pregnancy.

Its manifestations include cataracts, deafness, microcephaly, and heart defects.

Congenital toxoplasmosis. This syndrome is due to infection in the second half of gestation in a mother without previous exposure to *Toxoplasma gondii*. Its manifestations include psychomotor retardation, epileptic seizures, progressive hydrocephalus, and visual disturbances due to chorioretinitis. Imaging studies reveal intracerebral calcifications.

Congenital cytomegalovirus infection. Congenital CMV infection causes premature birth and low birth weight, microcephaly, hydrocephalus, seizures, periventricular calcifications, and abnormalities in organs outside the nervous system as well.

Congenital HIV infection. One-quarter of all fetuses with HIV-positive mothers are infected with HIV;

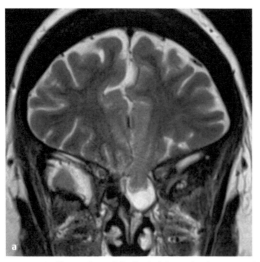
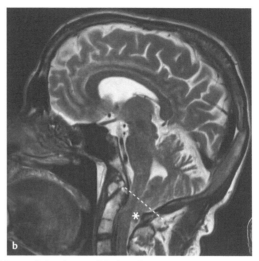

Fig. 6.3 Malformations of the brain (T2-weighted MR images). **(a) Encephalocele.** Part of the brain has prolapsed into an enlarged, CSF-filled ethmoidal cell at the base of the skull. **(b) Arnold–Chiari malformation.** The cerebellar tonsils (*) are displaced below the foramen magnum into the spinal canal. Their tips usually lie at least 5 mm above the level of the foramen magnum.

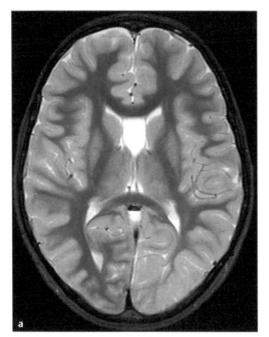
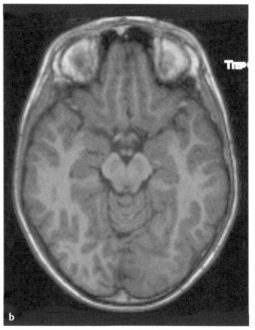

Fig. 6.4 Cortical dysplasia in an 11-year-old boy with occipital lobe epilepsy. The gyri of the left occipital lobe are abnormally thick in comparison to the normal ones in the right occipital lobe. **(a)** Axial T2-weighted spin-echo image. **(b)** Axial T1-weighted gradient-echo image.

cesarean section is recommended, as the virus is transmitted during delivery in two-thirds of all cases. Congenital HIV infection causes encephalopathy with psychomotor retardation, as well as immune deficiency, with its later complications.

Congenital syphilis. This entity is now rare. Its typical stigmata include a saddle nose, cutaneous

fissures at the corners of the mouth, and later crescentic defects of the teeth (Hutchinson's teeth), interstitial keratitis, and hearing loss.

6.1.10 Other Embryopathies

Alcohol embryopathy. Short stature, microcephaly, facial dysmorphism, and psychomotor retardation

| Table 6.4 |

The most important phakomatoses

Disease	Neurologic features	Further features	Remarks
Tuberous sclerosis (Bourneville disease)	Intellectual disability, autism, epileptic seizures, white depigmented cutaneous nevi, adenoma sebaceum	Intracranial calcifications; adenomas in the heart, kidney, and retina	Autosomal dominant inheritance
Encephalofacial angiomatosis (Sturge–Weber disease)	Epileptic seizures, intellectual disability, and sometimes hemiparesis; nevus flammeus on the face	Serpentine intracranial calcifications	Sporadic, no clear inheritance pattern
Encephaloretinal angiomatosis (von Hippel–Lindau disease)	Progressive cerebellar signs in middle age; signs of intracranial hypertension	Retinal angiomatosis; cystic hemangioblastoma of the cerebellum or spinal cord, tumors of other internal organs	Autosomal dominant inheritance
NF1 (von Recklinghausen disease)	Progressive radicular or peripheral nerve deficits (flaccid paresis, sensory deficits), possible spinal cord signs	Cutaneous neurofibroma, café-au-lait spots (**Fig. 6.5**), axillary/inguinal freckles, iris hamartoma (Lisch nodules), sphenoid wing dysplasia, long-bone pseudarthroses	Autosomal dominant inheritance, with frequent de novo mutations; mutation of the neurofibromin gene (a tumor suppressor gene)
NF2	Bilateral acoustic neuroma, meningioma	As in NF1 but less severe	Autosomal dominant inheritance; mutation of the neurofibromin-2 gene (also called the merlin or schwannomin gene), which is a tumor suppressor gene
Ataxia telangiectasia (Louis–Bar syndrome)	Progressive cerebellar ataxia from infancy onward, sometimes also chorea	Telangiectasias develop in later life, especially on the conjunctiva; frequent pulmonary and ear infections, immune deficit, tendency to develop malignant tumors	Autosomal recessive inheritance

Abbreviations: NF1, neurofibromatosis, type 1; NF2, neurofibromatosis, type 2.

are the main clinical features of alcohol embryopathy. This disorder is caused by maternal alcohol abuse during pregnancy.

Drug-induced embryopathy. Various drugs (licit and illicit) can cause congenital anomalies. Drugs of any kind should be avoided during pregnancy, especially in the first trimester. Only those that are considered nonteratogenic should be taken, if absolutely necessary. The tragic historic example of thalidomide (Contergan) illustrates why such a restrictive policy is advisable: this drug, used in Europe in the 1950s to treat nausea in pregnant women, caused severe malformations of the limbs and ears, as well as facial palsy.

6.1.11 Malformations of the Skull and Craniocervical Junction

Malformations of the skull come in various forms:

— Dysraphic malformations due to faulty closure of the cranial vault (**cranioschisis**).
— Premature closure of the cranial sutures (**craniosynostosis**); the most common types are illustrated in **Fig. 6.6**.

— **Anomalies of the craniocervical junction**, including:
• Basilar impression.
• Platybasia.
• Arnold–Chiari syndrome (described in section 6.1.3).
• Dandy–Walker syndrome (malformation of the posterior fossa with aplasia of the inferior portion of the cerebellar vermis, cystic enlargement of the fourth ventricle, and occlusive hydrocephalus).

6.1.12 Mental Disorders

The main types of congenital disorder that manifest themselves clinically during childhood are attention deficit–hyperactivity disorder (ADHD) and autism.

Attention Deficit–Hyperactivity Syndrome

This mental disorder, previously called "minimal cerebral dysfunction," generally arises in childhood. It persists into adulthood in one-third of cases.

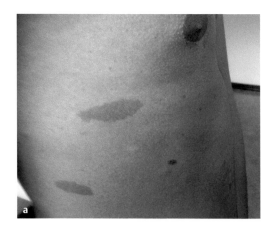

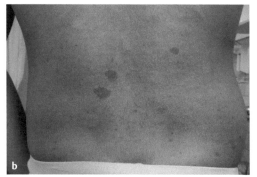

Fig. 6.5 Type I neurofibromatosis (von Recklinghausen-disease). (a) Café-au-lait spots on the chest. **(b)** Café-au-lait spots and a subcutaneous plexiform neurofibroma (seen here as a protrusion on the patient's right flank).

Epidemiology. ADHD affects an estimated 2 to 7% of all children and is considered the most common behavioral disorder among children and adolescents. Boys are more commonly affected than girls.

Etiology and pathogenesis. ADHD is of multifactorial origin; its causes include an inherited predisposition. Psychosocial and environmental factors are also of pathogenetic significance and can have a marked influence on the severity of the disorder.

Clinical features and complications. The main manifestations are impaired attention, impulsivity, and hyperactivity, causing emotional suffering in the affected children and in their family members as well. Interpersonal relationships can be impaired, and the affected children may do poorly in school (or, later, at work) and develop further emotional problems as a result.

Treatment. The affected children and adolescents should be treated with disorder-specific psychotherapy, including behavior therapy, with involvement of their families and their social environment. Supportive pharmacotherapy with methylphenidate (Ritalin) can be given.

Autism

Autism is an **impairment of social interaction and communication**; its severity is variable. Autistic persons generally fail to recognize nonverbal communicative signals and avoid eye contact with interlocutors. Their interests are limited, and their activities often stereotypical. Early-childhood autism (**Kanner syndrome**), generally associated with low intelligence, is considered distinct from adult autism (**Asperger syndrome**), in which intelligence is usually normal. Autistic persons may be highly gifted in special areas (as dramatized in the fictional motion picture *Rain Man*[1]). They suffer more frequently than normal persons from motor incoordination, epilepsy, and other mental disturbances, including anxiety disorders. The etiology of autism is multifactorial and partly genetic.

6.2 Traumatic Brain Injury

 Key Point

Traumatic injuries of the skull and the underlying brain can be of different types and varying severity, depending on the nature and intensity of the causative event. There may be a skull contusion, a skull fracture affecting the cranial vault or the base of the skull, a concussion, brain contusion, an injury to larger-sized blood vessels producing a traumatic hematoma, or any combination of these types of injury.

6.2.1 Overview

In more than half of all cases, traumatic brain injury occurs as a component of **multiple trauma**. The associated injuries commonly affect the face, limbs, spine, chest, abdomen, and pelvis (in descending order of frequency).

The **main clinical manifestation** of a traumatic brain injury is **impaired consciousness**, often associated with a **memory deficit** (retrograde and anterograde amnesia). These problems can be accompanied or followed by **neurologic deficits** and/or **epileptic seizures**.

Brain injuries are either **closed** (i.e., with the dura mater intact) or **open** (with a wound extending into the subdural compartment or deeper into the brain parenchyma). Their **severity** is judged clinically and rated numerically on the Glasgow Coma Scale (GCS). Traumatic hematomas can be located within the brain parenchyma (**traumatic intracerebral hematoma**) or in the **epidural** or **subdural** compartments.

---

1 A film (1988) by Barry Levinson, with Dustin Hoffman playing a gifted but autistic person.

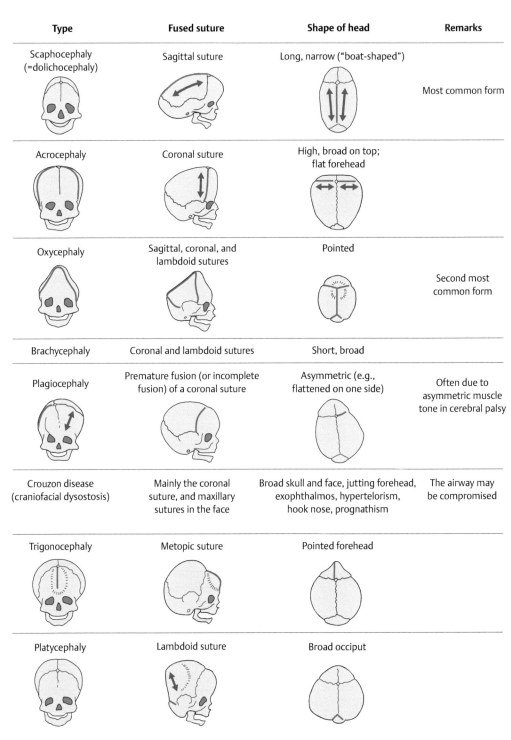

Type	Fused suture	Shape of head	Remarks
Scaphocephaly (=dolichocephaly)	Sagittal suture	Long, narrow ("boat-shaped")	Most common form
Acrocephaly	Coronal suture	High, broad on top; flat forehead	
Oxycephaly	Sagittal, coronal, and lambdoid sutures	Pointed	Second most common form
Brachycephaly	Coronal and lambdoid sutures	Short, broad	
Plagiocephaly	Premature fusion (or incomplete fusion) of a coronal suture	Asymmetric (e.g., flattened on one side)	Often due to asymmetric muscle tone in cerebral palsy
Crouzon disease (craniofacial dysostosis)	Mainly the coronal suture, and maxillary sutures in the face	Broad skull and face, jutting forehead, exophthalmos, hypertelorism, hook nose, prognathism	The airway may be compromised
Trigonocephaly	Metopic suture	Pointed forehead	
Platycephaly	Lambdoid suture	Broad occiput	

Fig. 6.6 Types of craniosynostosis.

Large traumatic hematomas, or extensive damage to the brain parenchyma with accompanying edema, may lead to a rapid rise of **intracranial pressure** (ICP), causing **brain compression** and possibly **brainstem herniation**.

Frequent **late complications** of severe traumatic brain injury include neuropsychological deficits, personality changes, and symptomatic epilepsy.

6.2.2 Clinical History and Neurologic Examination

 Key Point
In the initial phase after trauma, the recognition that a traumatic brain injury is present and its clinical and anatomic assessment (e.g., intracranial hematoma) are vital. The duration and type of the impairment of consciousness are especially important elements of the clinical history. Meticulous history-taking and directed physical examination point the way to proper diagnosis and treatment.

Relevant Aspects of the History
Particular attention must be paid to the following aspects of the history:
- **The duration of unconsciousness** (as reported by eyewitnesses).
- **The duration of amnesia** for events that occurred before the injury (**retrograde amnesia**) and after it (**anterograde amnesia**, perhaps accompanied by confusion).
- **Early epileptic seizures.**
- **Bleeding from the ear or nose** (indicating a basilar skull fracture).

Physical Examination
Important aspects of the initial physical examination in the emergency room are:
- The **vital signs**, especially **pulse and blood pressure** (is the patient in shock?).
- The **level of consciousness**: the depth of impairment of consciousness (up to and including deep coma) is assessed numerically with the **GCS** (**Table 6.5**). This assessment may need to be performed multiple times—in particular, with each change in the patient's circumstances and surroundings (before and after intubation, transport, arrival in the hospital, etc.).
- **Cranial injuries**: inspection and palpation of the skull, orbital rims, zygomatic arches, jaws.
- **Cervical spine injuries** and other accompanying bodily injuries.
- **Bleeding** and possibly **flow of CSF** from the nose or ears, or in the pharynx (a CSF leak is conclusive evidence of an open brain injury, while bleeding is not).
- **Periorbital hematoma**, a sign of basilar skull fracture.

Table 6.5

The Glasgow Coma Scale

Category	Points
Best verbal response:	
None	1
Unintelligible sounds	2
Inappropriate words	3
Disoriented	4
Oriented	5
Eye opening:	
None	1
To painful stimuli	2
To auditory stimuli	3
Spontaneous	4
Best motor response:	
None	1
Abnormal extension	2
Abnormal flexion	3
Withdraws (pulls away from pain)	4
Localizes (fends off painful stimulus)	5
Follows commands	6
Patient's overall score	...

Note: The overall score is the sum of the scores in the three categories.

- **Neurologic deficits** (impaired pupillary reflexes, visual impairment, nystagmus, deafness, weakness, pyramidal tract signs).

6.2.3 Assessment of Severity; Imaging Studies

 Key Point
Mild, moderate, and severe traumatic brain injury are distinguished on the basis of the type and duration of the impairment of consciousness.

Assessment of Severity
The severity of traumatic brain injury is assessed on the basis of the **clinical manifestations** and their classification on the **GCS** (**Table 6.6**).
Mild traumatic brain injury. In mild traumatic brain injury, consciousness is only mildly impaired (GCS score: 13–15) and the impairment lasts no longer than 1 hour. The patient may be confused. There may be amnesia for brief periods of time before and after the injury (retro- and anterograde amnesia).
Moderate traumatic brain injury. The impairment of consciousness is somewhat more severe (GCS score: 9–12) and longer-lasting. The patient may have neurologic deficits, such as weakness or cranial nerve deficits, and/or epileptic seizures.
Severe traumatic brain injury. The GCS score is 8 or lower and the patient is in coma for 1 day or longer.

Table 6.6

Traumatic brain injury: assessment of severity

	Mild	Moderate	Severe
Clinical features	Loss or impairment of consciousness lasting less than 1 hour, EEG changes lasting less than 24 h	Loss or impairment of consciousness lasting 1–24 h	Unconsciousness for more than 24 h, and/or brainstem signs
Score on Glasgow Coma Scale	13–15	9–12	3–8
Possible neurologic findings	Confusion, amnesia (generally encompassing the traumatic event itself, a short period before it, and the period of posttraumatic confusion)	Depending on the site and extent of brain injury: — Focal neurologic deficits — Cranial nerve deficits — Epileptic seizures — Manifestations of intracranial hypertension, up to and including herniation	

Neurologic deficits are generally seen, as well as signs of intracranial hypotension. Without appropriate treatment, transtentorial herniation of the midbrain and diencephalon may ensue (or, less commonly, herniation of the medulla through the foramen magnum).

Alternative classification. An alternative classification of traumatic brain injury, based on pathophysiology rather than clinical severity, consists of the following categories:

— Skull contusion.
— Commotio cerebri (brain concussion).
— Contusio cerebri (brain contusion).
— Compressio cerebri (brain compression).

Imaging Studies

Depending on the clinical situation, the following imaging studies can be performed:

Head CT. A head CT (often as a component of whole-body spiral CT) is generally obtained immediately on arrival of the injured patient in the emergency room for the prompt diagnosis of skull fractures, **intracranial hemorrhage**, brain contusions, cerebral edema, and intracranial air.

Cervical spine CT. Cervical spine CT with multiplanar reconstruction is used to diagnose fractures and dislocations of the cervical spine.

Whole-body spiral CT. A CT scan of the entire body is obtained in multiply and severely injured patients so that all of their injuries can be detected and classified according to the urgency of treatment.

MRI. MRI is more time-consuming than CT and thus plays only a limited role in the acute diagnostic evaluation of head-injured patients. It is a useful means of detecting intracranial hemorrhages and, in particular, diffuse axonal injury in the cerebral white matter, which may be present even in "mild" traumatic brain injury. MRI is preferable to CT for follow-up studies **after the initial, acute phase of traumatic brain injury** has passed.

Plain X-ray. There is no current indication for plain X-rays of the skull in traumatic brain injury. These have been entirely supplanted by CT for the diagnosis of skull fractures. Plain films of the cervical spine and other parts of the skeleton may be useful for various indications and are usually obtained with a whole-body, skeletal and soft-tissue, low-dose X-ray scanner, also called Lodox.

6.2.4　Pathophysiology and Clinical Features

 Key Point
The main pathophysiologic types of traumatic brain injury and their manifestations will be presented in this section. Traumatic hematomas will be discussed separately.

The pathophysiologic effects of brain trauma are divided into **primary and secondary brain injury**, as outlined in **Table 6.7**.

Open versus Closed Head Injuries

A head injury is said to be **open** only if there is an opening in the dura mater through which the intradural space communicates freely with the outside world, generally with leakage of CSF. Such injuries carry a high risk of **early and late infection** (meningitis, cerebritis, brain abscess). If the dura mater is intact, the head injury is **closed**. Thus, a skull fracture directly under a scalp laceration is not necessarily an open injury; it is one only if there is an underlying dural tear.

Skull Contusion

Patients with simple skull contusions have no evidence of a brain injury, that is, no loss of consciousness or amnesia and normal findings on neurologic examination. Some patients with this syndrome have scalp lacerations, or even skull fractures, and they may suffer from headaches afterward. Adequate

Table 6.7

Primary and secondary brain injury after trauma

Primary brain injury (immediate)	Secondary brain injury (delayed)
— **Injury of arteries or veins**, traumatic hematomas (see section 6.2.5) — **Focal brain injury** (e.g., brain contusion) — **Diffuse axonal injury**: shear injury of axons and their supplying blood vessels, leading to, e.g., axonal avulsion and the degeneration of fiber pathways	Mainly caused by **arterial hypotension** and **hypoxemia** as well as **intracranial hypertension**, leading to ischemia in brain tissue and, in turn, to: — Uptake of fluid in both the intra- and the extracellular compartments (cerebral edema) — Damage to cell membranes and DNA — Secretion of inflammatory mediators and invasion by inflammatory cells

therapy consists of a temporary restriction of activity and symptomatic medication, as required (analgesics, antiemetics).

Diffuse Axonal Injury

Even mild head trauma can be associated with **shearing forces** that are strong enough to damage axons in the cerebral white matter and the blood vessels that supply them. Axonal shear injuries in various regions of the brain can lead to the degeneration of neural pathways; their clinical neurologic effects may only be noticed weeks or months after the traumatic event.

Concussion

"**Concussion**" is often used as a near-synonym for mild traumatic brain injury. The concussion syndrome consists of a brief period of unconsciousness or impaired consciousness (generally no more than a few minutes), possibly followed by confusion. The periods of retro- and anterograde amnesia, if any, are only brief. Typical accompanying symptoms include headache, dizziness, nausea, and vomiting. There is **no neurologic deficit**, and it is thus often assumed that there is no underlying structural injury to the brain parenchyma. Nonetheless, T2-weighted MRI and diffusion tensor imaging (see section 4.2.3, Further MR Techniques) reveal evidence of axonal damage in some cases. Detailed neuropsychological testing may reveal subtle deficits even in patient who have "only" sustained a concussion; such deficits have been termed "minimal brain injury." Posttraumatic headache after concussion generally subsides over time.

The clinical distinction between concussion and brain contusion (see later) is not always easy to draw.

The treatment of concussion resembles that of a skull contusion, with transient restriction of activity and symptomatic medication as needed. The patient should not be immobilized any longer than necessary: as long as there is no contraindication (such as hemodynamic instability), the patient should stand up and walk with assistance on the day of injury or in the next few days at latest. Rapidly mobilized patients have less severe postconcussive symptoms with a lesser tendency toward chronification.

Brain Contusion

Brain contusion is, by definition, a direct injury of the brain parenchyma. It is associated with a long period of unconsciousness and retro- and anterograde amnesia; indeed, the patient may not remember anything for a period of several days surrounding the event. Examination in the acute phase often reveals **neurologic deficits**, which may persist. Residual anosmia is common (see section 12.1).

CT or MRI reveals **foci of contusion** (**Fig. 6.7**, **Fig. 6.8**) or intracranial hemorrhage, for example, an **acute epidural hematoma** (**Fig. 6.9**) or an **acute subdural hematoma**. Parenchymal injuries can be found both directly underlying the site of the external blow ("**coup**" injuries) and at the diametrically opposite location in the brain ("**contrecoup**" injuries). Injuries of the latter type are due to the violent, tissue-distorting force transmitted through the brain tissue at the moment of injury. The pathoanatomic findings in foci of brain contusion include ischemic and hemorrhagic **tissue necrosis**, small **hemorrhages**, **tears of brain tissue and blood vessels**, and secondary **brain edema**. Lumbar puncture (LP), if performed (generally contraindicated!), yields bloody or xanthochromic CSF.

MRI scans performed in surviving patients years after a traumatic brain injury with a brain contusion generally reveal a **loss of brain substance** (**Fig. 6.8**). **Neurologic and neuropsychological deficits** are usually demonstrable and may persist for life. These and other sequelae are discussed in section 6.2.7.

Cerebral Edema

Traumatic brain injury causes cerebral edema, whose extent depends on the severity of the injury. Immediately after the traumatic event, water and electrolytes enter the extracellular space (=cytotoxic edema); hours to days later, the blood–brain barrier collapses and vasogenic edema ensues. The result is brain swelling and intracranial hypertension, which, if severe enough, in turn leads to cerebral hypoperfusion and brainstem herniation (see also section 6.3).

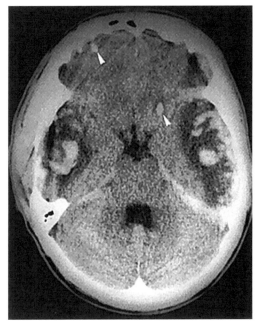

Fig. 6.7　Brain contusion (CT scan). There are extensive hemorrhagic contusions in both temporal lobes and smaller ones in both frontal lobes (arrowheads).

Brain Compression and Herniation

Large brain contusions and extensive traumatic hematomas, combined with the associated secondary brain edema, can cause very rapid and pronounced **increases in ICP**, leading to **brain compression** and **herniation** of the midbrain and diencephalon through the tentorial notch, and/or of the medulla through the foramen magnum. The clinical signs of brainstem herniation are: progressive **impairment of consciousness** leading to coma; a dilated pupil, initially only on the side of the expansive lesion; flexor and, later, extensor spasms; and, finally, impairment of autonomic regulatory functions (breathing, temperature control, cardiac activity, vascular tone), bilaterally fixed and dilated pupils, and death.

> **Practical Tip**
> The clinical severity of traumatic brain injury is correlated with the initially evident extent of structural damage to the skull and brain, but the correlation is not absolute. One patient may have an extensive skull fracture, but no neurologic deficit; another may sustain a relatively minor blow to the head that ruptures a bridging vein and produces a slowly growing subdural hematoma, which then compresses the brain, ultimately leading to coma and death.

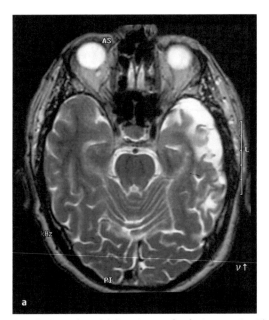
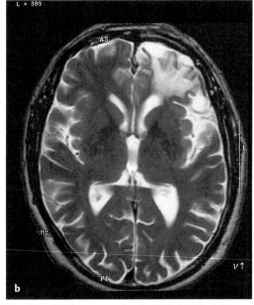

Fig. 6.8　Parenchymal defects 6 years after brain contusion. The T2-weighted MR images reveal cortical defects in the left temporal **(a)** and frontal lobes **(b)**, accompanied by signal changes in the underlying white matter.

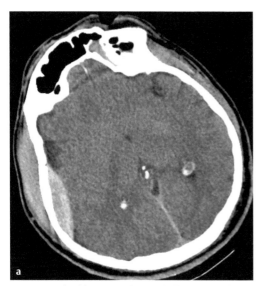 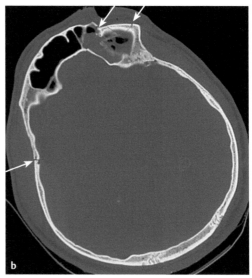

Fig. 6.9   Epidural hematoma (CT scan). There is an epidural hematoma on the right side **(a)** associated with marked extracranial soft-tissue swelling. **(b)** The bone window reveals a right-sided skull fracture over the hematoma as well as further fractures in the left frontal bone (arrows). This is the same patient seen in **Fig. 4.1**.

6.2.5 Traumatic Hematomas

 Key Point

Traumatic hematomas are due to tears in arteries or veins (see Fig. 6.11).

Traumatic Intracerebral Hematoma

Cause and localization. Traumatic intracerebral hematomas generally result from the tearing of small blood vessels, most often within contusions of the frontal or temporal lobes.

Clinical features. Intracerebral hematomas may exert considerable mass effect; combined with the surrounding **edema**, they may raise the ICP sufficiently to cause a **progressive decline of consciousness** and **increasingly severe neurologic deficits**.

Diagnostic evaluation. Intracerebral hematomas are seen as hyperdense areas in a CT scan of the brain.

Treatment. The neurosurgical evacuation of large hematomas can be considered, depending on their size and location.

Epidural Hematoma

Cause and localization. Epidural hematomas **(Fig. 6.9)** are generally produced by traumatic tearing of a **dural artery**, usually the **middle meningeal artery**. The tear itself is usually due to a temporoparietal **skull fracture**, but may occur in the absence of a skull fracture. The blood collection lies **between the periosteum and the dura mater**.

Clinical features. The **arterial hemorrhage** can **compress** the brain very rapidly. The following clinical features are typical of epidural hematoma:

- A patient who is initially unconscious because of a coexisting brain contusion may **fail to awaken** because an epidural hematoma has accumulated in the minutes or hours after the injury.
- On the other hand, an initially awake or only transiently unconscious patient may **rapidly lapse into coma** after a so-called "**lucid interval**" lasting minutes or hours.
- **The side of the hematoma** can often be determined by clinical examination: incipient uncal herniation compresses the ipsilateral oculomotor nerve, causing **ipsilateral pupillary dilatation**.
- **Hemiparesis**, if present, is generally **contralateral** to the hematoma.

Diagnostic evaluation. If an epidural hematoma is suspected, an immediate head CT is indicated. The hematoma is usually seen as a **hyperdense, biconvex zone** that is sharply demarcated from the underlying brain tissue.

Treatment. Immediate neurosurgical evacuation is necessary to prevent brainstem herniation and death. Patients often make an excellent recovery if they have no underlying brain injury and if the hematoma has been removed promptly.

Subdural Hematoma

Subdural hematomas can be **acute**, **subacute**, or **chronic**.

Localization. The blood collection lies between the dura mater and the arachnoid and comes about because of a tear in a bridging vein.

6

Acute Subdural Hematoma

Cause. An acute subdural hematoma is usually a component of a **severe traumatic brain injury** with extensive intraparenchymal contusions.

Clinical features. Clinical examination alone does not enable a clear-cut distinction between subdural and epidural hematomas: subdural hematoma, too, is characterized by a **rapidly progressive decline of consciousness**, **ipsilateral pupillary dilatation**, and **contralateral hemiparesis**.

Diagnostic evaluation. The diagnosis is established by **CT**: a subdural hematoma is typically seen as a **hyperdense or isodense area** (depending on the time elapsed since the traumatic event), either **crescent-shaped** or closely applied to the skull; unlike an epidural hematoma, a subdural hematoma is poorly demarcated from the underlying brain tissue. It may be spread over the entire cerebral hemisphere and may also be found as a layer of blood clot overlying the tentorium.

Practical Tip

Subdural hematomas may be spread over the entire cerebral hemisphere and may also be found as a layer of blood clot overlying the tentorium. Epidural hematomas are generally confined to the space between the cranial sutures.

Treatment. Immediate neurosurgical evacuation.

Chronic Subdural Hematoma

Cause. A chronic subdural hematoma may arise in the aftermath of a mild traumatic brain injury or even after a relatively trivial blow to the head, of which the patient may no longer have any recollection. Therapeutic anticoagulation is a risk factor for the development of a chronic subdural hematoma.

Clinical features. A few weeks or (rarely) months after the causative event, the patient begins to suffer from **increasingly severe headache, fluctuating disturbances of consciousness, confusion**, and ultimately **progressive somnolence**. Hemiparesis, if present, is usually mild, and signs of intracranial hypertension are usually absent.

Diagnostic evaluation. The diagnosis is established by **CT** or **MRI** (**Fig. 6.10**).

Treatment. The treatment is by **neurosurgical evacuation** through one or two burr holes (this is a relatively brief and uncomplicated procedure that can be performed under local anesthesia in cooperative patients).

6.2.6 The Treatment of Traumatic Brain Injury

Key Point

All patients with traumatic brain injury must be carefully clinically observed so that potentially fatal complications can be prevented, in particular, circulatory disturbances (hypotonia,

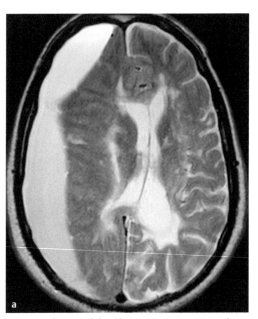
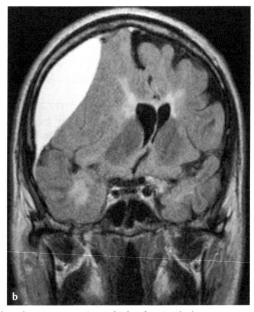

Fig. 6.10   Chronic subdural hematoma in a patient with secondary chronic progressive multiple sclerosis. The hematoma compresses the underlying brain tissue; note also the mainly periventricular signal changes due to MS. On the side of the hematoma, the cerebral sulci cannot be seen; the midline structures of the brain are markedly displaced toward the opposite side. **(a)** Axial T2-weighted spin-echo MR image. **(b)** Coronal FLAIR MR image.

hypoxemia) and intracranial hypertension. In some patients, pressure-measuring devices must be implanted in the brain for continuous, invasive monitoring.

Initial rescue measures. The initial rescue measures at the scene of injury include the following, depending on the severity of injury:
- **Circulatory stabilization** with the administration of isotonic fluids (e.g., normal saline; hypotonic fluids are contraindicated, as they can promote cerebral edema) and pressor drugs, if necessary, to sustain a systolic blood pressure of at least 120 mm Hg.
- **Intubation and artificial ventilation**: the airway must be secured, and, depending on the nature of the injury and the patient's state of consciousness, mask ventilation or intubation may be needed. Supplemental oxygen is given to achieve a saturation level of at least 95% and prevent hypoxia.
- **Analgesia, sedation, and relaxation**: opioids or short-acting general anesthetics such as propofol can be given to sedate the patient and relieve pain (these drugs may cause hypotension, which should be counteracted immediately).

The patient is transported to a trauma center, where imaging studies are performed on arrival to diagnose brain injuries and associated traumatic injuries.

Neurosurgical operations. The indications for a neurosurgical procedure include compressive hematomas causing neurologic deficits and/or incipient brain herniation, very extensive injuries to brain tissue, progressive worsening of deficits caused by the traumatic lesion, or otherwise intractable intracranial hypertension.

Mild traumatic brain injury. The treatment of mild traumatic brain injury mainly consists of **clinical observation**.

> **NOTE**
>
> Any head-injured patient with an impairment of consciousness immediately after the injury (GCS < 15) should be admitted to the hospital.

Patients are generally admitted to the hospital for **24 hours** for symptomatic treatment (analgesics and antiemetic drugs, as needed) and intravenous fluid administration until they are able to eat and drink.

Moderate and Severe Traumatic Brain Injury. After the initial measures have been taken (possibly including neurosurgical removal of compressive lesions), and depending on the patient's clinical state, further observation in an **intensive care unit** or dedicated neurotrauma unit may be needed, with

adequate analgesia and sedation, frequent checking of the **vital signs** and neurologic functions, and, possibly, invasive monitoring of the **ICP**. Optimal cardiovascular, respiratory, and metabolic conditions should be created, particularly **adequate oxygenation** and **blood pressure**, and **normoglycemia**. Enteral nutrition and antithrombotic prophylaxis increase the probability of survival.

Extensive parenchymal injuries and the associated brain edema usually elevate the ICP. Thus, **ICP-reducing measures** may need to be taken, including:
- Elevation of the head of the bed (generally to 30 degrees).
- Hyperventilation.
- Osmotherapy (mannitol).
- External drainage of CSF.
- Neurosurgical removal of compressive hematomas.

Patients with penetrating injuries of the brain or those who have already had an epileptic seizure in the early posttraumatic period should be given **anticonvulsant drugs**.

> **NOTE**
>
> All patients with traumatic brain injuries should be carefully clinically monitored. For comatose patients and those with impaired consciousness (particularly if their ICP is not being invasively monitored), regular checks of the size and reactivity of the pupils and of the other brainstem reflexes are mandatory, so that progressive intracranial hypertension can be detected and treated in timely fashion.

6.2.7 Complications

> **Key Point**
>
> This section deals with complications that arise later on by pathophysiologic mechanisms coming into effect some time after the initial injury. These include:
> - Early and late infections.
> - CSF leaks.
> - Neurologic deficits (brain and cranial nerves).
> - Posttraumatic epilepsy.
> - Malresorptive hydrocephalus.
> - neuropsychological deficits and personality changes.

A schematic overview of such complications is presented in **Fig. 6.11**.

Early Complications

Meningitis, empyema, cerebritis, brain abscess. Any open or penetrating brain injury (e.g., depressed

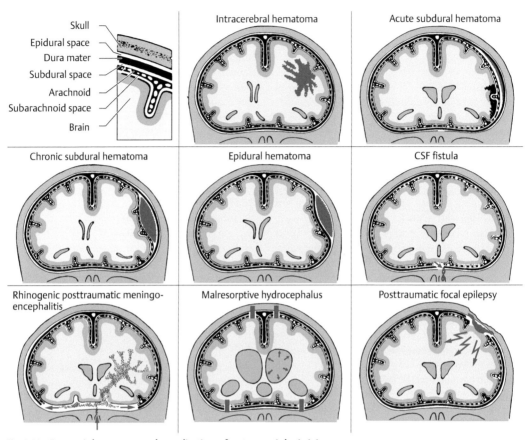

Fig. 6.11 Traumatic hematomas and complications after traumatic brain injury.

skull fractures, gunshot wounds) provides a route of access for **bacterial contamination** of the meningeal spaces and the brain. **Early posttraumatic meningitis, subdural empyema, cerebritis,** or a **brain abscess** may appear a few days or weeks after the traumatic event.

Early epileptic seizures. These may be present in the early phase and can also persist (late posttraumatic epilepsy).

Hydrocephalus. Particularly in patients with severe traumatic brain injury, an impairment of the CSF circulation may lead to hydrocephalus. Patients with hydrocephalus have a higher mortality; some of this excess mortality can probably be reduced by the timely insertion of an external ventricular drain.

Electrolyte disturbances. Dysfunction of the hypothalamic–pituitary axis can cause electrolyte disturbances—most commonly, diabetes insipidus because of insufficient secretion of antidiuretic hormone. Hypopituitarism may persist and necessitate hormone substitution.

Later Complications

CSF leak, meningitis, brain abscess. A skull base fracture associated with a dural tear may give rise to a **persistent CSF leak**, manifesting clinically as leakage of clear fluid out of the nose or ear (**CSF rhino- or otorrhea**) or down the pharynx. The diagnosis can be secured by detection of β2-transferrin in the leaking fluid. CSF leaks are sometimes accompanied by **orthostatic headache** due to intracranial hypotension (see section 14.2.4, Intracranial Hypotension). If the leak remains undiscovered or untreated, it can serve as a portal for bacterial infection. The patient may present with **meningitis** (often pneumococcal meningitis) and/or a **brain abscess**, possibly years after the initial trauma. The presence and exact location of a CSF leak can be demonstrated by MRI and thin-section CT, which may reveal a bony defect or fracture. CSF leaks should be **surgically repaired**.

Posttraumatic neurologic deficits. The commonest **cranial nerve deficit** after traumatic brain injury is **anosmia** (see section 12.1), which is permanent in two-thirds of patients, followed by **optic nerve dysfunction** (which only rarely improves) and **palsies of cranial nerves III, IV, and VI** (which usually resolve in 2–3 months). Fractures of the petrous pyramid(s) may cause **facial nerve palsy** as well as **deafness**, due to injury either to the vestibulocochlear nerve or to the cochlea itself; when caused by a transverse fracture, deafness is usually permanent. A fracture extending into the jugular foramen may cause a combined palsy of the glossopharyngeal, vagus, and accessory nerves (Siebenmann syndrome).

Focal brain lesions cause deficits according to their localization. **Diencephalic lesions** often cause diabetes insipidus. **Cerebellar lesions** cause ataxia, which does not always resolve. **Spasticity**, due to damage of the motor pathways in the central nervous system (CNS), may be uni- or bilateral.

Posttraumatic epilepsy. Posttraumatic epilepsy is seen within 2 years in 80% of the patients who develop it, but it can also arise many years after the initial trauma in rare cases. The seizures may be focal, secondarily generalized, or primarily generalized (cf. section 9.2).

neuropsychological deficits and personality changes. Posttraumatic neuropsychological deficits (variously designated as focal organic brain syndrome, psychoorganic syndrome, or posttraumatic encephalopathy) and personality changes are often the most disabling sequelae of traumatic brain injury for the patient and his or her family. The severity of these problems is positively correlated with the length of the initial loss of consciousness and with the duration of retrograde and anterograde amnesia around the time of the injury. Both short- and long-term memory are impaired and the attention span is shorter than normal. The patient has difficulty coping with complex tasks and situations and is easily fatigued. Impatience, irritability, diminished initiative, poor concentration, and lack of interest ranging to apathy characterize the patient's behavior.

> **NOTE**
>
> Traumatic brain injury often has very serious consequences for the patient's personal and professional life.

Rarer posttraumatic phenomena. There may be a persistent **Lhermitte sign** (paresthesia down the back on flexion of the neck, further described in section 8.2). **Malresorptive hydrocephalus** most commonly arises after a traumatic subarachnoid hemorrhage (in either the early or the late posttraumatic phase). It reflects impaired CSF flow and resorption (see section 6.1.3, **Table 6.3**, and section 6.12.6).

6.2.8 Prognosis

 Key Point
The prognosis after traumatic brain injury strongly depends on the severity of the injury on presentation. With an initial Glasgow coma score of 15, the mortality is near 0%; with a score of 3, it is over 80%.

Mild traumatic brain injury has a favorable prognosis; it usually causes **no lasting deficit** of any kind. After moderate traumatic brain injury, cognitive deficits and focal neurologic deficits (if present) can resolve significantly or even completely, but they can also persist. Survivors of severe traumatic brain injury generally have persistent neurologic deficits, including cognitive deficits. The severity of lasting impairment in such patients is highly variable, however, ranging all the way from the apallic syndrome (persistent vegetative state) to regained independence of function with only mild disability.

6.3 Intracranial Pressure

 Key Point
Intracranial masses rapidly elevate the ICP because the skull is a closed compartment. Intracranial hypertension may arise acutely, that is, in a few minutes or hours (especially in brain hemorrhage), or chronically (for example, when caused by a slowly growing brain tumor). Characteristic manifestations include impairment of consciousness (ranging from somnolence to coma), abnormal breathing, bradycardia, hypertension, opisthotonus, extensor spasms of the limbs, and pupillary dilatation.

Intracranial hypertension impairs cerebral perfusion and CSF circulation and may also result in **compression of intracranial structures** (e.g., compression of cranial nerves against the base of the skull, occlusive compression of the posterior cerebral artery) and **shifting of large portions of the brain within the skull** (e.g., herniation of the medial portion of the temporal lobe into the tentorial notch, or of the cerebellar tonsils into the foramen magnum).

6.3.1 Definition, Etiology, and Pathogenesis

Definition. Intracranial hypertension is defined as an ICP above 20 mm Hg; in normal individuals, the ICP is generally below 15 mm Hg. Another important quantity is the cerebral perfusion pressure (CPP), which is defined as the mean arterial pressure

(MAP) minus the ICP. In normal individuals, the CPP is above 50 mm Hg.

Etiology. The common causes of intracranial hypertension are:

- Tumor.
- Hemorrhage.
- Extensive stroke.
- Trauma.
- Venous sinus thrombosis.
- Hydrocephalus.

The **cerebral edema** that accompanies many of these conditions can exacerbate intracranial hypertension. The ICP can also be elevated by a variety of other conditions (cf. **Table 6.8**).

Pathogenesis. The rigid skull and the CSF protect the brain from external mechanical influences. At the same time, however, the skull limits the total volume available for the brain, CSF, cerebral vasculature, and any other intracranially introduced material. If a space-occupying lesion should arise, such as a hematoma or tumor, the ensuing rise in ICP can be counteracted, at least at first by a compensatory exit of venous blood and CSF from the cranial cavity. The amount of added intracranial material that can be tolerated without the development of neurologic symptoms is about 40 mL in younger persons and about 80 mL in the elderly (because of the brain atrophy that often occurs in old age). If volume compensation is exhausted or outpaced by a rapidly expanding lesion, a dangerous rise in ICP occurs. The CPP, which equals the MAP minus the ICP, accordingly falls, and the blood supply to the brain is compromised (or even, in the extreme case, abolished). The brain is damaged not just by the direct mechanical pressure, but also by the ensuing ischemia. Very high ICP leads to herniation of the temporal lobes through the tentorial notch or of the brainstem through the foramen magnum.

6.3.2 Clinical Features and Diagnostic Evaluation

Table 6.9 contains an overview of the clinical features and diagnostic evaluation of intracranial hypertension.

Table 6.8

Causes of intracranial hypertension

Category	Causes—particular entities	Clinical features; remarks
Intracranial mass	- Brain tumor - Subdural hematoma - Intracerebral hematoma - Extensive stroke (especially middle cerebral artery territorial infarction)	Focal neurologic and neuropsychological deficits, headache
Cerebral venous and venous sinus thrombosis	Infection, preexisting disease (e.g., coagulopathy). Venous sinus thrombosis most commonly arises without any identifiable cause	Impairment of consciousness, if the internal cerebral veins are involved; headache, epileptic seizures. Venous (sinus) thrombosis may be complicated by secondary intracranial hemorrhage
Infection	Encephalitis, meningitis, brain abscess	Fever, meningismus. Causes include herpes simplex encephalitis, neurobrucellosis, and syphilis
Traumatic brain injury	Contusion, brain edema, intra- or extracerebral hematoma	Progressively severe manifestations due to brain edema; focal seizures
Impairment of CSF flow or resorption	- Intraventricular tumors	Headache (possibly ictal), vomiting. Intracranial hypertension is intermittent
	- Aqueductal stenosis	Widened lateral ventricles and third ventricle; normal fourth ventricle
	- Malresorptive hydrocephalus	Spasticity of legs, urinary incontinence, psycho-organic syndrome. Often, prior history of subarachnoid hemorrhage or meningitis
Elevation of CSF protein concentration	For example, in polyradiculitis, spinal tumors (especially schwannoma)	Lumbar puncture yields CSF with elevated protein
Toxic processes	Lead poisoning, insecticide poisoning	Psycho-organic syndrome, anemia, lead line (on gums), sometimes other neurologic and systemic signs and symptoms
Iatrogenic	Steroids, oral contraceptives, tetracycline	
Altitude sickness	Rapid ascent, inadequate oxygen supply, pulmonary and cerebral edema	Headache, pulmonary edema, retinal hemorrhage, angina pectoris. Descend immediately
Idiopathic intracranial hypertension, pseudotumor cerebri	ICP elevation of no known cause	Usually affects obese young women; slit ventricles, sometimes papilledema. A diagnosis of exclusion

Abbreviations: CSF, cerebrospinal fluid; ICP, intracranial pressure.

Table 6.9

Manifestations of intracranial hypertension (symptoms, signs, and test findings)

Type of examination	Symptoms and signs	
Physical examination	Symptoms and signs of intracranial hypertension	— **Headache** (diffuse, persistent, most severe in the morning) — **Nausea and vomiting** (typically in the morning—paroxysmal dry heaves) — **Hiccups** — Progressive **impairment of wakefulness** and **consciousness** — With chronic elevation of intracranial pressure, **progressive lack of motivation, apathy**
	Signs of impending herniation	— Impairment of consciousness, ranging from somnolence to coma — Respiratory disturbance, bradycardia, hypertension (together called the **Cushing reflex**) — Opisthotonus and extensor spasms of the limbs — Dilated pupils
	Ocular findings	— **Papilledema** (absent if ICP rises very rapidly) — Occasionally retinal hemorrhage — Enlarged blind spot — Attacks of amblyopia with transient blindness — Occasionally oculomotor nerve palsy or abducens nerve palsy (the abducens nerve has the longest course in the subarachnoid space of any cranial nerve)
Skull X-ray	Abnormal only in chronic intracranial hypertension: increased digitate markings, enlarged sella turcica with demineralized dorsum sellae, diastasis of one or more cranial sutures in children and adolescents	
CT/MRI	Slit ventricles (when elevation of ICP is due to cerebral edema), compressed gyri, periventricular signal change; CT and MRI may reveal the causative lesion for intracranial hypertension (e.g., tumor, hemorrhage)	
EEG	Diffusely abnormal, nonspecific	
LP	**Contraindicated** if elevated ICP is suspected. If LP is nonetheless performed, the opening pressure generally exceeds 200-mm CSF but may be normal if CSF flow is blocked at the occipitocervical or spinal level	
Direct ICP measurement	Pressure gauge or ventricular drain in the lateral ventricle. Indicated for patients with impaired consciousness and suspected intracranial hypertension	

Abbreviations: CSF, cerebrospinal fluid; CT, computed tomography; EEG, electroencephalogram; ICP, intracranial pressure; LP, lumbar pressure; MRI, magnetic resonance imaging.

Practical Tip

An LP should, in general, not be performed if there is clinical suspicion of intracranial hypertension. It may be performed only if the imaging studies and ophthalmoscopic examination have yielded no evidence of acutely elevated ICP with impending brain herniation.

6.3.3 Complication: Herniation

The most important complication of intracranial hypertension is **brainstem herniation**. With increasing supratentorial mass effect, the mediobasal portion of the temporal lobe is pressed into the tentorial notch, with ensuing herniation and compression of the brainstem (see **Fig. 6.12**). The ipsilateral oculomotor nerve is compressed; the loss of its parasympathetic outflow leads to pupillary dilatation (mydriasis). The patient's consciousness is impaired. Unilateral herniation causes contralateral hemiparesis, and bilateral herniation causes quadriparesis. An infratentorial mass can compress the brainstem directly or cause brainstem herniation downward into the foramen magnum or upward into the tentorial notch.

6.3.4 Treatment

The treatment of intracranial hypertension consists of general measures to lower the ICP combined with specific treatment of the underlying cause.

General measures.
— **Elevation of the head of the bed to 30 degrees** (if the patient is not in shock and the blood pressure is adequate).
— **Adequate oxygenation** with monitoring of the O_2 saturation level.
— (Restoration of) **normoglycemia and normothermia**.
— **Fluid and electrolyte balance** (volume administration).

Specific measures.
— **Osmotic agents**, such as intravenous mannitol or hypertonic saline, and diuretics, for rapid (but transient) lowering of the ICP.
— **Sedation** if the ICP is severely elevated (GCS > 8), to lessen the brain's metabolic demand for oxygen.
— **Hyperventilation** (if the patient is intubated) to lower the Pco_2 and thereby transiently lower the ICP.
— **Corticosteroids** (e.g., dexamethasone, given intravenously) are used to counteract cerebral

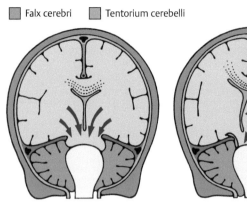

6

Falx cerebri   Tentorium cerebelli

Axial transtentorial
herniation

Uncal transtentorial and
subfalcine herniation

Fig. 6.12 Brainstem herniation. (Reproduced from Mattle H, Mumenthaler M. Neurologie. Stuttgart: Thieme; 2013.)

edema, particularly of the vasogenic type; they are mainly effective against peritumoral and inflammatory brain edema, but not at all against ischemic and traumatic brain edema, which are predominantly of the cytotoxic type.

- **External ventricular drainage** through a catheter inserted into the lateral ventricle; especially useful if intracranial hypertension is due partly or wholly to hydrocephalus.
- **Hemicraniectomy** is sometimes the only way to save the patient's life, for example, in traumatic brain injury or massive stroke with space-occupying edema.
- **Hypothermia** (cooling the patient) also lowers the ICP; its benefit after traumatic brain injury or stroke remains to be demonstrated.

6.4 Brain Tumors

  Key Point
Brain tumors are one of the more common causes of intracranial hypertension. They are subdivided into primary brain tumors, which arise from the brain tissue itself (either the neuroepithelial tissue or the neighboring mesenchymal tissues, e.g., the meninges), brain metastases, and tumors arising from the cells of the blood vessels. Brain tumors produce focal brain signs of different types depending on their location, as well as signs of intracranial hypertension that may progress more or less rapidly depending on the rate of tumor growth.

6.4.1 Overview

Epidemiology. The **incidence** of tumors of the brain or spinal cord is approximately 5 per 100,000 persons per year in children and adolescents, and 28 per 100,000 persons per year in adults. Brain and spinal cord tumors are the most common kind of solid tumor in children; in adults, they are much rarer than the most common kinds of cancer (prostate, breast).

The frequency of different kinds of brain and meningeal tumors is shown in **Fig. 6.13**. The spectrum of brain tumors **changes with age**. In children and adolescents, the most common tumors are pilocytic astrocytoma, glioma, and medulloblastoma; in adults, the most common tumors are meningioma, glioblastoma, and pituitary tumors. Among the elderly, meningioma and glioblastoma are most common.

| NOTE |

Meningioma, schwannoma, and pituitary tumors are among the most common benign tumors; glioblastoma and astrocytoma are among the most common malignant tumors.

Classification and grading. In the **WHO classification**, brain tumors are classified by their **histologic type** (for a simplified overview, see **Table 6.10**) and by their **degree of malignity**, ranked on a four-point scale (**Table 6.11**): tumors of WHO grades I and II are benign, while those of grades III and IV are malignant.

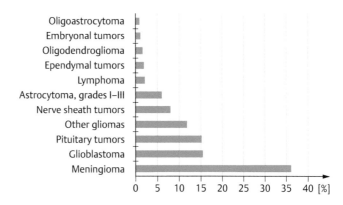

Fig. 6.13   The frequency of tumors of the brain and meninges.
(Data from www.cbtrus.org.)

6

Table 6.10

WHO histologic classification of tumors of the nervous system (2007, simplified)

WHO tumor type	Examples
Neuroepithelial tumors	Astrocytoma, glioblastoma
	Oligodendroglioma
	Mixed glioma
	Ependymoma
	Choroid plexus papilloma
	Gangliocytoma
	Pinealocytoma
	Medulloblastoma
Peripheral nerve tumors	Schwannoma (= neurinoma)
	Neurofibroma
Meningeal tumors	Meningioma
	Hemangioblastoma
Neoplasias of the hematopoietic system	Primary CNS lymphoma
	Malignant lymphoma
Germ-cell tumors	Germinoma
	Teratoma
Tumors of the sellar region	Pituitary adenoma
	Craniopharyngioma
Metastases	Carcinomas of the:
	— Lung
	— Breast
	— Kidney (renal cell carcinoma)
	— Colon

Abbreviation: CNS, central nervous system.

Etiology. Most brain tumors are of **no known cause**; in rare cases, they can be caused by a prior exposure to ionizing radiation or by a genetic syndrome. Examples include **Li–Fraumeni syndrome** (astrocytoma, primitive neuroectodermal tumors [PNET], sarcoma), **Turcot syndrome** (medulloblastoma, glioblastoma), and the **phakomatoses** (see section 6.1.8):
— Neurofibromatosis, type 1 (neurofibroma, iris hamartoma) and type 2 (meningioma, bilateral acoustic neuroma, retinal hamartoma).

— von Hippel–Lindau disease (hemangioblastoma of the cerebellum).
— Tuberous sclerosis (cortical hamartoma, giant-cell astrocytoma).
— Encephalofacial angiomatosis, that is, Sturge–Weber disease.

General clinical manifestations. The general manifestations of brain tumors are presented in **Table 6.12**. These can progress more or less rapidly depending on the type and growth rate of the tumor. **Malignant tumors** typically manifest a **"crescendo" course**, in which overt signs and symptoms arise soon after the onset of the illness, and then worsen steadily and rapidly. The signs and symptoms of **benign tumors**, on the other hand, often progress **slowly and insidiously**, perhaps over many years. Hemorrhage into a brain tumor (either benign or malignant) may cause symptoms to arise very suddenly.

Diagnostic evaluation. Neuroimaging studies are essential: the best is generally **contrast-enhanced MRI** (cf. **Table 4.2**). **CT** may provide useful complementary information in some cases, for example, calcifications or accompanying osseous changes, but may fail to reveal some tumors (especially low-grade gliomas). Sometimes **angiography** is indicated for visualization of a tumor's blood supply.

Brain tumors generally cannot be securely diagnosed by imaging studies alone; in most cases, at least some of the tumor must be surgically removed for **histologic examination**. If total resection is not possible because of the location of the tumor, or contraindicated for other medical reasons, then tissue can be obtained by a **stereotactic brain biopsy**. A secure histologic diagnosis is needed for the optimal planning of further treatment, such as chemotherapy or radiotherapy. Moreover, some "brain tumors" turn out, on biopsy, not to be tumors at all, but rather brain abscesses, foci of demyelination, etc. In such cases, diagnostic biopsies save the patient from needless and probably harmful treatment.

Table 6.11

WHO grading of brain tumors

Grade	Features	MRI	Representative examples
I	Slowly growing, not malignant, cells appear nearly normal, long survival	T2-hyperintense, hardly any mass effect, no enhancement	Pilocytic astrocytoma
II	Relatively slowly growing, occasional atypical cells, can transform into higher-grade tumors or recur as higher-grade tumors after treatment	T2-hyperintense, mass effect, no enhancement	Astrocytoma, oligodendroglioma
III	Malignant, with anaplastic cells; recur as high-grade tumors	T2-hyperintense, mass effect, variable enhancement (from none to highly complex)	Anaplastic astrocytoma
IV	Malignant, with anaplastic cells; rapid, aggressive growth	T2-hyperintense, mass effect, ring-shaped enhancement	Glioblastoma

Source: From Mattle H, Mumenthaler M. Neurologie. Stuttgart: Thieme; 2013.

Table 6.12

General manifestations of brain tumors

Symptoms	Signs
— **Headache** (diffuse, at night as well as in the daytime; an early symptom in half of all patients with brain tumors) — Possibly other **signs of intracranial hypertension** (vomiting, bradycardia) — **Epileptic seizures** (focal or generalized; the initial presentation of one quarter of all patients with brain tumors) — **Mental changes** (apathy, irritability, fatigability, impaired memory, and concentration)	— **Focal neurologic deficits** depending on the localization of the tumor — **Mental abnormalities and cognitive deficits** (memory loss, other neuropsychological deficits) — Sometimes **cranial nerve deficits** — Often **papilledema**

 Practical Tip

CSF examination is generally neither necessary nor helpful in the evaluation of brain tumors. CSF cytology is clinically useful only in case of meningeal spread (e.g., in carcinomatous meningitis) and when the presence of oligoclonal bands in the CSF helps to establish the correct diagnosis of a large multiple sclerosis plaque that resembles a brain tumor on imaging studies.

Tumor markers may be useful for diagnosis and treatment.

Additional Information

Mass lesions of the CNS that may be misdiagnosed as tumors include:
- Residual mass lesions after episodes of ischemia, inflammation, or thrombosis.
- Infections (bacterial abscess, tuberculosis, fungal or parasitic infection).
- Multiple sclerosis plaques (mainly of the "tumefactive" type).
- Sarcoidosis.

Treatment. Complete resection of the tumor is indicated whenever possible. The operability of brain tumors depends on their size, location, histologic grade, and relation to the surrounding brain tissue (infiltration vs. displacement). Not every tumor is neurosurgically accessible or fully resectable. Depending on the type of tumor, **radiotherapy and/ or chemotherapy** may have to be used, either as the primary form of treatment or as adjuvant therapy after surgery.

The **cerebral edema** that usually accompanies malignant tumors is treated with **corticosteroids** (usually **dexamethasone**). Dexamethasone is also given **preoperatively** to reduce swelling in all cases of brain tumor with mass effect and elevated ICP. Epileptic seizures, if they arise, are treated with anticonvulsants, for example, levetiracetam. In some circumstances, prophylactic anticonvulsant administration may be helpful as well.

 Practical Tip

Epileptic seizures are an important manifestation of brain tumors and can arise either before or after neurosurgical resection.

6.4.2 Astrocytoma and Glioblastoma

Astrocytoma is the most common type of primary brain tumor and is classed as a neuroepithelial tumor. Grade III and IV astrocytomas are called anaplastic astrocytoma and glioblastoma, respectively; these forms are highly malignant and lead rapidly to death. Grade I and II astrocytomas are more benign, growing slowly and progressively over a period of years. Pilocytic astrocytoma (grade I), a tumor seen mostly in children and adolescents, is the only type of astrocytoma that generally does not recur after total resection.

Grade IV Astrocytoma (Glioblastoma)

A distinction is drawn between **primary** and **secondary glioblastoma**. Primary glioblastoma is already a grade IV tumor at the time it arises (or is first discovered); secondary glioblastoma develops by **malignant progression** from a preexisting lower-grade astrocytoma or other type of glioma. Glioblastoma was historically called "glioblastoma multiforme;" the second word adds no information and has been dropped from modern classifications.

Epidemiology. Glioblastoma is the most common and most malignant type of primary brain tumor. It grows by infiltration into the brain tissue. Its highest incidence is in the **fifth and sixth decades of life**.

Localization and growth. Glioblastoma arises in a cerebral hemisphere and can spread to the contralateral hemisphere by way of the corpus callosum (**butterfly glioma**). Glioblastomas grow rapidly, causing rapidly progressive clinical manifestations; they are, therefore, usually diagnosed within a few weeks or (at most) months of the onset of symptoms.

Clinical features. Focal neurologic and/or neuropsychological deficits arise first, sometimes accompanied by epileptic seizures, soon followed by general signs of intracranial hypertension (see **Table 6.9**).

Diagnostic evaluation. The diagnosis can be made fairly securely from the typical appearance in neuroimaging studies (**Fig. 6.14**, **Fig. 6.15**), though this does not obviate the need for histologic examination of tumor tissue. Contrast-enhanced MRI or CT characteristically reveals **ringlike enhancement** with a **central nonenhancing area**, corresponding to necrosis in the interior of the tumor. Intratumoral hemorrhages may also be seen. Peritumoral brain

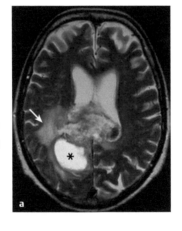
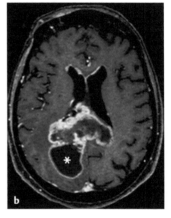

Fig. 6.14 Glioblastoma. The T2-weighted **(a)** and T1-weighted **(b)** MR images reveal a butterfly-shaped tumor in the splenium of the corpus callosum and adjacent regions of the two cerebral hemispheres. A cyst (*) in the right occipital lobe is part of the tumor; like the rest of the tumor, the cyst wall displays contrast enhancement **(b)**. Peritumoral edema is most marked in the right hemisphere (→) **(a)**.

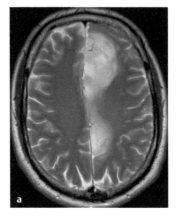
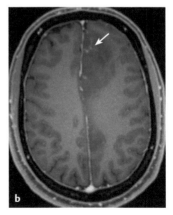

Fig. 6.15 Grade II–III astrocytoma. The tumor is hyperintense on T2-weighted MRI **(a)** and hypointense on contrast-enhanced T1-weighted MRI **(b)**. Its left frontal portion takes up contrast medium (→), probably because of malignant progression here to a grade III tumor.

edema is often extensive, causing mass effect and midline shift.

Prognosis. The survival of patients who have undergone the partial or gross total resection of a glioblastoma, with or without adjuvant radiotherapy and/or chemotherapy, is measured in **months** to a few years at most.

Grade III Astrocytoma (Anaplastic Astrocytoma)

Grade III astrocytoma occupies an intermediate position between grade II astrocytoma and glioblastoma with respect to malignant behavior.

Additional Information

Gliomatosis cerebri, defined as a glial tumor that grows diffusely into three or more lobes of the brain, is included in the category of grade III astrocytoma. It is inoperable and responds poorly to radiotherapy as well.

Grade II Astrocytoma

Epidemiology. Astrocytomas of the cerebral hemisphere(s) generally affect adults aged 30 to 40 years.

Growth. Though these tumors displace and infiltrate the surrounding brain tissue, they are **better demarcated** from it than glioblastoma; they often grow quite slowly, sometimes over many years.

Clinical features. These include focal or secondarily generalized **epileptic seizures**, often as the presenting manifestation, as well as **behavioral and neuropsychological changes**, increasingly severe **focal neurologic deficits** (e.g., hemiparesis), and signs of **intracranial hypertension**.

Treatment and prognosis. If epileptic seizures are the only manifestation, tumor resection may be useful for seizure control, if the location of the tumor permits. Totally resected tumors sometimes do not recur until years later.

Grade I Astrocytoma (Pilocytic Astrocytoma)

Epidemiology. This form of tumor usually arises in **children and adolescents**.

Localization and growth. Pilocytic astrocytoma is usually found in the cerebellar hemispheres or vermis and may extend into the pons. It grows slowly and is benign.

Clinical features. The symptoms and signs depend on the site of the tumor; thus, cerebellar manifestations are common.

Diagnostic evaluation. These tumors generally display **contrast enhancement** (and are the only nonmalignant type of brain tumor to do so).

Treatment and prognosis. Total resection often results in **cure**. Chemotherapy and radiotherapy are a treatment of second choice if radical surgery would endanger important structures.

Special Types of Brain Tumor

Brainstem astrocytoma, even if benign, is generally inoperable and incurable, though its symptoms and signs may improve with radiotherapy and chemotherapy.

6.4.3 Ependymoma

Epidemiology and growth. Ependymoma is a **benign tumor** usually seen in **children and adolescents**. It grows by expansion and displacement of brain tissue. It can be partly calcified and cystic.

Localization. Ependymomas develop from the neuroepithelium of the walls of the cerebral ventricles and the central canal of the spinal cord. They usually arise in the posterior fossa, most commonly near the **fourth ventricle**, and in the conus medullaris of the spinal cord (see **Fig. 7.8**).

Clinical features. Their main clinical manifestations are **focal (often cerebellar) neurologic deficits** and signs of **intracranial hypertension** resulting from compression of the CSF pathways and occlusive hydrocephalus. An **unusually persistent, continuous headache** in a child should arouse suspicion of an ependymoma or other mass in the posterior fossa.

Treatment and prognosis. The treatment is resection followed by radiotherapy of the entire neuraxis. Seventy percent of treated patients survive for 10 years or longer.

6.4.4 Medulloblastoma and Primitive Neuroectodermal Tumors

Epidemiology. Medulloblastoma mainly affects **children** (in three-quarters of cases). PNET, a rare type of tumor, is more common in children as well.

Localization and growth. These are **undifferentiated, highly malignant** tumors (WHO grade IV) characterized by rapid growth and **rapidly progressive clinical manifestations**. Medulloblastomas usually arise from the roof of the fourth ventricle, sometimes filling the entire ventricle, and grow into the inferior portion of the vermis. They grow by infiltration and often metastasize via the CSF into the spinal canal (**drop metastases**). PNET is mostly supratentorial.

Clinical features. The signs and symptoms resemble those of cerebellar astrocytoma (**headache, nausea, truncal ataxia**), possibly combined with manifestations referable to the **spinal cord and cauda equina**.

Treatment and prognosis. Medulloblastoma is treated by **resection** followed by radiotherapy (of the entire neuraxis, because of drop metastases) and/or chemotherapy. The prognosis after radical removal is not unfavorable (cure in 50% of cases), but often no more than an incomplete removal can be achieved, in which case tumor recurrence is the rule. PNET carries a worse prognosis than medulloblastoma.

6.4.5 Oligodendroglioma

Epidemiology. Oligodendroglioma tends to arise between the ages of 40 and 50 years.

Localization and growth. It is almost always found in the cerebral hemispheres, particularly the frontal lobes, and is usually a **relatively well-differentiated tumor** that grows slowly over the years and often becomes calcified.

Clinical features. Oligodendroglioma often presents with **epileptic seizures**; recurrent seizures affect 70% of patients.

Treatment. Oligodendroglioma is mostly radioresistant and is best treated by radical resection. If this can be achieved, radiotherapy is usually not given. Nonetheless, apparently radical resection can be followed by tumor recurrence, which may not take place until years after surgery.

> **Practical Tip**
>
> Gliomas of the optic nerve and chiasm arise almost exclusively in children, often as a component of neurofibromatosis.

6.4.6 Meningioma

Epidemiology and etiology. Meningiomas most often become clinically evident **between the ages of 40 and 50 years**. They arise sporadically in most cases, but there is a genetic predisposition toward meningioma formation in some tumor syndromes

(phakomatoses), above all **type II neurofibromatosis** (**Table 6.4**). **Radiation exposure** in early life also predisposes to meningioma formation.

Localization and growth. These **mesodermal tumors** arise from the **arachnoid** and are nearly always **benign**, well-demarcated lesions that displace rather than invade the adjacent neural tissue as they slowly grow. Histologic examination often reveals a layered architecture resembling an onion. Meningiomas tend to appear in certain **classic locations** with corresponding typical neurologic manifestations, as listed in **Table 6.13**.

Morphologic classification and WHO grading. The WHO grading of meningiomas depends on their gross and microscopic structure:

— **WHO grade I** (benign, including most meningiomas): meningotheliomatous, transitional, microcytic, secretory, fibromatous, psammomatous, and angiomatous meningiomas.

— **WHO grade II** (atypical, rapidly growing, with frequent recurrences): chordoid and clear-cell meningiomas.

— **WHO grade III** (malignant, anaplastic, infiltrative): papillary and rhabdoid meningiomas.

Clinical features. Meningiomas present with **epileptic seizures, focal neurologic deficits** (see **Fig. 4.24**), or, in rare cases, **signs of intracranial hypertension** (usually when the tumor lies far away from "eloquent" structures, e.g., in the right frontal lobe). The

Table 6.13

Common sites of meningiomas and associated clinical features

Site	Most common initial manifestations	Course	Special features
Olfactory groove	Anosmia	Epileptic seizures, headache, frontal-type personality change, possible involvement of optic nerve	
Convexity	Epileptic seizures	Hemiparesis	
Parasagittal and falx	Lower limb paresis, (sometimes) bilateral Babinski sign	Epileptic seizures	Rarely, paraparesis
Sphenoid wing	Loss of visual acuity, visual field defects (when medially located, adjacent to optic nerve); oculomotor disturbances	Exophthalmos, hemiparesis	Lateral tumors may be externally evident as temporal hyperostosis
Tuberculum sellae	Visual disturbances, pale optic discs	Progressive visual field defect	
Cerebellopontine angle	Deafness, vertigo	Facial and trigeminal nerve deficits, brainstem compression	Differential diagnosis: acoustic neuroma
Foramen magnum	Spastic quadriparesis, dysphagia, dysarthria	Lower cranial nerve deficits	
Intraventricular	Intermittent headaches and vomiting	Progressive hydrocephalus	Often found in trigone
Intraspinal	Progressive para- or quadriparesis	Paraplegia or quadriplegia	

neurologic deficits may evolve slowly over many years. Meningioma is also a common incidental finding.

Diagnostic evaluation. Meningiomas are diagnosed by MRI or CT scanning (see **Fig. 4.24**, **Fig. 6.16**). These reveal marked, homogeneous contrast enhancement.

Treatment. The indications for treatment must then be carefully considered: resection may be desirable in younger patients, but unnecessary in older ones. The need for resection also depends on the localization and growth rate of the tumor. Heavily calcified meningiomas grow very slowly or not at all. Radiotherapy is reasonable only for residual tumor after incomplete resection.

6.4.7 Lymphoma
Epidemiology. Lymphoma is typically seen in young, **immunocompromized** (e.g., HIV-infected) patients **aged 40 to 60 years** but can also affect **immunocompetent elderly persons**.

Localization and growth. Lymphoma may arise **secondarily** as a metastasis of a lymphoma elsewhere in the body or **primarily** at one or more sites in the CNS. Primary CNS lymphoma is a rare B-cell variant of **non–Hodgkin's lymphoma** and remains restricted to the CNS. These tumors grow rapidly.

Clinical features. CNS lymphoma presents with signs of intracranial hypertension, epileptic seizures, and focal neurologic and neuropsychological deficits. The cranial nerves and the eyes are often affected as well.

Diagnostic evaluation. CT and MRI generally show CNS lymphoma as a contrast-enhancing tumor near the ventricular wall.

Treatment. CNS lymphoma is treated with corticosteroids, **chemo- and immunotherapy** (methotrexate and rituximab), and radiotherapy.

> **NOTE**
>
> Primary CNS lymphoma in immunosuppressed persons is usually associated with the Epstein–Barr virus (EBV).

6.4.8 Pituitary Tumors
Pituitary tumors usually arise from the cells of the **anterior pituitary lobe**. Depending on their origin, they can produce hormones in excess or cause hormone deficiency. Thus, they present clinically with **endocrine disturbances** and/or **compressive effects** on the adjacent neural tissue.

Hormone-secreting pituitary tumors. These most commonly present **between the ages of 30 and 50 years**. Their presentation depends on the endocrine function of the cells from which they arise:

- **Basophil adenomas** produce excessive adrenocorticotropic hormone, causing **Cushing syndrome** (which, when caused by a pituitary tumor, is called **Cushing disease**).
- **Prolactinomas** cause **galactorrhea** and **secondary amenorrhea** in women and **impotence** in men.
- The rare **eosinophil adenomas** produce excessive growth hormone, causing **acromegaly**. They can also grow large enough to cause other symptoms by mass effect.

> **NOTE**
>
> Although basophil adenomas and prolactinomas rarely cause mass effect, eosinophil adenomas and, above all, the **hormonally inactive chromophobe adenomas** can **grow quite large**, causing compression and dysfunction of the normal pituitary tissue, clinically evident as **hypopituitarism** (multiple pituitary hormone deficiencies, including hypothyroidism and secondary hypogonadism).

Non–hormone-secreting pituitary adenomas. Inactive pituitary tumors are generally diagnosed only when they grow large enough to compress and functionally impair the neighboring structures. **Headache** can be a nonspecific symptom. They grow upward from the sella turcica and can compress the optic chiasm and cause **visual field defects**, usually

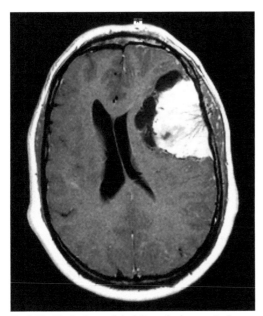

Fig. 6.16 Meningioma of the left cerebral convexity (contrast-enhanced MRI). Marked mass effect deforms the ventricles and shifts the midline structures rightward. There are cystic cavities at the tumor–brain interface. Blood vessels supplying the tumor are seen entering it from its "navel" on the outer surface.

bitemporal **upper quadrantanopsia** or **bitemporal hemianopsia** due to compression of the decussating optic nerve fibers (see section 12.2.1 and **Fig. 12.1**). If the nondecussating fibers are compressed as well, **visual acuity** may be impaired.

Treatment and prognosis. These tumors are removed **microsurgically**, by the transnasal-transsphenoidal route if they are not too large and otherwise through a frontolateral craniotomy. Residual and recurrent tumors are irradiated. Resection can often reverse visual impairment, as long as it is not complete or longstanding. Prolactinomas can often be treated **pharmacologically** with dopaminergic inhibitors of prolactin secretion, for example, cabergoline. All pituitary tumors require **lifelong follow-up**, even after initially successful treatment. **Hormone substitution** may be needed as well (with hydrocortisone, L-thyroxine, antidiuretic hormone, testosterone, estrogen, or combinations of these hormones).

6.4.9 Malformations and Hamartomatous Tumors

These include craniopharyngioma, dermoid and epidermoid tumors, and cavernoma.

Craniopharyngioma

Epidemiology. Craniopharyngioma is the most common suprasellar mass in **children and adolescents**.

Localization and growth. These tumors arise in or above the pituitary fossa, often growing upward toward the diencephalon and third ventricle. They are derived from epithelial remnants in Rathke's pouch and generally contain calcifications and cholesterol crystals.

Clinical features. Craniopharyngioma presents with **hypopituitarism**, **diencephalic manifestations** (diabetes insipidus), and/or **visual disturbances**. Like a pituitary tumor, it can cause hemi- or quadrantanopsia and impair visual acuity; it can also cause **occlusive hydrocephalus**.

Treatment. Craniopharyngioma is best treated by complete resection.

Other Hamartomatous Growths

Cavernoma (in the earlier and now superseded terminology, cavernous angioma or cavernous malformation) consists of a well-demarcated agglomeration of capillary blood vessels. Cavernomas can be multiple and familial (genetic locus on chromosome 7). They present with epileptic seizures and hemorrhage.

Epidermoid tumors are found at the base of the brain, are often calcified, and cause focal deficits or epileptic seizures. Their peak incidence is between the ages of 25 and 45 years.

6.4.10 Neurinomas

Growth and localization. **Neurinomas** (schwannomas) are benign neoplasms arising from Schwann cells (see **Fig. 7.8**). The most common type affects the **eighth cranial nerve** and is usually (though incorrectly) designated **acoustic neuroma** (**Fig. 6.17**). This tumor lies in the **cerebellopontine angle**.

Clinical features. Acoustic neuroma presents initially with **eighth nerve dysfunction**: progressive hearing loss, tinnitus, and disequilibrium. As it grows, it impinges on the other cranial nerves of the cerebellopontine angle, causing **facial palsy** and **trigeminal sensory deficits**. Further growth leads to compression of the cerebellum and brainstem, causing **cerebellar signs** (especially ataxia) and possibly **pyramidal tract signs**.

Diagnostic evaluation. Neurinomas are generally diagnosed by **sectional imaging** (CT or MRI). CSF examination is not necessary; if nonetheless performed in a patient with acoustic neuroma, it typically reveals **marked elevation of the CSF protein concentration**. Neurinomas that grow through a neural foramen (e.g., a spinal intervertebral foramen) have a typical **hourglass** shape.

Treatment. Until recently, the optimal treatment of all neurinomas was **complete resection**. Now many smaller acoustic neuromas can be treated safely and effectively with **stereotactic radiosurgery**.

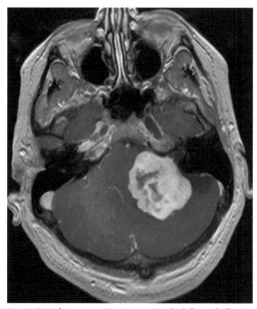

Fig. 6.17   A large acoustic neuroma in the left cerebellopontine angle. Its conical tip extends into the internal acoustic meatus, while the large tumor mass compresses and displaces the brainstem. Marked contrast enhancement on T1-weighted spin-echo images is typical of this type of tumor.

6.4.11 Brain Metastases

Epidemiology. Brain metastases account for approximately 15% of malignant brain tumors. The most common sources of brain metastases are **lung cancer** in men and **breast cancer** in women, followed in both sexes by **melanoma** and **renal cell carcinoma**.

Clinical features and diagnostic evaluation. The symptoms and signs of brain metastases depend on their localization. Brain metastases sometimes produce symptoms even before the primary tumor does; in such cases, multiple brain metastases are usually present, even if only a single one is apparent on the neuroimaging study. A case of multiple brain metastases of lung cancer is illustrated in **Fig. 6.18**.

Treatment and prognosis. Generally speaking, surgical resection is indicated only for **solitary metastases**, and the indication for surgery should always be carefully considered in the light of the extent of disease. Only approximately 20% of patients who undergo resection of a solitary brain metastasis, followed by radiotherapy, are still alive 5 years later, if they have not already died of the effects of their primary tumor. Brain metastases usually produce **extensive peritumoral edema** and often cause **epileptic seizures**; thus, **corticosteroids** and **antiepileptic drugs** can be given for palliation. This usually brings about a substantial, if only temporary, clinical improvement.

Additional Information

Neoplastic meningitis is the metastasis of tumor cells to the leptomeninges and subarachnoid space. It can arise with various types of primary tumor and accordingly designated, for example, carcinomatous, gliomatous, or lymphomatous meningitis. It is diagnosed by CSF cytology and carries a poor prognosis.

6.5 Cerebral Ischemia and Ischemic Stroke

Key Point
The term "stroke" encompasses both ischemic and hemorrhagic disturbances of the cerebral circulation that produce central neurologic deficits of acute or subacute onset. Ischemia accounts for 80 to 85% of stroke, and hemorrhage for 15 to 20%. Nontraumatic intracranial hemorrhage is discussed in section 6.6).

6.5.1 Overview

Roughly 2 per 1,000 persons per year sustain an ischemic stroke; the incidence of stroke rises markedly with age. Women are less commonly affected than men up to age 80, and equally commonly afterward.

Cerebral ischemia is critically impaired perfusion in an area of the brain.

Cerebral ischemia can be classified by

— **Etiology**: ischemia is mostly caused by the blockage of arteries by **emboli** (arterio-arterial emboli from atherosclerotic stenoses, as well as cardiogenic emboli), **macroangiopathy** (arteriosclerotic vascular occlusion), or **microangiopathy** (occlusion of smaller vessels by fibrinoid necrosis, also

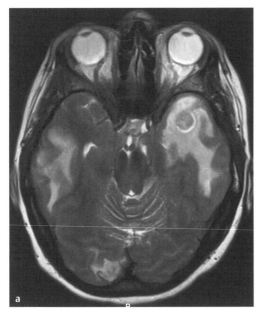
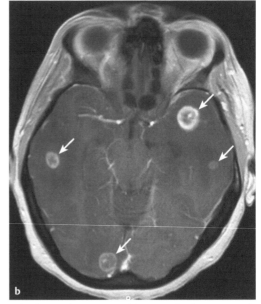

Fig. 6.18 Multiple brain metastases of lung cancer. (a) The T2-weighted spin-echo image reveals bitemporal and right occipital lesions with marked surrounding cerebral edema. **(b)** The T1-weighted image reveals four small contrast-enhancing nodules (→).

called "lipohyalinosis"). **Impaired venous outflow** is a less common cause.

- **Course**: transient ischemic attack (TIA) versus progressive or completed stroke.
- **Type of infarction**: territorial, watershed, border zone, lacunar.
- **The affected vessel** and the resulting vascular syndrome (e.g., middle cerebral artery [MCA] syndrome, posterior cerebral artery syndrome, basilar artery syndrome). Depending on the extent of tissue injury caused by ischemia, the ensuing **neurologic deficits** may be either transient or permanent.

Every ischemic event calls for **thorough diagnostic evaluation** to determine the cause, so that recurrences can be prevented. Moreover, **appropriate treatment** must be given immediately (above all, hemodynamic stabilization and surveillance, thrombolytic treatment where indicated, and recurrence prophylaxis). The diagnosis and treatment of stroke in a specialized institution (a so-called **stroke unit** or stroke center) is associated with a markedly better outcome.

6.5.2 Anatomy and Pathophysiology

Arterial Blood Supply of the Brain

To understand how the localization and extent of cerebral infarcts depends on the particular artery that is occluded, one must know the anatomy of the territories of the individual vessels, as well as their numerous **anastomoses**. The anastomotic arterial **circle of Willis**, at the base of the brain, provides a connection between the carotid and vertebral circulations and between the blood supplies of the right and left cerebral hemispheres (**Fig. 6.19**). The territories of the major cerebral arteries are shown in **Fig. 6.20**.

The Regulation of Cerebral Perfusion

Glucose is the brain's nearly exclusive source of energy. The brain accounts for only approximately 2% of body weight but receives approximately 15% of the cardiac output. Regulatory mechanisms ensure that the cerebral perfusion remains constant despite fluctuations in the arterial blood pressure, as long as the latter remains within a certain range. Thus, if the

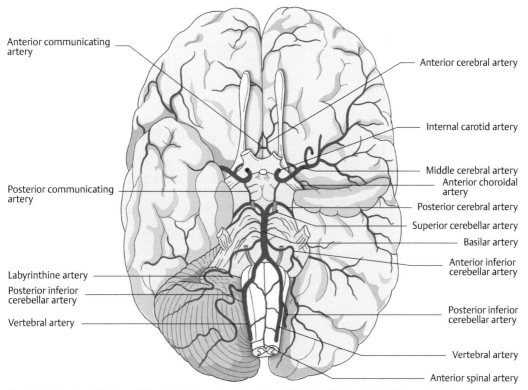

Anterior communicating artery

Anterior cerebral artery

Internal carotid artery

Middle cerebral artery
Anterior choroidal artery

Posterior communicating artery

Posterior cerebral artery

Superior cerebellar artery

Basilar artery

Anterior inferior cerebellar artery

Labyrinthine artery

Posterior inferior cerebellar artery

Vertebral artery

Posterior inferior cerebellar artery

Vertebral artery

Anterior spinal artery

Fig. 6.19   Arteries of the base of the brain. (Reproduced from Bähr M, Frotscher M. Duus' Topical Diagnosis in Neurology. 4th ed. Stuttgart: Thieme; 2005.)

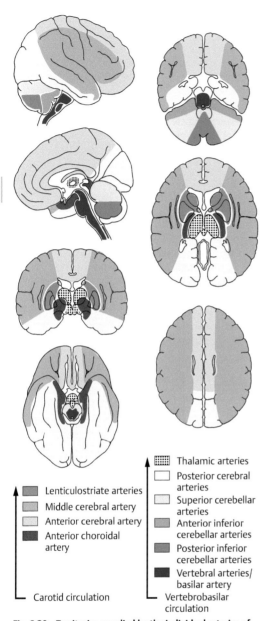

Thalamic arteries

Lenticulostriate arteries

Middle cerebral artery

Anterior cerebral artery

Anterior choroidal artery

Posterior cerebral arteries

Superior cerebellar arteries

Anterior inferior cerebellar arteries

Posterior inferior cerebellar arteries

Vertebral arteries/ basilar artery

Carotid circulation

Vertebrobasilar circulation

Fig. 6.20 Territories supplied by the individual arteries of the brain.

arterial blood pressure should fall, a **compensatory dilatation of the cerebral arteries** occurs to maintain cerebral perfusion, which is significantly reduced only when the systolic blood pressure falls below 70 mm Hg (or below 70% of the baseline value in hypertensive individuals). **Hyperventilation** and **intracranial hypertension** lessen cerebral perfusion, while **hypoventilation** (i.e., an elevated partial pressure of CO_2) increases it.

Consequences of Cerebral Hypoperfusion

Relative ischemia and penumbra. Normal cerebral perfusion is approximately 58 mL per 100 g of brain tissue per minute. Signs and symptoms of ischemia begin to appear when the perfusion falls below 22 mL per 100 g per minute. In this stage of **relative ischemia**, the functional metabolism of the affected brain tissue is impaired, but the **infarction threshold** has not yet been crossed and the tissue can regain its normal function as soon as the perfusion renormalizes. The longer the relative ischemia lasts, however, the less likely it is that normal function will be regained. The zone of tissue in which the local cerebral perfusion lies between the functional threshold and the infarction threshold is called the ischemic **penumbra** ("partial shadow"). Within the penumbra, brain perfusion is linearly related to the arterial blood pressure.

> **NOTE**
>
> The **penumbra** is of major importance in the diagnostic evaluation of stroke, as well as in therapeutic decision-making and prognostication:
> - Within the penumbra, perfusion is reduced, but diffusion is still normal (**perfusion–diffusion mismatch**). Thus, imaging studies (above all, MRI) can distinguish it from tissue that has already undergone infarction.
> - If the occluded vessel is promptly recanalized, the tissue in the penumbra can **largely survive** and regain its normal function. The penumbra thus represents the tissue at risk for further stroke that may be salvageable by revascularization. Imaging of the penumbra is an important aid to clinical decision-making.

The ischemic penumbra in a patient with an acute MCA occlusion is shown in **Fig. 6.21**. A normal cerebral angiogram was presented in an earlier chapter (see **Fig. 4.12**). An occlusion of the MCA is seen in **Fig. 6.24**.

Total ischemia causes irreversible structural damage of the affected region of the brain. If the blood supply of the entire brain is cut off, unconsciousness ensues in 10 to 12 seconds and cerebral electrical activity, as demonstrated by electroencephalogram (EEG), ceases in 30 to 40 seconds (**Fig. 6.22**). Cellular metabolism collapses, the sodium/potassium pump ceases to function, and interstitial fluid—that is, sodium and water—flows into the cells. The resulting cellular swelling is called **cytotoxic cerebral edema**. Later, when the blood–CSF barrier collapses, further plasma components, including osmotically active substances, enter the brain tissue; a net flow of fluid

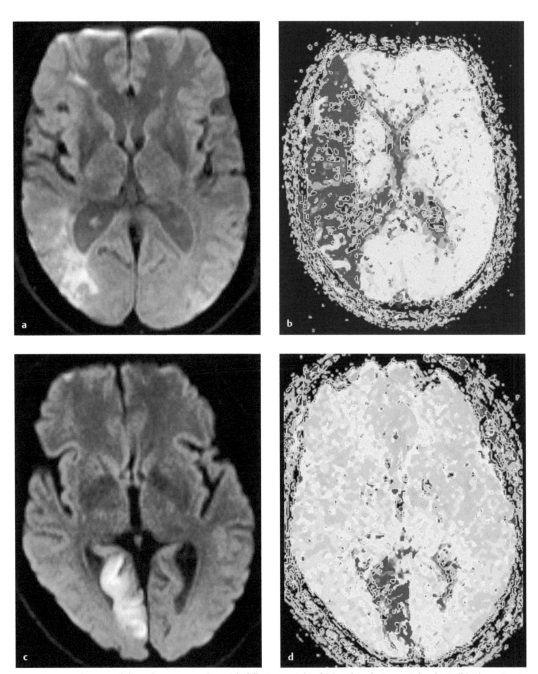

6

Fig. 6.21   Visualization of the ischemic penumbra with diffusion-weighted (a) and perfusion-weighted MRI (b). The patient is a 55-year-old man with acute left hemiparesis due to occlusion of the main stem of the right middle cerebral artery. For comparison, diffusion-weighted **(c)** and perfusion-weighted MRI scans **(d)** of a 58-year-old man with acute hemianopsia are also shown. **(a)** The diffusion-weighted image reveals a mottled hyperintense signal in the posterior portion of the right middle cerebral artery territory; most of the territory, however, has a normal diffusion signal. **(b)** The perfusion-weighted image is based on the time to peak uptake of contrast medium, which is delayed throughout the entire right middle cerebral artery territory. The penumbra is the area of tissue in which perfusion is diminished, but diffusion is normal. If the occluded vessel can be reopened early enough, bringing blood back into the hypoperfused area, the tissue in the penumbra will largely survive and regain its function. **(c)** Diffusion-weighted MRI for comparison. **(d)** Perfusion-weighted MRI for comparison. In this case, the area of abnormality is nearly congruent to that seen in (c); thus, there is no penumbra, i.e., the infarction is complete and no brain tissue can now be saved by recanalization.

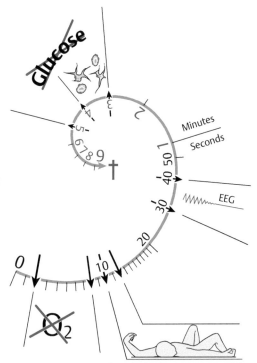

Fig. 6.22   Time course of cerebral ischemia. Diagram of the effect of sudden total deprivation of blood supply to the brain on tissue metabolism, consciousness, the EEG, neuronal morphology, and tissue glucose concentration.

from the intravascular space into the intercellular and intracellular spaces then produces **vasogenic cerebral edema**. In a vicious circle, these two varieties of edema lead to additional compression of brain tissue, thereby impairing the cerebral perfusion still further.

6.5.3 The Classification of Cerebral Ischemia by Severity

The severity of cerebral ischemia is correlated with its clinical course if untreated. Standardized scales and scores are available for its assessment. The most commonly used scale is the **National Institutes of Health Stroke Scale** (NIHSS, **Table 6.14**).

> **Practical Tip**
>
> The term "minor stroke" is commonly used to designate a stroke with only mild motor and/or sensory deficits, with an NIHSS score of 3 points at most (no more than 1 point on any item). Patients with a minor stroke are generally fully awake and alert and neuropsychologically intact. They have a good prognosis. A stroke with an NIHSS score of more than 15 points has a poor prognosis if untreated and is classified as a "severe stroke."

Table 6.14

NIHSS (National Institutes of Health Stroke Scale)

	Findings	0	1	2	3	4	Points
1a	Level of consciousness	Awake	Somnolent	Stupor	Coma	–	
1b	Orientation questions: Age? Month?	2 correct	1 correct	0 correct	–	–	
1c	Commands open and close (1) the eyes and (2) the nonparetic hand	2 correct	1 correct	0 correct	–	–	
2	Gaze paresis	None	Partial	Complete	–	–	
3	Visual field	Normal	Partial hemianopsia	Complete hemianopsia	Bilateral hemianopsia/ blindness	–	
4	Central facial palsy	None	Mild	Complete lower half of the face	Complete upper and lower halves of the face	–	
5a	Left arm motor function	No sinking when held up for 10 s	Sinks but does not touch underlying surface	Sinks onto underlying surface	No antigravity activity	No movement at all	
5b	Right arm motor function						
6a	Left leg motor function						
6b	Right leg motor function						
7	Limb ataxia	None	One limb affected	Two limbs affected	–	–	
8	Sensation	Normal	Partially impaired	Markedly impaired or lost	–	–	
9	Language	Normal	Moderate aphasia, communication possible	Severe aphasia, communication impossible	Global aphasia, mute	–	

Table 6.14

NIHSS (National Institutes of Health Stroke Scale) *(continued)*

	Findings	0	1	2	3	4	Points
10	Dysarthria	None	Slurred but intelligible speech	Unintelligible speech (or the patient is mute)	–	–	
11	Neglect, inattention	None	In one modality	In more than one modality	–	–	

Total = NIHSS score

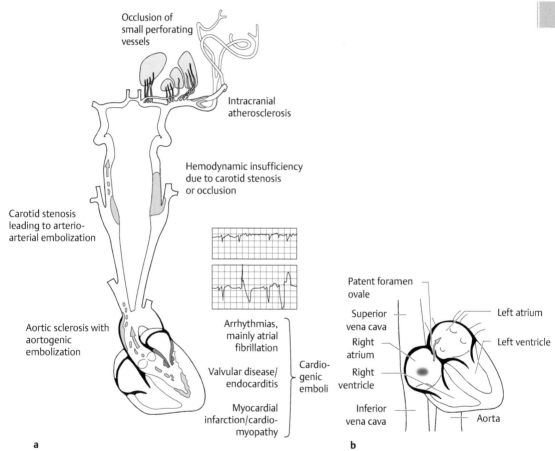

Fig. 6.23   The causes of stroke. (a) The most important causes of stroke. (Reproduced from Mattle H, Mumenthaler M. Neurologie. Stuttgart: Thieme; 2013.) **(b)** A paradoxical embolus through a patent foramen ovale.

6.5.4 Etiology, Risk Factors, and Primary Prophylaxis

Etiology
Ischemic stroke has multiple causes (**Fig. 6.23**). **Embolic events** and atherosclerotic **stenoses** of the major extra- and intracranial arteries play important roles, but there can also be hypertension-induced atherosclerotic changes of the midsized arteries or fibrinoid necrosis (lipohyalinosis) of the small arteries. A simplified classification by etiology divides ischemic strokes into five classes:

– **Macroangiopathy: atherosclerosis of large extra- and intracranial vessels**, leading to thrombosis in the region of an atherosclerotic plaque, hemodynamic insufficiency in the poststenotic circulation, or arterio-arterial embolism.

- **Cardiogenic and aortogenic embolism**, mainly due to atrial fibrillation, but also as a complication of myocardial infarction, valve replacement, endocarditis, or cardiomyopathy.
- **Microangiopathy: cerebral small-vessel disease/ arteriolosclerosis**, usually due to hypertension, most commonly seen in the elderly.
- **Other etiologies**, for example, vasculopathy, dissection, arteritis, coagulopathy, paradoxical embolism, right-to-left shunt.
- **Undetermined etiology**.

Table 6.15 may be a useful aid to the systematic search for the cause of stroke.

Risk Factors

Factors that increase the risk of stroke include the following:
- **Advanced age**.
- **Positive family history** with early onset of atherosclerotic disease (< 55 years).
- **Prior history of cardio- or cerebrovascular disease** or **peripheral arterial occlusive disease**.
- **Arterial hypertension**.
- **Sedentary habits**.
- **Obesity, truncal obesity, hypercholesterolemia**.
- **Diabetes mellitus**.
- **Sleep apnea syndrome**.
- **Cigarette smoking**.
- **Alcoholism**.
- **Estrogen use** (estradiol, mainly in combination with cigarette smoking).
- **Migraine** with aura.
- **Heart disease**, especially **atrial fibrillation** or **flutter**.
- **Stenosis of the cerebral vasculature**, especially the **internal carotid artery**.

| NOTE

The most important risk factors for stroke are **aterial fibrillation** and **arterial hypertension**.

Primary Prophylaxis in Patients with Risk Factors for Stroke

Cardiovascular risk factors should be prevented or treated if present. In particular, **atrial fibrillation** carries a high risk of stroke.

Atrial Fibrillation

Epidemiology. Atrial fibrillation becomes more common with increasing age; it affects approximately 8% of women and 10% of men older than 80 years and causes more than 10% of all cases of ischemic stroke. The risk of having a stroke due to atrial fibrillation increases with the number of other risk factors that are simultaneously present. The **CHA$_2$DS$_2$VASc score**

is an instrument for estimating the annual risk of stroke on the basis of multiple risk factors: age, sex, congestive heart failure, diabetes, arteriopathy, and prior stroke, TIA, or systemic embolism. In most patients, the estimated annual risk of stroke is 2 to 7%.

Pathogenesis of stroke. Atrial fibrillation leads to a disturbance of blood flow in the cardiac atria, which are usually enlarged as well. This, in turn, may lead to stasis and thrombus formation, most often in the left atrium. A loose thrombus or part of a thrombus can embolize into the systemic circulation and cause an infarction.

Clinical features. Patients with atrial fibrillation who suffer a stroke are older on average than the overall collective of stroke patients. Large territorial infarcts are common in this group and usually fatal. Thus, stroke due to of atrial fibrillation carries a high mortality and survivors are often severely disabled.

Stroke prevention.

| NOTE

Anticoagulation can prevent two-thirds of all strokes due to atrial fibrillation.

The new anticoagulants apixaban, edoxaban, and rivaroxaban (factor Xa antagonists) and dabigatran (a thrombin inhibitor) are particularly suitable for the anticoagulation of patients with atrial fibrillation. They are at least as effective as vitamin K antagonists (coumarins).

Dissection

Epidemiology. Arterial dissection, although rare, is the second most common cause of stroke in young adults, after atherosclerosis.

Pathogenesis of stroke. An intimal tear leads to splitting of the vascular wall layers. A mural hematoma can occlude the vessel or give rise to an arterio-arterial embolus.

Clinical features. Patients with an internal carotid artery dissection can present with the following symptoms and signs:
- Pain in the neck, head, or orbit (see also section 14.2.4).
- Horner syndrome (see section 12.3.5 and **Fig. 12.15**).
- Lower cranial nerve deficits.

In case of vertebral artery dissection:
- Nuchal and occipital pain.
- Medullary and cerebellar infarction.
- Rarely, basilar artery thrombosis and extensive brainstem infarction.

Table 6.15

Etiologic classification of ischemic stroke

Cause	
Atherosclerosis	▬ Major extra- and intracranial vessels, including aortic arch: thrombosis, arterio-arterial embolism, hemodynamic insufficiency
	▬ Aorta
	▬ Small vessels: lacunar infarction
Cardiogenic embolism	**Mural thrombus** due to myocardial infarction, cardiomyopathy, myocardial aneurysm
	Valvular heart disease including rheumatic heart-valve disease, bacterial and nonbacterial endocarditis, prosthetic valves
	Arrhythmia including atrial fibrillation, sick sinus syndrome, brady- and tachyarrhythmias
	Atrial myxoma
	Paradoxical embolism through an open foramen ovale or atrial septal defect
	Atrial thrombus in aneurysm of the atrial septum
Venous and venous sinus thrombosis	**Septic sinus thrombosis**
	Coagulopathy (e.g., polycythemia, antithrombin deficiency), pregnancy, drugs (oral contraceptives, glucocorticoids)
	Bland, i.e., without identifiable cause
Hematologic diseases	**Thrombophilia** due to protein C, protein S, or antithrombin-III deficiency, antiphospholipid antibodies, anticardiolipin antibodies, paroxysmal nocturnal hemoglobinuria
	Hemoglobinopathy, e.g., sickle-cell anemia, thalassemia
	Hyperviscosity syndrome due to polyglobulia, thrombocytosis, leukocytosis, macroglobulinemia, myeloma, polycythemia vera, myeloproliferative syndromes
Vasculitis	**Primary CNS vasculitis**, granulomatous angiitis of the CNS
	Systemic necrotizing vasculitis with CNS involvement, e.g., in periarteritis nodosa, Churg–Strauss syndrome, giant-cell arteritis (polymyalgia rheumatica, temporal arteritis), Takayasu's arteritis, Wegener granulomatosis, lymphomatoid vasculitis, hypersensitivity vasculitis
	Connective-tissue diseases and collagenoses with CNS involvement, e.g., systemic lupus erythematosus, scleroderma, rheumatoid arthritis, Behçet disease, mixed connective tissue disease
	Infectious vasculitis, e.g., due to HIV, tuberculosis, borreliosis, neurosyphilis, fungi, mononucleosis, CMV infection, herpes zoster, hepatitis B, rickettsia, bacterial endocarditis
Toxins	**Illicit drugs**, e.g., cocaine (also as crack), amphetamines, LSD, heroin
	Medications, e.g., sympathomimetic drugs, ergotamines, triptans, intravenous immunoglobulins
Nonatherosclerotic vascular diseases	**Dissections of the extra- or intracranial arteries supplying the brain** or of the **aorta**, spontaneous or due (e.g.) to trauma, Marfan syndrome, or fibromuscular dysplasia
	Posttraumatic thrombosis or avulsion of arteries supplying the brain
	Vasospasm after subarachnoid hemorrhage
	Arteriovenous malformations
	Hereditary vascular diseases, e.g., Osler–Weber–Rendu disease (hereditary telangiectasia), moyamoya,[a] CADASIL, and other familial cerebral vasculopathies; fibromuscular dysplasia in neurofibromatosis
	Pulmonary venous thrombosis
	Dolichoectasia[b]
	Amyloid angiopathy (β-amyloid deposition in the walls of cerebral blood vessels)
Various other causes	**Vasospasm**, e.g., in migraine, reversible cerebral vasoconstriction syndrome
	Metabolic diseases, e.g., homocystinuria, hyperhomocysteinemia, Fabry disease (lysosomal storage disease with ceramide trihexoside deposition in blood vessels), MELAS, and other mitochondrial encephalomyopathies
	Other sources of emboli, e.g., fat and air emboli, pseudovasculitic syndrome with cholesterol emboli, tumor emboli, distal emboli from giant aneurysms
	Collagenoses (e.g., in neurofibromatosis)
	Other **pulmonary diseases**
Iatrogenic stroke	Angiography and surgery on the carotid arteries, aorta, and heart
	Injection of steroid crystals, fat embolism, etc.
	Liposculpturing (liposuction and reinjection of adipose tissue)
Stroke of no identifiable cause	

Abbreviations: CADASIL, cerebral autosomal dominant arteriopathy with subcortical infarcts and leukencephalopathy; CNS, central nervous system; HIV, human immunodeficiency virus; LSD, lysergic acid diethylamide; MELAS, mitochondrial encephalomyopathy, lactic acidosis, and stroke-like episodes.
[a] A rare disease, most prevalent in Japan but also seen elsewhere, involving stenosis of the cerebral vessels due to fibrosis of the intima of the distal portion of the carotid artery. Collateral vessels form, resulting in the typical angiographic appearance of a puff of smoke (in Japanese, "moyamoya").
[b] Dilated macroangiopathy with widening and tortuosity of the cerebral blood vessels.

Table 6.16		
Classification of cerebral ischemia by temporal course		
Designation	Deficits and their duration	Remarks
TIA	**Transient** focal neurologic and/or neuropsychological deficits); transient visual disturbance in one eye (amaurosis fugax). **Duration usually 2–15 min**, rarely as long as 24 h[a]	The current definition of TIA requires the **absence of any visual damage to brain tissue** in imaging studies. Any such damage classifies the ischemic episode as a stroke whatever its duration
Stroke in evolution, progressive stroke	Stroke with neurologic deficits that **continue to worsen** for hours or days after onset	The **cause of progression** must be sought: progression may be due to repeated strokes, progression of a thrombosis or embolism, hemorrhagic transformation of an infarct, cerebral edema, hypotension, etc.
Completed stroke	Established neurologic deficit that is irreversible or only partly reversible	**Rehabilitation** enables the improvement or, at least, the retention of residual functional abilities

Abbreviation: TIA, transient ischemic attack.
[a]In earlier nomenclature, the term "reversible ischemic neurologic deficit" (RIND) designated transient ischemic attacks of longer duration (up to 7 days). This term is now hardly ever used.

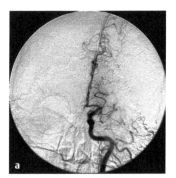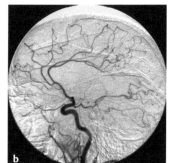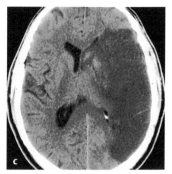

Fig. 6.24   Infarct in the territory of the left middle cerebral artery in a 60-year-old man with acute right hemiplegia. **(a)** The left carotid angiogram (anteroposterior view) reveals occlusion of the main stem of the middle cerebral artery at its origin. Only the anterior cerebral artery is visualized. **(b)** The lateral view shows only the pericallosal artery, with its branches, and the posterior cerebral artery, while the middle cerebral artery and its branches are not seen (cf. normal carotid angiogram, **Fig. 4.13**). **(c)** A CT scan obtained 2 days after the onset of symptoms reveals a massive infarct in the territory of the middle cerebral artery, extending from the cortex to the basal ganglia.

Treatment. Patients with local symptoms, such as pain, can be treated with heparin or acetylsalicylic acid (ASA) and symptomatic pain treatment. In case of stroke, the treatment is the same as for acute stroke of other causes (see section 6.5.9).

6.5.5 The Dynamic Time Course of Cerebral Ischemia

Cerebral hypoperfusion can cause a wide variety of clinical manifestations. In clinical practice, these are often classified by their **temporal course** and their degree of **reversibility or irreversibility** (Table 6.16). Although classification in this way is useful, it says nothing about the underlying etiology of the ischemic events. Moreover, the boundaries between the listed entities are not sharp.

6.5.6 Infarct Types

Three different basic types of ischemic stroke are distinguished from one another on the basis of the caliber of the vessels involved.

Territorial Infarction

Territorial infarcts are mainly produced by **occlusions of the main trunks or major branches of cerebral arteries (cerebral macroangiopathy)**, which may be due to thrombosis, embolism, or other causes. The infarct includes both cortex and subcortical white matter and sometimes the basal ganglia and thalamus (**Fig. 6.24, Fig. 12.2**). It is usually possible to infer which vessel has been occluded from the pattern of neurologic deficits that are produced, for example, in strokes involving the territory of the MCA (**Fig. 6.25**) or the posterior cerebral artery.

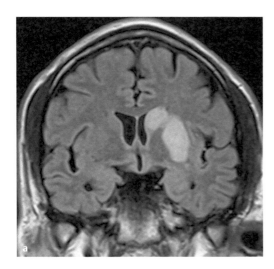

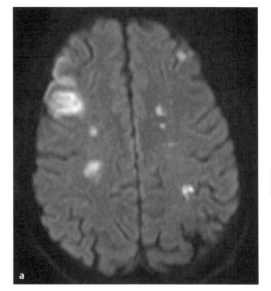

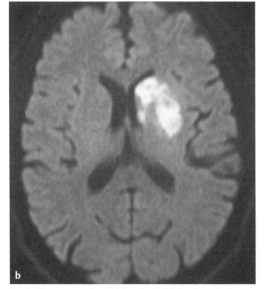

Fig. 6.25   Acute territorial infarct in the left basal ganglia due to occlusion of the main trunk of the middle cerebral artery. The affected areas include the striatum and the anterior portion of the internal capsule. **(a)** FLAIR sequence; **(b)** diffusion-weighted MR image.

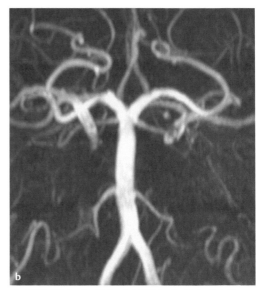

Fig. 6.26   Watershed infarct. (a) Watershed infarcts in the border area between the territories of the anterior and middle cerebral arteries, as seen on diffusion-weighted MRI. **(b)** A 37-year-old man with bilateral internal carotid artery occlusion due to dissection. In the center of the image, the vertebral arteries and the basilar artery are seen; they provide blood to the anterior circulation via collateral vessels. (Reproduced from Mattle H, Mumenthaler M, Neurologie. Stuttgart: Thieme; 2013.)

Watershed Infarction

Watershed infarcts (also called border zone infarcts) are infarcts of hemodynamic origin that are likewise due to **macroangiopathic processes.** Arterial narrowing **impairs perfusion in the vulnerable regions at the borders between the territories of two or more arteries** (**Fig. 6.26**). If the perfusion pressure is inadequate, infarction ensues.

Lacunar Infarction

Lacunar infarcts are caused by **microangiopathy,** usually **arteriolosclerosis** or **fibrinoid necrosis** (lipohyalinosis) due to hypertension. The infarcts (**lacunes**) are

less than 1.5 cm in diameter and often **multiple.** They are found mainly in the basal ganglia, thalamus, and brainstem, and sometimes in the cerebral cortex and subcortical white matter (**Fig. 6.27**). Their clinical presentation depends on their number and localization. Multiple subcortical infarcts due to hypertension are the hallmark of **subcortical arteriosclerotic encephalopathy,** which was once called Binswanger disease and is now generally designated in purely descriptive

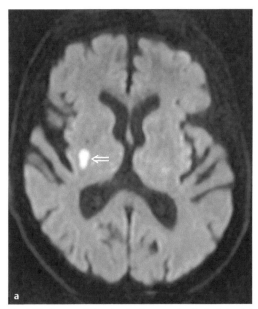 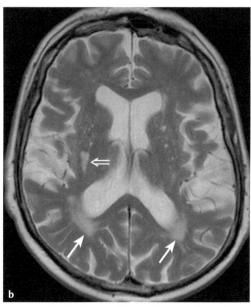

Fig. 6.27   Lacunar infarction in the posterior limb of the right internal capsule. This 72-year-old man with metabolic syndrome presented with an acute left hemisensory syndrome caused by cerebral microangiopathy. **(a)** The diffusion-weighted MR image shows a hyperintense area corresponding to the infarct (⇨). **(b)** The T2-weighted image reveals multiple further lesions as well as flatter, rather than rounded, lesions (→) behind the occipital horns that are typical of cerebral microangiopathy (vascular leukencephalopathy).

terms as **vascular leukencephalopathy**. This entity is associated with vascular dementia (see section 6.12.5).

> **NOTE**
>
> Ischemic stroke occurs when persistent ischemia or a complete interruption of the blood supply to a particular area of the brain produces irreversible destruction of brain tissue. The resulting neurologic deficits usually arise quite suddenly (whence the term "stroke") but in rare cases progress over a longer period of time ("stroke in evolution"). If untreated, they are irreversible, or at most only partly reversible.

6.5.7 Clinical Stroke Syndromes

The type of neurologic deficit caused by a stroke is predictably related to the site of the ischemic lesion, and thus **the site of the lesion can be inferred from the deficit**. We will now briefly summarize the clinical manifestations of the major cerebrovascular syndromes and the typical deficits produced by ischemia in circumscribed areas of the brain.

Territory of the Carotid Artery

Middle cerebral artery. About half of all strokes affect the territory of the MCA. The site of occlusion (main trunk vs. branch of the MCA) determines the clinical manifestations. As a rule, a mainly **brachiofacial hemiparesis and hemisensory deficit** are found, often accompanied by **homonymous hemi- or quadrant-anopsia** and, in the initial phase, a **horizontal gaze**

palsy toward the side of the hemiparesis. An MCA occlusion on the language-dominant (usually left) side additionally produces **aphasia** and **apraxia**, while one on the nondominant side produces **impairment of spatial orientation**. An occlusion of the main stem of the MCA causes ischemia not only of the cortex, but also of the basal ganglia and internal capsule, producing a more severe contralateral hemiparesis. An infarct involving a large percentage (or all) of the MCA territory can give rise to massive cerebral edema and intracranial hypertension; this is called "malignant MCA infarction." In the aftermath of the stroke, if the hemiparesis fails to improve over time, or does so only partially, a typical, permanent impairment of gait results: circumduction of the spastically extended lower limb, flexion of the paretic upper limb at the wrist and elbow, and absence of arm swing on the affected side (**Wernicke–Mann gait; Fig. 6.28**).

 Practical Tip

Hemiparesis, hemisensory deficit, and homonymous hemianopsia (all of them contralateral to the lesion), along with aphasia in lesions of the dominant hemisphere and hemineglect and impaired spatial perception in lesions of the nondominant hemisphere, constitute the full clinical picture of MCA infarction.

Anterior choroidal artery. This vessel is much less commonly the origin of stroke than the MCA. Ischemia

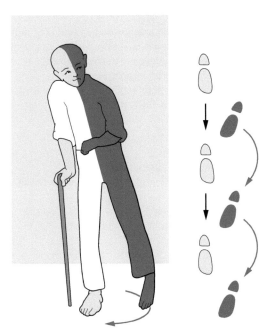

Fig. 6.28   Typical gait disturbance of a hemiplegic patient. Circumduction of the spastically paretic leg because of predominant extensor tone and flexion of the spastically paretic arm at the elbow because of predominant flexor tone.

in the territory of the anterior choroidal artery causes a **homonymous visual field defect**, a **hemisensory deficit**, and, less commonly, **hemiparesis**. The clinical manifestations resemble those of occlusion of the lenticulostriate arteries (branches of the MCA supplying the basal ganglia and internal capsule). There may also be extrapyramidal motor signs, such as hemiballism.

Anterior cerebral artery. Infarction in the territory of this artery, accounting for approximately 5% of all strokes, causes **contralateral hemiparesis mainly affecting the lower limb**, sometimes accompanied by contralateral ataxia and, if the lesion is left-sided, by apraxia. Occasionally, there may be apathy, abulia (pathologic lack of drive and motivation), and urinary incontinence.

 Practical Tip

Watershed infarction (cf. Fig. 6.26) in the border zone between the territories of the middle and anterior cerebral arteries typically produces contralateral motor and sensory deficits that are most prominent in the lower limb. If the perfusion is critical, these deficits can be more intense when the patient is standing. A tremor that is most prominent in the lower limb can also become apparent when the patient stands.

Ophthalmic artery. Transient ischemia in the territory of this vessel produces **amaurosis fugax** (transient monocular blindness), while longer-lasting ischemia causes **retinal infarction**. Retinal ischemia is often due to embolism of cholesterol crystals from ulcerating plaques in the internal carotid artery into the ophthalmic artery. Embolized crystals within the arteries of the retina can occasionally be seen by ophthalmoscopy.

Internal carotid artery. Stenosis or occlusion of the internal carotid artery can simultaneously cause ischemia of the eye with monocular visual loss (as in ophthalmic artery occlusion) and a large infarct in the territory of the middle cerebral artery. This **oculocerebral syndrome** is rare, however, as ischemia in the territory of the internal carotid artery usually presents with **either** monocular visual loss **or** variably severe hemiparesis and neuropsychological deficits.

Territory of the Vertebral Arteries and Basilar Artery

Posterior cerebral artery. This artery is involved in 10% of all ischemic strokes, often bilaterally (embolism). Proximal occlusion can lead to infarction in the cerebral peduncle, the thalamus, mediobasal portions of the temporal lobe, and the occipital lobe, with a similar constellation of clinical findings to MCA occlusion. The most prominent clinical sign of a distal occlusion (beyond the origin of the posterior communicating artery) is **contralateral homonymous hemianopsia**, possibly combined with neuropsychological deficits.

Thalamic infarction. Thalamic stroke results from occlusion of one of the perforating arteries supplying the thalamus. It usually presents with a **contralateral hemisensory deficit**, in addition to mild paresis and hemiataxia. The patient's **memory**, too, is often impaired.

Basilar artery. Occlusion of the main stem or of a branch of the basilar artery causes **brainstem, cerebellar**, and **thalamic** signs. Main stem thrombosis generally causes tetraparesis and is often fatal. Ventral pontine infarction can present clinically with **locked-in syndrome** (described in section 5.5.5).

The **basilar tip syndrome** reflects a bilateral midbrain and thalamic infarct, usually due to an embolus that becomes lodged in the distal portion of the basilar artery proximal to its bifurcation into the posterior cerebral arteries. Its typical manifestations are impaired consciousness and upward gaze palsy, sometimes accompanied by a uni- or bilateral hemisensory deficit, ataxia, uni- or bilateral hemianopsia, and neuropsychological deficits such as amnesia and cortical blindness.

Brainstem infarction. Brainstem strokes are usually lacunar. They arise in the territory of one or more small perforating arteries that branch off the basilar trunk and can be seen by MRI (**Fig. 6.29**). Their clinical presentation depends on the particular nuclei and fiber tracts that they affect. Brainstem stroke therefore takes many different clinical forms, corresponding to the wide variety of functions served by brainstem structures. As a rule, brainstem stroke causes **ipsilateral cranial nerve deficits** and a **contralateral hemisensory defect** and/or **hemiparesis**.

The large number of brainstem vascular syndromes that have been described and given eponymous names are only rarely seen in "pure" form in clinical practice. The most clinically relevant brainstem syndrome is **Wallenberg syndrome** (**Fig. 6.29**), which is due to occlusion of the posterior inferior cerebellar artery. Various brainstem syndromes reflecting involvement of different portions of the brainstem are listed in **Table 6.17**.

Territory of the Cerebellar Arteries

Cerebellar infarction. Occlusion of the **superior, anterior inferior, or posterior cerebellar artery** presents with vertigo, nausea, unsteady gait, dysarthria, and often acute headache. The neurologic examination reveals **ataxia**, **dysmetria**, and **nystagmus**. Often, simultaneous infarction of part of the brainstem produces additional brainstem signs. Not uncommonly, edema in and around the infarcted area rapidly leads to a life-threatening elevation of pressure in the posterior fossa, with progressive impairment of consciousness (with or without accompanying occlusive hydrocephalus). A typical MR image of cerebellar stroke is presented in **Fig. 6.30**.

6.5.8 Diagnostic Evaluation

Acute Diagnostic Evaluation

The acute diagnostic evaluation focuses on the following questions:

- Is the stroke ischemic or hemorrhagic in nature?
- What are its anatomic site and extent?
- What is its cause?

To answer these questions, the following are needed:

- **A precise history** including not only the present illness, but also the past medical history, with special attention to risk factors and systemic illnesses.
- **A thorough clinical neurologic examination** enabling localization of the lesion.
- **Physical examination of the cardiovascular system** (measurement of pulse and blood pressure and auscultation of the heart, the carotid arteries, and perhaps other vessels, depending on the

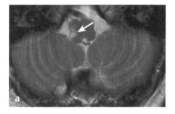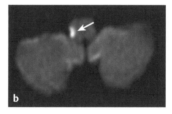

Fig. 6.29 Acute lacunar infarction of the medulla. This 63-year-old man presented with Wallenberg syndrome. **(a)** T2-weighted spin-echo MR image. **(b)** Diffusion-weighted MR image that reveals the lesion particularly clearly (→).

| Table 6.17 |

Selected brainstem syndromes

Name	Localization	Ipsilateral signs	Contralateral signs	Special features
Wallenberg syndrome	Dorsolateral medulla	Horner syndrome, vocal cord paresis, palatal and posterior pharyngeal paresis, trigeminal nerve deficit, hemiataxia	Dissociated sensory disturbance (loss of pain and temperature sensation on the trunk and limbs)	Nystagmus; this syndrome is caused by occlusion of the posterior inferior cerebellar artery
Benedikt syndrome (upper red nucleus syndrome)	Midbrain, red nucleus	Oculomotor palsy, sometimes vertical gaze palsy	Hemiataxia (sometimes), intention tremor, hemiparesis (often without Babinski sign)	Staggering gait
Weber syndrome	Midbrain	Oculomotor nerve palsy	Hemiparesis	
Millard–Gubler syndrome	Caudal pons	(Peripheral) abducens and facial palsy	Hemiparesis	

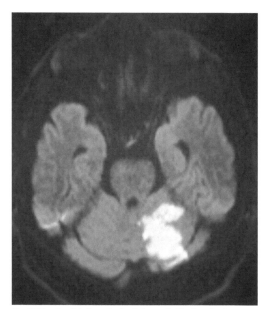

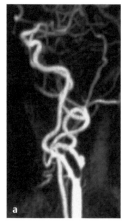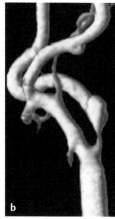

Fig. 6.31   High-grade stenosis of the left internal carotid artery. (a) Contrast-enhanced MR angiography of the cervical vessels shows atherosclerotic stenosis of the internal carotid artery at a typical site distal to its origin from the bifurcation of the common carotid artery. **(b)** The stenosis is seen even more clearly in the 3D reconstruction.

Fig. 6.30   Fresh infarct in the left cerebellar hemisphere, in the distribution of the superior cerebellar artery. Diffusion-weighted MR image.

clinical situation; particular attention should be paid to bruits and to any irregularities of the pulse that suggest arrhythmia).

Ancillary Testing in the Acute Phase

Any patient with a central neurologic deficit of acute onset is likely to have suffered a cerebrovascular event, probably of the ischemic variety. Nonetheless, **a CT or MRI** is indispensable to differentiate ischemia from hemorrhage and to rule out other, nonvascular etiologies.

> **NOTE**
>
> The history and physical examination alone cannot reliably differentiate ischemia from hemorrhage as the cause of the deficit; thus, a CT or MRI is needed. All stroke patients should be in a CT or MRI scanner no later than 25 minutes after their arrival in the hospital.

CT. Early CT reveals **acute brain hemorrhage** with high sensitivity (hyperdense lesion). Therefore, all patients with suspected stroke should have a CT scan in the acute phase to determine the further course of their treatment, even though ischemia only becomes evident a few hours later. A **perfusion CT** with contrast medium can demonstrate the core infarct zone and the penumbra, similarly to MRI. CT is less time-consuming than MRI.

MRI. MRI reveals the **infarct zone and perifocal edema** as soon as the patient begins to experience symptoms, and it displays brainstem and cerebellar infarcts more clearly than CT. **Diffusion-weighted MRI** clearly reveals the ischemic zone; **perfusion MRI**, in combination with diffusion-weighted MRI, reveals the penumbra (zone of potentially salvageable tissue; cf. **Fig. 6.21**).

Angiographic CT/MRI. These studies (**Fig. 6.31**) of the extra- and intracranial vessels can reveal stenosis, occlusion, or collateral circulation. They are generally most useful in the acute phase as an aid to the decision whether to attempt endovascular treatment.

Neurovascular ultrasound. This method, too, can reveal stenosis, occlusion, or collateral circulation; it is more commonly used in routine outpatient evaluation than in the emergency evaluation of acute stroke.

Electrocardiography. An ECG may reveal arrhythmia or regional myocardial dysfunction, pointing to a possible cardioembolic event, or else a prior or current (acute) myocardial infarction.

Laboratory tests. These are mainly used to identify risk factors, infectious/inflammatory disorders, metabolic disorders, and coagulopathies. The more important tests can generally be performed on an emergency basis.
- Electrolytes: sodium, potassium, calcium.
- Hemoglobin, complete blood count.
- Erythrocyte sedimentation rate, C-reactive protein → inflammation?

- Platelet count, prothrombin time, D-dimers if indicated → coagulopathy?
- Blood sugar, HbA$_{1c}$, liver enzymes, lipid profile → risk factors?
- Urea, creatinine → renal failure?
- Creatine kinase, troponin → cardiac problem?
- Syphilis serology.

Further Diagnostic Tests after the Acute Phase

Depending on the clinical situation, the following tests can also be performed after the acute phase:

- Angio-CT, angio-MRI (see **Fig. 4.8.**, **Fig. 4.9**, and **Fig. 6.31**), or neurovascular ultrasound (see **Fig. 4.32**, **Fig. 4.33**) if not already performed in the acute phase.
- **Echocardiography** (transthoracic or transesophageal) to reveal valvular disease and sources of emboli in the heart and aortic arch.
- **Long-term ECG** (24-hour ECG, perhaps event recording with an event or loop recorder, or long-term recording) to demonstrate arrhythmias that can give rise to emboli.
- **Cerebral angiography** (see **Fig. 4.13**, **Fig. 4.14**, **Fig. 4.15**, **Fig. 6.32**) to reveal stenosis or occlusion of the cerebral blood vessels or other, rarer types of vascular lesion that cannot be diagnosed by noninvasive means (also performed in the acute phase as a prerequisite to thrombolytic treatment).
- **Pulse oximetry** or apnea test.

6.5.9 Treatment of Ischemic Stroke

> **NOTE**
>
> Once an ischemic stroke has been diagnosed and an intracerebral hemorrhage has been excluded, the initial goal of treatment is to minimize the amount of brain tissue that will be irreversibly damaged. Brain tissue in the zone of relative ischemia (the penumbra) can be salvaged by prompt restoration of its blood supply. The sooner the lytic treatment can be provided, the better.

Practical Tip

All patients with suspected stroke should be immediately transported to an acute-care hospital with a specialized facility for the treatment of stroke (stroke unit or stroke center). Treatment in a stroke unit or stroke center markedly improves the clinical outcome.

Management in the Acute Phase Immediately upon Arrival

Monitoring. The vital signs and neurologic functions should be monitored continuously.

Maintenance of adequate perfusion pressure. The blood pressure must be kept relatively high (values up to 200–220 mm Hg systolic and 110 mm Hg diastolic are tolerable; reduction to 180 mm Hg systolic only before intravenous thrombolysis).

Optimization of O$_2$ delivery. The airways must be free; in case of hypoxia, supplementary oxygen must be administered and the cause treated. Pneumonia should be prevented or treated if present.

Stabilization of cardiovascular function. The patient must be adequately hydrated; heart failure and/or arrhythmia must be treated if present.

Thrombolytic treatment whenever indicated. The options include:

- **Intravenous (systemic) thrombolysis** with rtPA (recombinant tissue plasminogen activator) within 4.5 hours of symptom onset (3 is better, 5 the absolute limit), particularly in cases of peripheral rather than main stem vessel occlusion, with clinically mild to moderate stroke.
- **Intra-arterial (endovascular, interventional) thrombolysis**/recanalization up to 6 hours from symptom onset (**Fig. 6.32**), primarily in cases of clinically severe stroke.
- **Mechanical recanalization** within 8 hours of symptom onset.
- In cases of severe stroke, or if an interhospital transfer is needed before the patient can be treated, **combined intravenous and intra-arterial treatment** (so-called **bridging treatment**) is an option.
- If thrombolytic treatment and mechanical recanalization are contraindicated or not possible, **ASA** is the drug of first choice.

Before rtPA is given, contraindications such as anticoagulation, a fresh trauma, hemorrhage, recent surgery, or endocarditis should be ruled out. Even if rtPA is contraindicated, mechanical recanalization is usually still possible.

Treatment of cerebral edema. See the section on cerebral edema.

Treatment of fever and epileptic seizures. Pathologic oxygen- and nutrient-consuming metabolic processes such as fever or epileptic seizures must be treated if present.

Optimal blood sugar management. Prevention and, if necessary, treatment of hyper- or hypoglycemia.

6

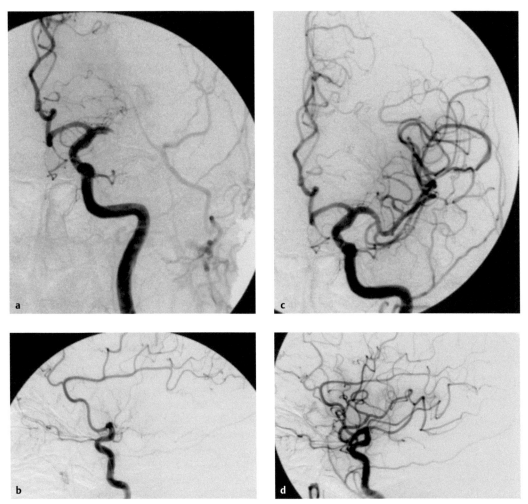

Fig. 6.32   Proximal occlusion of the middle cerebral artery before and after endovascular recanalization. (a,b) Images before recanalization; **(c,d)** images after recanalization.

Further Therapeutic Measures and Secondary Prevention

While the acute measures discussed earlier are being taken, the treatment team should begin to consider further therapeutic strategies to **prevent recurrent stroke**. Depending on the etiology of the patient's problem, these can include **rehabilitation** and **prophylactic measures**.

Early rehabilitation. Mobilization (decubitus prophylaxis), aspiration prophylaxis, physical and occupational therapy, and, if needed, speech therapy.

Prevention of recurrent stroke.

— General medical treatment:
- Minimization of vascular risk profile (optimal treatment of hypertension, diabetes mellitus, hypercholesterolemia, or sleep apnea syndrome, if present, and cessation of smoking).
- Treatment of heart failure and/or arrhythmia.

— **Antithrombotic therapy**: the type to be given depends on the etiology of the stroke. The following options are available:
- **Inhibition of platelet aggregation** (mainly aspirin, but also clopidogrel or aspirin with dipyridamole); the treatment begins immediately or 24 hours after intravenous thrombolytic therapy, and is usually continued indefinitely.
- **Full heparinization**: rare, for example, in cases of dissection or venous thrombosis.
- **Oral anticoagulation** (mainly after cardio- or aortoembolic stroke, venous thrombosis, venous sinus thrombosis, or dissections, possibly after ASA has already been given).
- **Surgical therapy**: endarterectomy for high-grade carotid stenosis (in symptomatic patients at any age or in asymptomatic patients younger than 75 years).

- **Endovascular therapy**: stent insertion for high-grade carotid stenosis if endarterectomy is contraindicated or too risky, or in cases of subclavian or intracranial stenosis (likewise in symptomatic patients at any age or in asymptomatic patients younger than 75 years).
- In younger patients with paradoxical embolism through a **patent foramen ovale**, interventional closure of the foramen ovale can be considered.

6.5.10 Special Types of Cerebral Ischemia

Transient Ischemic Attacks

Definition. TIAs are defined as transient focal neurologic manifestations or neuropsychological deficits (e.g., aphasia) **without any discernible abnormality** in imaging studies. A TIA can also present as a transient visual disturbance in one eye (**amaurosis fugax**). TIAs generally last **2 to 15 minutes**, although, by definition, they may persist for up to 4 hours.

> **NOTE**
>
> TIAs are not just small and clinically insignificant strokes. They are warning signs and harbingers of what may be a major stroke in the offing. Any patient with a TIA must be neurologically evaluated and treated without delay.

About 20% of all strokes are preceded by one or more TIAs; in about two-thirds of cases, the stroke follows within 3 to 4 days. Patients with vascular risk factors are at particular risk of having a stroke after a TIA, with a greater than 20% risk of stroke in the ensuing 7 days. Patients with TIAs, like stroke patients, should undergo a neurologic diagnostic evaluation and targeted prophylactic treatment as soon as possible, preferably on an emergency basis. These are performed according to the same criteria listed earlier for stroke (see sections 6.5.8 and 6.5.9).

 Practical Tip

Amaurosis fugax is often due to carotid stenosis. Patients with amaurosis fugax should be evaluated immediately with carotid ultrasound, angio-CT, or angio-MRI.

Venous Thrombosis and Venous Sinus Thrombosis

> **NOTE**
>
> Besides the much more common arterial disorders just discussed, obstruction to venous flow can also cause cerebral ischemia. Venous obstruction is usually due to thrombosis of the large venous channels draining the brain (venous sinus thrombosis) and of the veins that empty into them (cerebral venous thrombosis).

Etiology and frequency. Thromboses of the cerebral veins and venous sinuses are somewhat more common in young women than in men; they account for at most 1% of all cerebral ischemic events.

Localization. The **superior sagittal sinus** is most commonly affected, and the other sinuses and the cortical veins are less commonly affected.

Etiology. These thromboses are usually **bland**, that is, no specific etiology can be identified. They can arise in the postpartum period. A minority of cases are due to infection, either systemic or in the immediate vicinity of the sinus (e.g., chronic otitis); other causes include hypercoagulability states and systemic diseases (e.g., Behçet disease).

Pathogenesis. Damming of blood behind a venous obstruction leads to a secondary **reduction of arterial inflow** and thus to hypoperfusion and infarction. Smaller or larger diapedetic hemorrhages (diapedesis = migration of blood cells through endothelial gaps in the vascular wall because of built-up pressure behind an obstruction) can also occur in the infarcted area (**hemorrhagic infarction**).

Clinical features. The common signs and symptoms are **headache, focal or generalized epileptic seizures, papilledema**, and **sensory** and **motor deficits**, depending on the site of the thrombosis.

Diagnostic evaluation. Imaging studies reveal unilateral or bilateral hemorrhagic infarction; the thrombosis itself can usually be seen by **MRI**, or by **contrast-enhanced CT**. In rare cases, thrombosis is revealed only by angiography (**Fig. 6.33**). The diagnostic method of choice is **MRI**.

Treatment. Anticoagulation (heparin followed by oral anticoagulation), usually for a few months.

6.6 Nontraumatic Intracranial Hemorrhage

 Key Point

Nontraumatic intracranial hemorrhage is defined as a spontaneous hemorrhage into the brain parenchyma (intracerebral hemorrhage) or the CSF space (subarachnoid hemorrhage). Intracerebral hemorrhages cause acute signs and symptoms resembling those of cerebral ischemia and account for approximately 10% of strokes. One of the more common forms of intracerebral hemorrhage is hypertensive hemorrhage. The main symptom of subarachnoid hemorrhage is headache; its most common source is a ruptured aneurysm.

General manifestations of intracranial hemorrhage. Though the manifestations of intracranial hemorrhage and cerebral ischemia are similar, generally

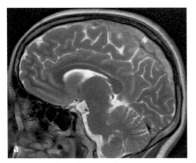
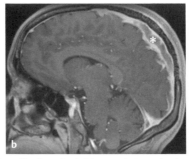
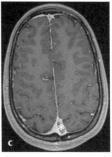

Fig. 6.33   Thrombosis of the superior sagittal sinus (* = thrombus). (a) Sagittal T2-weighted image. **(b)** The contrast-enhanced sagittal T1-weighted image shows the intraluminal thrombus, as does the axial image **(c)**.

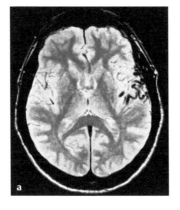
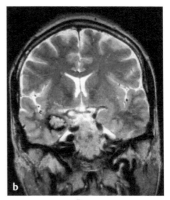

Fig. 6.34   Arteriovenous malformation and cavernoma. (a) Arteriovenous malformation in the left temporal lobe of a 68-year-old man with epileptic seizures. **(b)** Cavernoma in the right hippocampus of another patient (T2-weighted image).

speaking (sudden onset of focal neurologic deficits), there are several clinical signs and symptoms that are more characteristic of hemorrhage than of ischemia. These include:

— Acute headache.
— Often, vomiting.
— Rapidly or very rapidly progressive neurologic deficits (whose type depends on the site of hemorrhage).
— Progressive impairment of consciousness, possibly leading to coma.
— In many patients, epileptic seizures.

If these manifestations are present, an intracranial hemorrhage is the probable cause. The definitive diagnosis, however, can only be made with neuroimaging.

6.6.1 Intracerebral Hemorrhage

Etiology and pathogenesis. Most cases of intracerebral hemorrhage are due to the rupture of **vascular lesions of hypertensive origin** ("rhexis hemorrhages" of pseudoaneurysms of lipohyalinotic arterioles, generally in older patients) or of **vascular malformations** (aneurysms, arteriovenous malformations, and angiomas, which may affect younger patients) (**Fig. 6.34**, **Fig. 6.35**). Intracerebral hemorrhage may also be a complication of therapeutic (over-)

anticoagulation. Smaller hemorrhages, particularly those that are near the cortical surface, are often due to **amyloid angiopathy** (**Fig. 6.35**). There can also be bleeding into an infarct, a primary brain tumor, a metastasis, or a cavernoma. **Multifocal bleeding** should arouse suspicion of amyloid angiopathy (**Fig. 6.38**), a bleeding diathesis (anticoagulation, sepsis, leukemia), venous or venous sinus thrombosis, endocarditis, vasculitis, or trauma.

The more common etiologies of intracerebral hemorrhage are listed in **Table 6.18**.

The effects of intracranial hemorrhage include:

— Direct destruction of brain tissue at the site of the hemorrhage.
— Compression and possible damage of surrounding brain tissue.
— Elevation of ICP.
— Brain edema that additionally raises the ICP, possibly leading to a vicious circle of edema and intracranial hypertension (see Section 6.3 and **Table 6.9**).

Clinical features. The clinical picture mainly depends on the site and extent of the hemorrhage and to a much lesser extent on etiologic factors. Certain aspects of the clinical course can, however, suggest that one etiology is more likely than another:

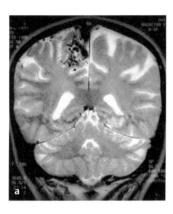
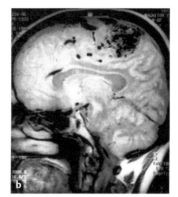

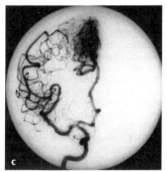
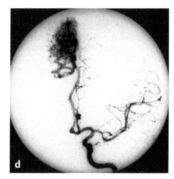

Fig. 6.35 Arteriovenous malformation.
(a) The T2-weighted spin-echo image reveals the feeding and draining vessels as signal-free areas ("flow voids").
(b) Analogous finding in a sagittal image.
(c) The right carotid angiogram shows that the malformation is fed by branches of the right middle cerebral and pericallosal arteries. **(d)** The left carotid angiogram shows that it also derives part of its blood supply across the midline from the left pericallosal artery.

Table 6.18

The main causes of nontraumatic intracerebral hemorrhage

Cause	Examples, remarks
Chronic arterial hypertension	Hypertension leads to microangiopathy with fibrinoid necrosis, pseudoaneurysms, and vascular leakage. When hemorrhage occurs, neighboring arterioles are torn, leading to further extension of the hemorrhage. Typical sites of hypertensive hemorrhage are the thalamus, basal ganglia, subcortical white matter, and pons
Aneurysm rupture	Typical sites are shown in **Fig. 6.40**. Aneurysms can rupture into the brain parenchyma as well as into the subarachnoid space
Hemorrhage into a preexisting lesion	For example, infarct, tumor
Vascular malformation	For example, cavernoma, arteriovenous malformation
Vascular fragility due to vasculopathy	For example, cranial arteritis, amyloid angiopathy
Bleeding diathesis	For example, hematologic disease, sepsis, therapeutic anticoagulation
Cerebral venous thrombosis and venous sinus thrombosis	Diapedetic hemorrhage
Drug abuse	Rare, e.g., cocaine
Acute hypertension (hypertensive crisis)	Rare

— **Chronic arterial hypertension** and advanced age (typically 60–70 years) make a **rhexis hemorrhage** more likely. These hemorrhages are ultimately caused by hypertension and are usually very large. Common sites are the **basal ganglia** (pallidum, putamen) and internal capsule (**Fig. 6.36**), with the corresponding clinical manifestations: **contralateral usually dense, hemiparesis** or hemiplegia, **horizontal gaze palsy**, and initially, in many cases, **déviation conjuguée and deviation of the head to the side of the lesion**. Less common sites are the subcortical white matter, brainstem, thalamus (**Fig. 6.37**), and cerebellum. Very large hemorrhages, particularly if located in the posterior fossa, can rapidly elevate the ICP, causing brainstem compression and, in turn, **impairment of consciousness** and coma.

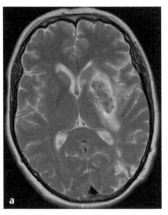 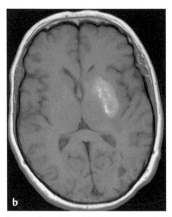 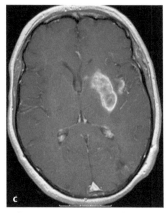

Fig. 6.36   A basal ganglionic hemorrhage that is a few days old. The MRI typically shows a heterogeneous signal, partly hyperintense, partly hypointense. **(a)** T2-weighted MR image. **(b)** T1-weighted MR image. **(c)** T1-weighted MR image after contrast administration; contrast enhancement at the edge of the hematoma.

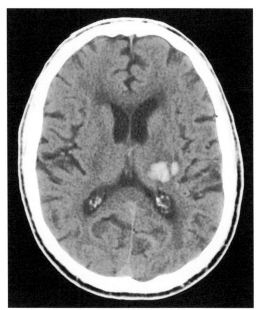

Fig. 6.37   A fresh left thalamic hemorrhage. CT scan of a 76-year-old patient with an acute right-sided hemisensory deficit.

- **Acute worsening** of more or less severe **preexisting signs and symptoms**, perhaps accompanied by **additional impairment of consciousness**, suggests **hemorrhage into an infarct or tumor**.
- Focal or generalized **epileptic seizures** preceding the acute event point toward a tumor, vascular malformation, or other **structural lesion of the brain** as the likely cause of hemorrhage.

Diagnostic evaluation. The diagnosis of intracranial hemorrhage is suggested by the characteristic clinical findings (see above) and then definitively

confirmed by the demonstration of blood on **CT** or **MRI**. CT reveals a hyperdense mass lesion; susceptibility-weighted T2* sequences are the most suitable MRI sequences for detecting hemorrhage. When these studies are performed in the acute phase, they may fail to reveal an underlying vascular malformation, which can be obscured by the hemorrhage; **angiography** may be necessary to complete the diagnostic workup. A complete **coagulation profile** should be obtained when indicated.

 Practical Tip
Old hemorrhages, such as those due to cerebral amyloid angiopathy, often cannot be seen in CT and may be visible only on MRI (Fig. 6.38).

Treatment. Patients suffering from an acute intracerebral hemorrhage require **close clinical observation**.

 Practical Tip
Progressive or recurrent intracranial bleeding or progressive cerebral edema often manifests itself with progressive signs of intracranial-hypertension: vomiting, impairment of consciousness, and sometimes anisocoria and papilledema. These signs demand prompt recognition and treatment.

Intracranial hypertension must be appropriately treated (see section 6.3.4). In addition, **stabilization of the vital functions** and the **treatment of epileptic seizures**, if present, are essential.
The clinical outcome of patients with acute intraparenchymal bleeding can be improved by rapidly **lowering the systolic blood pressure** below 140 mm Hg; this has been shown to lessen the likelihood of "early

6

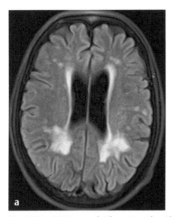 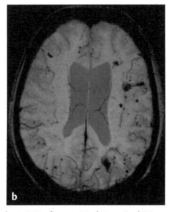 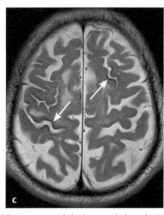

Fig. 6.38 MRI in amyloid angiopathy. This brain MRI of a cognitively impaired 74-year-old woman reveals leukoencephalopathy in the FLAIR image **(a)** and multiple old hemorrhages in the SWI image **(b)**, seen as signal voids caused by hemosiderin deposition. **(c)** This T2-weighted image obtained from an 80-year-old man reveals superficial siderosis (arrows) combined with leukoencephalopathy, indicating amyloid angiopathy.

progression," that is, further expansion of the hemorrhage within 6 hours of symptom onset, which occurs in about half of all cases.

The possible indication for **neurosurgical removal of the hematoma** or for **hemicraniectomy** should be carefully considered, in the light of the neurologic manifestations, the site of the hemorrhage, and the age and general condition of the patient. It is often helpful to remove hematomas located near the cortical surface of the cerebral hemispheres, but not deep hematomas, for example, in the basal ganglia. Cerebellar hemorrhage with mass effect generally confers a risk of brainstem compression and death and is often an indication for life-saving emergency surgery.

Prognosis. Although about one-third of all patients with an intracerebral hemorrhage will die of it, others go on to enjoy a more or less complete spontaneous recovery. Mortality rises with advancing age.

6.6.2 Subarachnoid Hemorrhage

> **NOTE**
>
> Nontraumatic subarachnoid hemorrhage, defined as spontaneous hemorrhage into the subarachnoid space **(Fig. 6.39)**, accounts for approximately 7% of all "strokes."

Epidemiology. Subarachnoid hemorrhage can occur at any age, with **peak incidence around age 50**. Children are very rarely affected.

Etiology. Subarachnoid hemorrhage is usually due to the **spontaneous rupture of a saccular aneurysm on an artery at the base of the brain**, usually one of the arteries forming the circle of Willis **(Fig. 6.39)**. Common sites of saccular aneurysms are shown in **Fig. 6.40**. Less frequent causes of subarachnoid hemorrhage include arteriovenous malformations,

vasculopathies, coagulopathies, and trauma. Perimesencephalic subarachnoid hemorrhages are usually of venous origin.

Clinical manifestations. Subarachnoid hemorrhage manifests itself with the following symptoms and signs:
— Sudden, extremely intense **headache**, often described as the "worst headache of my life;" the headache may have been preceded by an earlier, transient episode of headache or other minor symptoms (**"premonitory headache," "warning leak"**); it is most commonly diffuse or bioccipital.
— Often, at first, a brief and transient **impairment of consciousness**, which may be followed, at some point in the following hours or days, by a **recurrent impairment of consciousness** or coma.
— Often, **nausea and vomiting**.
— Rarely, cranial nerve palsies (caused by aneurysms at particular sites) or other focal neurologic deficits, reflecting, for example, bleeding into the brain parenchyma (see later).

Clinical grading. The clinical grading of a subarachnoid hemorrhage on the **Hunt and Hess, Fisher, or World Federation of Neurological Surgeons (WFNS) scale** is useful for prognostication and therapeutic decision-making.

Diagnostic evaluation. Physical examination reveals **meningismus** as the most prominent finding and sometimes other signs that may be useful for the localization of the lesion, for example:
— **Oculomotor nerve palsy** with aneurysms of the terminal segment of the internal carotid artery or the posterior communicating artery.
— **Abulia** with an aneurysm of the anterior communicating artery.
— **Hemiplegia** with an aneurysm of the MCA.
— **Brainstem and cerebellar signs** with aneurysms of the basilar artery.

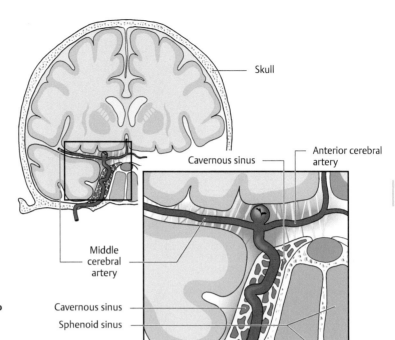

Skull

Cavernous sinus

Anterior cerebral artery

Middle cerebral artery

Fig. 6.39   Aneurysm rupture into the subarachnoid space: in this illustration, an aneurysm at the bifurcation of the internal carotid artery.

Cavernous sinus

Sphenoid sinus

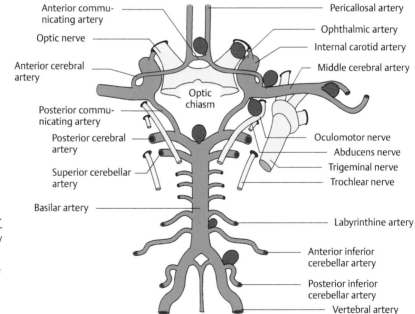

Anterior commu- nicating artery

Optic nerve

Anterior cerebral artery

Posterior commu- nicating artery

Posterior cerebral artery

Superior cerebellar artery

Basilar artery

Pericallosal artery

Ophthalmic artery

Internal carotid artery

Middle cerebral artery

Optic chiasm

Oculomotor nerve

Abducens nerve

Trigeminal nerve

Trochlear nerve

Labyrinthine artery

Anterior inferior cerebellar artery

Posterior inferior cerebellar artery

Vertebral artery

Fig. 6.40   The common locations of intracranial aneurysms. Saccular aneurysms are typically found at vascular bifurcations, on the vascular wall opposite the fork of the bifurcation (inside the "Y"). When such aneurysms rupture, the bleeding is usually into the subarachnoid space but may also be into the brain parenchyma. The figure also shows the relation of intracranial aneurysms to some of the cranial nerves.

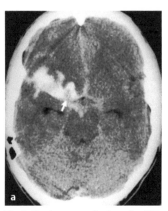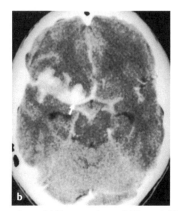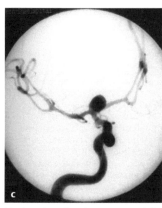

Fig. 6.41   Aneurysmal subarachnoid hemorrhage. (a) The nonenhanced CT reveals blood in the subarachnoid space, particularly along the course of the middle cerebral artery. The aneurysm (→) is also seen. **(b)** The lumen of the aneurysm, dark in **(a)**, turns bright after the administration of intravascular contrast (→). **(c)** Carotid angiography shows the aneurysm at the bifurcation of the internal carotid artery into the anterior and middle cerebral arteries.

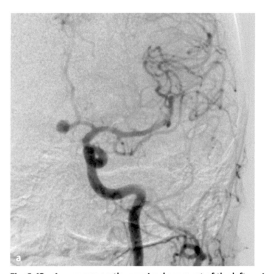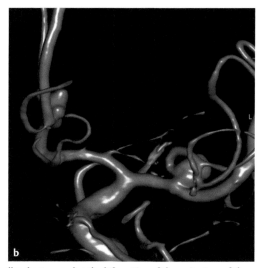

Fig. 6.42   Aneurysms on the proximal segment of the left pericallosal artery and at the bifurcation of the main stem of the left middle cerebral artery.

Whenever subarachnoid hemorrhage is suspected on clinical grounds, **neuroimaging** should be performed immediately. **CT** or **MRI with FLAIR (fluid-attenuated inversion recovery)** and **SWI (susceptibility-weighted imaging) sequences** can often reveal the presence of blood in the CSF space (**Fig. 6.41**). These studies can sometimes also reveal the source of hemorrhage (aneurysm or other) (**Fig. 6.41**, **Fig. 6.42**).

If CT and MRI fail to demonstrate any hemorrhage despite high clinical suspicion, an **LP** must be performed. Bloody CSF is found in patients with acute subarachnoid hemorrhage, and xanthochromic CSF (due to blood breakdown products) in those whose hemorrhage occurred a few hours or more before the LP.

 Practical Tip

A negative CT or MRI does not rule out subarachnoid hemorrhage. If clinical suspicion remains, an LP must be performed.

Once the diagnosis of subarachnoid hemorrhage is confirmed by imaging or LP, **cerebral angiography** should be performed as soon as possible to localize the source of the hemorrhage, usually an aneurysm. Angiography is only indicated, however, if the patient is clinically stable enough to undergo surgery or endovascular treatment.

Blood coming into contact with the outer walls of arteries that course through the subarachnoid space causes **vasospasm** (see Clinical course and prognosis, below), which can be detected with **transcranial Doppler or duplex ultrasonography**.

Blood coming into contact with arterial walls in the subarachnoid space causes **vasospasm**. Vasospasm often arises on the third to fifth day after subarachnoid hemorrhage; transcranial Doppler studies should be performed routinely so that it can be promptly detected and treated.

Treatment. Patients with aneurysmal subarachnoid hemorrhage must be admitted or transferred immediately to a hospital where neurosurgical and endovascular neuroradiologic treatment are available.

The main goal of treatment is **exclusion of the aneurysm from the circulation** as soon as possible (optimally within 34 hours) to prevent a potentially fatal recurrent hemorrhage.

The current methods of closing intracranial aneurysms are:
- Endovascular **coiling**: the introduction of platinum spirals (Guglielmi detachable coils) into the aneurysm through an endovascular catheter. The coils lead to thrombosis and thus occlusion of the aneurysm. At present, most aneurysms can be coiled.
- Surgical **clipping**: direct closure of the aneurysmal sac with a metal clip, via craniotomy.

The following **general measures** are also indicated:
- Strict bed rest.
- Stabilization of cardiovascular functions.
- Fluid and electrolyte administration.
- Analgesia and sedation.

A calcium-channel blocker (nimodipine) is given to prevent vasospasm.

Clinical course and prognosis. The clinical course of subarachnoid hemorrhage is often dramatic. **Recurrent hemorrhage** some time after the initial bleed is particularly worrisome and often fatal. Without treatment, approximately 25% of patients die in the first 24 hours and 40% in the first 3 months. The long-term risk of recurrent hemorrhage in untreated patients is approximately 3% per year.

After successful treatment to prevent recurrent hemorrhage (coiling or clipping), the course is often complicated by **vasospasm** arising 3 to 14 days after the initial hemorrhage (usually in the first 3 to 5 days). This may cause ischemia or infarction in the distribution of the spastic artery or arteries. Vasospasm may not resolve until 3 or 4 weeks later.

Malresorptive hydrocephalus (see sections 6.1.3 and 6.12.6) is a potential late complication; it is presumably caused by adhesions of the arachnoid villi, leading to an obstruction of CSF outflow.

Unruptured aneurysms. As neuroimaging becomes more common, asymptomatic (unruptured) aneurysms are being discovered ever more frequently. An unruptured aneurysm with a diameter of 5 to 7 mm or more has a bleeding risk of about 1% per year and therefore merits treatment; smaller aneurysms are better left unoperated. The indication for treatment also depends on the site of the aneurysm, the patient's age, and other factors.

6.7 Infectious Diseases of the Brain and Meninges

 Key Point
The CNS can be infected by bacteria, viruses, parasites, and other microorganisms. Different organisms tend to infect either the meninges or the brain substance itself. Thus, there are two main forms of intracranial infection, meningitis and encephalitis. Infectious diseases of the CNS can be classified, broadly speaking, into three basic clinical situations: a predominantly meningitic syndrome, which can be either acute or subacute to chronic, and a predominantly encephalitic syndrome. These three syndromes, and the organisms that cause them, will be discussed individually in this section. In addition, focal infections of the brain parenchyma can lead to the formation of brain abscesses, which will also be discussed.

6.7.1 Overview

Meningitis and encephalitis can also appear in mixed forms: a meningeal infection can spread to the brain (and/or spinal cord), or vice versa, causing **meningo-(myelo)encephalitis**. The latter term is only used if the patient unequivocally manifests clinical signs of both meningeal and cerebral involvement.

Localization and Nomenclature

The sites and nomenclature of infectious diseases of the CNS are summarized in **Fig. 6.43**.

The Meningitic Syndrome

The general features of the meningitic syndrome are as follows:
- Headache.
- Fever (though elderly and immune-deficient patients are often afebrile).
- Nausea and vomiting due to intracranial hypertension.

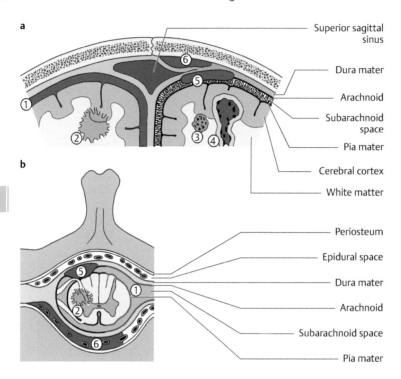

Brain:

1 = Meningitis
2 = Encephalitis
Brain abscess { 3 = Cerebritis (= early stage)
4 = Abscess (= late stage)
5 = Subdural empyema
6 = Epidural abscess

Spinal cord:

1 = Arachnoiditis
2 = Myelitis

5 = Spinal subdural abscess
6 = Spinal epidural abscess

Fig. 6.43 Sites and nomenclature of intracranial (a) and spinal (b) infections.

| Table 6.19 |

Meningitic syndromes

Syndrome	Leukocyte count	Protein	Glucose	Lactate
Acute bacterial meningitis	100 to 1,000, mainly multinucleated	High	Low or very low	High
Acute viral meningitis	100, more mono- than multinucleated	Normal or mildly elevated	Normal or mildly diminished	Normal
Chronic meningitis	100, mainly mononuclear	High or very high	Low or very low	Normal or high

— Meningismus, which, in severe cases, may be evident as a spontaneous extended posture of the neck, or opisthotonus.
— Positive meningeal signs, with the patient examined in the supine position:
  • **Lasègue** sign: passive elevation of an extended leg to 45 degrees (at most) induces shooting pain into the leg.
  • **Brudzinski** sign: passive neck flexion induces reflexive knee flexion.
  • **Kernig** sign: passive elevation of the extended legs induces reflexive knee flexion.

The clinical aspects of individual types of meningitis depend on the pathogen and the immune state of the host.

Meningitis can be classified as shown in **Table 6.19**.

The Encephalitic Syndrome

The **encephalitic**, rather than meningitic, syndrome is characterized by **focal neurologic and neuropsychological deficits** as well as a variably severe **impairment of consciousness**. Encephalitis, like meningitis, can be of viral, bacterial, fungal, protozoal, or parasitic origin. Prion diseases are a special category

Table 6.20

Diseases presenting with a mainly meningitic or encephalitic syndrome

Meninigitic syndrome	Encephalitic syndrome
Acute meningitis	**Viral encephalitis**
▬ Acute bacterial meningitis	▬ Herpes simplex encephalitis
▬ Acute viral meningitis	▬ ESME
Chronic meningitis	▬ HIV encephalitis
▬ Tuberculous meningitis	▬ Zoster encephalitis
▬ Fungal, protozoal, and parasitic meningitis	**Fungal, protozoal, and parasitic encephalitis**
▬ Meningitis due to sarcoidosis	**(Meningo)encephalitis due to spirochetal infection**
▬ Meningitis due to meningeal seeding with carcinoma or	▬ Neurosyphilis
sarcoma (carcinomatous meningitis)	▬ Neuroborreliosis (Lyme disease)
▬ Extradural (parameningeal) chronic infection	▬ leptospirosis
	Encephalitis in prion disease
	▬ Creutzfeldt–Jakob disease
	Encephalitis in slow viral disease
	Noninfectious encephalitis
	▬ Autoimmune encephalitis
	▬ Paraneoplastic encephalitis

Abbreviations: ESME, early summer meningoencephalitis; HIV, human immunodeficiency virus.

of encephalitis. Encephalitis can also arise on an autoimmune or paraneoplastic basis; in such cases, it mainly affects the limbic system (see section 6.8.8).

The infectious processes that cause encephalitis often also involve other structures in the nervous system besides the brain (e.g., the peripheral nerves and plexuses, nerve roots, spinal cord, and meninges). In particular, the three important clinical varieties of spirochetal infection (syphilis, borreliosis, and leptospirosis) often present initially with meningitic or polyradiculitic/polyneuritic manifestations.

The **general features of an encephalitic syndrome** are as follows:

- **Fever.**
- **Headache.**
- **Impairment of consciousness.**
- **Personality changes and neuropsychological abnormalities.**
- **Epileptic seizures.**
- **Focal neurologic deficits.**

The diseases covered in this section are listed in **Table 6.20**.

General Diagnostic and Therapeutic Measures in Cases of Suspected CNS Infection

History. The following should be specifically asked about:

- Contact with animals (e.g., certain viruses, leptospira, *Coxiella burnetii*).
- Tick bites, fleas, mites (borreliosis, early summer meningoencephalitis, rickettsiae).
- Swimming in ponds (amebiasis).
- Consumption of unpasteurized dairy products (listeriosis, brucellosis).
- Past medical history (immune deficiency, diabetes, surgery, endocarditis, or recent pneumonia,

mumps, or measles). The patient's past illnesses may predispose to CNS infection with certain types of pathogen.

Physical examination.

- Meningismus (abnormal response to passive movement of the neck), **neurologic examination**.
- **Inspection**: skin (petechiae, e.g., in meningococcal sepsis), oral cavity and throat (pharyngitis, tonsillitis, teeth, and gums).
- **Palpation**: lymph nodes, trigeminal exit points (sinusitis as the source of CNS infection).
- **Auscultation** of the heart and lungs.

Further procedure. If the clinical signs warrant, **blood cultures** should be drawn.

- **No intracranial hypertension or focal deficit**: CSF is obtained by **LP** and treatment is begun with **antibiotics** (directed against the most likely pathogen) and **glucocorticoids** (dexamethasone). The antibiotic treatment is tailored later based on the specific pathogen detected.
- **Presence of intracranial hypertension and/or focal deficits**: immediate initiation of treatment with **antibiotics** and **glucocorticoids** (dexamethasone), then **head MRI**. An LP should not be performed until the signs of intracranial hypertension have subsided.

6.7.2 Acute Bacterial Meningitis

Pathogens and routes of infection. The bacteria that cause bacterial meningitis can reach the meninges by any of three routes:

- **Hematogenous spread** (e.g., from a focus of infection in the nasopharynx).
- **Continuous extension** (e.g., from the middle ear or paranasal sinuses).
- **Direct contamination** (through an open wound or CSF fistula).

The organisms that most commonly cause acute, purulent meningitis are:
- In **neonates**, *Escherichia coli*, group B streptococci, and *Listeria monocytogenes*.
- In **children**, *Haemophilus influenzae* (HIB), pneumococci, and meningococci (*Neisseria meningitidis*).
- In **adults**, pneumococci, meningococci, and, less commonly, staphylococci and Gram-negative enterobacteria.

Practical Tip

If meningitis is suspected, the patient's vaccination status should be determined: infants have usually been vaccinated against HIB. The Centers for Disease Control and Prevention (CDC) in the United States and the Standing Committee on Vaccination (STIKO) in Germany recommend vaccination of all small children and high-risk adults against pneumococci and group C meningococci.

Clinical features.

> **NOTE**
>
> The clinical onset of purulent meningitis is usually acute or hyperacute, and patients very quickly become severely ill, usually with high fever and vomiting. The initiation of antibiotic therapy as rapidly as possible is essential for a good outcome.

The **course** of purulent meningitis is characterized by the meningitic signs and symptoms listed earlier, as well as by:
- Myalgia, back pain.
- Photophobia.
- Epileptic seizures (40%; these may occur if the infection is mainly located over the cerebral convexity with irritation of the underlying brain parenchyma).
- Cranial nerve deficits (10–20%, sometimes permanent deafness, particularly after pneumococcal infection).
- Variably severe impairment of consciousness.
- In infection with *N. meningitidis*, there may be petechial cutaneous hemorrhages and hemorrhagic necrosis of the adrenal cortex due to endotoxic shock (Waterhouse–Friderichsen syndrome).

Diagnostic evaluation. The most important and most urgent components of the diagnostic evaluation are **blood culture** (at least two sets of aerobic and anaerobic cultures from two different veins) and **CSF culture** after the CSF has been obtained by LP. Whenever acute meningitis is suspected, an LP should be performed **at once**, unless there is clinical evidence of intracranial hypertension.

Laboratory findings: the CRP and ESR are elevated, and the differential white blood count may reveal leukocytosis (with mainly segmented granulocytes). CSF examination enables confirmation of the diagnosis of meningitis and, in two-thirds of patients, demonstration of bacteria by **Gram stain** and **identification of the pathogen** by **CSF culture**.

> **NOTE**
>
> Typical CSF findings in bacterial meningitis:
> - Turbid CSF.
> - Florid granulocytic pleocytosis with **1,000 to several thousand cells/mm³**.
> - High protein concentration (>2,000 mg/L).
> - Low glucose concentration (ratio of CSF to serum glucose concentration <0.5).
> - High lactate concentration (>3.5 mval/L).

Treatment. The treatment begins with **antibiotic therapy**, with a single drug or multiple drugs, chosen for their effectiveness against the most likely causative organism(s) in the given clinical setting (= empiric treatment).
- Previously well children and adults with community-acquired meningitis are treated empirically at first with a **third-generation cephalosporin** (e.g., ceftriaxone) and **ampicillin** (which also covers *Listeria*).
- Nosocomial infections and infections in parts of the world where penicillin-resistant pneumococci are common are treated, for example, with a combination of **ceftriaxone and vancomycin**.

Corticosteroids (dexamethasone) are given as well, as they have been shown to improve the clinical course. Once the pathogen has been identified in the blood or CSF culture (with antibiogram), the empirically chosen antibiotics can be replaced with specifically tailored ones.

> **NOTE**
>
> The antibiotic treatment of bacterial meningitis must be started immediately after the blood draw for culture and the LP—sometimes even before these are done and before the CT or MRI. The elapsed time up to the initiation of treatment is the most important prognostic factor.

Course and Prognosis. Bacterial meningitis can have severe neurologic and general medical complications, including the following:
- Malresorptive hydrocephalus.
- Brain infarction and sinus vein thrombosis.
- Cerebral edema.
- Brain abscess.
- Cochlear damage resulting in hearing loss.

- Cranial nerve deficits.
- General medical complications: pneumonia, septic shock, consumption coagulopathy.

The prognosis depends on the **pathogenic organism**. The mortality in meningitis due to *Streptococcus pneumoniae* is over 50%. Survivors often suffer from **neurologic deficits** including deafness.

Pneumococcal Meningitis

Pneumococci (*S. pneumoniae*) are **Gram-positive diplococci**; they are the commonest cause of bacterial meningitis in **adults**. The diagnosis is established by Gram stain, blood or CSF culture, or **demonstration of the antigen** in the blood or CSF. **Vaccination** is possible for infants as well as adults; it is recommended for persons with immune deficiency or chronic disease and for persons older than 60 years.

Meningococcal Meningitis

Meningococci (*N. meningitidis*) are **Gram-negative diplococci**; they are the commonest cause of bacterial meningitis in **children and adolescents**. The meningococcal **antigen** can be detected in the CSF or blood. In Germany, **group B meningococci** are the most common type (65–70%).

> **NOTE**
>
> The course of meningococcal infection can be complicated by the following:
> - **Sepsis** (35%).
> - **Waterhouse–Friderichsen syndrome** (15%), also known as adrenal apoplexy: fulminant meningococcal sepsis leading to **adrenal dysfunction, petechiae** (also called **purpura**), extensive skin necrosis, and **disseminated intravascular coagulation**. If untreated, patients with this condition die within hours.

Patients must be **isolated** for 24 hours after the beginning of antibiotic treatment, and their **contacts** should be given antibiotics prophylactically (e.g., rifampicin). **Vaccination** against group C meningococci is recommended for all infants, and vaccination against groups A and C is recommended for travelers to Africa (recommendations of the German vaccination authority [STIKO]). There is as yet no vaccine against group B. Meningococcal meningitis is a **reportable illness**: all cases (even suspected ones) and fatalities must be reported. Nasopharyngeal colonization with meningococci without any sign of illness is not reportable.

6.7.3 Acute Viral Meningitis: Aseptic or Lymphocytic Meningitis

Pathogens and routes of entry. Several viruses can cause so-called **aseptic** or **lymphocytic meningitis**. The more common ones are **enteroviruses** (polio- and Coxsackie viruses), **arboviruses**, and **HIV**; other, rarer ones include **lymphocytic choriomeningitis virus, CMV, type II herpesvirus**, and the **mumps, Epstein–Barr**, and **influenza viruses**.

Clinical features. The illness begins acutely (less commonly, subacutely) after a nonspecific prodromal stage with flulike or gastrointestinal symptoms. The main clinical manifestations are **headache, fever, meningismus** (often mild), and **general symptoms** such as fatigue and myalgia.

Diagnostic evaluation. The causative virus is identified by **serologic testing**.

Treatment and course. The natural course of aseptic meningitis is usually favorable, provided the brain is not involved (i.e., provided there is no encephalitic component). Antiviral treatment is given if the causative virus is one for which an effective treatment exists (a virustatic agent, e.g., acyclovir for herpes simplex virus or varicella zoster virus). Residual neurologic deficits, such as deafness, are rare.

6.7.4 Chronic Meningitis

Chronic meningitis is caused by different organisms from the pus-forming bacteria that cause acute meningitis, and therefore takes a less acute and dramatic course, at least initially: the meningitic symptoms arise **gradually**, often fluctuate, and, depending on the causative organism, may progressively worsen over a long period of time. Fever and other clinical and laboratory signs of infection (elevated ESR and CRP, blood count abnormalities, general symptoms such as fatigue and myalgia) are common but may be absent. There may be variably severe neurologic deficits. The spectrum of causative organisms is very wide. By definition, chronic meningitis lasts **longer than 4 month**s. Fortunately, it is a rare condition.

Tuberculous Meningitis

Etiology and route of infection. *Mycobacterium tuberculosis* bacilli reach the meninges by hematogenous spread, either directly from a primary complex (**early generalization**) or from a focus of tuberculosis in an internal organ (**late generalization**). The site of origin may be clinically silent.

Clinical features and pathogenesis. **Meningitic symptoms** usually develop gradually. **Febrile bouts** and **general symptoms** are often but not always present. Because the infectious process typically centers on the base of the brain (so-called **basal meningitis; Fig. 6.44**), in contrast to bacterial meningitis, which is typically located around the cerebral convexities), **cranial nerve palsies** are common, particularly of the nerves of eye movement and the facial nerve. Moreover, **arteritis of the cerebral vasculature** may result

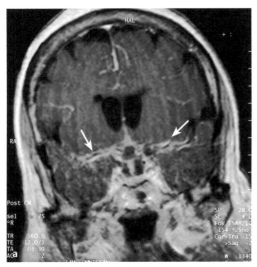
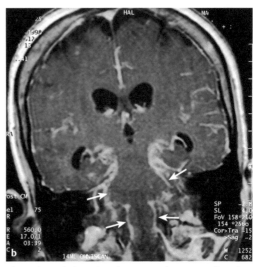

Fig. 6.44 Tuberculous meningitis. (a) This T1-weighted MR image shows the typical meningeal contrast enhancement along the course of the middle cerebral artery (→). **(b)** Typical contrast enhancement surrounding the brainstem (→).

in focal brain infarction. The protein concentration in CSF is typically markedly elevated, and gelatinous exudates in the subarachnoid space, including the basal cisterns, cause progressive fibrinous coating of the meninges and **malresorptive hydrocephalus**.

Diagnostic evaluation. The most important part of the evaluation is the **detection of the pathogen** in the CSF or other bodily fluids (sputum, tracheal secretions, gastric juice, urine). In the past, the detection of mycobacteria in the CSF often required weeks of culture; it can now be done relatively quickly with **PCR (polymerase chain reaction)**. Occasionally, a **Ziehl–Neelsen stain of the CSF** will directly and immediately reveal acid-fast bacilli (mycobacteria).

> **NOTE**
>
> CSF findings in tuberculous meningitis:
> - Initially granulocytic, then lymphocytic pleocytosis.
> - High CSF protein (1,000–5,000 mg/L), low glucose, high lactate.

Neuroimaging (CT, MRI) reveals pathologic lesions of multiple types (e.g., tuberculomas, infarcts, hydrocephalus, coated basal meninges).

Treatment and prognosis. The treatment generally begins with a **combination of four tuberculostatic drugs (isoniazid, rifampicin, pyrazinamide**, and **myambutol**), followed by a combination of three drugs, and then of two, for at least 12 months. Untreated tuberculous meningitis is lethal.

Tuberculosis (confirmed or suspected) is a **reportable illness**.

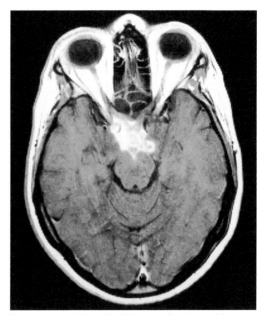

Fig. 6.45 Sarcoidosis. This MR image of a 31-year-old woman with sarcoidosis shows infiltration of the basal meninges. There is marked signal abnormality in the basal ambient cistern.

Other Causes

Several other organisms can rarely cause chronic meningitis, usually accompanied by variably severe encephalitis. These include:

- **Fungi**, mainly but not exclusively in immuno-deficient patients; the causative species include *Cryptococcus neoformans, Candida albicans*, and *Aspergillus*.

— **Protozoa**: *T. gondii.*
— **Parasites**: *Cysticercus, Echinococcus.*

The noninfectious causes of the chronic meningitic syndrome include **sarcoidosis**, which, like tuberculous meningitis, is mainly found around the base of the brain (**Fig. 6.45**), and **seeding of the meninges with metastatic carcinoma or sarcoma** (carcinomatous or sarcomatous meningitis).

6.7.5 Bacterial (Meningo)encephalitis: Spirochetal Infections

Neuroborreliosis (Lyme Disease)

Etiology. Borreliosis is called "Lyme disease" in North America (after the town of Lyme, Connecticut, in which an outbreak was described) and is caused there by *Borrelia burgdorferi*, a spirochete transmitted by bites of the tick *Ixodes ricinus*. *Borrelia afzelii* and *Borrelia garinii* cause borreliosis in Europe.

Clinical manifestations. Borreliosis can involve the nervous system, joints, cardiovascular system, liver, and skin. Its clinical manifestations are equally varied and run through three stages (**Table 6.21**). After transfer of the organism by a tick bite, some patients locally develop **erythema chronicum migrans**, a red, annular rash that expands centrifugally around the site of the tick bite, clearing in the central area as it grows outward. If the spirochetes are then disseminated systemically, headache, fever, arthralgia, and sometimes generalized lymphadenopathy will follow.

Fifteen percent of patients who reach the disseminated stage and do not receive treatment go on to develop **neurologic manifestations**, typically **lymphocytic meningitis** combined with **radiculoneuritis**, causing weakness, very unpleasant (often burning) dysesthesia, and severe pain in the distribution of the affected nerve roots (**Bannwarth syndrome**; **Fig. 6.46**). **Cranial nerve involvement** is also common and may cause **facial diplegia**, a condition that should always arouse suspicion of borreliosis. Less commonly, plexus neuritis, encephalitis, or myelitis can develop at this stage or later. Other possible complications of advanced borreliosis are **vasculitis of the cerebral vessels** and, outside the CNS, **myopericarditis**, **acrodermatitis chronica atrophicans**, **arthralgia**, and **liver involvement**. Arthralgia is typical in **Lyme disease**, which is therefore also known as "Lyme arthritis."

Diagnostic evaluation. A clinical suspicion of neuroborreliosis can be supported, though not definitively confirmed, by the demonstration of **specific immunoglobulin G (IgG)** and, above all, **IgM antibodies** in the **serum** and **CSF**.

> **NOTE**
>
> Serologic testing for *Borrelia* is positive in at least 10% of asymptomatic persons. Thus, the demonstration of antibodies against *Borrelia* is no reason to ascribe an unclear neurologic condition to florid borreliosis.

The diagnosis of neuroborreliosis can only be made if there is an **inflammatory CSF profile** (elevated cell count and protein concentration, positive **CSF Borrelia titer**). A normal CSF profile makes the diagnosis questionable, even if the serologic tests are positive.

Treatment. If borreliosis is suspected after a tick bite (overt erythema chronicum migrans, flulike symptoms), **doxycycline**, **amoxicillin**, or **cefuroxime axetil** is given orally. In all later stages of the disease, **third-generation cephalosporins** (e.g., ceftriaxone or cefotaxime) are given intravenously.

Table 6.21

The three stages of Lyme borreliosis

Stage	Manifestations
Local infection	**Erythema chronicum migrans**: a red, annular rash that expands centrifugally around the site of the tick bite, clearing in the central area as it grows outward
	General symptoms (headache, fever, pain in the limbs, exhaustion)
Dissemination	**General symptoms** (fever, headache, diaphoresis)
	Bannwarth syndrome (= **acute neuroborreliosis**: meningopolyradiculitis, facial palsy)
	Lymphadenosis benigna cutis (hyperplasia of lymphatic cells, often visible as a reddish swelling of the earlobes)
	"Migratory" **arthritis and myalgia** (affecting different joints one after another)
Late stage[a]	**Acrodermatitis chronica atrophicans** of Herxheimer (ACA)
	Chronic, recurrent **Lyme arthritis**
	Chronic **neuroborreliosis**: polyneuropathy, meningitis, encephalitis or encephalomyelitis, vasculitis of the cerebral vessels
	Further inflammatory manifestations (e.g., heart, liver, sensory organs)

[a]*If untreated; rare after antibiotic treatment.*

6

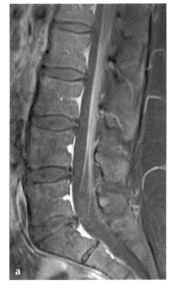

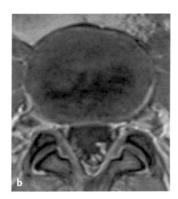

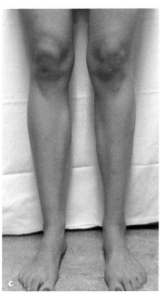

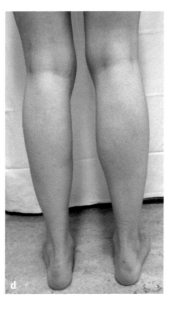

Fig. 6.46 Borrelia radiculitis. This 27-year-old woman complained of painful weakness of the left leg, mainly affecting the peroneal muscles. **(a, b)** T1-weighted MRI reveals contrast enhancement of the inflamed left lumbar and sacral nerve roots. **(c, d)** Atrophy of the left calf muscles as a late sequela.

Neurosyphilis

Etiology. Syphilis is caused by the sexually transmitted spirochete, *Treponema pallidum*.

Clinical features. Various neurologic changes arise in the secondary, tertiary, and quaternary phase of syphilis.

Secondary phase (6 weeks to 2 years after infection): hematogenous spread may lead to **meningeal irritation** or **early syphilitic meningitis** with cranial nerve palsies (basal meningitis).

Tertiary phase (usually 1 or 2 years after the primary infection and secondary seeding of treponemes): **cerebrospinal syphilis** (also called **meningovascular syphilis)** mainly affects the mesenchymal structures (blood vessels, meninges) of the brain and, often, the spinal cord. Inflammatory changes of vascular walls, particularly in the arteries of the skull base and the MCA, cause stenoses and **recurrent ischemic strokes**. **Meningitis**, mainly localized around the cranial base, presents with fluctuating headache and cranial nerve palsies. Occasionally, tertiary syphilis gives rise to polyneuropathic and polyradicular manifestations. In the rare gummatous variant of tertiary syphilis, large granulomatous masses (gummata) may form within the cranial cavity, producing mass effect and intracranial hypertension.

Quaternary phase (after a latency period of several years): the inflammatory process now involves the parenchyma of the brain and spinal cord, producing tabes dorsalis (spinal cord involvement) and/or progressive paralysis (chronic meningoencephalitis).

- **Tabes dorsalis** appears in 7% of untreated syphilitics 8 to 12 years after the primary infection. It is characterized, above all, by **progressive degeneration of the posterior columns and posterior roots**. Its clinical manifestations include progressively severe ataxia, lancinating pains, bladder dysfunction, diminished reflexes, loss of pupillary reactivity (see section 12.3.6), diminished sensitivity to pain, hypotonia of the musculature, and joint deformities.
- **Progressive paralysis** appears 10 to 15 years after the primary infection and is caused by **parenchymal meningoencephalitis** with formation of caseating granulomas. Its major clinical sign is **progressive dementia**, with typical features including impaired judgment, lack of social inhibition, and, in some patients, expansive agitation (megalomania, nonsensical and delusional ideas). In other cases, patients may develop flattening of drive and affect, become depressed, or manifest schizophreniform phenomena (hallucinations, paranoia).

The two late forms of neurosyphilis can also be present in combination.

Diagnostic evaluation. The diagnosis of neurosyphilis is established by various *serologic tests*:

- **TPHA** (*T. pallidum*) hemagglutinin test, a screening test).
- **FTA–ABS** (fluorescent treponemal antibody absorption) test, a confirmatory test for the demonstration of previous contact with *T. pallidum*.
- **VDRL** test for the assessment of current disease activity (this test detects anticardiolipin antibodies and is thus not specific for *T. pallidum*).
- **19-S-IgM–FTA–ABS** test to demonstrate treponeme-specific IgM antibodies, which indicate an active or florid infection.

Neurosyphilis also causes an **inflammatory CSF picture** with elevated leukocyte count and protein concentration, a positive CFS VDRL test, and an elevated CSF concentration of treponeme-specific IgG.

MRI of the brain, and of the spinal cord as well if indicated, is a further component of the diagnostic workup. It is used to detect inflammatory changes, hydrocephalus, and infarcts, and to rule out other conditions in the differential diagnosis.

Treatment and prognosis. All forms of neurosyphilis are treated with **penicillin G**; if the patient is allergic to penicillin, **tetracycline, erythromycin, or a cephalosporin** can be given instead. The success of treatment depends on its timing: improvement is less likely if the brain and spinal cord parenchyma are already damaged before treatment is begun. The prognosis of early syphilitic meningitis is good. In the later phases of neurosyphilis, progression can be prevented by appropriate treatment, but residual deficits are common.

Leptospirosis

Leptospirosis in its initial stage often causes **acute lymphocytic meningitis**. In a more advanced stage, there may be signs of **encephalitis** (epileptic seizures, delirium) or **myelitis**. The brain can also be damaged by **vasculitis of the cerebral vessels**. Outside the nervous system, leptospirosis can affect the liver (causing jaundice) and kidneys, and it can cause a bleeding diathesis.

6.7.6 Viral Encephalitis

Herpes Simplex Encephalitis

Etiology. Herpes simplex encephalitis is a serious infectious condition caused by the **herpes simplex virus, type I**.

Pathogenesis. This disease is characterized by **hemorrhagic–necrotic inflammation of the basal portions of the frontal and temporal lobes**, combined **with severe cerebral edema**. The inflammatory foci are found in both hemispheres, but one is usually more strongly affected than the other.

Clinical features. After a **nonspecific prodromal phase** with **fever**, headache, and other general symptoms, the disease presents overtly with the following:

- Progressive impairment of consciousness.
- Epileptic seizures (usually of complex partial type, with or without secondary generalization, because the infection affects the temporal lobe).
- Focal neurologic and neuropsychological deficits, particularly impairment of memory and orientation.

Aphasia and hemiplegia may ensue.

Diagnostic evaluation. CSF examination reveals up to 500 cells/mm^3, mainly lymphocytes but also granulocytes; the CSF is sometimes bloody or xanthochromic. **Viral DNA** can be identified in the CSF by the **PCR** in the first few days of illness and, for at least 2 weeks, **specific IgG for herpes simplex virus** can be detected in the CSF as well.

NOTE

CSF findings in herpes simplex encephalitis:
- Usually an initially lymphomonocytic pleocytosis.
- Protein elevated, glucose normal.

The **CT scan** is usually normal at first but, within a few days, reveals **temporal** or **frontal hypodense areas**, which may contain foci of hemorrhage. **MRI** may reveal corresponding signal changes even earlier (**Fig. 6.47**).

6

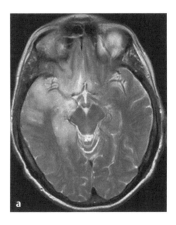
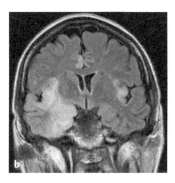

Fig. 6.47 Herpes simplex encephalitis. Herpes simplex encephalitis affecting both temporal lobes. **(a)** The axial T2-weighted MR image displays signal abnormalities in the right temporal lobe and in basal portions of both frontal lobes. **(b)** The coronal FLAIR image additionally shows typical bilateral involvement of the insular and cingulate cortex.

The **EEG**, in addition to nonspecific changes, may reveal **characteristic focal findings** over one or both **temporal lobes**.

Treatment. **Acyclovir** is given intravenously. **Corticosteroids** are given to combat cerebral edema and **anticonvulsants** to prevent seizures.

Prognosis. If untreated, herpes simplex encephalitis has a mortality of more than two-thirds, with neurologic damage in all surviving patients. Treatment with acyclovir lowers the mortality to 20%, but about half of the surviving patients have permanent deficits.

> **NOTE**
>
> Any one of the following findings is **adequate grounds for suspicion** of herpes simplex encephalitis:
> - Progressive impairment of consciousness, aphasia.
> - Epileptic seizures (particularly of the complex partial type).
> - An inflammatory CSF profile.
> - Uni- or bilateral frontotemporal signal changes in MRI.
> - Focal EEG abnormalities.
>
> If any of these are present, **intravenous acyclovir therapy** must be started **immediately**.

Early Summer Meningoencephalitis

Etiology and epidemiology. This disease is caused by an **arbovirus** (arthropod-borne virus) of the **flavivirus** group and is transmitted **by tick bites**. In endemic areas (e.g., Austria and southern Germany), it affects 1 in every 100 to 1,000 tick-bite victims. The family *Flaviviridae* includes several tick-borne viruses affecting humans, such as the European or Western tick-borne encephalitis virus, the Siberian tick-borne encephalitis virus, and the Far Eastern tick-borne encephalitis virus. In the United States and Russia, another tick-borne flavivirus, Powassan virus, is responsible for encephalitis in humans.

Clinical features and course. The course is biphasic: after an incubation period of 1 to 4 weeks, in which there is a **nonspecific prodrome** with fever and flu-like or gastrointestinal symptoms, approximately 20% of patients develop **headache**, **meningismus**, and **focal neurologic deficits** referable to the brain and spinal cord. **Peripheral nerve deficits** may also appear some time later. When the patient has recovered from the acute illness, residual paresis and, less commonly, neuropsychological deficits may remain.

Diagnostic evaluation. The essential diagnostic test is the demonstration of virus-specific IgM antibodies.

Therapy and prognosis. Only **symptomatic** treatment is possible. The overall mortality is 1%. Children have a markedly better prognosis than adults. Persons who recover from meningoencephalomyelitis generally have permanent residual deficits.

Prophylaxis. Early summer meningoencephalitis and other tick-borne flavivirus encephalitides can be effectively prevented by **exposure prophylaxis** (insect repellents and adequate clothing in endemic forest areas) and some also by **active immunization** (recommended for persons who are commonly exposed; boosters needed every 3–5 years).

HIV Encephalitis and Opportunistic CNS Infections

Nearly 50% of persons infected with HIV have a clinically evident infection of the brain or other parts of the nervous system at some point in the course of their illness. The nervous system can be infected with HIV itself, other opportunistic pathogens, or both. In severe cases, patients may suffer from **encephalitis**, **myelopathy**, **mono-** and **polyneuropathy**, and/or **myopathy**. Encephalitis presents with **neuropsychological abnormalities** including delirium, personality change, and dementia.

HIV encephalopathy. HIV encephalopathy arises when the HIV attacks the CNS, causing various neurologic deficits, primarily **cognitive deficits** (whence the term **HIV-associated dementia**). **High viral titers** are found in the CSF, and MRI reveals leukencephalopathy. The only effective treatment is properly administered HAART (highly active antiretroviral therapy).

Opportunistic infections. The main **AIDS-defining infections** of the CNS are toxoplasmosis, cryptococcosis, tuberculosis, nocardiosis (usually as a brain abscess: *Nocardia* live in the soil, are part of the normal oral flora, and pose no danger to immunocompetent persons), CMV encephalitis, PML (progressive multifocal leukencephalopathy due to the JC virus, **Fig. 6.48**, **Table 6.22**), and EBV-associated lymphoma. HIV patients are also prone to develop herpes zoster encephalitis and neurosyphilis. Treatment consists of antiretroviral therapy along with treatment of the opportunistic pathogen(s), if available.

Herpes Zoster Encephalitis

Herpes zoster encephalitis is accompanied by a **segmental vesicular rash** in the territory of a peripheral nerve (cranial nerve). CSF examination reveals lymphocytic pleocytosis up to 200 cells/mm³. The disease may appear in particularly severe form after a generalized herpes zoster infection. **Herpes zoster oticus** (involvement of the ear and auditory canal) and **herpes zoster ophthalmicus** (involvement of the dermatome of the ophthalmic nerve, in and around the eye) can cause severe neurologic complications, for example, postherpetic neuralgia.

Rarer Types

Other, rarer viruses causing meningoencephalitis, some of which are specific to particular regions, are listed in **Table 6.22** in addition to those already discussed.

Fig. 6.48 illustrates a case of **PML**, caused by JC virus, in an immunosuppressed patient.

6.7.7 Fungal Encephalitis

Etiology and clinical features. Some of the **fungi** mentioned earlier as causes of meningitis can also cause encephalitis.

 Practical Tip
Patients with neutropenia (mainly iatrogenic after bone marrow transplantation) are particularly susceptible to fungal infections.

In persons with **normal immune competence**, encephalitis can be caused by:
- *C. neoformans*.
- Coccidioides immitis.
- Histoplasma capsulatum.

- Blastomyces dermatitidis.

Persons with **reduced immune competence** due to disease or pharmacotherapy may develop encephalitis due to any of these or due to the following:
- *C. albicans* (especially meningitis).
- *Aspergillus* (cerebral aspergilloma and hemorrhagic stroke).
- *Zygomycetes* (e.g., Mucorales, with diffuse cerebral spread and abscess formation; more common in diabetics).

Diagnostic evaluation. The typical **CSF findings** of fungal infection are a lymphocytic pleocytosis (several hundred cells/µL) with elevated protein and lactate and low glucose concentrations. The fungi can be detected by direct microscopy of the CSF, by culture, or by capsular polysaccharides. Cryptococci can also be demonstrated by India ink staining.

Treatment. **Antimycotic drugs** (e.g., amphotericin B) are given for 6 months, tailored to the particular pathogen; abscesses must be **neurosurgically removed**.

6.7.8 Parasitic and Protozoal Encephalitis

Parasites, particularly *T. gondii*, and various types of **protozoa** (amebae, plasmodia, trypanosomes, cysticerci [**Fig. 6.44**], and echinococci) can also infect the brain.

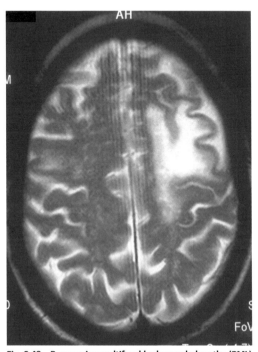

Fig. 6.48 Progressive multifocal leukencephalopathy (PML) due to JC virus in an immunosuppressed patient. The left frontal white matter is destroyed, with thinning of the overlying cortex. PML lesions generally do not take up contrast medium (except when there is immune reconstitution).

Table 6.22

Viruses that can cause meningoencephalitis

Virus	Route of infection	Season of peak incidence	Persons at risk	Clinical features	Special aspects of diagnostic evaluation
Echovirus	Fecal–oral	Summer/fall	Children and family members living with them	M, rash, gastrointestinal symptoms	Virology
Coxsackie A virus	Fecal–oral	Summer/fall	Children and family members living with them	M, rash, gastrointestinal symptoms	Virology
Coxsackie B virus	Fecal–oral	Summer/fall	Children and family members living with them	M, rash, pleuritis, pericarditis, myocarditis, orchitis, gastrointestinal symptoms	Virology
Mumps virus	Inhalation	Late winter/spring	Children, mainly boys	M, parotitis, orchitis, oophoritis, pancreatitis	Elevated amylase, CSF cell count, and CSF glucose
Adenovirus	Inhalation		Infants and children	M, pharyngitis, pneumonia	
Lymphocytic choriomeningitis virus	Mice	Late winter/spring	Laboratory personnel	M, pharyngitis, pneumonia	
Hepatitis viruses	Fecal–oral, sexual intercourse, blood transfusion		Mainly intravenous drug abusers, homo- and bisexuals, recipients of blood transfusions	M, jaundice, arthritis	Hepatic dysfunction
Epstein–Barr virus (infectious mononucleosis)	Oral		Teenagers and young adults	M, lymphadenopathy, pharyngitis, rash, splenomegaly	Atypical lymphocytes, Paul–Bunnell reaction, hepatic dysfunction
Echovirus				M, enanthem and exanthem	
ESME virus (early summer meningoencephalitis)	Tick bite, cutaneous	Early summer, fall	Persons who go into a forest in an endemic area	M, E, myelitis, meningoradiculitis	Serology
Varicella zoster virus	Inhalation		Children and persons who come in contact with them	M, radiculitis; M, E, and myelitis: pain, vesicular eruption	Demonstration of intrathecal antibodies, PCR
CMV			HIV-positive persons	E, epileptic seizures, radiculitis	Detection of HIV in the CSF or urine, PCR of CSF or EDTA blood, CMV-specific intrathecal IgG synthase, CMV retinitis
HSV type I	Person-to-person	All year	All persons	E, focal neurologic deficits, epileptic seizures, impairment of consciousness	MRI (Fig. 6.38), virus detection, PCR of the CSF, EEG with periodic steep waves, intrathecal HSV-specific IgG synthesis
HSV type II	Person-to-person	All year	Neonates and children, rarely adults	E in neonates; M in others	
Arboviruses (eastern equine, western equine, Venezuelan equine)	Mosquitoes		Children and adults in the Americas	E, rash	Virology
HIV	Sexual intercourse, blood transfusion	All year	Sexual partners of HIV-positive persons, mother–child, intravenous drug abusers, homosexuals	E, AIDS dementia, myelopathy, polyneuropathy, myopathy, opportunistic infections	Serology
Papovaviruses (e.g., JC virus)		All year	Immunocompromised persons (AIDS, lymphoma, natalizumab treatment for multiple sclerosis)	E, myelitis, clinical picture of progressive multifocal leukoencephalopathy (Fig. 6.48)	MRI with subcortical T2-hyperintensities, virology

Abbreviations: CMV, cytomegalovirus; CSF, cerebrospinal fluid; E, predominantly encephalitic manifestations; EDTA, ethylenediaminetetraacetic acid; EEG, electroencephalogram; HSV, herpes simplex virus; HIV, human immunodeficiency virus; IgG, immunoglobulin G; M, predominantly meningitic manifestations; MRI, magnetic resonance imaging; PCR, polymerase chain reaction.

CNS Toxoplasmosis

Toxoplasmosis is transmitted mainly by contact with cat feces and raw meat; it can be asymptomatic once acquired and only become evident later through endogenous activation when the individual is immunosuppressed. The disease is mainly dangerous for unborn children. In immunosuppressed persons (e.g., persons with AIDS), it can cause **multifocal necrotizing encephalitis** leading to a wide variety of neurologic manifestations (paresis, aphasia, epileptic seizures). The **CSF** is often normal (mild pleocytosis). Contrast-enhanced imaging (**CT**, **MRI**) reveals ring-shaped lesions. Toxoplasmosis is treated with a combination of multiple **antiparasitic drugs.** Co-trimoxazole can be given prophylactically to persons at risk.

Cysticercosis

Man is a definitive host for *Taenia solium* (the pork tapeworm). Cysticerci that are ingested orally with food (typically incompletely cooked pork) migrate through the bowel wall and travel to various organs, including the CNS, where they can cause manifest symptoms (cysticercosis) after an incubation period of weeks to years. A **chronic meningoencephalitis** ensues, with headache, signs of intracranial hypertension, focal deficits, and seizures. The pathogens and antibodies against them can be found in **CSF**; **CT** and **MRI** reveal granulomas, cysts, and calcifications (**Fig. 6.49**). Various **antihelminthic drugs** (e.g., albendazole) are given for treatment.

Echinococcosis

Man is an **accidental intermediate host** for the dog and fox tapeworms (*Echinococcus granulosus* and *multilocularis*). This organism affects the CNS, causing **intracerebral cysts** that can lead to **neurologic abnormalities** (focal deficits, epileptic seizures, signs

of intracranial hypertension). It can be detected by **serologic testing**. CT reveals the lesions (*E. granulosus*: round cysts, *E. multilocularis*: infiltrative growth). **Antihelminthic agents** are given.

6.7.9 Encephalitis in Prion Diseases: Creutzfeldt–Jakob Disease

Pathogens and routes of infection. Prions are **infectious particles composed of protein** that possess no genetic material (nucleic acids) of their own. They can arise in situ by mutation of the host's genetic material or else reach the body from outside and incorporate themselves into its cells, where they replicate. The replicating proteins have an abnormal steric configuration compared with the prion proteins that are normally found in the body.

Pathogenesis. Neurons in the brain that have been infected by prions may die after a latency period of years or even decades. The typical pathologic findings in prion infection are **vacuolization** and the formation of **amyloid plaques** (**spongiform encephalopathy, SEP**).

Epidemiology. The main prion diseases are **Creutzfeldt–Jakob disease** (subacute SEP), kuru, Gerstmann–Sträussler–Scheinker syndrome, familial progressive subcortical gliosis, and familial fatal insomnia. Creutzfeldt–Jakob disease, the most common prion disease in Europe and North America, is nevertheless rare, with an incidence of about one case per million individuals per year.

Clinical features. The disease presents initially with mental abnormalities, insomnia, and fatigability. Soon, progressive dementia develops, along with pyramidal tract signs, cerebellar signs, abnormalities of muscle tone, fasciculations, and myoclonus.

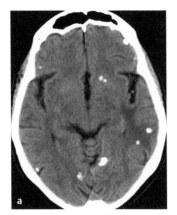
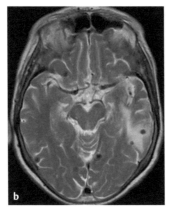
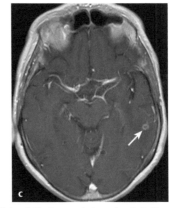

Fig. 6.49 Cysticercosis in a 74-year-old woman with epilepsy. (a) The CT shows multiple calcifications and a hypodensity in the left parietal lobe. **(b)** The T2-weighted MRI scan shows multiple nodular foci with low signal intensity in the area of the calcifications in the left parietal lobe. **(c)** A lesion within the edematous area takes up contrast medium (arrow), indicating an inflammatory reaction.

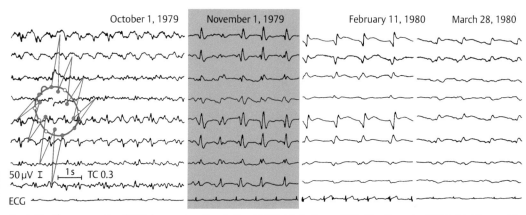

Fig. 6.50 The progression of EEG changes over time in Creutzfeldt–Jakob disease (CJD). The diagnosis of CJD in this 57-year-old woman was later confirmed by autopsy. Six weeks after the onset of the prodromal phase (October 1, 1979), only a hint of periodic activity is seen. It is fully developed 1 month later (November 1, 1979) and slowly declines in amplitude in the ensuing months. TC, time constant in seconds.

Diagnostic evaluation. In about two-thirds of patients, the **EEG** reveals characteristic, periodic triphasic and tetraphasic theta and delta waves (**Fig. 6.50**). T2-weighted **MRI** reveals hyperintensity of the basal ganglia and part of the occipital cortex (**Fig. 6.51**). The **14–3–3 protein** is found in the **CSF**.
Treatment, course, and prognosis. Only symptomatic treatment is available. The disease progresses rapidly, leading to a **decorticate state and death within months of onset**.

Additional Information

A previously unknown **variant of Creutzfeldt–Jakob disease** attracted considerable attention when it broke out in the late 1990s, particularly in the United Kingdom. This variant was contracted by eating beef derived from cows with **bovine spongiform encephalopathy ("mad cow disease")**.

6.7.10 Slow Virus Diseases

The slow virus diseases are characterized by **extremely long incubation periods, a protracted, chronically progressive course**, and little or no response to treatment.
Subacute sclerosing panencephalitis (SSPE). This disease usually arises in children who had **measles** in infancy. The virus persists in the CNS and, **years later**, gives rise to a disease of insidious onset and chronically progressive course, leading to death in 2 to 3 years. The initial presentation is with **mental abnormalities** such as irritability, fatigability, and impaired cognitive performance. **Involuntary movements** and **noise-induced myoclonus** appear a few weeks later. Finally, the child develops **generalized spasticity** and **severe, progressive dementia**. The EEG reveals **periodic, high-amplitude slow waves**. The illness is always fatal.

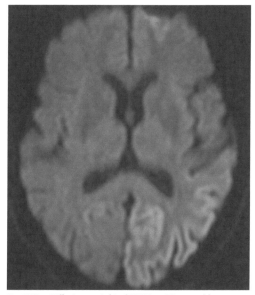

Fig. 6.51 Diffusion-weighted MRI in a 68-year-old woman with Creutzfeldt–Jakob disease. The left occipital cortex appears hyperintense; the insular cortex does as well, but to a lesser extent.

Rubella panencephalitis and other types of encephalitis. Other illnesses that probably share pathogenetic mechanisms with SSPE are progressive rubella panencephalitis and various types of encephalitis that can arise a few days or weeks after an infectious illness (measles, mumps, chickenpox, rubella).

> **NOTE**

Postvaccinial encephalitis: it has been hypothesized, but never proved, that encephalitis can rarely arise as a complication of vaccination against measles, rubella, or smallpox. This risk is no more than theoretical, but the associated anxiety in the general public is real and must be allayed by appropriately **educating** the parents of the children who are to be vaccinated. A child is at much greater risk of sustaining a severe complication from one of the supposedly trivial illnesses of childhood than from the vaccinations that prevent them. This is precisely the reason why the **universal vaccination** of infants and small children is recommended, and indeed required by law in many places.

6.7.11 Intracranial Abscesses

Key Pointbrainabscesses
Brain abscesses are caused by focal infection of the brain parenchyma leading to tissue destruction and pus formation. They can be solitary or multiple. A special form is focal encephalitis, in which systemic sepsis or the embolization of infectious material into the CNS gives rise to multilocular, disseminated microabscesses.

Solitary Brain Abscess

Pathogens and routes of infection. Brain abscesses are caused by one or more pathogens, mainly **streptococci** and **staphylococci** and, less commonly, *Pseudomonas*, *Actinomyces*, and fungi. Like the organisms that cause bacterial meningitis, these pathogens can reach the brain through **local extension of infection** (especially mastoiditis, sinusitis, and otitis), **hematogenous dissemination** from a distant infectious focus (usually pulmonary infections or endocarditis), or **direct contamination** (open brain injury). Immunocompromised patients are at increased risk.

Clinical features. A large **brain abscess** exerts **mass effect** and typically causes fever, leukocytosis, and rapidly progressive intracranial hypertension. Marked perifocal edema generally adds to the mass effect.

> **NOTE**
>
> The typical manifestations of a brain abscess are: signs and symptoms of intracranial hypertension, including papilledema and impaired consciousness, along with hemiparesis or other focal neurologic signs, and/or epileptic seizures. Fever, leukocytosis, and elevation of the erythrocyte sedimentation rate and the C-reactive protein level may be seen but are sometimes absent.

Alternatively, there may be a **subdural empyema** between the dura mater and the arachnoid, or an **epidural abscess** between the dura mater and the inner table of the skull. These processes usually arise as a complication of sinusitis or otitis, less commonly after trauma. Fever, headache, and meningismus,

accompanied by neurologic deficits, are their clinical hallmarks. The course of subdural empyema is often fulminant and life-threatening, while that of epidural abscess is usually more protracted.

Diagnostic evaluation. The diagnosis is suspected on the basis of the **typical clinical findings** and **relevant aspects of the past medical history** (such as traumatic brain injuries, known lung or heart disease, and immune suppression or diseases of the immune system).

Laboratory findings: serum inflammatory parameters (particularly the C-reactive protein level) are usually elevated.

CSF examination may reveal inflammatory changes (predominantly granulocytic pleocytosis, elevation of total protein).

Imaging studies: **CT or MRI** scanning reveals a **ring-shaped zone of contrast enhancement** (abscess wall) surrounding the hypodense interior of the abscess (**Fig. 6.52**). In the early stage of abscess formation ("cerebritis"), the enhancement may be diffuse rather than annular.

Treatment. Neurosurgical removal of the abscess (followed by microbiologic study of the abscess material) is the preferred form of treatment in most patients; **antibiotic therapy** is initiated immediately after surgery (in some cases, even beforehand) and continued thereafter for at least 6 weeks. A highly effective empirical combination of antibiotics consists of a third-generation cephalosporin (e.g., ceftriaxone), metronidazole, and an agent that is effective against staphylococci, such as flucloxacillin, rifampicin, or vancomycin. Cerebritis and abscesses measuring less than 3 cm in diameter can be treated with **antibiotics alone**. If clinically significant brain edema is present, it can be treated simultaneously with **corticosteroids**.

Practical Tip
It is important to find the source of the infection, that is, the original site from which bacteria made their way to the brain. The treatment of the original focus of infection is an important determinant of treatment success.

Focal Encephalitis

Pathogenesis. Focal encephalitis consists of **multilocular foci of infection in the brain parenchyma** (**Fig. 6.53**), which generally arise by one of two routes:
- **Metastatic focal encephalitis**, that is, seeding of the brain with bacteria in generalized sepsis, possibly arising from a single **focus of purulent infection** anywhere in the body.
  - **Embolic focal encephalitis**, that is, the embolization of multiple infectious microthrombi into the cerebral vasculature. The latter is usually a

complication of **subacute bacterial endocarditis**, which, in turn, is most often caused by *Streptococcus viridans*.

Streptococcal and staphylococcal infections are the usual causes.

Clinical features. The typical findings include **signs of generalized sepsis** (high fever, shaking chills)

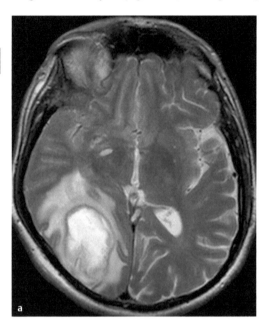

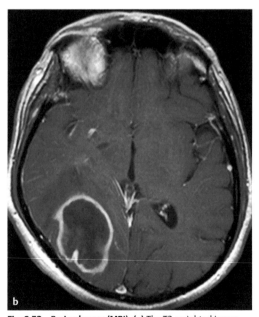

Fig. 6.52 Brain abscess (MRI). (a) The T2-weighted image reveals a right parieto-occipital mass with surrounding edema. **(b)** The T1-weighted image reveals ring-shaped contrast enhancement. (Reproduced from Mattle H, Mumenthaler M. Neurologie. Stuttgart: Thieme; 2013.)

combined with **focal brain signs**, **impaired consciousness**, and, not uncommonly, **psychosis**. The neurologic and psycho-organic signs **fluctuate** in severity. They manifest themselves in bouts, with remissions in between.

> **NOTE**
> A septic illness accompanied by fluctuating neurologic or psychiatric manifestations should raise suspicion of focal encephalitis.

Diagnostic evaluation. The diagnosis is suspected from the **clinical findings** and, possibly, **inflammatory CSF changes**, and confirmed by a **CT and/or MRI scan demonstrating multiple focal lesions in the brain**. Clinical evidence of **endocarditis** should always be sought (including listening for a heart murmur). **Blood cultures** may reveal the responsible pathogen; blood should be drawn for culture during the upward phase of the fever curve and during shaking chills.

Treatment. As in the treatment of brain abscesses, **antibiotic therapy** is indicated and should be tailored to the sensitivity profile of the responsible organism, if it can be identified. Infected heart valves may need to be surgically replaced.

6.8 Metabolic Disorders and Systemic Diseases Affecting the Nervous System

 Key Point

The intense metabolic activity of the nervous system (both central and peripheral) makes it vulnerable to damage by a wide variety of metabolic disorders, both congenital (inborn errors of metabolism, i.e., metabolic diseases in the narrower sense of the term) and acquired (e.g., toxic). These disorders manifest themselves clinically as metabolic encephalopathy and metabolic neuropathy, of which there are many different types. Similar manifestations arise when the nervous system is involved by systemic diseases (e.g., endocrinopathy or vasculitis) and paraneoplastic syndromes.

6.8.1 Congenital Metabolic Disorders

> **NOTE**
> Metabolic diseases are caused by hereditary enzyme defects. They usually present in early childhood but sometimes not until many years later. They can be roughly divided into disorders of lipid, amino acid, and carbohydrate metabolism. Wilson disease is due to a disturbance of copper metabolism.

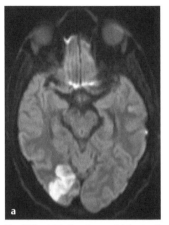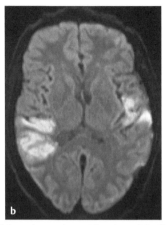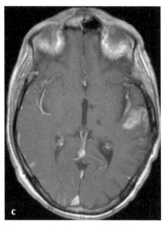

Fig. 6.53 **MRI showing multiple cerebral infarcts in a patient with endocarditis**. The diffusion-weighted images **(a, b)** show multiple fresh infarcts. The T1-weighted image **(c)** shows contrast enhancement in the left temporal infarct, but not in the right temporoparietal infarct; this implies that the two infarcts are of different ages, having arisen several days apart.

General clinical features. The following findings in children and adolescents suggest the presence of a metabolic disease:
— A positive family history.
— Delayed motor and cognitive development.
— A slowly worsening course.
— Progressive spasticity.
— Progressive dementia.
— Optic nerve involvement.
— Epileptic seizures.
— Accompanying polyneuropathy and myopathy.

General diagnostic evaluation. The diagnostic workup includes the following:
— The taking of a comprehensive personal and family history.
— A clinical neurologic (neuropediatric) examination.
— Amino acid screening of the urine.
— Measurement of the serum concentration of glucose, ammonia, lactate, and pyruvate, and screening for the lysosomal enzymes arylsulfatase A, hexosaminidase, and β-galactosidase.
— Light- and electron-microscopic examination of biopsied tissue samples, with routine and special stains.
— Radiologic examination of the skeleton.
— MRI of the brain.
— If indicated, specific genetic testing.

Disorders of Lipid Metabolism

Lipid storage diseases are due to faulty enzymatic degradation of individual lipid substances, leading to deposition of the intermediate products of lipid metabolism in various internal organs (liver, spleen, bone marrow) and in the nervous system. Disorders in which these nondegradable metabolites accumulate mainly in the neurons of the brain are characterized by degeneration of the cerebral cortex or of the subcortical nuclear areas (**lipidoses**); disorders in which they accumulate mainly in white matter are characterized by demyelination of the cerebral white matter and/or peripheral nerve sheaths (**leukodystrophies**). The **lipid storage diseases** affecting the nervous system are listed in **Table 6.23**. Two examples of the radiologic appearance of the brain in the leukodystrophies are shown in **Fig. 6.54**.

Disorders of Amino Acid and Uric Acid Metabolism

The more common disorders of these types include **phenylketonuria** (an autosomal recessive disorder of amino acid metabolism), **maple syrup urine disease**, **Hartnup disease**, and **homocystinuria** (**Table 6.24**).

Disorders of Carbohydrate Metabolism

These disorders include the **monosaccharides** (e.g., galactosemia), the **glycogenoses**, and the **mucopolysaccharidoses** (**Table 6.25**). **Myoclonus epilepsy**, a type of mucopolysaccharidosis, is characterized by generalized epileptic seizures, myoclonus, and dementia.

Disorder of Copper Metabolism: Wilson Disease

Etiology and pathogenesis. **Hepatolenticular degeneration** (Wilson disease), an autosomal recessive disorder whose genetic locus lies on the long arm of chromosome 13, involves a disturbance of copper metabolism. The concentration of the copper transport protein **ceruloplasmin** is abnormally low and, as a result, the serum free copper concentration is high and an abnormally large amount of copper is eliminated in the urine. Free copper is deposited in the

| Table 6.23 |

Lipidoses and leukodystrophies affecting the nervous system

Diseases	Clinical features	Particularities and treatment
Lipidoses		
GM1 gangliosidoses and **GM2 gangliosidoses**	Infantile progressive encephalopathy, progressive myopathy in adults; possibly myoclonus, convulsions, visual impairment, progressive spasticity, and dementia; muscle atrophy and progressive weakness	Galactosidase deficiency in GM1 gangliosidoses; hexosaminidase deficiency in GM2 gangliosidoses, including **Tay–Sachs disease** and **Sandhoff disease**, with characteristic cherry-red spot. The causes of these conditions are currently untreatable
Fabry disease (angiokeratoma corporis diffusum)	Onset of symptoms in childhood or adolescence; burning pain in the limbs, particularly in warm surroundings; deficient sweating; maculopapular, purplish-red skin changes; renal failure; frequent strokes	X-linked inheritance; α-galactosidase deficiency with intracellular accumulation of trihexosylceramides. Enzyme replacement therapy with agalsidase- α (a recombinant form of α-galactosidase) lessens limb pain and improves renal function
Gaucher disease, **juvenile and adult forms**	Diverse neurologic manifestations, gaze paresis, bulbar signs, spasticity, polyneuropathy, psychosis, dementia, myoclonus, epileptic seizures	Autosomal recessive inheritance, glucocerebrosidase deficiency; foam cells in bone marrow. Treatment possible with enzyme replacement therapy or inhibition of glucoceramide synthesis with miglustat. Bisphosphonate is given for bone stabilization
Niemann–Pick disease	Progressive developmental delay beginning in the first year of life; juvenile forms with encephalopathy or hepatomegaly, progressive dementia, spasticity, and ataxia as well as epileptic seizures and psychosis	Autosomal recessive inheritance; genetic defect on chromosome 18, more common in Ashkenazi Jews. Substrate reduction therapy with miglustat
Refsum disease (heredopathia atactica polyneuritiformis)	Onset of symptoms in middle age; night blindness due to retinitis pigmentosa, hearing loss, polyneuropathy with areflexia and gait ataxia; mental abnormalities	Lack of phytanic acid α-dehydrogenase, accumulation of phytanic acid in the body (liver, kidneys, nervous system). A low-phytanic-acid diet and plasmapheresis are effective treatments
Cerebrotendinous xanthomatosis (cholestanol storage disease)	Onset of symptoms in adolescence or later; intellectual disability; juvenile cataracts, progressive spasticity and ataxia; xanthomas, particularly on extensor tendons and Achilles tendons; polyneuropathy and muscle atrophy	Autosomal recessive inheritance; impaired synthesis of bile acids; accumulation of cholestanol in plasma and brain, tendon xanthomas. The administration of bile acids (chenodeoxycholic acid) combined with a statin can alleviate symptoms
Neuronal ceroid lipofuscinosis (Batten–Kufs disease)	Presentation in infancy and early childhood (Spielmeyer–Vogt type) or in adulthood (Kufs disease); ataxia, myoclonus, epileptic seizures, progressive visual loss, and mental deterioration	Waxy waste products (ceroid lipofuscins) are stored intracellularly and lead to cell death. Only symptomatic and palliative treatment is possible at present
Leukodystrophies		
Metachromatic leukodystrophy	*Late infantile type*: from the age of 1 year onward, spastic weakness progressing toward quadriplegia, loss of mental function, areflexia, bulbar and pseudobulbar signs, optic atrophy; *juvenile type*: onset at age 2–10 y, elevated CSF protein, white matter hypodensity in CT and hyperintensity in T2-weighted MRI	Autosomal recessive inheritance; lack of arylsulfatase A; accumulation of sulfatide in the brain, peripheral nerves, and other tissues; demonstration of low arylsulfatase A concentration in leukocytes and urine. Stem-cell transplantation can slow or arrest the progression of the disease
Globoid cell leukodystrophy (Krabbe disease)	Infantile, juvenile, and adult types; spasticity, optic atrophy, and polyneuropathy	Lack of galactocerebrosidase. The treatment is symptomatic and palliative; in late stages, stem-cell transplantation may be possible
Adrenoleukodystrophy (Fig. 6.54a)	Most patients are male; in the first two decades of life, they develop a spastic gait, visual impairment, and mental changes; adrenal insufficiency may arise in adulthood	X-linked deficiency of the enzyme lignoceroyl coenzyme A synthetase. The progression of the disease can be slowed or arrested with a diet low in fatty acids and by stem-cell transplantation. Patients with **adrenomyeloneuropathy** have these manifestations and polyneuropathy as well

Table 6.24

Disorders of amino acid and urate metabolism

Disease	Clinical features	Remarks
Phenylketonuria	Clinical manifestations from the age of 6 months onward, if untreated: intellectual disability, epileptic seizures, spasticity, tremor, hypopigmentation	Autosomal recessive inheritance; lack of hydroxylation of phenylalanine to tyrosine; neonatal screening (Guthrie test) The treatment is with a strictly low-phenylalanine diet
Maple syrup urine disease	Presentation in the neonatal period: impaired alertness, diminished muscle tone, intellectual disability	Impaired degradation of branched amino acids; sweet-smelling urine (like maple syrup) Treated with a protein-free diet and dialysis if indicated
Hartnup disease	Bouts of pellagra-like dermatitis, accompanied by episodes of ataxia, nystagmus, and gait unsteadiness, progressive dementia, and spasticity	Impaired tubular and intestinal reabsorption of tryptophan; aminoaciduria A high-protein diet may be beneficial
Homocystinuria	Arterial and venous thromboembolism, lens ectopy, intellectual disability	Impairment of methionine metabolism Low-methionine, high-cystine diet, and thrombosis prophylaxis with acetylsalicylic acid

Table 6.25

Disorders of carbohydrate metabolism

Disease	Clinical features	Remarks
Galactosemia	Onset in infancy: failure to thrive, retardation, jaundice, cataracts	Impaired enzymatic degradation of galactose; accumulation of the phosphorylated form in the liver, kidneys, lenses, and brain Treated with a lactose-free, low-galactose diet
Glycogenoses, types I–XI	Accumulation of glycogen in the liver, kidneys, muscles, and brain; clinically, hepatic dysfunction, possibly myopathy, intellectual disability, epileptic seizures	Impaired enzymatic degradation of glycogen Enzyme replacement therapy can slow the progression of type II glycogenosis (Pompedisease, α-glucosidase deficiency)
Mucopolysaccharidoses	– **Pfaundler–Hurler** syndrome: onset in infancy, corneal opacification, joint swelling, dwarfism, intellectual disability, possibly quadriparesis due to spinal cord compression – **Scheie syndrome**: juvenile type, with slow progression – **Progressive myoclonus epilepsy** (Lafora type): generalized epileptic seizures, myoclonus, progressive dementia, psychosis	In Pfaundler–Hurler syndrome and Scheie syndrome, acidic mucopolysaccharides are deposited in various tissues because of hydrolase deficiency In progressive myoclonus epilepsy, mucopolysaccharides are deposited in the form of Lafora bodies in the brain, muscles, and liver In rare cases, disease progression can be slowed by enzyme replacement therapy with iduronidase (Aldurazyme) or stem-cell transplantation

liver, the edge of the cornea (producing the typical **Kayser–Fleischer ring**), and the brain.
Clinical features. Hepatopathy or **hemolytic anemia** dominates the clinical picture in childhood and the **neurologic and psychiatric manifestations** come later; the most impressive of these is a **coarse postural and intention tremor of the limbs** (recognizable on extension of the arms to both sides, e.g., as a "flapping tremor"). **Dysarthria, dystonia**, and **rigidity** are common, as are mental abnormalities (depression, personality changes, or even psychotic episodes).
Diagnostic evaluation. The **Kayser–Fleischer ring**, a brown ring around the periphery of the cornea, helps establish the diagnosis. **MRI** reveals cortical atrophy, enlarged ventricles, and signal abnormalities in the basal ganglia.

Treatment. This disease is treated with **D-penicillamine** (a chelating agent) or **zinc sulfate** (a copper uptake inhibitor). A diet containing as little copper as possible is recommended (e.g., no organ meats, chocolate, nuts, or mushrooms). Caution: copper deficiency may arise. This initially manifests itself with anemia and leukopenia and may lead to myeloneuropathy and pancytopenia.

Other Metabolic Disorders

Several other metabolic disorders are mentioned here for completeness; some of them have no known cause. **Myoclonus epilepsy** and **adult polyglucosan body disease** (**Fig. 6.54b**) are polyglucosan storage diseases. Both are characterized by progressive spasticity, ataxia, and dementia.

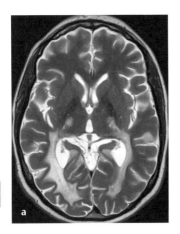
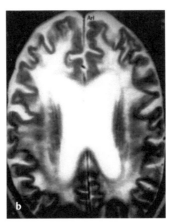

Fig. 6.54 T2-weighted MRI images of two patients with congenital metabolic disorders. (a) A 27-year-old man with quadriparesis, somewhat worse in the lower limbs, because of adrenoleukodystrophy. There are symmetric signal abnormalities in the white matter, particularly in the posterior zones of the cerebral hemispheres. **(b)** A 43-year-old man with polyglucosan body disease. Here, too, there are symmetric signal abnormalities in the white matter; the brain is atrophic as well.

Reye syndrome is probably of multifactorial origin. A few days after a viral illness, the patient becomes progressively somnolent, with nausea, delirium, and cerebral edema.

In the various types of α-**lipoproteinemia**, the serum cholesterol and triglyceride levels are abnormally low. These disorders are clinically characterized by ataxia, nystagmus, oculomotor disturbances, and polyneuropathy, in combination with retinitis pigmentosa. These manifestations are often accompanied by acanthocytosis (Bassen–Kornzweig).

6.8.2 Intoxications and Alcohol-Induced Disturbances of the Nervous System

> **NOTE**
>
> Medications, recreationally used substances, drugs of abuse, industrial toxins, and numerous other substances can exert a toxic influence on the nervous system. The effects of alcohol are presented separately because of their major clinical importance.

Intoxications and iatrogenic disturbances of the nervous system are classified according to their clinical features in **Table 6.26**.
Alcohol-induced disturbances of the nervous system are dealt with separately in **Table 6.27**.

6.8.3 Endocrine Diseases

> **NOTE**
>
> Neurologic manifestations often accompany dysfunction of the endocrine glands, particularly the thyroid gland, the parathyroid glands, the pancreatic islet cells, and the adrenal gland.

Thyroid Diseases

Hypothyroidism. Hypothyroidism causes **cretinism** in infants, and **intellectual disability** and **short stature** in children. In adults, it can cause **ataxia, dysarthria, nystagmus**, a mainly **sensory polyneuropathy**, and muscle weakness with characteristically delayed relaxation of muscle fibers after elicitation of the deep tendon reflexes. **Mental abnormalities** may also be present (apathy, depression, dementia, delirium).

Hyperthyroidism. In addition to its characteristic **general manifestations** (nervousness, insomnia, tremor, sweating, tachycardia, diarrhea, heat intolerance), hyperthyroidism can produce a variety of neurologic deficits:

- **Cerebral manifestations**: irritability, psychotic episodes, tremor, choreoathetosis, spastic elevation of muscle tone, pyramidal tract signs.
- **Ocular manifestations**: diminished frequency of blinking (Stellwag sign), ophthalmoplegia, diplopia, optic neuropathy; in Graves disease, lid retraction (Graefe sign), weakness of convergence (Möbius sign), exophthalmos.
- **Muscular manifestations**: thyrotoxic myopathy with mainly proximal weakness, myasthenia gravis, and thyrotoxic periodic paralysis.
- Partial and generalized **epileptic seizures**.
- Rarely, **polyneuropathy**.

Parathyroid Diseases

Hypoparathyroidism. A deficiency of parathyroid hormone causes **hypocalcemia**, leading to tetany, epileptic seizures, intracranial hypertension with headache and papilledema, hypomotor and hypermotor movement disorders, and neurastheniform mental manifestations and delirium.

Hyperparathyroidism. An excess of parathyroid hormone manifests itself clinically mainly in **behavioral disturbances** (emotional lability, agitation, fatigability, and confusional states) and **dementia-like cognitive impairment**, in addition to muscle weakness, ataxia, dysarthria, and sometimes spasticity and epileptic seizures.

Table 6.26

Neurologic manifestations of toxic or iatrogenic origin

Neurologic signs and symptoms	Causes
Headache	Nearly all headache preparations when overused; withdrawal of caffeine, ergotamine, or amphetamine; oral contraceptives and other hormone preparations (pseudotumor cerebri); nitrates, aminophylline, tetracycline, sympathomimetics, IV immunoglobulins, tamoxifen, H_2-antagonists, dipyridamole, interferons, cyclosporine, vitamin A
Aseptic meningitis	Intravenous immunoglobulins, nonsteroidal anti-inflammatory drugs, amoxicillin, trimethoprim-sulfamethoxazole, cephalosporins, azathioprine, sulfasalazine, allopurinol
Ischemic stroke	Oral contraceptives and other hormone preparations, antihypertensive agents, ergotamine, amphetamines, cocaine, sympathomimetics, intravenous immunoglobulins, intra-arterial methotrexate, angiography, interventional intra-arterial procedures, cardiovascular surgery, radiotherapy, fat injection ("liposculpturing"), chiropractic manipulation, steroid infiltration of the nasal mucosa
Spinal infarction	Transforaminal epidural steroid infiltration, root infiltration with steroids
Hemorrhage (intra-cerebral, extracerebral, spinal)	Anticoagulants, fibrinolytic agents, inhibitors of platelet aggregation, amphetamines, cocaine, sympathomimetics; vessel perforation in endovascular procedures; reperfusion injury after treatment of stenosis
Epileptic seizures	Antibiotics (penicillin, isoniazid), general and local anesthetics (e.g., lidocaine), insulin, radiologic contrast media, withdrawal of benzodiazepines or other sedatives, anticonvulsant withdrawal, phenytoin overdose, antidepressants, aminophylline and theophylline, phenothiazines, pentazocine, tripelennamine, cocaine, meperidine, cyclosporine, antineoplastic agents, other
Coma	Insulin, barbiturates, benzodiazepines and other sedatives, analgesics, other
Neurasthenic symptoms, acute and chronic encephalopathy	Heavy metals, lithium, aluminum, heroin pyrolysate, cyclosporine, anticholinergics, dopamine agonists, benzodiazepines and other sedatives, antihistamines, antibiotics, anticonvulsants, corticosteroids, H_2-antagonists, disulfiram, methotrexate, organic solvents, hallucinogens, radiotherapy, dehydration, water intoxication, dialysis encephalopathy, other
Extrapyramidal movement disorders (acute dystonia, dyskinesia, akathisia, drug-induced parkinsonism, tardive dyskinesia)	Neuroleptics (phenothiazines, thioxanthenes, butyrophenones, dibenzazepines), antiemetics containing metoclopramide or phenothiazines, dopamine agonists, levodopa, antihypertensive agents (e.g., reserpine, captopril), flunarizine, cinnarizine, MPTP, lithium, valproate
Cerebellar ataxia	Phenytoin, carbamazepine, barbiturates, lithium, organic solvents, heavy metals, acrylamide, 5-fluorouracil, cytosine arabinoside, procarbazine, hexamethylmelamine, vincristine, cyclosporine, ciguatera fish poisoning
Central pontine myelinolysis	Too rapid correction of hyponatremia
Malignant neuroleptic syndrome	Neuroleptic agents
Malignant hyperthermia	Succinylcholine, halothane, other general anesthetics
Polyneuropathy	See section 11.3
Optic neuropathy	Tobacco, ethanol, methanol, myambutol, vigabatrin (retinal degeneration)
Deafness	Aminoglycosides, cytostatic agents
Disorders of neuro-muscular transmission	Penicillamine, muscle relaxants, procainamide, magnesium, quinine, aminoglycosides, interferon-α
Myopathy and rhabdomyolysis	Ethanol, cocaine, heroin and other opiates, pentazocine, benzene, corticosteroids, thyroxines, antimalarial agents, colchicine, antilipid agents (fibrates and statins), zidovudine, cyclosporine, diuretics (via hypokalemia), ipecac

Disturbances of Insulin Metabolism

Hypoglycemia. Hyperinsulinism is one of the possible causes of hypoglycemia, which in turn causes the neurologic manifestations listed in **Table 6.28**.

Hyperglycemia. The most prominent neurologic manifestation of the **insulin deficiency** of diabetes mellitus is **polyneuropathy** (see section 11.3); in addition, diabetic arteriopathy may secondarily harm the nervous system (ischemic stroke, mononeuropathies of peripheral or cranial nerves).

6.8.4 Gastrointestinal Diseases

NOTE

Gastrointestinal diseases can cause toxic damage to the nervous system (e.g., in hepatic dysfunction). The nervous system can also be harmed by secondary nutritional deficiencies and hypovitaminoses (e.g., in stomach diseases and intestinal malresorptive disorders).

Table 6.27

Effects of alcohol on the nervous system

Clinical condition	Features	Remarks
Acute alcohol intoxication	Euphoria, dysphoria, disinhibition, ataxia, somnolence, stupor	Respiratory arrest may cause death
Alcohol withdrawal syndrome, delirium tremens	Diaphoresis, tachycardia, insomnia, tremor, hallucinations, epileptic seizures, psychomotor agitation, possibly delirium	— When the patient's alcohol intake is cut off, the blood alcohol level falls and the patient passes through the stages of alcohol withdrawal syndrome, from mild autonomic symptoms to predelirium and delirium — **Delirium tremens** is the most severe form of the alcohol withdrawal syndrome — Treated with clomethiazole
Alcoholic dementia	Chronic alcohol abuse with systemic effects on the liver and peripheral nervous system	**Brain atrophy**, visible in CT and MRI, reversible with abstinence
Wernicke encephalopathy	Memory impairment, confusion, oculomotor dysfunction (abducens palsy, nystagmus, conjugate gaze palsy), ataxia, dysarthria	— Signal abnormalities around the cerebral aqueduct and third ventricle in T2-weighted MRI — Caused by **thiamine deficiency** and malnutrition — Often combined with Korsakoff psychosis
Korsakoff syndrome	Acute amnestic syndrome with anterograde and retrograde amnesia, confabulation, reduced drive, and reckless behavior	**Thiamine deficiency**; also seen in nonalcoholics
Marchiafava–Bignami syndrome	Acute confusion, epileptic seizures, impairment of consciousness; demyelination of corpus callosum and centrum semiovale; patients who survive the acute phase are often abulic and demented	Predominantly seen in Italian drinkers of red wine
Alcoholic cerebellar degeneration	Progressive limb ataxia mainly affecting the lower limbs, with gait impairment	
Central pontine myelinolysis	Confusion, followed within a few days by dysphagia, dysarthria, quadriparesis with pyramidal tract signs, and oculomotor disturbances (bilateral abducens palsy or horizontal conjugate gaze palsy); progressive impairment of consciousness, later development of the locked-in syndrome	— Seen in malnourished chronic alcoholics — Also as an iatrogenic process after excessively rapid correction of hyponatremia — Also in liver disease
Alcoholic polyneuropathy	Mainly sensory polyneuropathy, often painful; distal sensory deficit in the lower limbs, areflexia	
Fetal alcohol syndrome (alcohol embryopathy)	Short stature, psychomotor retardation, microcephaly, facial dysmorphism (stub nose, thin lips, micrognathism)	Caused by maternal alcoholism

Hepatic Encephalopathy

Neurologic manifestations are commonly seen in hepatic diseases, particularly **chronic hepatopathy** with **portal hypertension** and **portacaval shunting**. Ammonia and other toxic substances bypass the portal circulation, enter the systemic circulation, and are transported to the brain, where they cause **hepatic encephalopathy**. This disorder is characterized at first by **somnolence and apathy**, and later by **progressive impairment of consciousness** and **delirium**. As in renal insufficiency, **asterixis** can be seen (see section 6.8.9). In addition, there may be **spasticity**, with exaggerated deep tendon reflexes and pyramidal tract signs.

Other Gastrointestinal Diseases That Can Involve the Nervous System

In **celiac disease (sprue)**, impaired intestinal absorption can cause malnutrition, which in turn causes polyneuropathy and cerebellar ataxia (**vitamin B$_{12}$ deficiency**). The **gliadin antibodies** that are present in sprue are also often associated with ataxia.

Crohn disease may be accompanied by myelopathy and muscle weakness, while **ulcerative colitis** may be accompanied by peripheral neuropathy.

Gastrointestinal manifestations and myopathy are combined in the so-called **MNGIE syndrome**, an abbreviation for myo-neuro-gastrointestinal encephalopathy

Table 6.28

Clinical manifestations of hypoglycemia

Type of manifestation	Symptoms, signs
Autonomic	– Dizziness, headache, diaphoresis, nausea, pallor – Palpitations, precordial pressure – Abdominal pain, hunger – Anxiety
Cerebral	– Paresthesiae, blurred vision, diplopia, tremor, unusual or abnormal behavior – Epileptic seizures: simple partial, complex partial, or generalized – Impairment of consciousness ranging from somnolence to coma – Focal neurologic deficits, e.g., hemiparesis, hemianopsia, aphasia, apraxia
Permanent neurologic deficits (after prolonged or recurrent hypoglycemia)	– Cognitive deficits, dementia – Focal cognitive deficits, focal neurologic deficits – Mainly distal muscular atrophy due to damage of anterior horn cells and axons

(for details see section 15.5.2, Examples of Mitochondrial Myopathies).

6.8.5 Hematologic Diseases

NOTE

Hematologic diseases can alter the viscosity and coagulability of the blood, putting the patient at risk of thrombosis or hemorrhage. They can also alter its transport properties (quantitative and structural anomalies of the blood cells or plasma proteins). Finally, some hematologic diseases involve malignant neoplasia of certain types of blood cells. All of these phenomena can damage the nervous system.

Anemia. Anemia reduces the oxygen-carrying capacity of the blood and can lead to **hypoxic (ischemic) cerebral dysfunction**. The vitamin B_{12} deficiency of untreated **pernicious anemia** causes funicular myelosis (see section 7.6.4) and polyneuropathy (cf. **Table 11.1**).

Polycythemia vera. This is associated with headache, dizziness, and paresthesiae, as well as TIAs, ischemic stroke, and extrapyramidal manifestations.

Leukemia. Leukemia often causes cerebrovascular complications (hemorrhage, infarct, venous sinus thrombosis). One-third of leukemia patients have a meningeal leukemic infiltrate (**leukemic meningitis**). Leukemic infiltrates can cause various kinds of focal deficits of the central and peripheral nervous system.

6.8.6 Collagen Diseases and Immune Diseases

NOTE

Collagenoses affect not only the skin, joints, and internal organs, but also the nervous system. Secondary damage of nervous tissue (ischemia and/or hemorrhage) occurs because of inflammatory changes of the blood vessels of the brain, spinal cord, and peripheral nerves (vasa nervorum). These vascular changes are mostly produced by autoimmune mechanisms.

In this section, we will merely list the neurologic manifestations of the main types of collagen disease. More detailed discussions can be found in textbooks of internal medicine.

Practical Tip

Though collagen diseases and vasculitis are only briefly discussed in this book, the clinician must keep them in mind when formulating the differential diagnosis of practically any condition with neurologic manifestations.

– **Periarteritis nodosa.** In the nervous system, this disease causes polyneuropathy and mononeuropathies and, less commonly, focal deficits of the CNS or epileptic seizures.
– **Churg–Strauss syndrome.** The main clinical manifestations of this disorder, closely related to periarteritis nodosa, are bronchial asthma and marked eosinophilia; painful polyneuritis is the main neurologic manifestation.
– **GANS (granulomatous angiitis of the CNS)** is a vasculitic disorder, restricted to the cerebral vessels, that causes multiple thrombotic strokes.
– **Temporal arteritis.** Intractable **headache** is the main symptom of this disease. The temporal artery is thickened (at least on one side) and, in advanced disease, no longer pulsates. A more extensive discussion of this disease can be found in section 14.2.4, Cranial Arteritis.
– **Wegener granulomatosis** is a systemic, necrotizing vasculitis that mainly involves the kidneys and the upper airways, but can also cause mononeuritis (of the cranial nerves as well) and focal manifestations in the CNS.

- **Systemic lupus erythematosus** only rarely presents with neurologic deficits, but more than half of all patients develop neurologic and/or psychiatric manifestations as the disease progresses. The most common ones are headache, neuropsychological deficits and behavioral abnormalities, focal neurologic deficits, and spinal cord transection syndromes, followed by neuritis and myopathy.
- **Sarcoidosis** (Boeck disease) is characterized by the formation of multiple granulomas in the lungs and other internal organs. Depending on their location, granulomas in the nervous system can cause chronic meningitis (see section 6.7.4), encephalitic manifestations (diabetes insipidus, hemiparesis, ataxia), cranial nerve palsies, or mononeuritis multiplex (see section 11.3.1, Mononeuropathies and Mononeuritis Multiplex).

Diagnostic evaluation. Collagen and immune diseases are diagnosed by their typical clinical manifestations, the demonstration of specific (auto) antibodies in the serum, and further evidence derived from angiography or from biopsies of tissue and/or blood vessels.

Treatment. These diseases generally require immunosuppressive treatment for weeks or months (occasionally longer).

6.8.7 Paraneoplastic Syndromes

| NOTE |

Cancer can impair the functioning of the nervous system by direct tumor invasion, metastasis, or **long-distance humorally mediated effects** (paraneoplastic syndromes).

Etiology. The paraneoplastic effects of cancerous growths are, by definition, those that do not arise directly (e.g., tissue compression or infiltration), but rather indirectly, for example, through the mediation of cytokines, hormones, or immune reactions. They can, in principle, occur in any type of malignancy, but are especially common in **small-cell bronchial carcinoma**.

Clinical features. Paraneoplastic syndromes often become clinically evident while the primary tumor is still asymptomatic. They can affect the **CNS**, the **spinal nerve roots**, the **peripheral nerves**, or the **muscles**.

Diagnostic evaluation. These syndromes are diagnosed from their clinical findings, combined with the **identification of the responsible tumor**; the diagnosis can be confirmed, in many patients, by the demonstration of more or less **specific antineuronal antibodies**. Nonetheless, paraneoplastic syndromes are still, in general, **diagnoses of exclusion**.

Practical Tip

If a typical paraneoplastic syndrome arises, an underlying cancer should be suspected and looked for—generally with diagnostic imaging.

Some of the paraneoplastic syndromes affecting the nervous system are listed in **Table 6.29**, together with the primary tumors that cause them.

6.8.8 Limbic Encephalitis

Etiology and pathogenesis. This disease was first described as a type of **paraneoplastic encephalitis**, but it can also occur as an **autoimmune encephalitis** in the absence of cancer.

Clinical features. As the name implies, limbic encephalitis manifests itself mainly in symptoms and signs that are referable to the **limbic system** (see section 5.5.4). It usually begins with a disturbance of explicit memory that progresses over the course of several weeks, or else with partial or generalized epileptic seizures. Further manifestations include personality change, affect disturbances, confusion, and sometimes agitation and hallucinations.

Diagnostic evaluation. The **CSF** displays inflammatory changes, and **MRI** reveals mesiotemporal signal abnormalities. Serologic tests often reveal **antibodies against neuronal intracellular antigens** (anti-Hu, anti-Ma, anti-GAD) or against **cell-membrane antigens** (VGKC, NMDA, AMPA, GABA, glycine receptors). Histopathologic examination reveals **inflammatory infiltrates**, **neuron loss**, and **reactive gliosis**, mainly in the limbic and insular cortex. The responsible tumor is often a small-cell cancer of the lung and less commonly a cancer of the breast, ovary, uterus, or testis. The neurologic manifestations usually arise before the tumor itself becomes clinically evident.

Treatment. The treatment is by **immune modulation or suppression**. Steroids or immunoglobulins often lead to clinical improvement. If these fail, rituximab, cyclophosphamide, or other immunosuppressants can be tried. If an underlying tumor is discovered, it should be removed.

6.8.9 Renal Failure and Electrolyte Disturbances

Electrolyte disturbances can become symptomatic through either of the following:

- **Brain dysfunction** (impairment of consciousness and/or cognition, generalized epileptic seizures).
- **Disturbances of neuromuscular transmission** (overexcitability, e.g., in tetany due to hypocalcemia; underexcitability, e.g., in disorders of potassium metabolism with episodic paralysis; see section 15.4.2).

Table 6.29

Paraneoplastic syndromes affecting the nervous system

Syndrome/structure affected	Clinical features	Remarks
Paraneoplastic encephalomyelitis	Affects the cerebral hemispheres, limbic system, brainstem, cerebellum, and spinal cord; limbic system involvement is prominent; confusion, agitation, hallucinations, anxiety, depression, epileptic seizures, pyramidal tract signs	– Occurs in small-cell bronchial carcinoma, less commonly in carcinoma of the breast, ovary, uterus, testis, and other organs – There are subtypes that preferentially affect individual nervous structures, e.g., paraneoplastic myelitis, paraneoplastic retinopathy, opsoclonus-myoclonus syndrome, and stiff person syndrome
Paraneoplastic cerebellar degeneration	Rapidly progressive cerebellar ataxia (weeks), disabling truncal and appendicular ataxia, dysarthria, nystagmus, and sometimes other neurologic deficits	– The most common paraneoplastic syndrome – Seen in small-cell bronchial carcinoma, ovarian carcinoma, Hodgkin's lymphoma; also in carcinoma of the lung, breast, or uterus – Actually a subtype of paraneoplastic encephalomyelitis
Paraneoplastic polyneuropathy	Sensory or, less commonly, sensorimotor polyneuropathy or mononeuropathy	– Mainly in lung carcinoma
Paraneoplastic syndromes of the neuromuscular junction: myasthenia gravis and Lambert–Eaton syndrome	Myasthenic syndrome preferentially affecting the extraocular and bulbar musculature (in myasthenia gravis) or the limb muscles (in Lambert–Eaton syndrome)	– Thymoma (myasthenia gravis) – Mainly small-cell bronchial carcinoma (Lambert–Eaton syndrome)
Dermatomyositis, polymyositis	Progressive muscle weakness; also skin changes in dermatomyositis	– Tumors of the breast, lung, stomach, ovary, and intestine

 Practical Tip

Electrolyte disturbances should be included in the differential diagnosis of any impairment of consciousness, epileptic seizure, or paralysis.

Electrolyte disturbances, particularly those affecting sodium concentration, are often caused by **renal failure** or by **side effects of diuretic drugs**. In renal disease, the pathologic retention of substances normally excreted in the urine can have further toxic effects.

Acute Renal Failure

Acute renal failure causes **uremic encephalopathy**, which is characterized by progressive **loss of concentration and short-term memory**, followed by **impairment of consciousness and delirium**. These abnormalities of mental state are often accompanied by **dysarthria**, **gait unsteadiness**, and **ataxia**. Nearly all affected patients have **myoclonus** and **asterixis** (bilateral, irregular back-and-forth movements of the fingers when the arms are extended; sometimes, analogous motor phenomena in other parts of the body as well).

Chronic Renal Failure

Chronic renal failure may lead to **polyneuropathy** and **restless legs syndrome** (see section 10.2.2). Patients undergoing dialysis may develop the **dialysis disequilibrium syndrome** (nausea, agitation, delirium, convulsions). Those who have been treated with dialysis for a long time are at risk for **dialysis encephalopathy** (dialysis dementia), with dysarthria, ataxia, and convulsions.

Electrolyte Disturbances

NOTE

Disturbances of sodium concentration alter the serum osmolality and are the type of electrolyte disturbance most commonly causing neurologic dysfunction. The neurologic condition in such cases can be considered a type of **metabolic encephalopathy**.

Hyponatremia and hypo-osmolality. These can cause **cerebral edema**, which presents clinically with headache, nausea, impaired attention and concentration, epileptic seizures, and a progressive decline of consciousness.

Hypernatremia and hyperosmolality. These lower the water content and thus also the volume of the brain; they cause **cognitive impairment** and a **progressive decline of consciousness**. The generalized hypercoagulable state characterizing these conditions may lead to venous sinus thrombosis. Alternatively, as the brain shrinks from loss of water, bridging veins may be torn, producing a subdural hematoma.

Rapid rise of serum sodium concentration. A rapid return of the sodium concentration from below normal (hyponatremia) toward normal values is considered to be the cause of **central pontine myelinolysis**, that is, bilaterally symmetric demyelination of the white matter of the base (ventral portion) of the pons. Clinically, the disorder presents with impairment of consciousness, dysphagia, dysarthria, and spastic quadriparesis, and sometimes oculomotor dysfunction (horizontal gaze paresis). In severe cases, it manifests itself as the locked-in syndrome (described in section 5.5.5) or decerebrate rigidity. **Further Electrolyte Disturbances.**

> **NOTE**
>
> **Disturbances of potassium, calcium, and magnesium balance**, as well as **hypophosphatemia**, can affect **muscle function**, sometimes dramatically.

— **Hypokalemia or hyperkalemia** can cause flaccid **paresis** of peripheral neurogenic type, as well as disturbances of myocardial excitability.
— **Hypocalcemia** and **hypomagnesemia** cause **tetany**.
— **Hypercalcemia** and **hypermagnesemia** cause metabolic encephalopathy with slowing, confusion, and impairment of consciousness. **Hypophosphatemia** causes peripheral **paresis**.

6.9 Parkinson Disease and Other Hypertonic–Hypokinetic Syndromes

 Key Point
The common feature of diseases of the basal ganglia is a movement disorder in which there is either too much or too little movement, that is, an excess or deficiency of movement impulse, movement automaticity, and/or muscle tone (see section 5.5.2).
In general, such diseases are characterized by the following:
— Disturbances of the process or movement (always).
— Abnormally increased or diminished muscle tone (usually).
— Involuntary movements (often).
— Associated neuropsychological manifestations (sometimes).

Increased muscle tone is often associated with **paucity of movement**, and, conversely, diminished muscle tone with **excessive movement**. Thus, there are two main classes of extrapyramidal syndrome:
— **Hypertonic–hypokinetic extrapyramidal syndromes** (above all, parkinsonian syndromes and related neurodegenerative disorders, which will be discussed in this section).
— **Hypotonic-hyperkinetic extrapyramidal syndromes** (e.g., chorea, athetosis, ballism, and dystonia, which will be discussed in the next section).

6.9.1 Overview

> **NOTE**
>
> In hypertonic–hyperkinetic syndromes, elevated muscle tone is typically manifest as **rigidity**. Paucity of movement, depending on its severity, is termed either **hypokinesia** (= diminished movement) or **akinesia** (= complete lack of movement). A third so-called "cardinal manifestation," **tremor**, is also commonly present. This clinical triad, called the **parkinsonian syndrome** (or parkinsonism), is typically found in idiopathic Parkinson disease. Often, postural instability (= **tendency to fall**) occur as a fourth cardinal manifestation.

Parkinson disease, however, is only one possible cause of parkinsonism; there are many others besides. Parkinsonism may be due to an underlying illness or condition other than idiopathic Parkinson disease (**symptomatic parkinsonian syndromes**). In addition, several **systemic neurodegenerative diseases** cause parkinsonism. These rare diseases are marked by a loss of neurons not only in the basal ganglia, but also in other areas of the CNS, and thus are clinically characterized not only by extrapyramidal manifestations, but also by neurologic deficits localizable to other regions of the brain. The most important diseases in this category, multisystem atrophy (MSA) and corticobasal degeneration (CBD), will be discussed further in this chapter. Lewy body dementia belongs in this category as well but will be discussed later in the subsection on dementia (section 6.12).

6.9.2 Parkinson Disease (Idiopathic Parkinson Syndrome)

Definition. Parkinson disease is defined by its clinical manifestations (characteristic body posture and gait, with hypokinesia, rigidity, and, usually, rest tremor) and their pathologic correlates in the brain: Lewy bodies containing α-synuclein and degeneration of dopaminergic neurons in the pars compacta of the substantia nigra (a pigmented nucleus in the midbrain).

Epidemiology, Etiology, and Pathogenesis
Epidemiology and etiology. Parkinson disease has an overall prevalence of 0.15%. Its age-specific prevalence rises with increasing age, to 1% in persons older than 60 years and 3% in persons older than 80 years. Most cases are **idiopathic**, that is, **without any identifiable cause**.
Familial clustering of Parkinson disease is seen in 5 to 15% of cases (so-called **hereditary Parkinson disease**); patients who develop Parkinson disease at an **unusually young age** are particularly likely to have a

problem of this type. To date, 18 genetic loci (PARK1 through PARK18) and at least 7 genes have been identified whose mutations can cause a hereditary parkinsonian syndrome. The mode of inheritance can be autosomal dominant with variable penetrance or autosomal recessive. A special type is the familial Parkinson–dementia complex seen on the island of Guam. The combination of parkinsonism and dementia also sometimes exhibits familial clustering.

Pathogenesis. The neuropathologic hallmark of idiopathic Parkinson disease is **degeneration of the dopaminergic neurons of the substantia nigra** and the **locus ceruleus.** Hyaline inclusion bodies, called **Lewy bodies**, are found within the degenerated neurons. The loss of dopaminergic neurons leads to a **degeneration of the (inhibitory) nigrostriatal dopaminergic pathway** and, therefore, to **dopamine deficiency in the striatum.** This, in turn, leads to enhanced activity of the striatal glutamatergic neurons, which produces the clinical manifestations of the disease.

Additional Information

In the **Braak system** of Parkinson disease there are **six neuropathologic stages** that trace the temporal progression of intraneuronal Lewy body formation from lower to higher neural centers in the brain. In stages 1 and 2, before any clinical manifestations of the disease have arisen, Lewy bodies are present only in certain areas of the brainstem and the olfactory system. The first symptoms arise in stages 3 and 4 when Lewy bodies begin to appear in the substantia nigra. Finally, in stages 5 and 6, Lewy bodies are found in diffuse areas of the cerebral cortex.

Clinical Features

The clinical picture of idiopathic Parkinson disease and of hereditary parkinsonian syndromes (**Fig. 6.55**) is typically characterized by:

- **Hypokinesia**, i.e., slowing of movement.
- **Increased muscle tone (rigidity).**
- **Abnormal body posture** (stooped head and trunk, flexion at the knees).
- **Impaired postural reflexes**, sometimes leading to **falls.**
- Often **tremor.**
- Later, **neuropsychological deficits** and certain **vegetative/autonomic disturbances** such as oily (seborrheic) face and bladder dysfunction.

 Practical Tip
The motor signs are often only unilateral, or more marked on one side, when the disease first appears. They can be aggravated by emotional stress.

Hypokinesia. Hypokinesia manifests itself as **paucity of facial expression** (mask-like facies), **reduced frequency of blinking**, and **speech disturbances** (dysphonia, i.e., slow, monotonous, unmodulated speech, and repetitions). There is little spontaneous movement, and the normal accessory movements (e.g., arm swing during walking) are diminished or absent. The patient's handwriting becomes progressively smaller (**micrographia**). Repeated or alternating movements (e.g., finger-tapping) are performed slowly and with smaller excursions (dysdiadochokinesia; cf. **Fig. 3.19**). Axial movements, such as turning around while standing or turning over in bed, are difficult to perform. Very severe hypokinesia is sometimes called **akinesia.**

Gait. A parkinsonian gait is characterized by a mildly **stooped posture**, with the head jutting forward, and a **small-stepped, often shuffling gait, without accessory arm movements** (**Fig. 6.56**). To turn around while standing, the patient makes **many small turning steps.**

Increased muscle tone. This is primarily evident as **rigidity** (**Fig. 3.24**), felt by the examiner during large-amplitude, passive flexion and extension of the joints. Rigidity is sometimes easier to detect when the patient voluntarily contracts the muscles on the opposite side of the body. Often, during passive movement, the examiner may feel a small, brief, periodically recurring diminution of muscle tone, known as the **cogwheel phenomenon**, which is usually most evident at the wrist (**Fig. 3.25**). The patient's **postural tone**, too, is elevated; if, for example, the head is lifted off the bed and let go, it may remain suspended in midair for some time (the Wartenberg sign; the classic literature spoke of a "*coussin psychique*," i.e., a virtual pillow).

 Practical Tip
Another test for the objectification of rigidity is the so-called swinging test: the examiner grasps and shakes the patient's forearm back and forth. Rigidity markedly diminishes the swinging (pendular) motion of the wrist. The test can also be performed at the elbow or knee joint.

Tremor. Three-quarters of patients with Parkinson disease have tremor sooner or later in the course of their disease, typically a **distal rest tremor at a frequency of 5 Hz.** A **pronation–supination ("pill-rolling") tremor** is highly characteristic. The tremor is present at rest and generally disappears on voluntary movement; it is sometimes increased by mental exertion, deep concentration, or walking. Some patients have **postural** and **intention tremor** in addition to rest tremor (see **Fig. 3.22**).

The risk of falling. An impairment of postural reflexes, combined with hypokinesia, has the consequence that changes of body posture and orientation in space can no longer be compensated for by reflexive, rapid corrective movements. The most obvious manifestations of this problem are **pro- and retropulsion**. If the patient is pushed while standing still, or stumbles over an obstacle, the movements made to regain balance are too small and too slow, and a **fall** may result.

Practical Tip

The patient's postural reflexes and possible tendency to fall can be tested with the pull test and the push-and-release test. In the former, the examiner stands behind the patient and pulls back on both shoulders; in the latter, the patient is propped up in a standing position from behind by the examiner's hands, which are then suddenly released. (Obviously, when performing these tests, the examiner must make sure that the patient can be caught in case of a fall.)

Impaired olfaction. An impaired sense of smell is almost universal in patients with idiopathic Parkinson disease but rare in patients with symptomatic parkinsonism.

neuropsychological deficits. When the first symptoms of Parkinson disease arise, the patient's cognitive functions are generally normal or only mildly impaired. As the disease progresses, however, neuropsychological deficits almost always arise. Memory is impaired, cognitive processes are slowed (bradyphrenia), and there is a tendency toward perseveration. Rapid changes in thought content are difficult to achieve, and the planning and execution of actions and behaviors is impaired (so-called dysexecutive syndrome).

Psychiatric manifestations. Depression affects one-third to one-half of all patients over the course of the disease and is treatable. Isolated apathy (without depression) can also arise. Impulse-control disorders, such as compulsive shopping, gambling, or hypersexuality, are usually side effects of dopaminergic drugs. The patient's perceptions and thought processes can become abnormal over the course of the disease, because of either the disease itself or its dopaminergic treatment; hallucinations and overt psychoses can result.

Disturbances of autonomic and vegetative function. Such disturbances arise partly as a by-product of hypokinesia and partly because of direct involvement of the autonomic nervous system. These include **seborrhea** (an oily face, caused by excessive fat production in the skin), hypersalivation, cold intolerance, a tendency toward **orthostatic hypotension** and **constipation**, **urinary urgency** (possibly causing incontinence), and sexual dysfunction (altered libido, **erectile dysfunction**). Insomnia and behavioral disturbances during REM sleep (see section 10.4) are often seen early on in the course of disease; the patient's sleep can also be disturbed by restless legs syndrome (see section 10.2.2) or spontaneous **pain in the limbs**.

The nonmotor manifestations of Parkinson disease are summarized in **Table 6.30**.

Classification and grading of manifestations. The manifestations described are present to variable extents in different patients with Parkinson disease. Generally speaking, the disease has three main clinical variants:

- The **akinetic-rigid type** (without tremor).
- The **tremor-dominant type** (with little hypokinesia and rigidity).
- The **mixed or "equivalence" type** (with roughly equal severity of all three cardinal manifestations —rigidity, hypokinesia, and tremor).

Individual clinical manifestations can be graded on pseudoquantitative scales, if this is desired for long-term follow-up or for research purposes, for example, with the **Webster Rating Scale** (**Table 6.31**) or the very detailed **Unified Parkinson's Disease Rating Scale** (UPDRS), which is not reproduced here. Cognitive function can be assessed with the MOCA test or the Mini-Mental State Examination (MMSE; see **Table 3.11**).

The Neurologic Examination and Other Diagnostic Tests

NOTE

The diagnosis of Parkinson disease is based on the typical clinical manifestations and **characteristic findings on neurologic examination**.

History. Important points to be addressed in clinical history-taking include the following:

- Has the patient had difficulty with fine motor activities such as writing, getting dressed, or eating?
- Is the patient's gait less steady than before, perhaps with stumbling or falls?
- Has the patient noticed any difference between the right and left sides of the body?
- Does the patient suffer from pain or disturbed sleep?
- Has there been any impairment of the sense of smell or any difficulty swallowing?

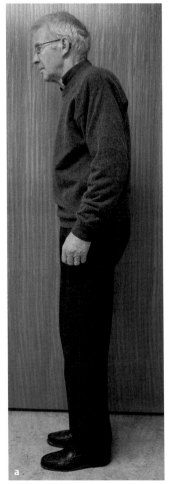
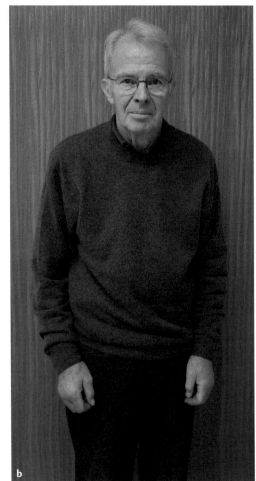

Fig. 6.55   Parkinson disease. (a) Typical posture with stooped head and upper body and lightly flexed elbows, hips, and knees. **(b)** Hypomimia (paucity of facial expression) and the asymmetry of manifestations that is typical in idiopathic Parkinson disease (the right elbow is somewhat more strongly flexed than the left).

Neurologic examination. In addition to hypokinesia, **rigidity**, **tremor**, and **propulsion/retropulsion**, the examination generally reveals the following:
- **Weak convergence** (movements to focus the eyes are slowed).
- A **persistent glabellar reflex** (i.e., lack of habituation of the reflex after repeated glabellar tapping).
- **Saccadic ocular pursuit movements**.
- **Impaired olfaction**.

The intrinsic muscle reflexes are normal, however, as are all somatosensory modalities.

For numerical grading, see the preceding paragraphs and **Table 6.31**.

Imaging studies. CT and MRI of the head reveal no abnormalities and are generally performed only to rule out competing diagnoses, for example, symptomatic parkinsonian syndromes. The loss of **dopaminergic afferent input to the striatum** can be demonstrated with **positron emission tomography**

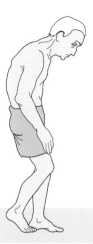

Fig. 6.56   Typical parkinsonian posture while walking: inclined head, slightly stooped upper body, flexed elbows, and lightly flexed hips and knees.

Table 6.30

Nonmotor manifestations of Parkinson disease

Autonomic/vegetative	Cognitive	Psychiatric
— Hyperhidrosis — Hypersalivation — Seborrhea — Obstipation — Cold intolerance — Circulatory dysregulation, orthostatic hypotension — Sexual dysfunction (loss of libido, abnormally increased libido, erectile dysfunction) — REM-sleep behavioral disorder — Insomnia — Daytime somnolence, sleep attacks — Pain, paresthesiae — Hyposmia, anosmia	— Slowed thinking (bradyphrenia) — Perseveration — Impaired planning, strategy, and execution (dysexecutive syndrome) — Cognitive impairment, ranging from mild to severe frontal dementia in advanced disease	— Depression — Apathy — Hallucinations, illusions — Psychosis (mainly as a drug effect) — Impulse-control disorder (compulsive shopping, gambling, or sexual behavior; mainly as a drug effect)

Table 6.31

Simplified scale for evaluating the severity of individual signs of Parkinson disease

1. Bradykinesia of hands, including handwriting	0 = normal 1 = mild slowing 2 = moderate slowing, handwriting severely impaired 3 = severe slowing
2. Rigidity	0 = none 1 = mild 2 = moderate 3 = severe, present despite medication
3. Posture	0 = normal 1 = mildly stooped 2 = arm flexion 3 = severely stooped; arm, hand, and knee flexion
4. Arm swing	0 = good bilaterally 1 = unilaterally impaired 2 = unilaterally absent 3 = bilaterally absent
5. Gait	0 = normal, turns without difficulty 1 = short steps, slow turn 2 = markedly shortened steps, both heels slap on floor 3 = shuffling steps, occasional freezing, very slow turn
6. Tremor	0 = none 1 = amplitude < 2.5 cm 2 = amplitude > 10 cm 3 = amplitude > 10 cm, constant, eating and writing impossible
7. Facial expression	0 = normal 1 = mild hypomimia 2 = marked hypomimia, lips open, marked drooling 3 = mask-like facies, mouth open, marked drooling
8. Seborrhea	0 = none 1 = increased sweating 2 = oily skin 3 = marked deposition on face
9. Speech	0 = normal 1 = reduced modulation, good volume 2 = monotonous, not modulated, incipient dysarthria, difficulty being understood 3 = marked difficulty being understood
10. Independence	0 = not impaired 1 = mildly impaired (dressing) 2 = needs help in critical situations, all activities markedly slowed 3 = cannot dress him- or herself, eat or walk unaided

Source: Webster DD. Critical analysis of the disability in Parkinson disease. Mod Treat 1968;5(2):257–282.
Note: The sum of the scores indicates the degree of severity of Parkinson disease: 0–10 mild, 10–20 moderate, 20–30: severe.

(PET) or **single-photon emission computed tomography (SPECT)** after the administration of ^{18}fluorodopa (**Fig. 6.57**). **Cerebral ultrasonography** can reveal early changes in the substantia nigra.

> **NOTE**
>
> Idiopathic Parkinson disease is always a diagnosis of exclusion, that is, all varieties of symptomatic parkinsonism must be **ruled out** before this diagnosis can be made.

Testing of olfaction. Impairment of the sense of smell early on in the course of disease is supporting evidence for idiopathic or genetically triggered Parkinson disease. Smell is tested with small samples of various substances (coffee, etc.).

Genetic testing. In young patients with a positive family history, genetic testing can help secure the diagnosis and enable a more accurate prognosis.

Treatment, complications, and prognosis. Effective treatment alleviates the manifestations of the disease, moving the symptomatic progression curve to the right by some 3 to 5 years, but does not affect the disease process as such. The putative **early neuroprotective effect** of certain antiparkinsonian drugs has not yet been confirmed.

Pharmacotherapy. The goal of drug therapy is to **replace the missing dopamine** in the striatum.

> **NOTE**
>
> The most important antiparkinsonian drug is still **levodopa (L-DOPA)**, which is metabolized to dopamine in the CSF. At the beginning of treatment, only small doses are needed to alleviate the clinical manifestations; later on, however, higher doses are needed, and side effects such as dyskinesia and on–off motor fluctuations commonly arise. Therefore, efforts are often made to delay the administration of L-DOPA to younger patients by giving alternative drugs first.

- **MAO-B inhibitors** are increasingly used as drugs of first choice because of their putative neuroprotective effect. These include selegiline and rasagiline (a long-acting selegiline derivative). They inhibit the degradation of dopamine to homovanillic acid and thereby ameliorate parkinsonian manifestations.
- **Amantadine**, an NMDA-receptor antagonist, is sometimes used very early in the course of disease; it is thought to enhance dopamine release from nerve terminals.
- If these agents are no longer sufficiently effective, nonergot **dopamine agonists** (e.g., ropinirole, pramipexole, or rotigotine) can be used in younger patients; their effectiveness, however, matches that of L-DOPA only in the early stages of the disease.

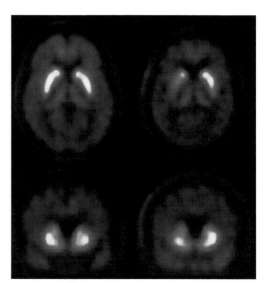

Fig. 6.57 An ^{18}F-DOPA-PET scan in a normal person (left, top and bottom) and in a patient with incipient Parkinson disease, worse on the left side of the body (right, top and bottom). The basal ganglia are seen in axial and coronal section (upper and lower rows of images, respectively). The patient with Parkinson disease has a more than 20% reduction in the activity of dopamine decarboxylase in the right putamen (particularly in its dorsal aspect), with relatively normal activity in the caudate nucleus. (Image provided courtesy of Dr. F. Jüngling, PET/CT-Zentrum NW-Schweiz, St. Claraspital, Basel, Switzerland.)

- In older patients, **L-DOPA** is used from the outset. This agent, unlike dopamine itself, crosses the blood–brain barrier; it is converted to dopamine in the CSF.
- L-DOPA is always given in combination with a **decarboxylase inhibitor** (e.g., **benserazide** [HCl] or **carbidopa**) to prevent its premature degradation in the periphery.
- The combination of L-DOPA with a **COMT inhibitor**, such as **entacapone** or **tolcapone**, can further increase dopamine bioavailability. Tolcapone, however, is occasionally hepatotoxic and is therefore reserved for otherwise intractable cases. Entacapone is sold as a combination drug together with L-DOPA and a decarboxylase inhibitor.
- **Anticholinergic drugs**, such as **biperiden**, are mainly effective against tremor. *Note:* their anticholinergic effect can also induce or worsen confusion and/or dementia.

> **NOTE**
>
> The following should be borne in mind as rules of thumb for the dosing of antiparkinsonian drugs, particularly L-DOPA:
> - Give as much as necessary and as little as possible.
> - The drug regimen should be as simple as possible to promote compliance.

Drug side effects and complications. Prolonged treatment with L-DOPA and other antiparkinsonian drugs can cause several problems:

— **Fluctuations in drug effect (on–off fluctuations, end-of-dose akinesia)** can often be improved by the use of sustained-release L-DOPA preparations, division of the daily dose into smaller individual doses at more frequent intervals (perhaps with the use of water-soluble L-DOPA preparations), and/or the addition of dopamine agonists or COMT inhibitors. Water-soluble L-DOPA takes effect very rapidly and can shorten off-phases or prevent imminent off-phases. Deep brain stimulation is another therapeutic possibility (see later).

— **Drug-induced dyskinesias**, for example, **peak-dose dyskinesia** or **hyperkinesia** (often involving choreiform involuntary movements; see section 6.10), are seen in 40% of patients after 6 months of L-DOPA treatment, in 60% after 2 years, and in nearly all after 6 years. They are usually more disturbing to patients' families than to the patients themselves, but they can be disabling if severe and may be untreatable except by deep brain stimulation.

— **Painful foot dystonia** can be managed with the use of sustained-release preparations in the evening and perhaps with apomorphine injections.

— **"Freezing,"** that is, sudden arrest of movement, is not directly related to the serum concentration of L-DOPA. Various mental techniques can help (carrying a briefcase, stepping over real or imagined obstacles, etc.).

— **Psychosis** and other psychiatric disturbances (e.g., hypersexuality, illusions, hallucinations, delusions, compulsive gambling, food cravings) usually arise as side effects of drugs, especially **dopamine agonists** (ropinirole, pramipexole). They may respond to a reduction of the dose or to the addition of an atypical neuroleptic drug (clozapine, risperidone).

— An **akinetic crisis** is a prolonged phase of extreme rigidity causing **complete immobility** and accompanied by hyperthermia, hyperhidrosis, other autonomic disturbances, and dysphagia. Such crises can be precipitated, for example, by abrupt discontinuation of antiparkinsonian drugs, errors in drug-taking or drug-prescribing, the use of neuroleptic drugs, surgical procedures, or infection. They can be treated with water-soluble L-DOPA (given by nasogastric tube), amantadine (by intravenous infusion), or apomorphine (by subcutaneous injection).

— Further side effects that can be induced by any dopaminergic drug include **nausea** (especially at the beginning of treatment; it can be counteracted with an antiemetic dopamine antagonist that has a purely peripheral effect, such as domperidone), fatigue, and orthostatic hypotension.

> **NOTE**
>
> Movement disorders that are caused by **L-DOPA:**
> **On-dyskinesia** (also called peak-dose or plateau hyperkinesia); choreatiform movements that arise as the serum L-DOPA concentration increases (see section 6.10).
> **Off-dystonia** (also called early-morning dystonia): painful dystonia, for example, in one or both feet, that arises as the serum L-DOPA concentration falls.

Deep brain stimulation. Neurosurgical treatment, consisting of the **stereotactic implantation of stimulating electrodes** into the thalamus (nucleus ventrointermedius), globus pallidus, or subthalamic nucleus for chronic electrical stimulation, can markedly alleviate the manifestations of the disease; its indication depends on their severity and intractability in the individual patient. Each stimulating electrode has multiple metallic contacts, at which the intensity, pulse width, and frequency of the applied current can be independently controlled to optimize the clinical effect. This method has now largely replaced earlier destructive methods involving the creation of permanent lesions. It was once considered a treatment of last resort but is now increasingly used for patients in intermediate stages of the disease. An overview of the expected effects of deep brain stimulation in each of the three currently used target structures is provided in **Table 6.32**.

Further types of treatment. Aside from drugs and surgery, **physical therapy** and regular exercise (sports, walking, hiking) can help improve and maintain mobility. **Speech therapy** may be helpful as well. Moreover, adequate **psychological support** for patients and their families is important. **Self-help groups** can be valuable in this regard.

Course and prognosis. **L-DOPA treatment** can shift the symptomatic progression curve to the right by 6 to 7 years. It is hard to predict which patients will eventually become dependent on the help of others or on around-the-clock nursing care. This tends to occur after approximately 20 years of illness.

The **tremor-dominant type** has a relatively favorable prognosis. The prognosis is worse for older patients, men as opposed to women, and patients with severe disease (in terms of both motor and nonmotor manifestations). Parkinson disease can shorten the patient's life span.

Table 6.32

Current target structures for deep brain stimulation in the treatment of Parkinson disease, and the expected effects of stimulation at each structure

Target structure	Best effect	Remarks
Subthalamic nucleus	Reduction of hypokinesia, less frequent and less intense off-phases	The L-DOPA dose can be markedly reduced. Dyskinesia and tremor improve as well
Globus pallidus internus	Reduction of dyskinesia during on-phases	Hypokinesia and rigidity improve as well, but less than with stimulation in the subthalamic nucleus
Nucleus ventrointermedius of the thalamus	Reduction of tremor	Little effect on hypokinesia or dyskinesia

> **NOTE**
>
> Parkinson disease is a progressive disease whose manifestations can be alleviated by drugs, deep brain stimulation, and physiotherapy.

Differential Diagnosis

Tremor, hypokinesia, and rigidity can also be expressions of diseases other than Parkinson disease, including symptomatic parkinsonian syndromes.

> **NOTE**
>
> The main differential diagnoses of idiopathic Parkinson disease are: **neuroleptic side effects** and **other neurodegenerative systemic diseases** causing abnormal movements: Lewy body dementia, MSA, progressive supranuclear palsy (PSP), malresorptive **hydrocephalus**, and **subcortical arteriosclerotic encephalopathy**.

Neuroimaging now enables the recognition of some of these entities by their **typical MRI findings**:
- Ventricular enlargement in malresorptive hydrocephalus (also called "normal pressure hydrocephalus").
- "Hot-cross-bun" sign in MSA.
- Midbrain atrophy with the "Mickey Mouse" and/or "hummingbird" signs, along with frontal atrophy, in PSP.

An overview of these and other differential diagnoses is provided in **Table 6.33**.

6.9.3 Symptomatic Parkinsonian Syndromes

There are several clinical conditions that resemble idiopathic Parkinson disease but have a different underlying cause or pathophysiologic mechanism. The clue to such a condition may be a history of a **precipitating event** (e.g., **intoxication, drug use, trauma, or infection**) or a **structural abnormality of the basal ganglia** or other brain areas (e.g., **multiple arteriosclerotic changes, hydrocephalus**) revealed by CT or MRI. A further characteristic of symptomatic parkinsonism is its **relative resistance to treatment with L-DOPA**, in contrast to idiopathic Parkinson disease, which usually responds very well to L-DOPA, at least at first. Moreover, some forms of symptomatic

parkinsonism present with symmetric manifestations, while idiopathic Parkinson disease generally presents asymmetrically.

6.9.4 Progressive Supranuclear Palsy

This disease is also known as Steele–Richardson–Olszewski syndrome.

Etiology and pathology. A polymorphism in the tau protein gene (chromosome 17) causes deposition of an abnormally phosphorylated tau protein in the cells of the basal ganglia. This "tauopathy," in turn, leads to cellular degeneration in the substantia nigra, globus pallidus, subthalamic nucleus, periaqueductal area of the midbrain, and other brain nuclei.

Clinical features. The clinical features of PSP include the following:
- Paucity of movement.
- **Gait disturbance** early in the course of the disease.
- Predominantly **axial rigidity**, often with a **permanently extended cervical spine** (head turned upward).
- **Frequent falls** with a tendency to fall backward.
- Progressive **dementia**.
- Impaired vertical gaze movements (particularly downward), with **nystagmus**.

Diagnostic evaluation. PSP is diagnosed from its typical clinical features. MRI reveals **midbrain atrophy**.

Treatment and course. This disease presents between ages 50 and 70 years, mainly in men. Its manifestations tend to respond only weakly to L-DOPA, or not at all. PSP progresses rapidly and causes death within a few years.

6.9.5 Multisystem Atrophy

This term subsumes a collection of **rare diseases** that were previously described as separate entities:
- Olivopontocerebellar atrophy (**OPCA**), now also called **MSA-C** (cerebellar type).
- Striatonigral degeneration (**SND**), now also called **MSA-P** (parkinsonian type).
- Shy–Drager syndrome (**SDS**).
- Mixed forms of these.

6

Table 6.33

The differential diagnosis of idiopathic Parkinson disease

Cause of parkinsonism	Examples
Arteriosclerotic parkinsonism	– For example, in cerebral microangiopathy and subcortical arteriosclerotic encephalopathy
Drug-induced parkinsonism	– Neuroleptic agents (most common cause) – Antiemetic drugs (mainly dopamine agonists such as metoclopramide) – Lithium – Valproic acid – Reserpine – Calcium antagonists such as flunarizine
Parkinsonism of infectious origin	– Postencephalitic parkinsonism (after encephalitis lethargica) – Cerebrospinal syphilis – AIDS encephalopathy
Normal pressure hydrocephalus (also called malresorptive hydrocephalus)	
Toxic parkinsonism	– Carbon monoxide poisoning – Manganese poisoning – MPTP (1-methyl-4-phenyl-1,2,3,6-tetrahydropyridine, a by-product of the synthesis of the designer drug MPPP) – Cyanide – Methanol
Trauma	– Recurrent blunt trauma to the head (e.g., in boxers) – Midbrain trauma – Chronic subdural hematoma
Metabolic diseases	– Hypo- and pseudohypoparathyroidism with basal ganglionic calcification – Idiopathic basal ganglionic calcification, Fahr disease
Neurodegenerative diseases (see also **Tab. 1.1**)	– Progressive supranuclear palsy – Multisystem atrophy – Corticobasal degeneration – Lewy body disease – Frontotemporal dementia – Alzheimer disease with parkinsonian manifestations
Hereditary diseases that can have prominent parkinsonian manifestations	– Wilson disease – Pantothenate kinase–associated neurodegeneration – SCA3 spinocerebellar ataxia – Fragile-X-tremor-ataxia syndrome (FXTAS) – Westphal variant of Huntingtonchorea – Prion diseases
Further causes	– Brain tumor – Polycythemia vera – Acanthocytosis – Hemiparkinson-hemiatrophy syndrome

Pathology. The neuropathologic lesion consists of intracellular inclusion bodies (with α-synuclein; synucleinopathy) in glial cells as well as cellular degeneration and gliosis in the substantia nigra, striatum, pons, inferior olive, and cerebellum.

Clinical features. The main clinical features of MSA are present to varying extents in its different forms of MSA, each of which has its own characteristic initial presentation:

– **Parkinsonism**: **bradykinesia, akinesia, rigidity**, and **rest tremor** (seen early in the course of MSA-C and MSA-P).
– **Autonomic dysfunction**, including orthostatic hypotension, incontinence, and erectile dysfunction in men (seen early in the course of SDS).
– **Ataxia** and other **cerebellar signs** (prominent in OPCA, i.e., MSA-C).

– **Pyramidal tract signs** such as pathologic reflexes and spasticity.
– In some cases, dementia and/or frontal signs.

Diagnostic evaluation. These conditions are diagnosed from their **clinical features**. The diagnosis of MSA may be supported by an **MRI** finding of focal brain atrophy, for example, cerebellar atrophy or a loss of fiber connections in the pons (the "hot-cross-bun" sign with cross-shaped hypointensity in the pons).

Treatment. MSA generally responds poorly to treatment; dopamine agonists tend to be more effective than L-DOPA. The disease usually leads to severe disability and death within a few years of onset.

6.9.6 Corticobasal Degeneration

Pathology. The neuropathologic lesion in this disease consists of cellular degeneration and gliosis in the substantia nigra and in the pre- and postcentral gyri. The cerebral peduncles are correspondingly diminished in size. Like PSP, CBD is a type of tauopathy.

Clinical features. The manifestations of CBD, which are asymmetrically distributed, include:

- **Impaired fine motor control of an arm** (early in the course of the disease).
- Progressive **rigidity** and **akinesia**.
- **Weakness**.
- Central **sensory disturbances**.
- (Sometimes) apraxia.
- (Sometimes) dystonia.

Treatment and course. L-DOPA is generally not very effective and patients usually become severely disabled within a few years of the onset of the disease.

6.9.7 Lewy Body Dementia

This disease is described later in the section on dementia (section 6.12.3).

6.10 Chorea, Athetosis, Ballism, Dystonia: Hyperkinetic Syndromes

Key Point

These disturbances, unlike Parkinson disease, are characterized by "too much" movement, often in combination with diminished muscle tone. The different clinical types of hyperkinesia include chorea, athetosis, ballism, and dystonia, and mixed forms. Each of these movement disturbances may be due to a variety of underlying diseases. Thus, the hyperkinetic extrapyramidal syndroms are a diverse group both in their clinical features and in their causes.

An overview of the hyperkinetic extrapyramidal syndroms is provided in **Table 6.34**. The more important ones are described in greater detail in the text that follows.

6.10.1 HuntingtonChorea

Etiology. Huntington disease (chorea major) is a genetic disorder of autosomal dominant inheritance caused by an unstable CAG trinucleotide repeat expansion on the short arm of chromosome 4.

Pathology. The neuropathologic correlate of the disease is loss of small ganglion cells, mainly in the putamen and the caudate nucleus.

Clinical features. The disease generally becomes symptomatic between the ages of 30 and 50 years. As a rule, **choreiform movements** appear first, followed by **progressive dementia**. Patients who **inherited the defective gene from their father** tend to develop overt disease at an earlier age, sometimes

with rigidity and pyramidal tract signs as the initial manifestations.

 NOTE

Chorea consists of irregular, sudden, **involuntary movements that are usually more pronounced at the distal end of the limbs**.

- In some patients, these movements are of low amplitude and look almost normal, resembling nonpathologic "fidgetiness;" in others, they are massive and highly disturbing.
- Chorea can be unilateral ("hemichorea," **Fig. 6.58**) or bilateral.
- Muscle tone is normal or diminished.
- There is no weakness or sensory deficit, and pyramidal tract signs are absent.
- The intrinsic muscle reflexes are normal, except that they may have a second extension phase (**Gordon phenomenon**) if elicited at the same time as an incipient choreiform movement.

Practical Tip

Chorea, like other hyperkinesias (see later), is typically enhanced by goal-directed movement, mental stress, or concentration, and subsides in sleep and under general anesthesia.

Treatment, course, and prognosis. Huntingtonchorea **progresses chronically**, generally ending in **death** 10 to 15 years after the onset of symptoms. There is no treatment other than palliative, symptomatic management. The abnormal movements can be alleviated to some extent with **perphenazine, tetrabenazine, tiapride**, and other neuroleptic drugs. Depression can be treated with an **SSRI** or **sulpiride**; anxiety, agitation, and insomnia with **benzodiazepines**; and psychosis with **neuroleptic drugs**, preferably atypical ones such as olanzapine.

6.10.2 Chorea Minor (Sydenham Chorea)

Epidemiology. Chorea minor is the most common disease associated with choreiform movements. It mainly strikes **school-aged girls**.

Etiology and pathogenesis. This disease arises after an infection with **β-hemolytic group A streptococci** and is caused by an autoimmune reaction in which **antibodies** are generated that **cross-react** with neurons.

Clinical features. Within a few days or weeks after an attack of "strep throat," or within a few weeks or months of an attack of rheumatic fever, the patient develops **choreiform motor unrest** (mainly in the face, pharynx, and hands), combined with **irritability** and other **mental abnormalities**.

6

Table 6.34

The diagnostic evaluation of hyperkinetic extrapyramidal syndromes

Syndrome	Etiology	Remarks
Chorea: sudden, usually rapid, distal, brief, irregular involuntary movements; hypotonia		
Chorea minor	Autoimmune; streptococcal infection	Often a sequela of streptococcal pharyngitis, most commonly in girls aged 6 to 13 y
Chorea mollis	Autoimmune; streptococcal infection	Hypotonia is prominent
Chorea gravidarum	Third to fifth month of pregnancy	Usually during first pregnancy, often with prior history of chorea minor
Chorea due to antiovulatory drugs	Antiovulatory drugs	Rare, reversible with discontinuation of the drug
Huntington disease	Autosomal dominant	Onset usually at age 30 to 50 y; associated with progressive dementia
Benign familial chorea	Autosomal dominant	Onset in childhood, no further progression, no dementia
Choreoacanthocytosis	Autosomal recessive	Mainly orofacial, tongue-biting, elevated CK, hyporeflexia, acanthocytosis
Postapoplectic chorea	Vascular (prior stroke)	Sudden hemichorea and hemiparesis, often combined with hemiballism
Senile chorea	Vascular and degenerative	Occasional presenile onset, often more severe on one side, occasionally with dementia
Athetosis: slow, exaggerated movements against resistance of antagonist muscles, mainly distal; seem uncomfortable and cramped		
Status marmoratus	Perinatal asphyxia	Soon after birth, increasingly severe athetotic hyperkinesia, often cognitive impairment, sometimes also spasticity
Status dysmyelinisatus	Kernicterus of the newborn	Onset immediately after birth, often with other signs of perinatal brain damage; further progression
Pantothenate kinase–associated neurodegeneration	autosomal recessive disorder of pigment metabolism	Choreoathetotic movements beginning at age 5 to 15 y, rigidity, dementia, and retinitis pigmentosa in one-third of cases; progressive, with characteristic joint hyperflexion/hyperextension; death by age 30 y
Hemiathetosis	Focal lesion of pallidum and striatum	Unilateral, may come about some time after the causative lesion
Ballism/hemiballism: unilateral, lightning-like, high-amplitude flinging movements of multiple limb segments	Ischemic or neoplastic lesion of the subthalamic nucleus	Sudden onset, usually with hemiparesis as well
Dystonic syndromes		
Torsion dystonia: slow, tonic contractions of muscles or muscle groups, of shorter or longer duration, usually against the resistance of antagonist muscles	Familial types	Often in Ashkenazi Jewish families, onset before age 20 y with focal dystonia; later, rotatory movements of the head and trunk, as well as limb movements and athetotic finger movements
	Symptomatic types	For example, in Wilson disease, Huntington disease, pantothenate kinase–associated neurodegeneration
L-DOPA-sensitive dystonia: usually arises in childhood with dystonia of variably localization and fluctuation over the course of the day; progresses over the years	Sometimes due to familial tyrosine hydroxylase deficiency	Responds well to L-DOPA; can be difficult to distinguish from juvenile Parkinson disease with dystonia
Spasmodic torticollis: slow contraction of cervical and nuchal musculature against antagonist resistance, with rotatory movements of the head	Idiopathic, occasionally after cervical spine trauma and various other causes	One-third spontaneous recovery, one-third no change, one-third progression to torsion dystonia
Localized dystonia (see section 6.10.5)		For example, writer's cramp, faciobuccolingual dystonia, oromandibular dystonia

Abbreviation: CK, creatine kinase.

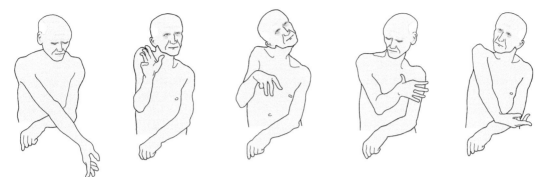

Fig. 6.58 Senile hemichorea. Drawings from video stills.

Treatment, course, and prognosis. The treatment is with high-dose **penicillin** for at least 10 days. The manifestations resolve spontaneously in a few weeks or months.

6.10.3 Athetosis

Pathology. The neuropathologic basis of athetosis is loss of neurons in the striatum, the globus pallidus, and, less commonly, the thalamus.

Etiology and types of athetosis. Congenital and peri-natally acquired lesions of the basal ganglia (status marmoratus, status dysmyelinisatus, severe neonatal jaundice = kernicterus) cause bilateral athetosis (**athétose double**), sometimes in conjunction with other signs of brain damage. Choreoathetosis and dystonia are prominent manifestations of iron deposition in the basal ganglia in **pantothenate kinase–associated neurodegeneration. Focal brain lesions**, too, for example, an infarct, can produce hemiathetosis.

Clinical features. Athetosis generally consists of **slow, irregular movements mainly affecting the distal ends of the limbs**, causing extreme flexion and extension at the joints and correspondingly bizarre postures, particularly of the hands (**Fig. 6.59**). The interphalangeal joints may be hyperextended to the point of subluxation ("**bayonet finger**"). Athetosis is often found in combination with chorea ("choreoathetosis").

  Practical Tip

Athetosis can be hard to distinguish from dystonia and is often designated as such. Athetosis can be considered a form of dystonia that is most prominent at the distal end of the limbs.

6.10.4 Ballism

Pathology. The neuropathologic substrate of ballism is a lesion of the contralateral subthalamic nucleus (corpus Luysii) and/or its fiber connections to the thalamus.

Etiology. Ballism is usually due to **focal ischemia**, and less commonly due to a **space-occupying lesion**. It

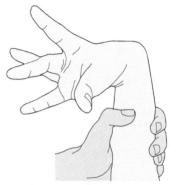

Fig. 6.59 Hand posture in athetosis.

may also be the result of severe neonatal jaundice or of a hereditary degenerative disease; it is typically bilateral in such patients.

Clinical features. Rapid, propulsive, large-amplitude, unbraked flinging movements of the limbs are seen on one side of the body (hemiballism) or both. Unlike chorea, these movements occur mainly in the **proximal** joints. The limbs may be hurled against walls, etc., causing injury.

Treatment. Haloperidol and **chlorpromazine** can alleviate ballism. Stereotactic neurosurgical procedures are sometimes necessary.

6.10.5 Dystonic Syndromes

Pathology and etiology. There are no characteristic neuropathologic abnormalities in dystonia. To date, only a few of the disorders that cause dystonia have a known pathophysiologic basis (e.g., L-DOPA-sensitive dystonia). Precipitating factors of symptomatic dystonia are likewise only rarely identifiable. Often, the etiology of dystonia remains unclear.

Clinical features. Dystonia consists of **slow, long-lasting contractions of individual muscles or muscle groups**. The trunk, head, and limbs assume uncomfortable or even painful positions and maintain them for long periods of time. The various clinical types of dystonia are classified as either **focal**, that is, affecting isolated, individual (small) muscle groups, or **generalized**.

Treatment. In the treatment of generalized dystonia, baclofen, carbamazepine, and trihexyphenidyl are used, either as monotherapy or in combination, often with only limited success. For some types of dystonia, a trial of L-DOPA treatment may be worthwhile. Focal dystonias can be successfully treated with **botulinum A toxin injections**. In some cases of dystonia, deep brain stimulation can be highly effective; the preferred target structure is the globus pallidus internus.

Types of Generalized Dystonia

Torsion dystonia. This category of dystonia is characterized by **slow, forceful, mainly rotatory movements of the trunk and head**, usually accompanied by athetotic finger movements. Muscle tone is diminished at the onset of the disease. In some cases, hyperkinesia gradually ceases and gives way to hypertonia with a rigidly maintained dystonic posture (**myostatic type**). The various types of primary torsion dystonia are mostly of **autosomal dominant** inheritance, with low penetrance, and have been localized to genes on various chromosomes. The early-onset form is particularly common among Jews of Ashkenazi (Eastern European) ancestry and is due to a genetic defect at the 9p34 locus.

L-DOPA-sensitive dystonia (Segawa disease). This is an **autosomal recessive** disorder due to a genetic defect on chromosome 14q. It usually presents in **young girls** as a **gait disturbance** characterized by dystonic postures or movements of the legs that fluctuate widely in severity over the course of the day. It is liable to misdiagnosis as a psychogenic disorder. It typically responds to low doses of L-DOPA (250 mg, or a little more, per day). A therapeutic test of L-DOPA is worthwhile in any young patient with dystonia, even if no other family members are affected.

Focal Dystonia

Focal dystonia is much more common than generalized dystonia. The abnormal movements are restricted to individual parts of the body or muscle groups. The main types of focal dystonia are the following:

Spasmodic torticollis. In this disorder, slow contraction of individual muscles of the neck and shoulder girdle produce **tonic rotation of the head** to one side or the other (**Fig. 6.60**). It is usually the contralateral sternocleidomastoid muscle that is most strongly contracted. Only one-third of all patients with "wry neck" due to spasmodic torticollis undergo spontaneous remission; a further third go on to develop other dystonic manifestations. The etiology usually remains unclear; there are probably multiple causes.

Blepharospasm. This consists of bilateral tonic contraction of the orbicularis oculi muscles, often with **very long-lasting involuntary eye closure**, during which the patient cannot voluntarily open his or her eyes. Blepharospasm tends to affect older patients, mainly women. Eye closure may be forceful, with visible contraction of the orbicularis oculi muscle, or weak, with a relatively normal external appearance. Cases of the latter type are alternatively designated **lid-opening apraxia**. Misdiagnosis as a psychogenic disturbance is, unfortunately, common.

Dystonia affecting multiple muscles of the head. The various types of focal dystonia that come under this heading are not rare when taken together; they include **facio-bucco-lingual dystonia, oromandibular dystonia**, and **Brueghel** or **Meige syndrome**. There may also be a relatively isolated **dystonia of the mouth, pharynx, and tongue**, particularly in patients who have been treated with neuroleptics. An acute form can appear as a complication of antiemetic drugs such as metoclopramide.

Isolated dystonia. Isolated dystonias have been described for practically every muscle group in the body. Dystonia of this type may be idiopathic or may arise in connection with **occupational overuse** of the muscle group in question. Well-known examples include **writer's cramp**, **hand dystonia** in musicians, and **foot dystonia** in certain other occupations. **Spastic dysphonia** is a focal dystonia of the laryngeal musculature.

6.10.6 Essential Tremor and Other Types of Tremor

Types of tremor. The main **phenomenological** distinction is between the following:
- Rest tremor.
- Action tremor.

Action tremor, in turn, is subdivided into the following:
- Postural tremor.
- Isometric tremor (appearing when a muscle is contracted against constant resistance).
- Kinetic tremor (appearing only during movement). Intention tremor is a kinetic tremor that worsens as the limb nears its target.

Tremor can also be classified **etiologically** as shown in **Table 6.35**.

Essential tremor. This is the **most common type of tremor** and often **runs in families**. Genetic defects causing familial essential tremor have been found on chromosomes 2p22– p25 and 3q. It usually arises between the ages of 35 and 45 years. It is a predominantly **postural** and sometimes also **kinetic** tremor

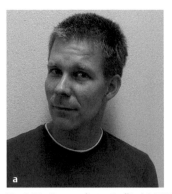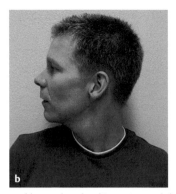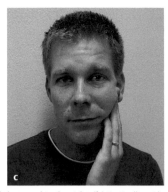

Fig. 6.60   Spasmodic torticollis. (a) A 32-year-old man whose head is spontaneously lightly turned to the right. **(b)** Torticollis with tonic, involuntary head rotation to the right. Note the hypertrophic left sternocleidomastoid muscle. **(c)** The patient can bring his head back to the neutral position by pressing gently on the lower jaw with a fingertip.

of the hands; a pure **intention tremor** is seen in 15% of patients (see **Fig. 3.22**). It may also affect the **head** in isolation (nodding or shaking tremor of the "yes" or "no" type), sometimes including the chin and/or vocal cords.

 Practical Tip
Essential tremor typically improves after the consumption of a small amount of alcohol and worsens with nervousness or stress.

"**Essential tremor plus**" is a combination of this entity with another neurologic disorder (e.g., Parkinson disease, dystonia, myoclonus, polyneuropathy, restless legs syndrome).

Diagnostic evaluation. Thorough history-taking and a precise neurologic examination often yield important clues to the etiology of tremor; further studies (e.g., imaging studies) are only rarely necessary. In some cases, **electrophysiologic testing** is needed to pinpoint the correct diagnosis (e.g., in suspected orthostatic tremor). Laboratory testing may also be needed to exclude underlying disease.

Treatment. If the tremor is severe enough to interfere with the patient's everyday activities, a **β-blocker** such as propranolol can be tried; this drug is particularly effective against essential tremor. **Primidone, benzodiazepines**, and **clozapine** are further alternatives. A tremor accompanied by dystonia may respond well to botulinum toxin injections. **Deep brain stimulation** through an electrode that has been stereotactically implanted in the nucleus ventrointermedius of the thalamus is highly effective but is reserved for severe, medically intractable cases.

Differential diagnosis. Involuntary movements arising from diseases of the basal ganglia must be differentiated from a variety of other movement disorders, which are listed in **Table 5.3**.

6.11 Cerebellar Diseases and Other Conditions Causing Ataxia

 Key Point
Cerebellar disturbances present clinically with disequilibrium, truncal and/or appendicular ataxia, impaired coordination, and diminished muscle tone (see also section 5.5.6).

6.11.1 Overview
Classification. The different clinical types of ataxia can be classified in several ways:
— By the affected neural structure(s):
  • Cortical cerebellar ataxia.
  • Olivopontocerebellar ataxia.
  • Spinocerebellar ataxia.
— By etiology (see also **Table 6.37**, **Table 6.38**):
  • Hereditary (autosomal recessive, autosomal dominant, x-chromosomal) or sporadic.
  • Acquired (= symptomatic).

Clinical features. Ataxia is characterized by **impaired coordination of movement** and a dysfunctional interplay of agonist and antagonist muscles. Thus, it typically manifests itself as **poorly controlled movements that tend to overshoot their target**. The additional manifestations of the individual diseases causing ataxia depend on their etiology and the particular neural structure involved.

| NOTE
Ataxia can be caused not only by cerebellar disease, but also by disease of the afferent and efferent pathways leading to and from the cerebellum, or of any afferent somatosensory or special sensory pathways. The underlying lesion may be in the cerebellum, but it may also be in the brainstem, spinal cord, peripheral nerves, sensory cortex, or thalamus.

Table 6.35

Types of tremor

Designation	Characteristics
Physiologic tremor	Seen in normal individuals; intensified by pain, anxiety, cold, caffeine ingestion, etc.
Thyrogenic tremor	Hyperthyroidism also intensifies physiologic tremor through the mediation of catecholamines. The tremor appears as a fine trembling of the hands
Essential tremor	See text. This hereditary condition is sometimes misdiagnosed as Parkinson disease
Orthostatic tremor	Similar to essential tremor bur arises only when the patient is standing, manifesting itself as shaking of the legs; mainly seen in the elderly. Other muscle groups can be similarly affected when under tonic stress
Parkinsonian tremor	See the discussion of Parkinson disease (see section 6.9.2). Usually consists of rest tremor, e.g., of the hand or fingers when resting on a solid surface, or of the hand when the arm is dependent
Psychogenic tremor	Sudden attacks of tremor, e.g., in acute stress disorder; often highly variable in intensity; coarse; of demonstrative quality
Holmes tremor	Unilateral, low-frequency rest, postural, and intention tremor (becomes stronger as the movement nears its target)
Cerebellar tremor	Intention tremor arising after cerebellar injury (becomes stronger as the movement nears its target)
Dystonic tremor	Tremor and movement disturbance due to dystonia (section 6.5.10)
Asterixis ("flapping tremor")	Sudden loss of postural tone, mainly seen in hepatic encephalopathy but also in other liver diseases, e.g., Wilson disease
Alcohol-related tremor	Fine rest and intention tremor, worse during alcohol withdrawal, improves after consumption of alcohol (but note: essential tremor often improves with alcohol as well)
Tremor induced by drugs, hormones, or toxic substances	Resembling physiologic tremor, but more intense

An initial, clinically based classification of ataxia distinguishes **symmetric** from **focal, asymmetric** types (**Table 6.36**). The table can serve as an overview and guide to the differential diagnosis of ataxia.

Diagnostic evaluation. When ataxia is suspected, the **age at onset** and the **family history** are diagnostically relevant:

- If ataxia arises in childhood or adolescence in a patient with a positive family history, the diagnosis is probably an **autosomal recessive ataxia**. The most common of these is Friedreich ataxia.
- If a parent is similarly affected, then the diagnosis is probably an **autosomal dominant ataxia**, for example, spinocerebellar ataxia.
- Ataxia arising after age 40 years is less likely to be hereditary and may be an **acquired ataxia**, for example, of toxic origin (such as alcohol-induced cerebellar degeneration).

Individual types of ataxia can be diagnosed by molecular-genetic testing, imaging studies, or laboratory analysis.

Treatment. The symptom complex called "ataxia" has no specific treatment, although coordination may be improved by **physiotherapy**. Certain types of ataxia of known cause can be correspondingly treated: examples include vitamin E administration in ataxia due to vitamin E deficiency and in Aβ-lipoproteinemia, a diet that is low in phytanic acid in Refsum disease, and a low-copper diet combined with chelators or zinc in Wilson disease.

6.11.2 Selected Types of Ataxia

 Key Point

Disturbances of the cerebellum, like those of the cerebral hemispheres, are usually due either to vascular processes (ischemia, hemorrhage) or to tumors. Multiple sclerosis is a further common cause. In this section, we will also discuss other diseases that may present primarily with cerebellar dysfunction, including infectious, parainfectious, (heredo-)degenerative, toxic, and paraneoplastic conditions, as well as cerebellar involvement in general medical diseases.

A thorough description of each ataxia syndrome would be beyond the scope of this textbook, and we therefore discuss only the more important ones briefly. Friedreich ataxia is described in greater detail in a later chapter (section 7.6.2) among the other hereditary diseases of the spinal pathways.

Cerebellar Heredoataxias

Cerebellar heredoataxias are of genetic origin. The enzymatic defects and pathophysiologic mechanisms underlying each have not yet been determined,

Table 6.36

The differential diagnosis of symmetric and focal asymmetric ataxias

Symmetric ataxia	Focal asymmetric ataxia
– Acute or chronic intoxication	– Ischemic stroke
– Electrolyte disturbance	– Cerebellar hemorrhage
– Acute viral cerebellitis	– Subdural hematoma
– Miller Fisher syndrome	– Abscess
– Postinfectious, ADEM	– Neoplasia (primary brain tumor, metastasis)
– Alcoholic-nutritional cerebellar damage	– Demyelinating plaque, multiple sclerosis
– Vitamin B_1 deficiency	– Arteriovenous malformation, arteriovenous fistula
– Vitamin B_{12} deficiency	– Arnold–Chiari or Dandy–Walker malformation
– Paraneoplastic cerebellar disease	– Psychogenic ataxia
– Antigliadin antibody syndrome	
– Hypothyroidism	
– Creutzfeldt–Jakob disease	
– Hereditary cerebellar degeneration	
– Familial episodic ataxia	
– Multisystem atrophy	
– Tabes dorsalis	
– Psychogenic ataxia	

Abbreviation: ADEM, acute disseminated encephalomyelitis.

except in a few cases. The main types are listed in **Table 6.37**. **Spinocerebellar ataxias** involve both the cerebellum and the spinal cord and are associated with cognitive deficits as well (see sections 7.6.1 and 7.6.2).

NOTE

The most common hereditary ataxia is **Friedreich ataxia**, an autosomal disorder with onset usually in the first or second decade of life that generally leads to death between the ages of 30 and 40 years. Its typical manifestations are the following:

– Unsteady gait, particularly with eyes closed; areflexia, pyramidal tract signs.
– Dysphagia, cerebellar dysarthria, oculomotor disturbances (gaze-evoked nystagmus, square-wave jerks, abnormal suppression of the vestibulo-ocular reflex, **Fig. 12.6**).
– Optic nerve atrophy.
– Early loss of proprioception and vibration sense.
– Distal muscle atrophy, typical foot deformity (pes cavus), kyphoscoliosis.
– Cardiac manifestations (conduction abnormalities, cardiomyopathy), diabetes mellitus.
– Cognitive disturbances.
– Dementia.

Symptomatic Types of Ataxia and Cerebellar Degeneration

Aside from hereditary and idiopathic types of ataxia and cerebellar degeneration, there are also types that reflect particular underlying illnesses, including a wide variety of cerebellar and systemic diseases (**Table 6.38**). The clinical manifestations vary depending on the cause. Other systems and organs are often involved.

Additional Information

Intermittent cerebellar manifestations are found mainly in the following diseases:
– Pyruvate dehydrogenase deficiency.
– Hartnup disease.
– Familial periodic paroxysmal ataxia.
– Multiple sclerosis.

The differential diagnosis of cerebellar ataxia must also include disease processes that cause ataxia but do not involve the cerebellum:
– (Contralateral) **frontal lobe lesions**.
– **Paresis** of any cause.
– Lesions of the **afferent sensory pathways** (e.g., polyneuropathy or posterior column lesion).
– Lesions of the **parietal sensory cortex**.
A **prolonged beridden state** ("bed ataxia") and **psychogenic mechanisms** are further possible causes.

6.12 Dementia

 Key Point
Unlike the terms "intellectual disability" and "oligophrenia," which refer to congenital disturbances, the term "dementia" refers to an acquired degeneration of intellectual and cognitive abilities that persists for at least several months or takes a chronically worsening course, leading to major impairment in the patient's everyday life. The clinical picture is dominated by personality changes as well as neuropsychological and accompanying neurologic (particularly motor) deficits. Reactive changes, including insomnia, agitation, and depression, are common.

Table 6.37

Types of cerebellar ataxia

Disease	Clinical features	Remarks
Autosomal recessive hereditary ataxias		
Friedreich ataxia	– Lumbering, broad-based, unsteady gait, progressive from the first or second decade onward – Later, clumsiness of the hands, explosive speech – Typical Friedreich foot (see **Fig. 7.15**) – Scoliosis, hypotonia	GAA triplet expansion on chromosome 9; impaired synthesis of the protein frataxin
Refsum disease (heredopathia atactica polyneuritiformis)	– Ataxia of gait and limbs beginning in childhood or adulthood – Polyneuropathy with areflexia and sensory loss – Hearing impairment – Retinitis pigmentosa – Mental abnormalities	Lack of phytanic acid α-dehydrogenase
Aβ-lipoproteinemia (Bassen–Kornzweig syndrome)	– Progressive ataxia, nystagmus, ophthalmoplegia, polyneuropathy – Acanthocytosis, low cholesterol and triglyceride levels, vitamin E deficiency	Low serum lipoprotein, cholesterol, and triglyceride levels
Ataxia telangiectasia (Louis–Bar syndrome)	– Onset in infancy with ataxia and choreoathetosis – Frequent lung, ear, nose, and throat infections – Slow eye movements – Telangiectases in conjunctiva and joint creases	One of the chromosomal fragility syndromes
Spinocerebellar ataxia (different varieties, e.g., deficiencies of hexosaminidase, glutamate dehydrogenase, pyruvate dehydrogenase, ornithine transcarbamylase, or vitamin E)	– Onset usually before age 10 y – Ataxia with variable accompanying deficits, e.g., intellectual disability, visual or hearing impairment, polyneuritis, myoclonus – Speech may be loud, deep, and harsh ("lion's voice") – If hereditary, generally autosomal recessive	
Autosomal dominant hereditary cerebellar ataxias (ADCA)		
Cerebellar cortical atrophy (Holmes type = Harding type III)	– Onset at age 20 y or later – Cerebellar signs	Genetically heterogeneous, SCA 5 and SCA 6
Olivopontocerebellar atrophy (Menzel type = Harding type I)	– Onset at age 20 y or later – Cerebellar and noncerebellar signs including optic nerve atrophy, basal ganglionic dysfunction, pyramidal tract signs, muscle atrophy, sensory deficits, and sometimes dementia	Genetically heterogeneous, SCA 1–SCA 4; SCA 3 = Machado–Joseph disease
Cerebellar atrophy (Harding type II)	– Onset after age 20 y with cerebellar signs and retinal degeneration	Corresponds to SCA 7
Autosomal dominant hereditary episodic ataxias		
Familial periodic paroxysmal ataxia	– Degenerative cerebellar ataxia with onset in childhood – Manifests itself in attacks (paroxysms)	– Gene defect on chromosome 19p – Responds to acetazolamide
Sporadic, nonhereditary ataxias		
"Atrophie cérébelleuse tardive à prédominance corticale"	– Onset in late adulthood with slowly progressive gait and truncal ataxia, later arm ataxia – Rarely, nystagmus, muscle hypotonia, and pyramidal tract signs	Symmetric degeneration of Purkinje cells, predominantly in the vermis; alcohol may be a precipitating factor in persons with an underlying genetic predisposition

Abbreviation: SCA, spinocerebellar ataxia.

Table 6.38	

Causes of symptomatic ataxia and cerebellar degeneration

Cause or precipitating factor	Examples and remarks
Local disease: mass lesion or ischemia	Malformation, cerebellar tumor, infarct, hemorrhage, inflammation, trauma or other physical causes
Infection	Often in the aftermath of an **infectious disease**, e.g., mononucleosis **Acute cerebellar ataxia in childhood** arises a few days or weeks after a chickenpox infection, less commonly after another viral illness. The patient is usually a preschool-aged child. Unsteady gait, ataxia, tremor, and nystagmus are the characteristic signs; they usually resolve spontaneously in a few weeks. **Acute cerebellitis** is similar to the foregoing and affects both children and adults. In older patients, the manifestations can persist
Systemic diseases	For example, **multiple sclerosis**, macroglobulinemias
Toxic conditions	**Tardive cerebellar atrophy** in **chronic alcoholism**, other toxic causes (diphenylhydantoin, lithium, organic mercury, piperazine, methotrexate, 5-fluorouracil, DDT)
Metabolic and hormone-associated conditions	Familial AVED (an autosomal recessive condition that clinically resembles Friedreich ataxia), vitamin B deficiency Hypothyroidism and myxedema Malresorption syndrome, gluten intolerance (gluten-induced ataxia with or without gastro-intestinal manifestations)
Paraneoplastic conditions	Subacute cerebellar cortical atrophy
Further causes	— Heatstroke — Miller Fisher syndrome (see section 11.2.3) — Cranial polyradiculitis (see section 11.2.3) — Creutzfeldt–Jakob disease (see section 6.7.9): ataxia is sometimes the first sign of this disease

Abbreviations: AVED, ataxia with vitamin E deficiency; DDT, dichlorodiphenyltrichloroethane.

In this chapter, we will first provide an overview of the general aspects of the dementia syndrome and then describe the main types of degenerative brain disease that cause dementia in greater detail.

6.12.1 Overview: The Dementia Syndrome

Etiology and classification
Unlike the various types of neuropsychological disturbance caused by focal brain lesions, the dementia syndrome is caused by a **diffuse loss of functional brain tissue**. Neuroimaging usually discloses **extensive brain atrophy** or **multifocal brain lesions**.
Primary brain atrophy. The loss of functional tissue is often due to primary (degenerative) brain atrophy, which mainly affects the cerebral cortex, progresses chronically, and causes irreversible cognitive impairment. In such cases, dementia is the direct consequence and most obvious expression of the causative pathologic process. Primary brain atrophy characterizes **dementing diseases** in the narrow sense of the term:
— Alzheimer disease.
— Lewy body disease.
— Focal cortical atrophies.
Symptomatic dementia. In principle, however, any disease that damages the structure or function of the brain can produce the dementia syndrome. Dementia, in such cases, is often a **possible but not universal accompaniment** of the main features of the disease

in question, and is generally not the only manifestation. It is important to realize that nearly 10% of all cases of dementia are due to diseases that can be reversed, or at least kept from progressing further, by appropriate treatment. The timely diagnosis and treatment of such patients is crucial for the prevention of further deterioration.
Cortical and subcortical dementia. In **cortical** types of dementia, **dementia is the main manifestation** of the disease (classic example: Alzheimer disease). In contrast, **movement disorders** are typically prominent in patients with **subcortical** dementia.
Overview of causes. **Table 6.39** contains an overview of the causes of dementia, with an indication of which among these conditions are irreversible and which are at least partly treatable.

NOTE

All patients with dementia deserve a thorough diagnostic evaluation, because a treatable cause may be discovered.

Epidemiology
One percent of persons aged 60 to 64, and more than 30% of persons older than 85 years, suffer from dementia. The most common cause is **Alzheimer disease**, which accounts for 40 to 50% of all patients. The second most common cause, and the most common cause of symptomatic dementia, is **vascular (i.e., multi-infarct) dementia** (15%); the third most common cause is **alcoholism**.

General clinical features

The dementia syndrome is characterized by neuropsychological deficits, personality changes, and behavioral abnormalities. In particular, the following are seen:

- Impairment of short-term and long-term memory:
  - For new content (faulty generation of engrams), and/or
  - For old content (faulty recall).
- **Impairment of thinking**, particularly with respect to:
  - Judgment.
  - Problem-solving.
  - Symbol comprehension.
- Impairment of visuospatial and spatial-constructive functions.
- Aphasia and apraxia.
- Impairment of attention and concentration.
- Reduced drive, initiative, and motivation; easy fatigability.
- Affect lability and impaired affect control.
- Impairment of emotionality and social behavior.
- In some patients, confusion and impairment of consciousness.

General diagnostic evaluation

The diagnosis of the dementia syndrome is based on thorough **history-taking** from the patient and family members, a comprehensive **general medical and neurologic examination**, and **neuropsychological testing**.
Screening tests. The following can be used as screening tests for dementia, although they are not very informative or specific:

- Mini-Mental State Examination (**Table 3.1**).
- Clock test (the patient is asked to draw a clock face indicating a particular time).
- Montreal Cognitive Assessment (MoCA) test: this test simultaneously assesses various cognitive skills with a sequence of simple tasks that can be scored on a point system. It takes approximately 10 minutes to administer. See www.mocatest.org.

Imaging studies and electrophysiology. Neuroimaging (usually **MRI**) should be performed in every case as part of the search for the underlying etiology. **PET**, **SPECT**, and **EEG** can be performed as well.
Laboratory tests. Depending on the specific clinical situation and the suspected causes, **targeted laboratory testing** should be performed, including, for example, complete blood count, electrolytes, hepatic and renal function tests, thyroid hormones, vitamin B$_{12}$, folic acid, TPHA test, HIV serology, and CSF examination.

Differential Diagnosis at the Syndrome Level

The dementia syndrome may be hard to differentiate from certain other psychopathologic states, especially the following:

- Nonpathologic **cognitive decline in old age** (can be diagnosed on the basis of history obtained from family members and clinical testing).
- Depression with severely reduced drive, so-called **depressive pseudodementia** (neuropsychological and psychiatric examination).
- An isolated **neuropsychological disturbance**, especially aphasia, apraxia, and/or agnosia (clinical testing, neuropsychological examination).
- **Congenital intellectual disability**, that is, oligophrenia (history).
- Cognitive impairment by **medications or drugs of abuse** (history, general physical examination, laboratory testing).
- **Status epilepticus** with partial complex seizures or absences (EEG).
- Cognitive impairment due to **endogenous psychosis** (neuropsychological and psychiatric examination).

General Aspects of Treatment

Cause-directed treatment. If the dementia syndrome is found to be due to a treatable condition, **cause-directed treatment** can be given, leading to a cure or, at least, the prevention of further progression. In all other cases, however, dementia responds poorly to treatment, if at all. The current medications for Alzheimer disease provide only modest clinical benefit, often at the cost of side effects.
Accompanying manifestations. Various manifestations that accompany dementia can be treated **symptomatically**, with major benefit to the patient and his or her family, including depression, delusions, insomnia, and agitation. **Training of (temporarily) preserved cognitive abilities** is also advisable to keep the patient functionally independent for as long as possible.
Nursing care. In advanced stages of disease, patients often require **home nursing visits**, or care in a suitable **day clinic**; removal from the home to a permanent care facility should be deferred for as long as this is practically achievable. The patient's family is an important component of treatment. Family members should receive early and thorough information about the patient's disease and, where appropriate, counseling in the ways they can help care for the patient.

6.12.2 Alzheimer Disease (Senile Dementia of Alzheimer Type)

NOTE

Alzheimer disease is the paradigmatic example of cortical (as opposed to subcortical) dementia, with dementia itself as the main clinical manifestation. It is the most common cause of dementia in the elderly.

Table 6.39

Causes of dementia

Type	Treatability	Diseases
Degenerative diseases of the nervous system	Partly treatable[a]	— Alzheimer disease — Parkinson disease — Progressive supranuclear palsy — Progressive myoclonus epilepsy
	Irreversible	— Frontotemporal dementia (Pick disease) — Frontal lobe degeneration — Pantothenate kinase–associated neurodegeneration — Heredoataxias — Lewy body disease — Corticobasal degeneration — Fragile-X syndrome
Cerebrovascular diseases	Partly treatable[a]	— Multi-infarct syndrome — "Strategically placed" infarcts or hemorrhages — Subcortical arteriosclerotic encephalopathy (previously called Binswanger disease)
	Irreversible	— Amyloid angiopathy — CADASIL
Infectious dementias	Treatable[b]	— Syphilis (progressive paralysis) — Brain abscesses — Whipple disease (intestinal lipodystrophy)
	Partly treatable[a]	— HIV, AIDS-dementia complex — Other viral encephalitides and postviral encephalopathies

	Irreversible	— Prion diseases:
		  • Kuru
		  • Creutzfeldt–Jakob disease
		  • Gerstmann–Sträussler–Scheinker syndrome
		  • Familial fatal insomnia
		  • Familial progressive subcortical gliosis

Metabolic disorders affecting the brain	Treatable[b]	— Wilson disease (hepatolenticular degeneration)
	Partly treatable[a]	— Disorders of lipid, protein, urea, and carbohydrate metabolism
	Irreversible	— Leukodystrophies — Polyglucosan body disease
Neoplasia	Partly treatable	— Primary brain tumors, metastases
	Irreversible	— Status post radio- and chemotherapy for brain tumor
Autoimmune encephalopathies	Treatable[b]	— Hashimoto encephalopathy
	Partly treatable[a]	— Paraneoplastic encephalopathies — Limbic encephalitis — Primary CNS vasculitis
Epilepsy	Treatable[b]	— Status epilepticus
	Partly treatable[a]	— Progressive myoclonus epilepsy — Frequent seizures
Mental illnesses	Treatable[b]	— Depression — Schizophrenia — Hysteria
Hydrocephalus	Treatable[b]	— Occlusive hydrocephalus — Malresorptive hydrocephalus
Trauma	Partly treatable[a]	— Closed head trauma with contusion or subcortical shearing injury — Dementia pugilistica (chronic traumatic encephalopathy of boxers)
	Irreversible	— Open head trauma with destruction of brain tissue
Demyelination	Partly treatable[a]	— Multiple sclerosis

Abbreviations: AIDS, acquired immunodeficiency syndrome; CADASIL, cerebral autosomal dominant arteriopathy with subcortical infarcts and leukoencephalopathy; CNS, central nervous system; HIV, human immunodeficiency virus.
[a]For example, preventable, occasionally curable, or amenable to symptomatic treatment in some cases.
[b]Usually curable or responsive to treatment.

Synonyms

Senile dementia of Alzheimer type; Alzheimer dementia.

Epidemiology. Women are more commonly affected than men, and the prevalence rises with age. The mean age at the onset of Alzheimer disease is 78 years. Persons under age 65 with the disease are said to have "presenile dementia."

Etiology and genetics

Genetic factors are clearly contributory, as first-degree relatives of Alzheimer patients are much more likely to develop the disease than persons with no family history of it. Yet, as most affected persons have no such history, **environmental factors** must also play a role. It seems that the likelihood of developing the disease is higher in persons of low educational attainment and those whose intellectual abilities are not regularly put to use; hypercholesterolemia, diabetes mellitus, and other brain diseases also increase the risk.

Genetics. Hereditary cases of Alzheimer disease (which are often early-onset cases) are associated with defects in:

- Chromosome 21q, which contains the amyloid precursor protein (APP) gene.
- Chromosome 14: mutation of the presenilin-1 gene.
- Chromosome 1: mutation of the presenilin-2 gene.

Familial clustering of Alzheimer disease is associated with defects in:

- Chromosome 19q: mutation of the apolipoprotein E locus (ApoE-4).

Persons with **trisomy 21** (Down syndrome) are generally demented after age 30 years.

Pathogenesis and Pathology

NOTE

The neuropathologic lesion in Alzheimer disease consists of **neuronal loss in the cerebral cortex**, particularly in the **basal temporal lobe** (hippocampus) and the **temporoparietal region**. Histologic examination reveals **cell necrosis** and an accumulation of **neuritic ("senile") plaques** and **Alzheimer neurofibrillary tangles. Amyloid angiopathy** is often present as well.

Amyloid and tau protein deposition. In Alzheimer disease, degradation of the membrane protein APP (amyloid precursor protein) leads to the increased production of a neurotoxic protein called **β-amyloid** (more precisely, Aβ1–42, which is longer than the physiologic degradation product). This pathologic protein forms **perivascular deposits** and **cortical amyloid plaques**. In addition, hyperphosphorylated **tau protein** also accumulates within neurons in **Alzheimer fibrils and tangles**. Amyloid and tau protein deposition has multiple consequences:

- **Neuron degeneration**, mainly temporobasal (hippocampal) and temporoparietal.
- **Axon degeneration** and **loss of synapses**.
- A **cholinergic deficit** in the cerebral cortex.
- In the late stage of the disease, **immune reactions** of glial cells to plaques, resulting in further cell loss.

Cholinergic deficit. Neuron degeneration is regularly seen in the **nucleus basalis of Meynert**, which sends a diffuse cholinergic projection to the frontal cortex. This and the **diminished amount of acetylcholine** found in the brain of persons with Alzheimer disease suggest that the **cholinergic system** plays a role in the pathogenesis of the disease. These observations provide the motivation for treatment with cholinergic drugs (as described later).

Clinical Features, Course, and Diagnostic Evaluation

Clinical features and course. The nonspecific **early manifestations** can include depression, insomnia, agitation, anxiety, and excitability. Early signs of dementia include impairments of memory, word-finding ability, and spatial orientation.

 Practical Tip

Persons who have a demonstrable memory deficit that impairs their performance of complex everyday tasks (but not of simpler ones) are said to have "mild cognitive impairment." This can be an early manifestation of Alzheimer disease.

Within a year, patients manifest gradually worsening **forgetfulness, fatigability, poor concentration**, and **lack of initiative**. Nonetheless, motor functioning, including erect body posture, remains normal for a long time, so that the superficial appearance of good health is preserved.

There are often also **focal neuropsychological deficits** such as aphasia, apraxia, impaired temporal and spatial orientation, and the applause sign (described in section 5.5.1). The patient loses the ability to think abstractly or grasp complex situations, and confusion, lack of interest, and the progressive loss of language ultimately lead to the **loss of functional independence** and the **need for nursing care**.

Diagnostic evaluation. Early recognition and interpretation of the psychopathologic deficits described earlier is crucial for the diagnosis of the disease. Often, the diagnosis is further supported by typical **neuroimaging findings** (MRI: **cortical brain atrophy**, especially in the temporal lobe, and **ventriculome-galy**; see **Fig. 6.61**). Neuroimaging is also mandatory because it can rule out some of the other causes of the dementia syndrome (cf. **Table 6.39**).

Further studies (**hematologic biochemical, and serologic blood tests, CSF examination, EEG**) may be indicated, depending on the specific differential diagnostic considerations in the individual patient.

A differential diagnostic overview of the main clinical and radiologic features of Alzheimer disease and other conditions resembling it is provided in **Table 6.40**.

6.12.3 Treatment and Prognosis

Treatment. Cholinomimetic drugs (acetylcholinesterase inhibitors: donepezil, galantamine, rivastigmine) and **antiglutamatergic NMDA-receptor antagonists** (memantine) improve neuropsychological deficits symptomatically but do not halt the progression of dementia.

A possible beneficial effect of acetylsalicylic acid is currently being studied, as patients with Alzheimer disease often have concomitant small-vessel disease as a contributory cause of dementia.

No clear benefit has been shown for high-dose vitamin E, *Ginkgo biloba* preparations, calcium antagonists, or nootropic drugs (= drugs that putatively improve brain performance), such as piracetam.

The most important aspect of treatment in all patients is the management of the **accompanying manifestations**:

— **Depression** (preferably with selective serotonin reuptake inhibitors).

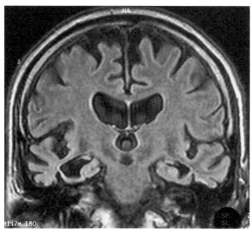

Fig. 6.61 **Brain atrophy in dementia.** High-grade, symmetric, mainly frontal atrophy of the cerebral hemispheres in a 64-year-old man. Note the marked atrophy of the temporal lobes as well. The lateral ventricles, including the temporal horns, are markedly dilated, as is the third ventricle. Both external hydrocephalus and internal hydrocephalus are present ("ex vacuo," i.e., as a result of brain atrophy).

— **Psychosis** (preferably with clozapine or olanzapine).

— **Insomnia, agitation, and aggressiveness** (preferably with low-potency neuroleptic agents such as pipamperone, melperone, and clomethiazole).

Patients with advanced Alzheimer disease, and their families, can benefit from referral to **special outpatient and day care facilities**.

Prognosis. Alzheimer disease always **progresses**. The average life expectancy from the time of diagnosis is 8 to 9 years.

6.12.4 Dementia with Lewy Bodies

Epidemiology. Vascular dementia is the second most common type of dementia after Alzheimer disease, but the second most common neurodegenerative dementing disease is Lewy body dementia.

> **NOTE**
>
> Lewy body disease overlaps with **Parkinson disease** (section 6.9) in its neuropathologic and clinical features but differs in having dementia as a prominent early manifestation, appearing at the same time as the motor disturbances or even before them.

Pathology. The neuropathologic hallmark of this disease is the presence of **Lewy inclusion bodies** (deposits of **α-synuclein**) in the neurons of the cerebral cortex and brainstem.

Clinical features. In these patients, **progressive dementia** (of a combined **cortical and subcortical** type; cf. **Table 6.38**) is accompanied by certain other characteristic findings: there are **fluctuating** deficits of attention and concentration, as well as frequent, objective **visual hallucinations** and **motor parkinsonism** (particularly in patients with early disease onset). Patients often suffer from repeated falls, syncope, brief episodes of unconsciousness, and hallucinatory experiences.

Diagnosis and treatment.

— SPECT and PET reveal diminished perfusion and metabolism in the occipital lobes.

— An L-DOPA challenge test may alleviate motor parkinsonism in patients with this disease (although it often does not), while tending to intensify the hallucinations. Neuroleptic drugs make all manifestations worse.

— Acetylcholinesterase inhibitors can improve both dementia and hallucinations.

6.12.5 Frontotemporal Dementia (Pick Disease)

Classification. Frontotemporal dementia (Pick disease) is the commonest type of **focal cortical atrophy**. The dementing diseases belonging to this

Table 6.40

Distinguishing features of different types of dementia

	Alzheimer dementia	Lewy body dementia	SAE (vascular dementia)	Frontotemporal dementia (Pick disease)
Type of dementia	Cortical	Both cortical and subcortical	Subcortical	Frontal
Main cognitive manifestations	Disturbance of recent memory, visuospatial orientation, word-finding. Typical: normal "façade"	Combined manifestations of cortical and subcortical dementia	Slowing, forgetfulness, impaired concentration and drive	Personality change, loss of drive, sometimes aphasia
Accompanying neurologic or other bodily manifestations	Sometimes hyposmia, otherwise no particular bodily manifestations at first. Physical impairment only in the late stage	Fluctuating attention and wakefulness, visual hallucinations, parkinsonism	Increased muscle tone, hypokinesia, small-stepped and broad-based gait (lower-body parkinsonism), dizziness, falls, sometimes TIAs, urinary incontinence	Early urinary incontinence, sometimes parkinsonism
Mental disturbances	Depression, later restlessness, anxious agitation, paranoia, insomnia	Insomnia, visual hallucinations, delusions	Sometimes depression, irritability, "lazy" speech	Variable; personality change, abnormal behavior, progressively "lazy" speech
Neuroimaging	CT, MRI: cortical brain atrophy, ventriculomegaly	SPECT, PET: low dopaminergic activity in occipital lobes	CT, MRI: marked SAE lesions and multiple lacunar infarcts	CT, SPECT, PET: frontal hypoperfusion and hypometabolism

Abbreviations: CT, computed tomography; MRI, magnetic resonance imaging; PET, positron emission tomography; SAE, subcortical arteriosclerotic encephalopathy; SPECT, single-photon emission computed tomography; TIAs, transient ischemic attack.

category, all of them much rarer than Alzheimer disease, are characterized by **localized atrophy of circumscribed areas of the cerebral cortex**. They are classified among the system atrophies. Histopathologic examination reveals **gliosis** and **spongiform changes**.

Additional Information

Aside from frontotemporal dementia, focal cortical atrophy can also be of the following kinds:

- In **primary progressive aphasia**, the language disturbance may precede the development of generalized dementia by several years.
- In **posterior cortical atrophy**, dementia may be accompanied by the specific neuropsychological deficits of Gerstmann syndrome (see section 5.5.1, Parietal Lobe Syndrome).

Frontotemporal dementia is also classified by some authors as a type of **frontal lobe degeneration**.

Etiology and epidemiology. Some cases are hereditary, with an autosomal dominant inheritance pattern. Most patients are less than 65 years old; in this age group, frontotemporal dementia is, in fact, nearly as common as Alzheimer disease. Overall, however, the focal cortical atrophies account for only approximately 5% of all cases of dementia.

Clinical features. See also **Table 6.40**. Patients with frontotemporal dementia often manifest frontal

personality changes and abnormal social conduct (see section 5.5.1). They may have reduced drive, **aphasia**, and difficulty initiating speech, as well as an affect disturbance. The type of cognitive deficit depends on the particular area of cerebral cortex that is affected. Patients often develop **urinary incontinence** early in the course of this disease.

6.12.6 Vascular Dementia: SAE-Associated Dementia and Multi-Infarct Dementia

SAE stands for subcortical arteriosclerotic encephalopathy. On this topic, see also the discussion of lacunar infarction in section 6.5.6.

Etiology and epidemiology. Vascular dementia, the second most common etiologic category of dementia, is caused either by multiple subcortical lacunar infarcts due to cerebral microangiopathy (SAE) or, less commonly, by multiple cortical and subcortical infarcts due to **macroangiopathy** or **recurrent embolic stroke** (multi-infarct dementia). These two mechanisms often operate in combination. The site and extent of the infarcts determine the severity and rate of progression of the dementia syndrome.

Clinical features. See **Table 6.38**. Vascular dementia often strikes patients with **preexisting arterial hypertension** and/or other **vascular risk factors**. There may be a history of **transient neurologic deficits** in the past, due to TIAs or minor strokes. **Dementia** can

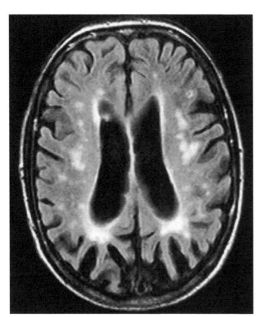

Fig. 6.62   Vascular encephalopathy as seen by MRI. There are multiple focal signal abnormalities in the deep white matter, the subcortical region, and the cerebral cortex. The ventricles and subarachnoid space are dilated ("hydrocephalus ex vacuo").

arise suddenly or progress in spurts. There may be accompanying neuropsychological deficits, such as aphasia, as well as marked incontinence of affect: involuntary laughing and crying are common. The **neurologic findings** include enhanced perioral reflexes, signs of pseudobulbar palsy (e.g., dysarthria and dysphagia), a tripping, small-stepped gait (old person's gait, "marche à petits pas"), and, sometimes, pyramidal and extrapyramidal signs. The **psychopathology** of subcortical vascular dementia includes apathy, depression, and slowness. Patients can recall old information more easily than they can store new information.

Diagnostic evaluation. Neuroimaging reveals brain atrophy and evidence of **multiple focal lesions**, often old lacunar infarcts; these are usually found in the **subcortical white matter** (**Fig. 6.62**).

Treatment. The intermediate goal of treatment is **vascular risk reduction** (treatment of arterial hypertension, cardiac arrhythmias, diabetes mellitus, and hypercholesterolemia, if present; inhibition of platelet aggregation with aspirin and/or other to lower the risk of thrombosis). Generally speaking, the treatment is the same as that discussed earlier for the prevention of ischemic stroke (section 6.5.9). The symptomatic and supportive measures are the same as for Alzheimer disease: **cholinomimetic drugs** (donepezil, galantamine, rivastigmine) and the

antiglutamatergic drug **memantine** alleviate the cognitive disturbances.

Course and prognosis. Vascular dementia is a progressive illness, typically with stepwise progression. The rate of progression is variable, however, as it depends on the type and extent of the underlying arteriopathy.

6.12.7 Dementia due to Malresorptive Hydrocephalus

Synonym. This disorder is often incorrectly called (idiopathic or secondary) **normal pressure hydrocephalus**.

Epidemiology. The peak incidence is between the ages of 50 and 70 years.

Etiology. This disorder can arise in the aftermath of meningitis, aneurysmal or traumatic subarachnoid hemorrhage, or venous sinus thrombosis; as a consequence of elevated CSF protein concentration; or spontaneously, that is, without any known risk factor. The common pathophysiologic mechanism is **impaired CSF outflow through the arachnoid granulations** and nerve root pouches, leading to a buildup of CSF and ventricular dilatation (see **Fig. 6.2**).

Clinical features. The classic clinical triad of malresorptive hydrocephalus includes a **progressively severe gait disturbance**, **urinary incontinence**, and **psycho-organic syndrome**. Neurologic examination reveals paraparesis, ataxia, impaired memory, and, in advanced stages, **dementia**. Some patients also have headache.

Diagnostic evaluation. **CT or MRI** characteristically reveals **enlarged lateral ventricles**, while the subarachnoid space appears tight (**Fig. 6.2c**). The CSF pressure measured via **LP** is normal or, at most, mildly elevated (hence the alternative name of this condition, "normal pressure hydrocephalus").

Practical Tip

The removal of CSF via LP can bring about prompt, but transient, improvement of the patient's gait and memory. The "sticky" and small-stepped gait can suddenly become much more fluid. A good response to CSF removal (the "CSF tap test") supports the diagnosis of malresorptive hydrocephalus and implies a likely benefit from treatment with a shunt (see later).

Treatment. If the patient responds well to the CSF tap test, a **ventriculoperitoneal shunt** is neurosurgically implanted. This generally leads to an improvement of the symptomatic triad.

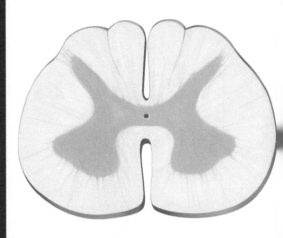

Chapter 7

Diseases of the Spinal Cord

A Fall Brings the Answer

The patient, a 74-year-old retiree, had never been seriously ill before. Two years before admission, he began to have trouble walking. His legs felt stiff and he could not lift his feet fully off the ground, so that he shuffled while walking and sometimes fell. He thought this might be normal for his age and did not seek medical attention. He secretly feared he might have Parkinson disease, of which his father had died at age 75 years.

His gait rapidly worsened in the months before admission. He could no longer feel the soles of his feet when walking barefoot, and he had a strange sensation of walking on cotton. He fell more often. He also developed more frequent minor injuries on his feet, some of which he failed to notice. Finally, a fall led to a comminuted forearm fracture, and he was admitted to the hospital.

The orthopaedists repaired the fracture surgically and consulted a neurologist, who took a thorough history and performed a neurologic examination. The patient said that he had fallen more often in recent months and also (in response to a specific question) that he had sometimes failed to get to the toilet on time. His bladder control was poor at the moment, "but, after all, I have prostate trouble, too." Further questioning brought out the family history of Parkinson disease.

On examination, there were no abnormalities of the head, cranial nerves, spine, or upper limbs, and there was no rigidity or tremor. Rapid alternating movements were dexterous. There was, however, a marked diminution of sensation to light touch and, to a lesser extent, of pain, from the level of the umbilicus downward. The lower limb extensors were spastically hypertonic. The knee- and ankle-jerk reflexes were brisk, with pathologic spreading. Babinski signs were present bilaterally.

The patient's symptoms, age, and family history had made the orthopaedists think of Parkinson disease. The classic triad of hypokinesia/akinesia, rigidity, and tremor was missing, but repeated falls are indeed common in atypical parkinsonian syndromes. Yet the neurologic examination clearly showed that the cause had to lie elsewhere. The neurologist diagnosed an incomplete spinal cord transection syndrome at the T8 level. A sensory level (i.e., a band around the trunk below which multiple, or all, sensory modalities are impaired), spastic paraparesis with gait impairment, and bladder dysfunction are all typical findings of an incomplete spinal cord transection syndrome.

The slow progression of the deficits led the neurologist to suspect a slowly growing, and therefore probably benign, tumor compressing the spinal cord. The magnetic resonance imaging (MRI) scan that she ordered revealed the tumor, which was then completely resected by a neurosurgeon. Within a few months, the patient's deficits resolved completely.

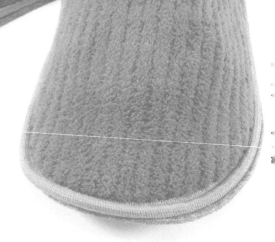

7.1 Overview

Key Point

Diseases of the spinal cord have manifestations in the limbs and trunk and sometimes affect micturition, defecation, and sexual function. Their symptoms and signs depend on the level of the lesion and the affected structures—conducting pathways, anterior horn cells, or the entire cross-sectional extent of the spinal cord.

7.1.1 Anatomy

The spinal cord is the component of the **central nervous system** (CNS) that connects the brain to the peripheral nerves; its anterior horn cells, though located in the CNS, are functionally a part of the **peripheral nervous system**. The spinal cord contains the following:

— In the **white matter**, fiber pathways leading from the brain to the periphery and vice versa.
— In the **gray matter**, an intrinsic neuronal system consisting of:
  • **Interneurons**, that is, relay neurons for the conducting pathways and reflex loops.
  • **Motor neurons** in the anterior horns.
  • **Autonomic neurons** in the lateral horns.

The somatosensory neurons are located outside the spinal cord, in the spinal ganglia.

The topographic relations of the spinal cord, vertebral column, and nerve roots are shown in **Fig. 7.1**, and the major ascending and descending pathways of the spinal cord are shown in **Fig. 7.2**. The **blood supply of the spinal cord** is described later.

7.1.2 The Main Spinal Cord Syndromes and Their Anatomic Localization

Key Point

The clinical manifestations of spinal cord lesions depend on their level and extent. Thus, the first step in diagnostic evaluation is topographic localization, that is, the deduction of the level and extent of the lesion from the patient's constellation of neurologic deficits. The next step is the determination of the etiology, usually based on further criteria (accompanying nonneurologic manifestations, temporal course, findings of ancillary tests).

Spinal Cord Transection Syndrome

NOTE

Spinal cord transection syndrome is the pattern of neurologic deficits resulting from damage of the entire cross-section of the spinal cord at some level. In an **incomplete spinal cord transection syndrome**, only part of the cord is damaged.

Most acutely arising cases of spinal cord transection syndrome are of either **traumatic** or **ischemic** origin; rare cases are due to inflammation or infection (transverse myelitis) or nontraumatic compression (e.g., by a hematoma or tumor).

The clinical features of the spinal cord transection syndrome are:

— Dysfunction of all of the **ascending sensory pathways** up to the level of the lesion, and of the posterior horns and posterior roots at the level of the lesion: there is a **sensory level** below which all sensory modalities of sensation are impaired or absent.
— Bilateral **pyramidal tract** dysfunction: **spastic paraparesis or paraplegia**, or, with cervical lesions, **spastic quadriparesis or quadriplegia** (immediately after a trauma, in the phase of "spinal shock" [diaschisis], there is usually flaccid weakness, which subsequently becomes spastic).
— **Bladder dysfunction**.
— Dysfunction of the **motor neurons of the anterior horn** at the level of the lesion: possibly, **flaccid paresis** in the myotome(s) supplied by the cord at the level of the lesion, corresponding **loss of reflexes** and, later, **muscle atrophy**.

Practical Tip

Partial and incomplete transection syndromes are more common than complete transection syndrome.

To understand the pathogenesis of spinal cord syndromes, one needs to know the anatomic course of the **pyramidal tract** (cf. **Fig. 5.1**) and of the **sensory afferent pathways** (the posterior columns and lateral spinothalamic tract, cf. **Fig. 5.2**). Only the essential structures for clinical purposes are shown in **Fig. 7.2**.

NOTE

— As the **pyramidal tract** descends, it crosses in the medulla and then travels down the **anterolateral column** of the spinal cord. A lesion of the pyramidal tract in the spinal cord causes ipsilateral **paresis**.
— The **somatosensory afferent fibers** in the **posterior columns** ascend ipsilaterally and terminate in the nucleus gracilis and nucleus cuneatus of the medulla. A lesion of the posterior columns thus impairs fine sensation (touch, stereognosis), proprioception, and vibration sense **ipsilaterally** (**Fig. 7.2**).

7

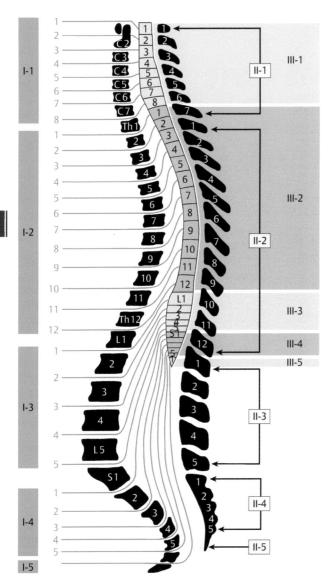

Fig. 7.1   Topographic relations of the vertebral column and nerve roots to the spinal cord. The growth of the spinal cord during embryonic development lags behind that of the spinal column; therefore, more caudally lying nerve roots traverse greater distances in the spinal subarachnoid space to reach their exit foramina. In the conventional numbering system, the cervical spinal nerves exit the spinal canal above the correspondingly numbered vertebra, while all spinal nerves from T1 downward exit below the correspondingly numbered vertebra. The conus medullaris generally ends at the upper L1 vertebral level but can also end more caudally, sometimes as far down as L3.

I-1	Cervical roots C1–C8
I-2	Thoracic roots T1–T12
I-3	Lumbar roots L1–L5
I-4	Sacral roots S1–S5
I-5	Coccygeal root

II-1	Spinous processes C1–C7
II-2	Spinous processes T1–T12
II-3	Spinous processes L1–L5
II-4	Spinous processes S1–S5
II-5	Coccyx

III-1	Spinal cord segments C1–C8
III-2	Spinal cord segments T1–T12
III-3	Spinal cord segments L1–L5
III-4	Spinal cord segments S1–S5
III-5	Spinal cord segment C01

– Nociceptive fibers from the periphery enter the spinal cord through the dorsal roots, **cross to the other side on the same segmental level** in the anterior commissure of the spinal cord, and then ascend in the lateral **spinothalamic tract** (**Fig. 7.2**). A lesion impairs pain and temperature sensation **contralaterally**.

See also the overview of the anatomic basis of sensory and motor function in Chapter 5.

Hemisection Syndrome (Brown-Séquard Syndrome)

The symptoms and signs of spinal cord hemisection are described in **Table 7.1** (see also **Fig. 7.2b**). An anatomic or functional disconnection of one half of the spinal cord exactly to the midline is a rare event. **Incomplete unilateral lesions** present with a subset of these manifestations; the most common type of unilateral lesion preferentially affects the **anterolateral column**.

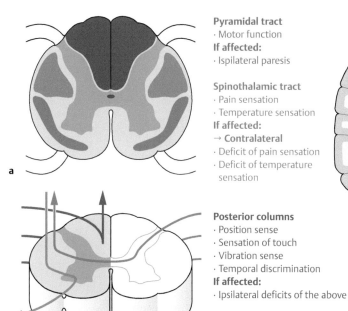

Pyramidal tract
· Motor function
If affected:
· Ispilateral paresis

Spinothalamic tract
· Pain sensation
· Temperature sensation
If affected:
→ Contralateral
· Deficit of pain sensation
· Deficit of temperature
  sensation

a

Posterior columns
· Position sense
· Sensation of touch
· Vibration sense
· Temporal discrimination
If affected:
· Ipsilateral deficits of the above

b

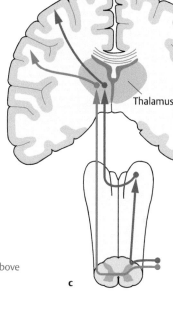

Thalamus

c

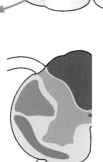

Pyramidal tract
· Ipsilateral paresis

Spinothalamic tract
→ Contralateral
· Deficit of pain sensation
· Deficit of temperature
  sensation

Posterior columns
· Deficit of position sense
· Deficit of touch sensation
· Deficit of vibration sense
· Deficit of temporal discrimination

d

Fig. 7.2   Major fiber tracts of the spinal cord and the consequences of hemisection. a Clinically important structures are shown in cross-section, with color-coded descriptions of function. **b** The course of the nerve fibers and pathways, superimposed on a cross-sectional image. **c** The course of the somatosensory fibers and pathways in a coronal longitudinal section from the posterior root to the cortex. **d** Diagram of Brown-Séquard syndrome caused by hemisection of the spinal cord on the right side at one level. Strength, sensation to touch, position sense, and vibration sense are impaired ipsilaterally from the level of the lesion downward; pain and temperature sensation are impaired bilaterally at the level of the lesion and contralaterally below it.

Central Cord Syndrome

| NOTE |

Central cord syndrome reflects damage to the decussating nociceptive fibers in the anterior commissure of the spinal cord (second neuron of the lateral spinothalamic tract). A dissociated sensory deficit is found in the corresponding segment(s).

Central cord syndrome is the classic presentation of **syringomyelia** (see **Fig. 7.11**) but can also be due to an intramedullary hemorrhage or tumor. Its clinical features are:

— Pyramidal tract dysfunction: **spasticity** of the limbs below the level of the lesion; cervical lesions tend to affect the upper limbs more than the lower limbs.
— Interruption of the pain and temperature fibers of the anterior spinal commissure: bilateral impairment of pain and temperature sensation at the level of the lesion, with preservation of touch (**segmentally restricted dissociated sensory deficit**); in analogous fashion, concomitant involvement of the posterior horn(s), if present, causes segmental impairment of touch sensation, either uni- or bilaterally, depending on whether one or both posterior horns are affected.

Table 7.1	
Brown-Séquard syndrome	
Involved structure	Deficits
Ipsilateral deficits	
Pyramidal tract	Paresis
Vasomotor fibers of the lateral columns	Initially, warmth and redness of the skin; sometimes absence of sweating
Posterior columns	Loss of proprioception and vibration sense, finely localized sensation of touch and pressure, two-point discrimination
Anterior horns and anterior roots	Segmental muscular atrophy and flaccid weakness
Entering posterior roots	Segmental anesthesia and analgesia
Contralateral deficits	
Lateral spino-thalamic tract	**Contralateral** diminution or loss of pain and temperature sensation (dissociated sensory deficit)

— Dysfunction of the lateral horn/intermediolateral tract: **autonomic and trophic disturbances** (disturbances of sweating, nail growth, and bone metabolism; hyperkeratosis and edema; all disturbances more pronounced in the upper limbs).
— Possible concomitant involvement of the spinothalamic tracts: (bilateral) deficit of pain and temperature sensation below the level of the lesion, with intact touch sensation.
— Possible concomitant involvement of the motor neurons of the anterior horns at the level of the lesion: segmental flaccid weakness, loss of reflexes, and muscle atrophy.
— Sparing of the posterior horns and spinocerebellar tracts: touch, vibration sense, and proprioception usually remain intact.
— **Bladder dysfunction**.

Bilateral Lesion of the Anterolateral Region of the Spinal Cord

In this situation, the posterior columns are intact, and there is thus no impairment of sensation to touch, proprioception, or vibration sense.

The most common cause is ischemia or infarction in the territory of the anterior spinal artery (see section 7.4.2).
— Pyramidal tract dysfunction: depending on the level of the lesion, spastic **quadriparesis** (**quadriplegia**) or **paraparesis** (**paraplegia**), with enhanced intrinsic muscle reflexes and pyramidal tract signs.

— Involvement of the spinothalamic tracts and the pain and temperature fibers crossing in the anterior spinal commissure: **dissociated sensory deficit** in the entire region of the body **at and below the level of the lesion**; less commonly, the spinothalamic tracts are spared and there is a segmentally restricted dissociated sensory deficit.
— Intact posterior columns: no impairment of touch or proprioception.
— **Bladder dysfunction**.

Lesions of Both Posterior Columns

NOTE

Sensations to touch, proprioception, and vibration sense are impaired, but the anterolateral columns are intact and there is thus no deficit of muscle strength or of pain and temperature sensation. The patient's stance and gait are markedly ataxic.

A typical example is **funicular myelosis** due to vitamin B_{12} deficiency (see section 7.6.4).
— Below the lesion, impaired proprioception, vibration sense, fine touch and pressure sensation, and two-point discrimination.
— **Sensory ataxia** that worsens in the dark or when the patient's eyes are closed; positive Romberg test.
— Sometimes, the **Lhermitte sign** is present (see section 8.2).

Isolated or Combined Long Tract Processes

NOTE

In these situations, only some of the ascending or descending long tracts (or a single one) are affected.

The clinical syndromes vary correspondingly and include:
— **Pure spastic paraparesis** (isolated lesion of the pyramidal tracts, e.g., in spastic spinal paralysis).
— **Impaired touch and position sense** (posterior column lesion).
— **Ataxia** (lesion of the spinocerebellar tracts and/or posterior columns).
— **Combinations** of the above (e.g., pyramidal tract and posterior column dysfunction in funicular myelosis, dysfunction of these tracts and the spinocerebellar tracts in Friedreich ataxia).

Anterior Horn Lesions

> **NOTE**
>
> Isolated involvement of the motor anterior horn cells causes weakness and atrophy without any sensory deficit.

This group of diseases includes spinal muscular atrophy and acute poliomyelitis and is characterized by:
- **Flaccid weakness** of various muscles and **muscle atrophy** (as well as fasciculations in chronic processes).
- **Diminution or loss or reflexes**.
- No sensory impairment or bladder dysfunction.

Combined Anterior Horn and Long Tract Lesions

> **NOTE**
>
> For example, muscle atrophy may be combined with pyramidal tract dysfunction.

This type of problem is seen, for example, in **amyotrophic lateral sclerosis** (ALS; see section 7.7.3), with simultaneous involvement of the anterior horn ganglion cells and of the pyramidal and corticobulbar tracts due to upper motor neuron degeneration. The patient has **weakness**, **muscle atrophy**, and **fasciculations**, but also **brisk reflexes**.

Epiconus Syndrome

> **NOTE**
>
> This syndrome affects the segment of the spinal cord above the conus medullaris, that is, levels T11 and/or T12.

Sacral and (sometimes) lumbar spinal functional deficits are seen, including:
- Weakness of the muscles supplied by the affected lumbar and sacral segments.
- Partial or total sensory loss in the affected lumbar and sacral dermatomes.
- Usually, diminished lower limb reflexes (because the lesion destroys the sensory arm of the reflex loop as well as its motor arm); the Babinski sign is usually absent.
- Bladder dysfunction.
- Bowel dysfunction, sphincter weakness.
- Sexual dysfunction.

 Practical Tip

Epiconus syndrome is clinically indistinguishable from cauda equina syndrome (Fig. 7.3).

Conus Medullaris Syndrome

> **NOTE**
>
> The conus medullaris is the lower end of the spinal cord and lies in the spinal canal at the L1 level (**Fig. 7.3**).

An isolated conus lesion typically produces:
- Bladder dysfunction.
- Bowel dysfunction with sphincter weakness.
- Sexual dysfunction.
- Possibly a dissociated sensory deficit or complete loss of sensation in the cutaneous distribution of the sacral and coccygeal spinal cord segments (saddle anesthesia).
- usually, intact motor function and absence of pyramidal tract signs.

Cauda Equina Syndrome

> **NOTE**
>
> Cauda equina syndrome (**Fig. 7.3**) results from compression of the nerve roots coursing through the spinal canal below the conus medullaris, that is, below the L1 level. Unlike conus medullaris syndrome, it involves a variably severe impairment of sensory and motor function in the lower limbs (see also Radicular Syndromes, section 13.1).

Its clinical manifestations are:
- Flaccid weakness and areflexia of the lower limbs, without pyramidal tract signs.
- Impairment of all sensory modalities in multiple lumbar and/or sacral dermatomes, usually most pronounced in the "saddle" area.
- Impaired urination, defecation, and sexual function, with sphincter weakness.

An epiconus lesion can present with the same signs and symptoms as the cauda equina syndrome.

 Practical Tip

A complete cauda equina syndrome can arise as the result of massive posteromedial intervertebral disk herniation (Fig. 7.4). This condition demands immediate surgical treatment.

7.1.3 Further Diagnostic Evaluation of Spinal Cord Lesions

The further diagnostic evaluation of spinal cord lesions involves imaging studies (MRI, sometimes computed tomography [CT]) and laboratory testing of the cerebrospinal fluid (CSF) and blood. Electrophysiologic studies may also help determine the etiology. For details, see Chapter 4.

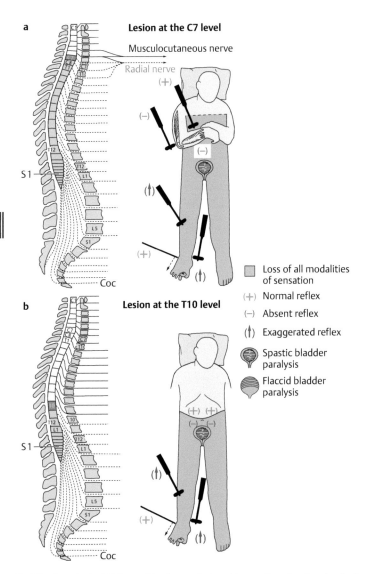

Fig. 7.3 **Neurologic deficits resulting from spinal cord transection at various levels.** Regarding the position of the conus medullaris, cf. legend to **Fig. 7.1**. **a** lesion at C7; **b** lesion at T10.

7.2 Spinal Cord Trauma

 Key Point

Traumatic spinal cord lesions are usually due to fractures and dislocations of the spine causing displacement of fragments of bone and/or intervertebral disk. The spinal cord can also be compressed by a traumatic hemorrhage in the spinal canal or sustain a direct traumatic contusion in the absence of a fracture. Spinal cord trauma is often a component of polytrauma.

The signs and symptoms of spinal cord trauma depend on the level and severity of the lesion, as shown schematically in **Fig. 7.3**.

Like traumatic brain injury, spinal cord trauma can be **classified by severity**:

Spinal concussion. Immediately after blunt trauma to the spine, a more or less complete spinal cord transection syndrome arises, usually at a cervical or thoracic level. The neurologic deficits regress completely within minutes.

Spinal contusion. The traumatic event has caused extensive structural damage and contusion of the spinal cord, usually with hemorrhage. There is a **partial or complete spinal cord transection syndrome** (depending on the extent of the lesion), including bladder dysfunction (see section 7.1.2) and an initially flaccid paraparesis (paraplegia) or quadriparesis (quadriplegia) (phase of **spinal shock**, also called

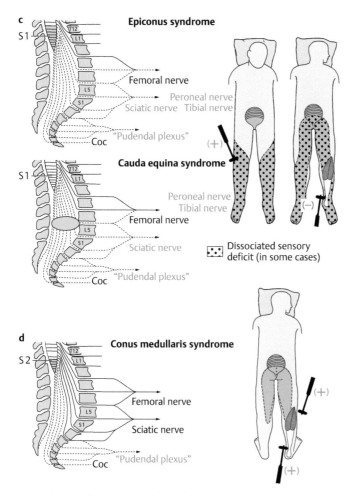

Fig. 7.3   *(continued)* **c** epiconus syndrome and cauda equin syndrome, **d** conus medullaris syndrome.

diaschisis). The transection syndrome usually improves no more than partially, if at all.

Sometimes the level of a high spinal cord lesion can be inferred from visual inspection of the patient alone (**Fig. 7.5**).

> **NOTE**
>
> **Spinal shock** in the acute phase of severe spinal cord trauma: motor, sensory, and autonomic function are lost below the level of the lesion, and the muscle tone (including that of the bladder) is **flaccid**.
>
> Function may (partially) return after a few days or weeks. The initially flaccid paresis becomes progressively **spastic**.

Spinal cord compression. In traumatic spinal fractures and dislocations, the spinal cord can be compressed by fragments of bone or intervertebral disk, or by hemorrhage within the spinal canal. Compression can also be partly or even entirely due to

enlargement of the cord from within by edema or hemorrhage in a severe contusion. As long as the acute spinal cord compression is not severe enough to choke off the cord's blood supply and cause infarction, the neural tissue may be able to recover its function again once the external compressing elements have been surgically removed, the traumatic spinal cord edema has subsided, and any hemorrhage within the cord has been resorbed.

Practical steps. In acute spinal cord trauma, these include the following:

— **Keep the airway free** (to permit breathing and prevent aspiration), stabilize and monitor circulatory function, stop any ongoing hemorrhage.

— **Safely transport the patient** to a trauma center (e.g., hard collar, back board, vacuum mattress).

— **Perform a gentle, nontraumatic neurologic examination** to determine the level of the lesion.

— **Order targeted neuroimaging studies**, usually CT possibly followed by MRI, to identify spinal

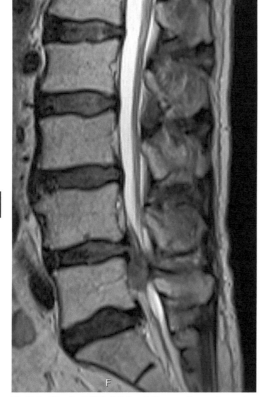

Fig. 7.4   **Massive L4/L5 disk herniation** causing acute cauda equina syndrome.

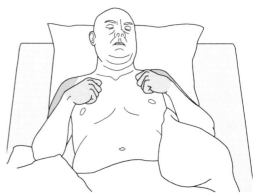

Fig. 7.5   **A patient with a traumatic spinal cord lesion at the C7 level.** The nerve supply to the elbow flexors, derived from the C6 root, is still intact; the triceps muscles, supplied by C7, are weak, as are the extensors of the wrist and finger joints.

fractures and dislocations of the vertebral column and assess damage of the intraspinal structures, including the spinal cord; objectively correlate the image findings with the clinically determined level, extent, and type of spinal cord injury.
- **Insert a bladder catheter.**
- **Surgically decompress the spinal cord** if indicated, in case of bony lesions, hematomas, etc.
- **Prevent decubitus ulcers** from the beginning, with frequent repositioning of the patient.
- High-dose steroids (given routinely in the past) are currently not recommended, as recent studies suggest that their complications may outweigh their modest benefit.

Patients should be transferred as soon as possible to a **rehabilitation** hospital specializing in spinal cord trauma where they can receive appropriate **physiotherapy**, ergotherapy, and psychological support.

7.3 Slowly Progressive Spinal Cord Compression

 Key Point
Spinal cord compression may develop acutely or by slow progression. Acute spinal cord compression is usually due to trauma (see earlier)

or hemorrhage (e.g., epidural hematoma). Slowly progressive compression is usually due to a tumor.

Less common causes include abscess, granuloma, spinal deformities (kyphoscoliosis, ankylosing spondylitis), degenerative narrowing of the spinal canal (especially in the cervical region), and massive intervertebral disk herniation.

Clinical features. Typical features of slowly progressive spinal cord compression include:
- Increasing stiffness or fatigability of the lower limbs.
- More or less rapidly progressive gait impairment.
- Bladder dysfunction.
- Impaired sensation in one or both lower limbs.
- Band-like paresthesiae around the chest or abdomen.
- Back pain.

Diagnostic evaluation. Neuroimaging usually provides definitive evidence of spinal cord compression; **MRI** is generally superior to CT for this purpose.

General aspects of treatment. The treatment is determined by the nature of the compressive lesion and is generally analogous to the treatment of corresponding lesions affecting the brain.

7.3.1 Spinal Cord Tumors

 Practical Tip
A tumor must be included in the differential diagnosis of any patient with progressive spinal cord dysfunction.

Tumors in the spinal canal can arise from:
- The spinal cord tissue itself (**intrinsic spinal cord tumors**).
- The spinal meninges (**meningioma**).
- The Schwann cells of the spinal nerve roots (**neurinoma**).

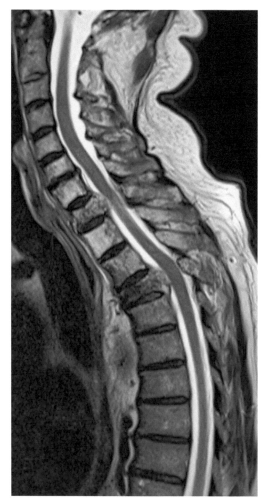

Fig. 7.6   Metastatic adenocarcinoma. Destruction of the T1 and T4 vertebral bodies by tumor, with tumor projecting into the spinal canal at these levels and compressing the spinal cord.

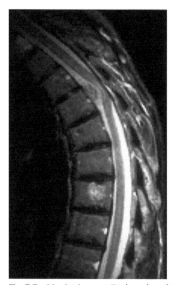

Fig. 7.7   Meningioma at T4, based on the ventral dura mater. Spinal cord compression is clearly visible on this T2-weighted MR image. The increased signal in the T7 vertebral body reflects an incidental, asymptomatic hemangioma.

Tumors (particularly **metastases**) can also project into the spinal canal from the vertebral and paravertebral regions.

Intrinsic spinal cord tumors are **intramedullary**; leptomeningeal tumors are usually **extramedullary**, though still intradural (cf. **Fig. 4.17**). Tumors growing into the spinal canal from the surrounding structures are extramedullary **and** extradural. Some highly invasive tumors arising in an extramedullary location can infiltrate the substance of the spinal cord, thereby becoming partly intramedullary.

The more common varieties of spinal cord tumor are briefly described in the following paragraphs.

Extramedullary Tumors

Metastases. Metastases to the spine are usually derived from **cancers of the lung and breast**, followed by cancer of the **prostate**.

Metastases usually grow from the vertebral bodies into the spinal canal. Their initial symptom is usually **pain**, which may be restricted to the site of the tumor or else radiate in a radicular distribution. **Paraparesis** can arise quite rapidly thereafter, followed by **bladder dysfunction**. Clinical examination reveals the corresponding **neurologic deficits** (pyramidal tract signs, possible sensory level, radicular segmental deficits) and, often, **focal tenderness of one or more spinous processes to percussion**.

Neuroimaging studies are essential for the definitive diagnosis (**Fig. 7.6**).

Meningiomas. Meningiomas arise from the spinal **arachnoid** and account for one-third of all intraspinal masses. They are usually found in the **thoracic and lumbar** regions. They produce very slowly progressive **gait impairment** and **spastic paraparesis**, often over the course of several years.

MRI reveals meningiomas as well-demarcated, dural-based lesions with homogeneous contrast enhancement (**Fig. 7.7**).

Neurinomas. Neurinomas (also called schwannomas) are nearly as common as meningiomas and, like them, are usually found in the **thoracic and lumbar regions**. They arise from the **Schwann cells** of the **spinal nerve root sheaths**. They nearly always present with **radicular pain and radicular deficits**. A neurinoma that arises from a nerve root and straddles an intervertebral foramen, so that it has both intra- and extraspinal portions, is called a **dumbbell** or **hourglass** tumor (**Fig. 7.8**).

Meningeal carcinomatosis and leukemic meningitis. These can cause clinically evident spinal cord

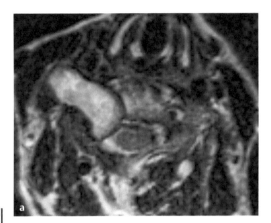

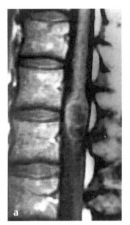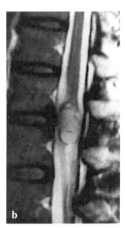

Fig. 7.9 Intramedullary ependymoma in the conus medullaris, as seen in T1-weighted (**a**) and T2-weighted (**b**) MR images.

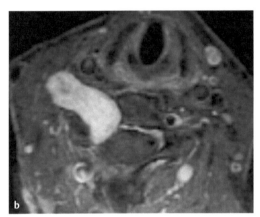

Fig. 7.8 Neurinoma of the right C5 root straddling the intervertebral foramen, with a small intraspinal portion and a large extraspinal portion. **a** The tumor has heterogeneous signal characteristics in this T2-weighted image. **b** Neurinomas are typically hyperintense in T1-weighted contrast-enhanced images.

compression, in addition to **pain** (the most common symptom) and **polyradicular neurologic deficits**.

Intramedullary Tumors

Intramedullary tumors are less common. Their symptoms and signs depend on their location. The two most common types are **astrocytoma** and **ependymoma**; imaging studies are essential for definitive diagnosis (**Fig. 7.9**).

7.3.2 Myelopathy due to Cervical Spondylosis

| NOTE |

Cervical myelopathy is usually due to degenerative narrowing of the spinal canal and its lateral recesses, with resulting spinal cord compression. Patients are generally elderly and typically present with symptoms in the hands and legs that progress very slowly, over months to years.

Patients with inflammatory diseases of the spine, such as rheumatoid arthritis, are at elevated risk.

Clinical features. The initial presentation is often with **(poly)radicular deficits** due to narrowing of the intervertebral foramina; as the central spinal canal becomes increasingly stenotic, clinically evident **spinal cord compression** develops. Patients typically complain at first of paresthesiae in the fingers and impairment of the sense of touch (examination reveals astereognosia). The intrinsic muscles of the hands may become atrophic. Ultimately—or, rarely, as the sole manifestation—involvement of the **long white matter tracts** produces spastic paraparesis, enhanced reflexes, and pyramidal tract signs.

Diagnostic evaluation. Neuroimaging is essential for the establishment of the diagnosis; **MRI** is best (**Fig. 7.10**), as it reveals not only spinal cord compression, but also **intramedullary signal abnormalities**.

Treatment. Decompression of the spinal canal, often with spinal stabilization (fusion) at the same procedure, halts the progression of the neurologic deficits.

7.3.3 Syringomyelia and Syringobulbia

 Key Point

Syringomyelia, a condition coming under the general heading of spinal dysraphism, is sometimes seen in combination with other congenital defects such as the Arnold–Chiari syndrome or spina bifida. It is characterized by the formation of a cavity inside the spinal cord.

Pathogenesis. Syringomyelia is defined by the pathologic finding of a tubelike or cleft-like, fluid-filled **cavity (syrinx) within the spinal cord**, often lined by ependyma and usually extending over several spinal segments. The cavity may reach all the way up to the medulla or even the midbrain (**syringobulbia**, syringomesencephaly). Mere widening of the central canal of the spinal cord is called **hydromyelia**.

Clinical features. The symptoms and signs of syringomyelia depend on the location of the syrinx within the spinal cord and on its vertical extent; they usually arise in the patient's second or third decade. The typical clinical features are summarized in **Table 7.2**.

Diagnostic evaluation. Syringomyelia can be diagnosed from its typical symptoms and physical findings, from which the presence of an **intramedullary lesion** can be inferred. The characteristic picture is of a **dissociated sensory deficit** combined with **trophic disturbances**. The diagnosis must be confirmed with neuroimaging, specifically **MRI** (**Fig. 7.11**).

Clinical course and treatment. Syringomyelia is usually slowly progressive. Neurosurgical treatment is occasionally successful. The options include the **Puusepp operation** (opening the posterior aspect of a large syrinx into the subarachnoid space), drainage of the syrinx with a shunt, or operation of an accompanying Arnold–Chiari malformation (**Fig. 6.3b**) at the craniocervical junction.

7.4 Spinal Cord Ischemia and Hemorrhage

 Key Point

Vascular lesions of the spinal cord, as of the brain, are of two main types: hemorrhage and ischemia. The latter is due to blockage of either the arterial blood supply (e.g., because of thrombosis or embolism) or the venous outflow.

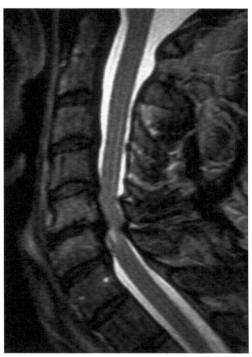

Fig. 7.10   Myelopathy in cervical spondylosis. The T2-weighted MR image reveals narrowing of the spinal canal at C4/C5 and C5/C6 both anteriorly and posteriorly because of degenerative spondylotic changes. A signal abnormality in the spinal cord below C5/C6 indicates a lesion induced by compression.

7

Table 7.2

Common symptoms and signs of syringomyelia

Symptoms/signs	Localizing significance	Remarks
Spastic paraparesis/quadriparesis	Pressure of syrinx cavity on the pyramidal tracts	May be unilateral or asymmetric
Muscle atrophy	Loss of anterior horn ganglion cells	Segmental, usually unilateral
Sensory level	Pressure of syrinx cavity on all ascending sensory pathways	Differential diagnosis: extramedullary lesion compressing the spinal cord
Uni- or bilateral dissociated sensory deficit below a given level	Uni- or bilateral involvement of the ascending spinothalamic tract	Highly characteristic
Segmental loss of all modalities of sensation	Syrinx involving posterior root entry zone	Usually unilateral or asymmetric; predisposes to burns and other types of mutilating injury
Pain	Involvement of entering sensory fibers or ascending spinal cord pathways	
Segmental dissociated sensory deficit	Syrinx involving the anterior spinal commissure, thereby interrupting the decussating fibers of the lateral spinothalamic tract	Segmental, bilateral, less commonly unilateral
Autonomic disturbances	Involvement of the intermediolateral tract in the upper thoracic spinal cord or of the lateral horns	Impaired sweating, edema, osteolytic bone lesions, arthropathy
Trophic disturbances	As above	Severe spondylosis, mutilation of the fingers
Kyphoscoliosis	Secondary to weakness of the paravertebral muscles	Usually a late finding, rarely congenital
Associated anomalies	Part of a disorder of prenatal development	Basilar impression, Arnold–Chiari malformation, spina bifida, hydrocephalus

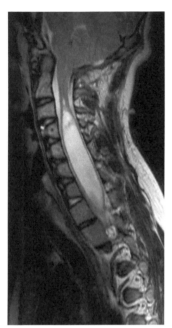

Fig. 7.11　Syringomyelia. The T2-weighted MR image reveals a cavity in the spinal cord from the C2/C3 level down to at least T1/T2. The spinal canal (and thus the syrinx) could not be included in the lower third of the image because of the patient's scoliosis.

7.4.1　Blood Supply of the Spinal Cord

The spinal cord receives arterial blood from three vessels:

— The unpaired **anterior spinal artery**, which runs down the anterior median fissure of the cord and supplies the anterior two-thirds of its cross-sectional area.

— The paired **posterolateral spinal arteries**.

Each of these spinal arteries is made up of a series of individual segments that are linked with one another along the longitudinal axis cord and receive arterial blood from various sources. At cervical levels, the anterior spinal artery receives blood mainly from the **vertebral artery** and the **costocervical and thyrocervical trunks**; further down the spinal cord, it is supplied by **segmental arteries** arising from the **aorta** (spinal branches and radicular arteries, each of which has an anterior and a posterior branch). In the embryo, there is a radicular artery for each spinal segment; postnatally, only six to eight such arteries are still present. The largest of these, called the **great radicular artery** or the **artery of Adamkiewicz**, usually enters the spinal canal at some level from T10 to L2, more commonly on the left side.

The anatomy of the spinal vessels is shown in **Fig. 7.12**, and the intramedullary blood supply of a cross-section of the cord is shown in **Fig. 7.13**.

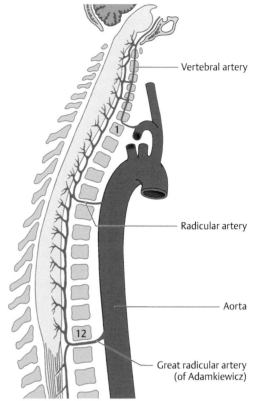

Vertebral artery

Radicular artery

Aorta

Great radicular artery (of Adamkiewicz)

Fig. 7.12　Blood supply of the spinal cord (longitudinal view).

The **venous outflow** of the spinal cord is through radicular veins and into the vena cava.

> **NOTE**
>
> The arterial blood supply of the spinal cord is derived from a small number of radicular arteries. An anastomotic vascular network links the territories of these vessels both vertically and ventrodorsally.

7.4.2　Arterial Hypoperfusion

> **NOTE**
>
> Arterial hypoperfusion of the spinal cord can give rise to symptoms **acutely** (suddenly) or in a **stuttering, progressive course** over several hours or days. It can affect the entire cross-section of the spinal cord or only a part of it.

Global (Arterial) Myelomalacia

Infarction of the entire cross-section of the spinal cord at a particular level may be due to the **occlusion of a local spinal artery or of a radicular artery**, or due to extraspinal vascular pathology, such as an **aortic aneurysm**. The clinical presentation is usually an

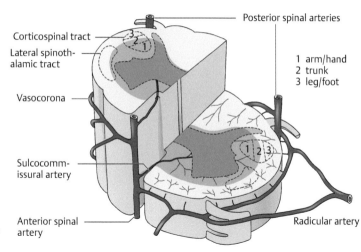

Corticospinal tract
Lateral spinoth-
alamic tract
Vasocorona
Sulcocomm-
issural artery

Posterior spinal arteries

1 arm/hand
2 trunk
3 leg/foot

Fig. 7.13 Blood supply of the spinal cord (diagram, cross-sectional view). Occlusion of the anterior spinal a. produces infarction in the area shaded in blue.

Anterior spinal artery

Radicular artery

7

acute spinal cord transection syndrome (complete or partial, see section 7.1.2), although, in some patients, symptoms develop subacutely over the course of a few days or with stepwise progression. The affected patients usually remain paraplegic, particularly if the ischemic lesion is very extensive.

Anterior Spinal Artery Syndrome
Thrombotic or embolic occlusion of the anterior spinal artery causes infarction in the anterolateral aspect of the spinal cord over one or more segments. The characteristic clinical features were described in section 7.1.2. An occlusion more distally along the course of the anterior spinal artery, for example, in a sulcocommissural artery (cf. **Fig. 7.13**), may cause a **partial Brown-Séquard syndrome** (**Table 7.1**), with preservation of the sense of touch.

Central Cord Infarction
Infarction of the spinal cord, whether it involves the entire cross-section of the cord or only a part of it, is usually not restricted to a single cord segment in the vertical dimension, but rather tends to involve multiple segments, with **loss of the motor neurons of the anterior horn**. This causes **flaccid paresis** and **areflexia** at the level of the lesion. In a few weeks' time, the flaccid muscles become **atrophic**. The clinical picture is, therefore, that of a **"peripheral" paralysis at the level of the transection**.

Other
- **Intermittent spinal ischemia** is very rare and causes a type of spinal intermittent claudication with fluctuating spastic paraparesis.
- **Chronically progressive vascular myelopathy** can cause slowly progressive spastic paraparesis, as well as muscle atrophy owing to involvement of the anterior horns.

7.4.3 Impaired Venous Drainage

| NOTE |

Spinal cord ischemia due to impaired venous drainage is a rare cause of infarction. It is usually due to a **spinal arteriovenous fistula** or **arteriovenous malformation**.

Spinal **arteriovenous malformations** are usually found in the thoracolumbar region, while **arteriovenous fistulae** are usually found at lower lumbar levels (cf. **Fig. 4.16**). Both types of vascular anomaly are **more common in men**.
Patients generally become symptomatic between the ages of 10 and 40 years, often with **(band-like) pain** as the initial symptom. **Neurologic deficits** referable to the spinal cord are often only intermittent at first and are (partially) reversible at this stage; later, they take a chronic, progressive course and become permanent. A **dural arteriovenous fistula**, for example, can cause chronically progressive spastic paraparesis. These vascular anomalies also occasionally present with **spinal subarachnoid hemorrhage**.
MRI is the most important diagnostic study for the visualization of the vascular malformation and the congested veins distal to it. **Spinal angiography** can provide useful additional anatomic detail.

7.4.4 Hemorrhage in or adjacent to the Spinal Cord

| NOTE |

Intramedullary, subdural, and (most commonly) **epidural** hemorrhage can arise spontaneously in an anticoagulated patient or can be caused by a ruptured vascular malformation or trauma.

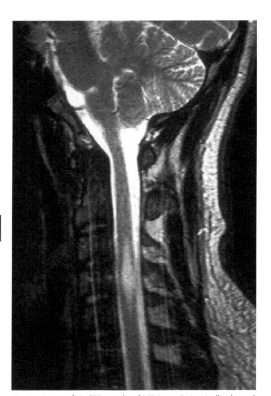

Fig. 7.14 Myelitis (T2-weighted MR image). A spindle-shaped signal anomaly extends from C3 to C5 and expands the spinal cord (which is wider here than the normal cervical enlargement).

The typical initial symptom of hemorrhage in or adjacent to the spinal cord is **intense pain** (possibly radiating in a radicular pattern), followed by a **partial or complete spinal cord transection syndrome** depending on the level and extent of the hemorrhage. Such hemorrhages **always** require immediate diagnostic evaluation with MRI or CT, sometimes followed by **surgical decompression** or interventional neuroradiologic treatment.

7.5 Infectious and Inflammatory Diseases of the Spinal Cord

  Key Point

The spinal cord and spinal nerve roots, like the brain, can be infected by bacteria, viruses, and other pathogens. Combined infection of the brain and intraspinal structures is common: simultaneous manifestations of encephalitis, meningitis, myelitis, and radiculitis (section 13.1) can be caused by spirochetes (borrelia, leptospira, treponemes; cf. section 6.7.5) and by many viruses. Acute anterior poliomyelitis, on the other hand, affects only the motor neurons of the anterior horns of the spinal cord.

7.5.1 Myelitis

NOTE

Any infectious or inflammatory disease of the spinal cord, whatever its etiology, is called **myelitis**. The causes of myelitis include direct infection, secondary autoimmune processes in the wake of an infectious disease, and chronic autoimmune inflammatory diseases of the CNS, such as multiple sclerosis and neuromyelitis optica.

Acute Myelitis

Etiology. The main causes of acute myelitis are **viruses** (measles, mumps, varicella zoster, herpes simplex, HIV, flaviviruses), rickettsiae, and leptospira. Postvaccinal and postinfectious myelitis have also been described, as has myelitis in the setting of granulomatous disease.

Clinical features and diagnostic evaluation. The manifestations range from progressive spastic paraparesis to partial spinal cord transection syndrome. Myelitis can be visualized by MRI (**Fig. 7.14**).

Multiple sclerosis or neuromyelitis optica can manifest itself as acute myelitis, sometimes with marked changes in the spinal cord (cf. **Fig. 8.6b**).

Treatment and prognosis. The treatment of myelitis is directed at its etiology (e.g., antibiotic or antiviral drugs). Patients who cannot walk because of myelitis need prophylactic treatment against deep venous thrombosis and thromboembolism, as well as physiotherapy.

Transverse Myelitis

Transverse myelitis is usually of **parainfectious** origin. It affects the entire cross-section of the spinal cord, producing a **complete spinal cord transection syndrome**.

Etiology and clinical features. Transverse myelitis has a variety of causes; often, the cause cannot be determined (idiopathic transverse myelitis). In distinction to acute myelitis, transverse myelitis is thought to arise, in most cases, from an immune reaction (e.g., a parainfectious reaction after contact with a pathogen). The neurologic manifestations are often preceded by **nonspecific flulike symptoms** 1 to 3 weeks before onset. The **spinal cord deficits** usually arise acutely or subacutely and become maximally severe within a few days. **Fever**, **back pain**, and **myalgia** accompany the acute phase.

Diagnostic evaluation. The **CSF** displays inflammatory changes (lymphocytic pleocytosis, elevated immunoglobulin G, and total protein concentrations), but contains CSF-specific oligoclonal proteins less commonly than in multiple sclerosis (cf. **Fig. 8.7**). A

neuroimaging study (usually MRI) must be performed to rule out a mass or ischemic event.

Treatment and prognosis. The pathogen is treated specifically if it can be identified; otherwise, only symptomatic treatment can be given (e.g., analgesic drugs, prednisone). The spinal cord transection syndrome resolves completely in only one-third of all patients. High transverse myelitis can also cause respiratory paralysis and death.

Acute Anterior Poliomyelitis

Etiology and epidemiology. This disease, caused by a **poliovirus**, almost exclusively affects the motor neurons of the anterior horn of the spinal cord. Its incidence in countries with a well-developed public health system has been reduced nearly to zero by prophylactic vaccination. It is transmitted by the fecal–oral route under conditions of poor sanitation.

Clinical features. After an incubation period ranging from 3 to 20 days, **nonspecific prodromal manifestations** arise, consisting of fever, flulike symptoms and, in some patients, meningeal signs. The prodrome may resolve without further consequence or be followed, within a few days, by a **paralytic phase** (likewise accompanied by fever): over the course of a few hours or days, **flaccid paralysis** arises in various muscles or muscle groups. The weakness is asymmetric, often mainly proximal, and of variable extent and severity. There is **no sensory deficit**, but the affected muscles may be painful and tender.

Diagnostic evaluation. The diagnosis is based on the typical course and physical findings, combined with an **inflammatory CSF pleocytosis**: at first, there are several hundred cells per microliter, often mainly polymorphonuclear granulocytes. Later, there is a transition to a predominantly lymphocytic picture. The responsible pathogen (poliovirus) can be identified in the patient's **stool**.

Treatment. There is no specific etiologic treatment; the most important aspect of treatment is the **management of respiratory failure** (if present).

Prognosis. Brain stem involvement and respiratory paralysis confer a poor prognosis; in the remainder of patients, **paralysis may regress partially or completely** in a few weeks or months. There is usually some degree of **residual weakness**.

Postpolio syndrome. This term is used variously to refer to two very different syndromes.

- Some authors use it for a **symptom complex seen a few years after the acute illness** in polio patients with residual weakness, characterized by fatigability, respiratory difficulties, pain, and abnormal temperature regulation (with negative polio titers).
- Others use it for a syndrome with **progressive worsening of residual weakness** occurring

decades after the acute illness. Before this problem can be ascribed to the earlier polio infection, other possible causes of weakness must be ruled out, for example, compression of the spinal cord or spinal nerve roots because of secondary degenerative disease of the spine.

7.5.2 Spinal Abscesses

Localization. Spinal abscesses are most often **epidural**, less often subdural, and only rarely intramedullary.

Etiology. The most common pathogen is **_Staphylococcus aureus_**, which reaches the spinal canal from a site of primary infection outside it by way of the bloodstream (hematogenous spread).

Clinical features. Patients typically have **general signs of infection** (fever, elevated erythrocyte sedimentation rate, leukocytosis, sometimes shaking chills), **pain**, and **neurologic deficits** referable to the spinal nerve roots or spinal cord, depending on the specific anatomic situation.

Treatment. Spinal abscesses usually require prompt **surgical treatment**, followed by high-dose antibiotics for several weeks.

7.6 Diseases Mainly Affecting the Long Tracts of the Spinal Cord

 Key Point

The diseases described in this section are those that remain confined to the white matter and primarily involve one or more of its long tracts. Many of these diseases are of genetic origin (e.g., the spinocerebellar ataxias); some are of metabolic (e.g., vitamin B_{12} deficiency), endocrine, paraneoplastic, or infectious origin.

7.6.1 Overview

Hereditary diseases.

> **NOTE**
>
> Hereditary diseases can affect ascending or descending pathways, or both, and can thus manifest themselves with spasticity, sensory dysfunction, and/or incoordination.

The genetic basis of most of the hereditary **cerebellar and spinocerebellar atrophies** (cf. **Table 6.37**) has been thoroughly studied. For example, the disease previously known as olivopontocerebellar atrophy, now called **SCA1 and SCA2**, has been traced to an extended CAG trinucleotide repeat at 6p22–p23. **Friedreich ataxia**, the most common type of hereditary ataxia, will be described in greater detail later as a prominent member of the class of diseases with degeneration of the **spinocerebellar tracts**.

Aside from the spinocerebellar ataxias, there are other diseases that cause degeneration of specific fiber tracts in the spinal cord. The pathogenesis of these diseases is only partly understood. For example, the pyramidal tract degenerates in **familial spastic spinal paralysis**, which will also be described in greater detail later.

Adrenoleukodystrophy (see **Table 6.23**) and certain other congenital metabolic disorders can affect individual fiber tracts of the spinal cord.

Nonhereditary diseases. The tracts of the spinal cord can also become dysfunctional more or less acutely because of vitamin B_{12} deficiency or toxic, autoimmune (e.g., **paraneoplastic**), or metabolic processes. The clinical features resemble those of the hereditary disorders. An important member of this class, described in greater detail later, is **funicular myelosis** due to vitamin B_{12} deficiency.

7.6.2 Friedreich Ataxia

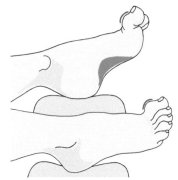

Fig. 7.15   **The typical foot deformity in Friedreich ataxia** ("Friedreich foot").

> **NOTE**
>
> This autosomal recessive disease, the most common hereditary form of ataxia, is due to a defect on chromosome 9 (an extended repeat of the triplet GAA).

Pathogenesis. The main **pathologic findings** include cell loss in the **dentate nucleus** and **combined degeneration** of the spinocerebellar tracts, pyramidal tracts, and posterior columns.

Clinical features and diagnostic evaluation. The disease usually manifests itself in the second decade, initially with **signs of posterior column degeneration** and then with **spasticity** and **cerebellar signs**.

Typical findings early in the course of disease include:
- **Progressive (spinal) ataxia** with disequilibrium, particularly when walking with the eyes closed.
- Diminution or **loss of intrinsic muscle reflexes**.
- Impaired proprioception.

In advanced stages of the disease, **cerebellar dysarthria** is found as well.

The diagnosis is based on the typical symptoms and signs, including:
- A typical **deformity of the foot** due to the pathologic increased muscle tone (**Fig. 7.15**).
- **Intracardiac conduction abnormalities**.
- Often **kyphoscoliosis**.
- Sometimes **optic nerve atrophy** and nystagmus.
- Pyramidal tract signs, distal muscle atrophy.
- Cognitive deficits tending toward **dementia**.

Course. Friedreich ataxia is chronically progressive and causes invalidism within a few years of onset. It sometimes takes a protracted course.

Treatment. No effective treatment is known.

7.6.3 Familial Spastic Spinal Paralysis

Synonyms. Hereditary spastic paraplegia, spastic paraplegia.

Etiology. This **genetically heterogeneous syndrome** can be inherited in X-linked, autosomal dominant, or (most commonly) autosomal recessive fashion.

Pathogenesis. Its pathophysiologic hallmark is **degeneration of the pyramidal tracts**, more severe at caudal levels, due to diffuse loss of neurons in the primary motor cortex. This condition is thus caused by **isolated disease of the first (upper) motor neuron**, as opposed to the spinal muscular atrophies, which involve isolated disease of the second (lower) motor neuron (as will be described further in section 7.7.2).

Clinical features and course. Spastic spinal paralysis is characterized by **spastic paraparesis, usually beginning in childhood and then progressing slowly over many years**, with brisk reflexes, pyramidal tract signs, and increasing gait impairment ("scissors gait" due to adductor spasticity).

Treatment. Only symptomatic treatment is now available, consisting mainly of physiotherapy.

7.6.4 Funicular Myelosis

Synonym. Funicular spinal disease.

Etiology and pathogenesis. Funicular myelosis is caused by **vitamin B_{12} deficiency**. The latter, in turn, may be due either to inadequate dietary intake or to impaired resorption because of insufficient **gastric intrinsic factor** (e.g., in atrophic gastritis, or after gastrectomy). The pathologic findings include **demyelination of the posterior columns**, **posterior roots**, and **pyramidal tracts**; in later stages of the disease, other tracts of the spinal cord, and the cerebral white matter, can be affected as well.

Clinical features. There is often, but by no means always, an accompanying **hyperchromic, megaloblastic anemia** with macrocytosis, and the patient's skin is pale yellow. Neurologic examination reveals an ataxic gait, impaired proprioception, and, rarely, other sensory deficits. These abnormalities may arise subacutely (over a few weeks) or acutely (over a few days). The **intrinsic muscle reflexes are diminished** because of posterior root involvement, **pyramidal tract signs** are common, and **cognitive and emotional disturbances** may be seen, ranging to dementia.

Diagnostic evaluation. The diagnosis rests on the demonstration of vitamin B_{12} deficiency in patients with typical clinical features.

Treatment and course. Vitamin B_{12} must be given as rapidly as possible, by the intramuscular route. The neurologic deficits will then resolve at least in part, but not always completely.

7.7 Diseases of the Anterior Horns

 Key Point

The anterior horns of the spinal cord contain the motor neurons whose axons exit the spinal cord in the ventral roots and travel via the peripheral nerves to innervate the skeletal musculature. The pyramidal and extrapyramidal motor pathways terminate in the anterior horns, which also mediate the proprioceptive muscle reflexes (deep tendon reflexes). Diseases of the anterior horns thus manifest themselves in flaccid paresis, attenuation or loss of reflexes, progressive muscle atrophy, and fasciculations.

7.7.1 Overview

Although the best-known acute anterior horn disease is **acute anterior poliomyelitis** (see section 7.5.1), most diseases in this class are of **genetic** origin and take a **chronic progressive course**. The typical clinical features of diseases involving chronic loss of anterior horn cells are summarized in **Table 7.3**. Some of these diseases are described in further detail in this section.

The best-known degenerative disease affecting the anterior horns is **amyotrophic lateral sclerosis**, in which there is simultaneous degeneration of the anterior horn cells and of the first motor neurons that give rise to the corticospinal and corticobulbar tracts. It thus has spastic manifestations as well: brisk reflexes and pyramidal tract signs.

> **NOTE**
>
> The **first motor neuron** has its cell body in the motor cortex and sends its axon down the pyramidal tract to terminate in the anterior horn of the spinal cord.
>
> The **second motor neuron** has its cell body in the anterior horn and sends its axons down the spinal nerve roots and peripheral nerves to innervate the skeletal musculature.

Table 7.3

Diseases with chronic involvement of the anterior horn ganglion cells

Disease	Affected structures	Symptoms and signs	Remarks	Etiology
Infantile SMA (Werdnig–Hoffmann)	Anterior horn ganglion cells of the spinal cord (and bulbar motor neurons)	Muscle atrophy and weakness, hypotonia, fasciculations of the tongue	Affects infants and small children; rapidly fatal	Autosomal recessive inheritance; mutation of the SMN-1 gene on chromosome 5q13.2
Pseudomyopathic SMA (Kugelberg–Welander)	Anterior horn ganglion cells of the spinal cord	Muscle atrophy and fasciculations, progressive gait disturbance, no bulbar involvement	Children and adolescents, proximal, usually begins in the lower limbs, slowly progressive	Autosomal dominant inheritance due to a heterozygous mutation in the DYNC 1H1 gene on chromosome 14q32.31
Adult SMA (Aran–Duchenne)	Anterior horn ganglion cells of the spinal cord	Muscle atrophy, weakness, and fasciculations	Young adults; begins distally (hands)	Usually sporadic, of unknown etiology; occasionally due to syphilis
Proximal SMA of the shoulder girdle (Vulpian–Bernhardt)	Anterior horn ganglion cells of the spinal cord	Muscle atrophy, weakness, and fasciculations in the shoulder girdle	Adults; slowly progressive	Unknown; occasionally due to syphilis
ALS (sometimes including true bulbar palsy)	Anterior horn ganglion cells of the spinal cord, perhaps also motor cranial nerve nuclei, pyramidal tracts, and corticobulbar tracts	Muscle atrophy and weakness, fasciculations, bulbar palsy with dysarthria and dysphagia, spasticity, pyramidal tract signs	Adults, rapidly progressive and lethal; juvenile (familial) cases are less common and have a relatively benign course	Usually sporadic, rarely familial

Abbreviations: ALS, amyotrophic lateral sclerosis; SMA, spinal muscular atrophy.
Note: Several rarer neurologic diseases affect the anterior horn ganglion cells as one component of a wider disease process: these include, but are not limited to, Creutzfeldt-Jakob disease, orthostatic hypotension, diabetic amyotrophy, recurrent hypoglycemia due to an insulin-secreting tumor, metacarcinomatous myelopathy, and organic mercury poisoning.

- Only first neuron (pyramidal tract) affected: **familial spastic spinal paralysis**.
- Only second neuron affected: **spinal muscular atrophy (SMA)**.
- First and second motor neurons affected: **amyotrophic lateral sclerosis (ALS)**.

7.7.2 Spinal Muscular Atrophies

| NOTE

These diseases are due to a **genetic defect on chromosome 5** that causes isolated degeneration of the second (lower) motor neurons, that is, the motor neurons of the anterior horn cells and the cranial nerve nuclei. The result is the typical clinical syndrome of **anterior horn degeneration**:
- Flaccid weakness.
- Diminution or loss of reflexes.
- Progressive muscle atrophy.
- Fasciculations.

All types of SMA are genetically linked to **chromosome 5q11.2–13.3**.

The main clinical types of SMA are classified according to their **age of onset** and the **pattern of motor deficits** that they cause:

Werdnig–Hoffmann type (early childhood type). **Neonates and infants** with this disease suffer from rapidly progressive muscle weakness, beginning in the **muscles of the pelvic girdle**. They can survive for no more than a few years.

Kugelberg–Welander type (pseudomyopathic spinal muscular atrophy). The clinical onset is between the 2nd and 10th years of life. The **pelvic girdle** is most severely affected at first, as in the early childhood type, but the **weakness and atrophy progress more slowly**, and the overall prognosis is much more favorable. The first signs of disease are progressive quadriceps weakness, loss of the patellar tendon reflex, and, sometimes, pseudohypertrophy of the calves.

Generalized types. Types that become symptomatic from the third decade onward tend to be generalized, though the initial presentation tends to be either **mainly distal (Aran–Duchenne)** or **mainly proximal (Vulpian–Bernhardt)**. The Aran–Duchenne type often presents with atrophy of the intrinsic muscles of the hand, and the Vulpian–Bernhardt type with scapulo-humeral atrophy. The latter is now considered a subtype of familial ALS (see later); it affects not only the muscles of the limbs, but also those of the trunk and respiratory apparatus (**Fig. 7.16**).

7.7.3 Amyotrophic Lateral Sclerosis

| NOTE

ALS is characterized by combined degeneration of the anterior horn cells and the corticospinal (pyramidal) and corticobulbar tracts. Loss of the anterior horn cells causes **muscle atrophy, weakness**, and **fasciculations**, while loss of the upper-motor-neuron tracts causes **brisk reflexes** and **pyramidal tract signs**.

Synonyms. This disease is also known as myatrophic lateral sclerosis, as motor neuron disease, and (in North America) as Lou Gehrig disease, after a prominent sufferer.

Epidemiology and Etiology. Three-quarters of patients are men, most of them between the ages of 40 and 65. More than 90% of cases are **sporadic**; the rare **familial** cases are thought to be due to a defect of the Cu/Zn superoxide dismutase gene.

Pathogenesis. The neuropathologic hallmark of this disease is loss of anterior horn cells, combined with degeneration of the pyramidal and corticobulbar tracts and of the Betz's pyramidal cells in the precentral gyri.

Clinical features. The following are typical:
- **Weakness and atrophy** of the muscle groups of the limbs and trunk (including the **respiratory**

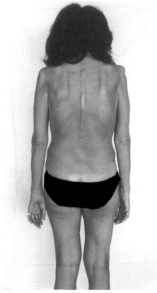

Fig. 7.16   Spinal muscular atrophy in a 46-year-old woman. There is marked atrophy of the muscles of the shoulder girdles, arms, and hands, as well as of the paravertebral musculature.

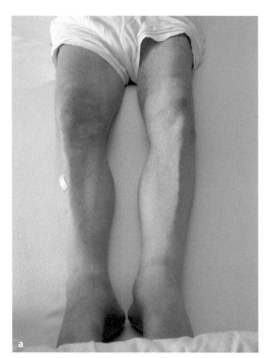
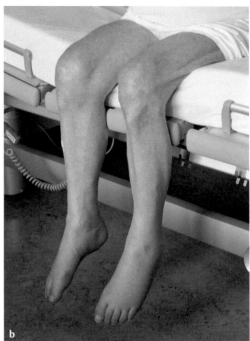

7

Fig. 7.17   Muscle atrophy and dorsiflexor weakness in ALS. a A 72-year-old man with bilateral atrophy of the thigh and calf muscles, more marked on the left. **b** When the patient sits, his feet hang limply because of weakness of the foot and toe dorsiflexors.

apparatus) and/or the bulbar muscles (tongue, throat), progressing slowly over months.

— **Fasciculations**.
— **Brisk reflexes**.
— (In some patients) pyramidal tract signs.
— Intact sensation.
— Often **muscle cramps** and **pain**.

Course. At first, there is circumscribed, asymmetric, **mainly distal muscle atrophy**, which is usually most apparent in the **intrinsic muscles of the hands**. There may be accompanying **pain** or **fasciculations**, which are often evident only on prolonged observation. As the disease progresses, muscle atrophy spreads proximally (**Fig. 7.17**). **Spasticity** gradually appears as well; it is usually only mild at first and may indeed remain so over the ensuing course of the disease. The **intrinsic muscle reflexes** are usually **brisk**, more so than one would expect in view of the concomitant atrophy and weakness, but pyramidal tract signs are not necessarily demonstrable. The **bulbar muscles** are also involved in approximately 20% of patients, as manifested by **atrophy, weakness, and fasciculations of the tongue** (**Fig. 7.18**), dysarthria, and dysphagia (**true bulbar palsy**). Involvement of the corticobulbar tracts leads to **brisk nasopalpebral, perioral** and **masseteric reflexes**, and, frequently, **involuntary laughing and crying**. Further progression often leads to frontal dementia.

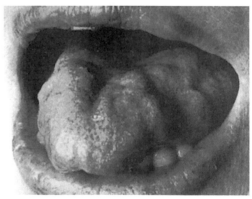

Fig. 7.18   Atrophy of the tongue due to true bulbar palsy in a 65-year-old woman with ALS.

Rarely, the course of ALS deviates from the typical one just described. For example, spasticity may dominate the clinical picture for several months at first, or a patient with a slowly progressive SMA may not develop signs of a corticospinal lesion until years after the onset of disease.

Diagnostic evaluation. ALS can generally be recognized by its **typical clinical features**. Ancillary tests are important mainly for the **exclusion of competing differential diagnoses**.

7

- **EMG**: Electromyography reveals pathologic **spontaneous activity**, both in the paretic muscles and in those that still seem normal.
- **Motor evoked potentials** (MEP, see section 4.3.3) are used to demonstrate dysfunction of the upper motor neuron.
- **Pulmonary function tests** typically reveal **alveolar hypoventilation** with low vital capacity.
- **Laboratory tests**: Creatine kinase (CK) activity is mildly elevated. Further laboratory values of interest include vitamins B_{12} and D, immune electrophoresis, thyroid hormones, and parathyroid hormone.
- **Lumbar puncture** for the exclusion of other diseases. The CSF is normal in ALS.
- **Imaging studies**: For example, MRI of the head and spine can be used to rule out cervical spinal cord compression as the cause of the patient's problem.

The El Escorial criteria for ALS are a selection of important clinical, neurophysiologic, and neuropathologic criteria that can be used to characterize the diagnosis of ALS as definite, probable, possible, or presumptive.

Treatment and prognosis. ALS takes a **chronically progressive course**. Death usually ensues within one or two years, although a minority of patients survives longer. The treatment of ALS consists of numerous symptomatic measures, which vary as the disease progresses.

- **Riluzole** is a sodium-channel blocker with an antiglutamatergic effect. It marginally slows the progression of ALS.

- **Adequate nutrition** is important to prevent **weight loss** and **dehydration**. Dysphagic patients will need to be fed via gastrostomy. This measure should be discussed and implemented early in the course of disease.
- When **hypoventilation** causes hypercapnia and daytime somnolence, **mask ventilation** may improve the patient's quality of life. When bulbar palsy is present, adequate ventilation requires a **tracheostomy**, which can prolong the patient's life. This should be discussed with the patient and his or her family before respiratory failure occurs. If a tracheostomy is performed in this situation, the patient may survive until progressive weakness finally results in a locked-in state. The patient and his or her family should be aware of this possibility, and the patient's instructions should be recorded in an advance care directive.
- Patients with severe **dysarthria** can be helped to communicate with **electronic communication aids**.
- **psychological care** of the patient and family is important at all times, optimally by the same person for the entire duration of the illness.

Additional Information

Fasciculations are a typical feature of ALS but should only be interpreted as a sign of disease when accompanied by other abnormalities (e.g., weakness, atrophy). Fasciculations can be seen in patients with other neurologic diseases and even in **healthy medical students and hospital staff**.

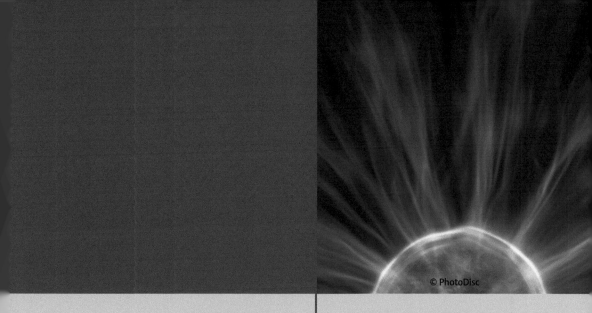
© PhotoDisc

Chapter 8

Multiple Sclerosis and Other Autoimmune Diseases of the Central Nervous System

Ups and Downs

In the spring of 1970, the patient, who was then 30 years old, noticed a tingling in her left big toe. Over the next 3 days, this sensation spread into her entire left leg and then into her right leg as well, and she then developed numbness all over her trunk. Her gait was unsteady, she very rapidly became fatigued, and she had trouble holding her urine from the moment she felt the urge to urinate. These problems all resolved spontaneously in the ensuing weeks, and she ascribed no special importance to them. Six months later, however, her right eye began to hurt, and the vision in that eye became blurry. Once again, the problem resolved spontaneously in about 10 days, and she did not consult a doctor.

In 1973, she had marked difficulty walking for 2 months; practically as soon as this problem improved, she began to see double and was dizzy. These problems, too, got better in about a month, but, in the meantime, she had finally seen a doctor. In the light of her current problems, her past history, and the clinical and laboratory findings (in particular, the visual evoked potentials and the cerebrospinal fluid [CSF] findings), the doctor diagnosed multiple sclerosis (MS).

Over the following years, she had multiple episodes of sensory disturbance on the upper or lower limbs, unsteady gait, and (once) double vision. She often felt uncommonly tired. She sought psychiatric treatment twice for depression. As a rule, each episode resolved within a few weeks or, at most, months, sometimes spontaneously and sometimes after infusions of adrenocorticotropic hormone or corticosteroids.

In the late 1980s, her gait gradually worsened. She no longer experienced any improvement between episodes or any asymptomatic periods, as she had in the past. She became depressed again and gave up her job as a schoolteacher. In 1987, she could still walk 500 m unaided; from 1995 onward, she needed a cane at all times. She was hospitalized twice for urinary tract infections with high fever. Each time, during the febrile phases, her gait transiently worsened to the point that she was totally unable to get out of bed and walk. Two or three years later, she could no longer leave the house without her husband's help, and was dependent on a wheelchair. Now, in 2015, the patient is 75 years old and can help her husband cook dinner from a seated position in her wheelchair. She can pull herself from bed into the wheelchair with difficulty, but she needs help to get dressed and undressed, or to use the toilet.

This case illustrates the typical clinical features and long-term course of MS arising in a young woman. At first, relapsing and remitting disturbances of sensory and motor function and coordination are characteristic, as is transient cranial nerve dysfunction. Phases of abnormal fatigue and depression are common as well. Over time, "classic" relapses become less frequent and are replaced by the slow progression of neurologic deficits—usually a gradually worsening gait impairment. Only half of all patients can still walk 25 to 30 years after the onset of the disease. If the first symptoms arise when the patient is older, less time generally elapses before the phase of secondary progression begins. At present, the most important ancillary diagnostic study for MS is magnetic resonance imaging (MRI). Immune-modulating treatment lessens the frequency and severity of relapses. Over the long term, the result is less severe permanent disability and a better quality of life.

8.1 Fundamentals

Key Point

MS is the most common autoimmune-mediated disease of the central nervous system (CNS). Other autoimmune diseases are much rarer; these include neuromyelitis optica (NMO) and acute disseminated encephalomyelitis (ADEM). The latter primarily affects children and is usually precipitated by a viral infection.

Systemic autoimmune diseases can also affect the CNS and manifest themselves with neurologic symptoms and signs. Further important differential diagnoses of MS include **vascular leukoencephalopathy** (see section 6.5.6, Lacunar Infarction, and section 6.12.5) and the **leukodystrophies** (see **Table 6.23**).

8.2 Multiple Sclerosis

Key Point

MS typically arises in young adults (women more often than men). It is a chronic disease of the CNS (i.e., the brain and spinal cord) that causes the loss of axons and neurons. If untreated, it almost always leads to severe disability. Autoimmune processes involving autoreactive lymphocytes play a major role in its pathogenesis. The disease often manifests itself in episodically occurring neurologic deficits that arise over a few hours or days, and then subside: this is the typical relapsing–remitting course of MS. As the disease progresses, the episodes often leave residual deficits behind, and these accumulate over time. The relapsing MS usually undergoes a transition to secondary progressive MS, in which there is progressive disability, with or without discrete episodes of worsening. A primary progressive course—usually involving spasticity and paralysis—is rarer. The symptoms and signs of MS are highly diverse because of the involvement of many different areas of the CNS and the variable dynamics of disease progression.

 "**Disseminated encephalomyelitis**" is a synonym for MS. In French, the disease is called "sclérose en plaques," as it was named by Charcot; related terms are used in the other Romance languages.

Epidemiology. The incidence of MS in temperate zones is 4 to 6 new cases per 100,000 persons per year and the prevalence is approximately 120 per 100,000. The disease becomes **more common with increasing distance from the equator** and is thus particularly common in northern Europe, Russia, the northern United States., Canada, New Zealand, and southern Australia. **Women** are affected twice as commonly as men. Relatives of MS patients have an elevated risk of developing the disease; the risk is 3% for siblings and 30% for monozygotic twins. The initial attack usually occurs in the **third decade**, and only rarely in a child or older adult. The primary progressive form of MS is of later onset, usually after age 40 years.

NOTE

In developed countries, MS is the most common disease of the nervous system that arises in young adults and causes permanent disability. For older adults, the most common cause of permanent neurologic disability is ischemic stroke.

Pathologic anatomy. There are **disseminated foci of demyelination in the CNS**, which are associated with the destruction and loss of myelin sheaths, axons, and neurons. Local, reactive gliosis is found at the sites of older foci. Thus, "sclerosis" develops at "multiple" locations, giving the disease its English name.

Etiology and pathogenesis. The cause of MS is unknown; genetic factors, environmental influences, and disturbances of the immune system all play a role in its pathogenesis. It is not currently known whether MS is a heterogeneous disease with a complex pathogenesis or, alternatively, a unitary disease whose complex pathogenesis gives it a heterogeneous appearance. It has often been hypothesized that viruses are etiologic factors for MS, precipitating the disease either by infecting neurons directly or by serving as antigens that call forth an uncontrolled immune response. It is clear, in any case, that **autoimmune processes** with **autoreactive T-lymphocytes and monocytes** play a role in the pathogenesis of the disease and cause episodes of inflammation and demyelination.

Experimental allergic encephalomyelitis (EAE) in mice is a laboratory model for MS. In EAE, the inflammatory cells form nitrogen oxides that act as toxic free radicals, promoting apoptosis and leading to the destruction of neurons, axons, and glia. After numerous prolonged episodes of inflammation, more and more neurons, myelin sheaths, axons, and glia are lost. The body's intrinsic repair mechanisms cannot keep up with the destructive process.

In the early stages of MS, **foci of inflammation and demyelination** arise in the cerebral white matter and, to a lesser extent, in the gray matter as well. In the first few years of the disease, these inflammatory cellular autoimmune mechanisms play the most important role. The more active these mechanisms are, the more axons and neurons are lost, and the

8

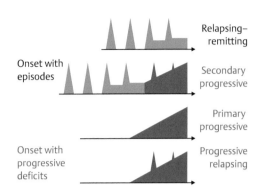

Fig. 8.1   The temporal course of multiple sclerosis: four major types. (Reproduced from Mattle H, Mumenthaler M. Neurologie. Stuttgart: Thieme; 2013.)

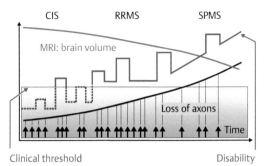

Fig. 8.2   Increasing brain atrophy as multiple sclerosis progresses, with increasing disability. CIS, clinically isolated syndrome; RRMS, relapsing–remitting multiple sclerosis; SPMS, secondary progressive multiple sclerosis. (Reproduced from Mattle H, Mumenthaler M. Neurologie. Stuttgart: Thieme; 2013.)

more **sclerotic glial scarring** takes their place. Cumulative scarring over the course of the disease leads to progressive atrophy of the brain and spinal cord, with increasing involvement of the cerebral gray matter (see **Fig. 8.4**).

Course. The temporal course of MS (**Fig. 8.1**) can be of four main types:

- **Relapsing (or "relapsing–remitting") type**: characterized by the episodic appearance of new neurologic deficits, which can then remit completely or almost completely, leaving residual deficits of greater or lesser severity, without any progression of disease between the episodes.
- **Secondary progressive type**: episodic worsening at first, followed by steady progression (possibly punctuated by further episodes).
- **Primary progressive type**: steady progression from the beginning, most commonly seen in older patients with spastic-paraparetic MS.
- **Progressive relapsing type**: steady progression with interspersed episodes of acute worsening, from the onset of the disease onward.

NOTE

In the initial years of the disease, **autoimmune inflammatory processes** are the most important factors causing the clinical manifestations and relapsing episodes; in the later years and decades, **degenerative processes**, with loss of axons and neurons, play the main role (**Fig. 8.2**).

Clinical features and neurologic findings. The general clinical features of MS are summarized in **Table 8.1**. The neurologic deficits present in each individual patient depend on the number and location of the demyelinating foci. The following are among the more characteristic disease manifestations and physical findings:

Table 8.1

Clinical features of multiple sclerosis

Symptoms and signs	Remarks
Repeated episodes	- At varying temporal intervals - After each episode, either complete recovery or residual deficit
Diverse sites in CNS affected	- Multiple, distinct CNS sites can be involved in a single episode - Different episodes generally involve different sites - Rarely, successive episodes may have similar clinical manifestations (particularly with spinal cord lesions)
Progressive neurologic impairment	- In relapsing–remitting type, cumulation of residual deficits - In primary progressive type, steady progression without episodes (particularly in late-onset disease)

Abbreviation: CNS, central nervous system.

Retrobulbar neuritis is usually **unilateral**. Over the course of a few days, the patient develops an **impairment of color vision** (red desaturation), followed by **impairment of visual acuity**. **Orbital pain** is often present and the patient may **see flashes of light** on movement of the globe. These problems begin to improve in 1 or 2 weeks and usually resolve completely. The temporal side of the optic disc becomes pale 3 or 4 weeks after the onset of symptoms because of nerve fiber degeneration (**Fig. 8.3**). Retrobulbar neuritis rarely affects both eyes, either at the same time or in rapid succession. If retrobulbar neuritis is an isolated event in a patient otherwise free of neurologic disease, the probability that other clinical signs of MS will appear in the future is roughly 50%. The probability is greater if abnormalities are found in the CSF (see later) or on an MRI scan (see **Fig. 8.6**).

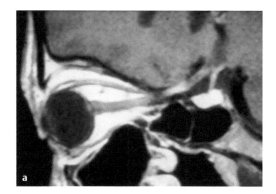

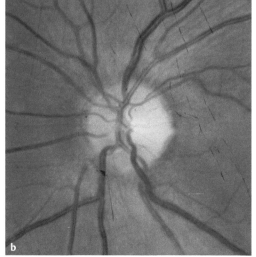

Fig. 8.3   Retrobulbar neuritis. (a) MRI: behind the apex of the orbit, the inflamed optic nerve takes up contrast medium, and a short segment of it therefore appears hyperintense (bright). **(b)** Funduscopy after an episode of left retrobulbar neuritis: the temporal side of the optic disk is pale up to its edge.

Oculomotor disturbances: Diplopia, particularly due to **abducens palsy**, is a common early symptom. Later, typical findings are **nystagmus** (often dissociated) and **internuclear ophthalmoplegia** (see section 12.3.3, Internuclear Ophthalmoplegia), often without any subjective correlate. Internuclear ophthalmoplegia in a young patient is relatively specific for MS.

Lhermitte sign (positive neck-flexion sign): Active or passive forward flexion of the neck induces an "electric" or tingling paresthesia running down the spine and/or into the limbs.

Sensory disturbances are present in half of all MS patients early on in the course of the disease, often as an initial manifestation. **Vibration sense in the feet** is impaired in practically all patients from some point in the course of the disease onward. **Pain** is common, and there is occasionally a **dissociated sensory deficit**.

NOTE
Retrobulbar neuritis, oculomotor disturbances, Lhermitte sign, and sensory deficits are common early findings in MS.

Pyramidal tract signs and brisk intrinsic muscle reflexes may also be present early in the course of the disease. The abdominal cutaneous reflexes are absent. Later on, in almost all patients, spastic paraparesis or quadriparesis develops.

Cerebellar signs are practically always present in advanced MS, including impaired coordination, ataxic gait, and, often, a very characteristic intention tremor (cf. **Fig. 3.22**).

Gait impairment often becomes severe early in the course of the disease. Typically, the combination of spastic paraparesis and ataxia results in a spastic-ataxic, uneven, uncoordinated, and stiff gait (cf. **Fig. 3.2**).

Bladder dysfunction is present in about three-quarters of all patients (generally in association with spasticity); disturbances of defecation are much rarer. Bladder dysfunction is sometimes an early manifestation of the disease. Urge incontinence is highly characteristic, that is, a sudden, almost uncontrollable need to urinate, perhaps leading to involuntary loss of urine. Patients often do not mention bladder dysfunction unless they are directly asked about it.

Ictal phenomena of various types are not uncommon. Epileptic seizures are somewhat more common than in healthy individuals, but less common than in persons with cerebrovascular disease. About 1.5% of persons with MS suffer from trigeminal neuralgia, which may alternate from one side to the other. Acute dizzy spells can occur, as can paroxysmal dystonia, dysarthria, or ataxia. The characteristic so-called tonic brainstem seizures consist of paroxysmal, often painful, tonic stiffness of the muscles on one side of the body. The lower limb is hyperextended and the upper limb flexed (Wernicke–Mann posture). The patient remains fully conscious. Tonic brainstem seizures are often provoked by a change of position; they last less than 1 minute and are followed by a refractory period of a half hour or more in which no further seizures can occur. Tonic brainstem seizures and most other MS-associated ictal phenomena respond to treatment with carbamazepine or other antiepileptic drugs.

Mental disturbances are not severe early in the course of the disease, although sometimes unusually severe fatigue is the main symptom. Later on, however, many patients develop psycho-organic changes, including psychoreactive and depressive disturbances, as a consequence of progressive brain atrophy (**Fig. 8.4**). Psychosis is very rare.

8

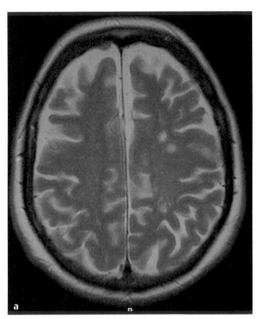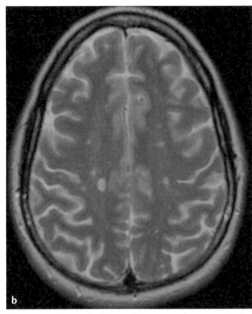

a b

Fig. 8.4 Brain atrophy in multiple sclerosis. The progressive loss of neurons and axons leads, over the years, to brain atrophy that is visible in MRI. In these two axial T2-weighted images obtained from two different patients, the subarachnoid space is wider in **a** than in **b** as a result of brain atrophy in **a**.

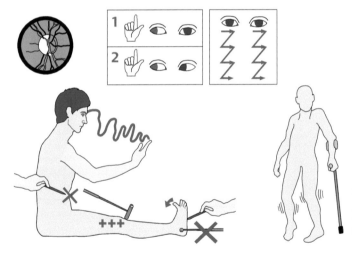

Fig. 8.5 Common physical findings in multiple sclerosis. Optic disk atrophy, internuclear ophthalmoplegia nystagmus, intention tremor, spasticity with absent abdominal skin reflexes, brisk intrinsic muscle reflexes, Babinski signs, and ataxia.

The typical clinical findings in MS are shown schematically in **Fig. 8.5**.

The initial manifestation of multiple sclerosis: clinically isolated syndrome. **Sensory disturbances**, **visual disturbances** due to optic neuritis, **diplopia** due to oculomotor dysfunction, and **weakness** are very common initial manifestations of MS. Such manifestations, occurring initially before MS has definitively declared itself (i.e., before it has become "multiple"), are now called clinically isolated syndrome (CIS) (see **Fig. 8.2**). Not all patients with CIS go on to develop MS. Around 30 to 40% of patients with CIS develop MS within 2 years. Among patients with CIS whose MRI scan shows more than one lesion, more than 80% develop MS within 10 years; if the MRI shows only a single lesion, only 10% do. The presence of oligoclonal bands (see later) in the CSF is also associated with a higher risk of developing MS. CIS converts into MS, by definition, as soon as a second neurologic symptom arises that differs from the first one.

If the MRI at the time of the initial presentation shows contrast-enhancing lesions that do not explain the neurologic deficit(s) present at that time,

Table 8.2

The Expanded Disability Status Scale for MS (simplified)

Score	Findings/neurologic deficits
0	Normal
1	No impairment, minimal positive findings
2	Minimal impairment
3	Moderate impairment, fully able to walk
4	Impaired ability to walk, but can walk at least 500 m
5	Can walk at least 200 m; restricted everyday activities
6	Can walk 100 m with aid
7	Cannot walk any more than 5 m; wheelchair-dependent; can transfer independently
8	Mostly bedridden or in wheelchair, needs help with transfers
9	Bedridden and helpless
10	Death due to MS

Abbreviation: MS, multiple sclerosis.

as well as further, non–contrast-enhancing lesions, this indicates that **foci of demyelination of different ages** are present. The disease process displays multiplicity in both space and time and thus meets the definition of relapsing MS.

Tumefactive multiple sclerosis and the concentric sclerosis of Baló. Rarely, individual MS plaques can be very large and, together with the surrounding edema, exert **mass effect**; they are then called tumefactive. Tumefactive plaques typically consist of sequentially demyelinated layers around a central core; such plaques are the hallmark of the "concentric sclerosis" described in 1928 by Baló. Their clinical presentation depends on their location. This disease is treated in the same way as relapsing–remitting MS (see later).

The severity of MS. Various scales are in use to characterize the severity of MS. The Expanded Disability Status Scale is most commonly used (**Table 8.2**).

Diagnostic evaluation. The diagnosis is based on the **history**, the typical **physical findings** (see earlier), and the findings of **ancillary tests** (see later). To determine whether a patient is suffering from a relapse (also called an episode or attack) of MS, the following definition of a relapse should be applied.

NOTE

In a relapse of MS, neurologic symptoms and deficits newly appear, or old ones are reactivated. These criteria must be met:

— Duration of **at least 24 hours**.
— Interval of **at least 30 days** since the last relapse.
— The episode is **not** a **pseudorelapse**, that is, a reversible exacerbation of manifestations in the setting of infection or otherwise elevated body temperature (the **Uhthoff phenomenon**).

The following **ancillary tests** are also useful:

— **Neuroimaging studies**, particularly **MRI**, typically reveal abnormal white matter signal in the periventricular regions and the corpus callosum and elsewhere in the cerebrum, cerebellum, and spinal cord. Active MS plaques take up contrast medium (**Fig. 8.6**).
— **CSF** examination reveals a mild elevation of the total protein concentration, mild lymphocytic and plasma cell pleocytosis, and, in more than 90% of patients, CSF-specific oligoclonal bands (demonstrable by isoelectric focusing, **Fig. 8.7**). Moreover, many patients with MS have an elevated antibody synthesis index (CSF divided by serum concentration) for measles, rubella, and/ or varicella zoster virus (the so-called MRZ reaction).
— **Electrophysiologic testing**: delayed latency of the visual evoked potentials (see **Fig. 4.26**) is typical, as a result of demyelination of axons in the visual pathway.
— **Laboratory tests** are mainly useful for the exclusion of competing differential diagnoses.

NOTE

The **McDonald criteria** are now used for the diagnosis of MS. The diagnosis is considered definitive if the history, physical findings, and ancillary tests document CNS involvement that is **disseminated in both space and time**.

Differential diagnosis. Generally speaking, when a patient presents with an **isolated neurologic deficit** that would be typical of MS, the differential diagnosis must include all other conditions that could produce that deficit. Even recurrent and relapsing neurologic deficits that are **referable to more than one area of the CNS** (the typical clinical picture of MS) do not by themselves establish the diagnosis.

NOTE

Important differential diagnoses of MS include **autoimmune diseases** (mainly systemic lupus erythematosus, Wegener granulomatosis, vasculitis of various types), **leukodystrophies**, mitochondriopathies, infections (e.g., borreliosis), neurosarcoidosis, and **vascular leukoencephalopathy** (section 6.5.6, Lacunar Infarction, and section 6.12.5).

Vascular leukoencephalopathy is a microangiopathy that mainly affects elderly persons with arterial hypertension or (less commonly) diabetes mellitus. An important differential-diagnostic clue to this entity is the involvement of **other organs** (e.g., the heart—coronary heart disease, the limbs—peripheral

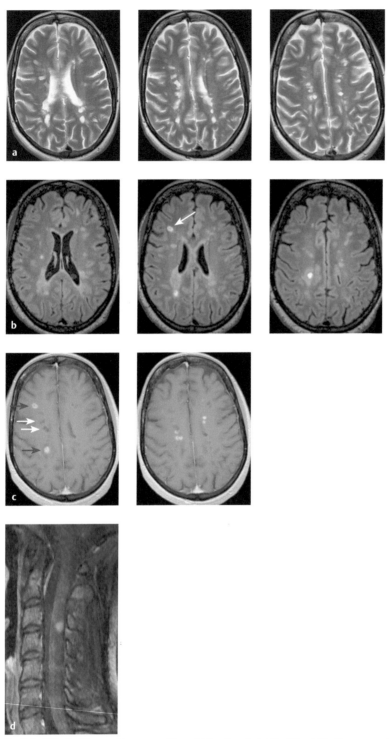

Fig. 8.6   MRI of a 46-year-old woman with multiple sclerosis. (a) The T2-weighted image reveals multiple lesions, mainly in the periventricular zones and on the periphery of the corpus callosum. **(b)** The FLAIR sequence reveals subcortical lesions that are also typical of MS (arrow). **(c)** T1-weighted image in the same plane as **a**: note the lesions of different ages. The hypointense, non–contrast-enhancing lesions (white arrows) are older, while the foci of contrast enhancement (red arrows) indicate fresh inflammation. **(d)** The T1-weighted image of the cervical spinal cord likewise reveals a typical contrast-enhancing lesion.

arterial occlusive disease). A further difference concerns lesions in the spinal cord, which are common and visible on MRI in MS, but rare in vascular leukoencephalopathy. Further important differential diagnoses of MS are summarized in **Table 8.3.**

Treatment. Individual acute episodes (relapses) are treated with **high-dose steroids**, for example, methylprednisolone 500 mg IV per day for 5 days, followed by oral prednisone, initially 100 mg per day and then in tapering doses, for 2 weeks (e.g., 100 mg per day

for 3 days, then 50 mg per day for 3 days, then 25 mg per day for 3 days, and finally 12.5 mg per day for 3 days).

As soon as the diagnosis of MS has been established, or even in the CIS stage, patients should be given **immune-modulating** or **immunosuppressive treatment** (**Table 8.4**). The earlier such treatment is started, the better the long-term outcome, with a lower probability of disability (**Table 8.2**, **Fig. 8.8**).

The **injectable drugs interferon-β-1a** and **glatiramer acetate** are of well-tested efficacy and long-term safety. Newer **oral drugs** are effective as well; most of them are well tolerated, but their long-term safety is not as well documented as that of the injectable drugs. All of these drugs inhibit activated T- or B-lymphocytes that cross the blood–brain barrier or become active in the CNS; they do so by a variety of mechanisms. Inflammatory reactions are thus prevented, and little or no neural tissue is destroyed.

If the disease activity is very high, or if the injectable and oral drugs do not adequately suppress relapses, **intravenous drugs** are used. These are generally more effective but can have more serious side effects as well, for example, progressive multifocal leukoencephalopathy (see section 6.7.6, Rarer Types, and **Fig. 6.48**). Alemtuzumab can be used to treat extremely active MS. It suppresses B- and T-lymphocytes and, in a certain sense, reprograms the body's immune memory.

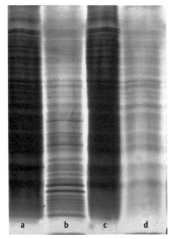

Fig. 8.7   Oligoclonal bands in the serum (a) and CSF (b) of a patient with multiple sclerosis; compare with the serum (c) and CSF (d) of a normal control subject.

Table 8.3

The differential diagnosis of multiple sclerosis (other than vascular leukoencephalopathy)

Clinical manifestation	Possible alternative diagnoses	Useful criteria for differential diagnosis
Lhermitte sign	− Status posttraumatic brain injury or radiotherapy − Pathologic process in the thoracic spinal cord, the dorsal cervical spinal cord, or the junction of the spinal cord and medulla − Vitamin B$_{12}$ deficiency	History and physical findings
Intermittent visual loss	− Amaurosis fugax, e.g., in carotid stenosis − Amblyopic attacks in papilledema − Glaucoma	− Age, risk factors for arteriosclerosis − Duration of episodes − Signs of intracranial hypertension − Cervical bruit
Optic disc pallor	− Optic nerve compression by a mass − Glaucoma	− Slowly progressive visual impairment − CT/MRI findings
Paresis of extraocular muscles	− Diabetic mononeuritis − Compression of one or more cranial nerves by a mass, e.g., at the skull base or in the region of the cavernous sinus	− Diabetes − Pain − Tumor or aneurysm on CT or MRI
Nystagmus	Disease affecting the cerebellum	Other cerebellar signs, e.g., ataxia
Progressive spastic paraparesis	− Spinal cord compression − Arteriovenous fistula − Spastic spinal paralysis − Parasagittal mass	− Slow progression, sensory level − Relapsing course − No relapses or remissions; purely motor deficit − Possibly, headache
Intermittent paraparesis	− Vascular spinal cord lesion (e.g., arteriovenous malformation) − Benign spinal cord tumor (e.g., lipomatosis after prolonged steroid treatment)	− Very rapid or sudden worsening − Look for a sensory level

Abbreviations: CT, computed tomography; MRI, magnetic resonance imaging.

Table 8.4

Immune-modulating and immunosuppressive drugs for multiple sclerosis

	Drug	Dosage	Side effects
Injectable drugs	Interferon-β-1b (Betaferon)	250 µg SC every other day	Flulike symptoms, side effects of injection (mainly redness, swelling, and/or itch at the injection site), elevated liver enzymes
	Interferon-β-1a (Avonex)	30 µg IM 1x/week	Flulike symptoms, side effects of injection, elevated liver enzymes
	Interferon-β-1a (Rebif)	44 µg SC 3x/week	Flulike symptoms, side effects of injection, elevated liver enzymes
	Glatiramer acetate (Copaxone)	20 mg SC qd	Side effects of injection, immediate systemic postinjection reaction
Orally administered drugs	Fingolimod (Gilenya)	0.5 mg/d p.o.	(Brady)arrhythmia, reduction of forced expiratory volume, macular edema
	Teriflunomide (Aubagio)	14 mg/d p.o.	Diarrhea, nausea, hair loss
	Dimethyl fumarate (Tecfidera)	2 × 240 mg/d p.o.	Gastrointestinal symptoms, diarrhea, cutaneous flushing
Drugs for intravenous infusion	Alemtuzumab (Lemtrada)	12 mg IV/ qd for 5 d in the first year and for 3 d in the second year	Infusion reactions, secondary autoimmune diseases (thyroiditis, autoimmune thrombocytopenia, Goodpasture syndrome)
	Natalizumab (Tysabri)	300 mg IV every 28 d	Allergic reactions, PML
	Mitoxantrone (Ralenova)	12 mg/m² BSA IV approximately every 3 mo; maximal cumulative dose 140 mg/m² BSA	Nausea, vomiting, alopecia, leukemia, cardiotoxicity

Abbreviations: BSA, body surface area; IM, intramuscular; IV, intravenous; PML, progressive multifocal leukoencephalopathy; p.o., per os; qd, daily; SC, subcutaneous.

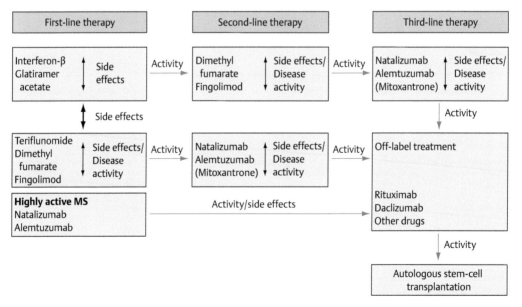

Fig. 8.8   Treatment algorithm for relapsing–remitting multiple sclerosis. First-line therapy employs injectable drugs (e.g., interferon-β) or orally administered drugs (e.g., teriflunomide). Intravenous drugs such as natalizumab are given to treat highly active MS. The choice of the drug and route of administration are based on the side effects and, later, on the observed effects on disease activity.

Anti-MS drugs are most effective in the relapsing–remitting stage of the disease. They are effective to some extent in patients with secondary progressive MS who still have superimposed attacks, but no drug has yet been found effective against primary progressive MS. In patients with CIS, injectable and oral drugs (as far as these have been studied) lessen the risk of a second episode and thus the risk of developing relapsing–remitting MS, and they probably also lessen the long-term risk of disability. Generally speaking, anti-MS drugs **slow the progression of the disease**, but cannot cure it.

General measures remain very important: patient education and psychological support, symptomatic treatments (antispasmodic drugs, treatment of bladder infections, paroxysmal phenomena, pain, etc.), physical therapy, and rehabilitation.

Prognosis. Unfavorable prognostic factors include advanced age at the onset of disease, but only if the disease takes a primary or secondary progressive course. Further unfavorable prognostic factors include cerebellar and brainstem signs and frequent relapses early on in the course of the disease course. An MS patient's condition 5 years after the onset of the disease (particularly with respect to cerebellar and pyramidal tract signs) is closely correlated with his or her condition 5 and 10 years later. About half of all untreated patients can walk only 100 m or less or are wheelchair-bound 20 to 25 years after onset. The course of MS is, however, highly variable. About one-third of patients have no relevant impairment after the first episode of the disease, and a small percentage still has none 25 years later. The life expectancy of an MS patient is now normal or nearly so with current forms of treatment, and the progression of the disease can be stopped or, at least, markedly slowed.

> **NOTE**
>
> Half of all patients with MS have relevant difficulty walking 20 to 25 years after the onset of the disease. This fact underscores the importance of early immune-modulating treatment.

8.3 Other Autoimmune Diseases of the CNS

  Key Point

Aside from MS, there are other autoimmune diseases that affect the CNS, among them NMO, which consists of optic neuritis combined with acute myelitis, and ADEM, which is characterized by rapidly progressive neurologic deficits. Moreover, various types of autoimmune vasculitis, such as Behçet disease, can affect the CNS, and sarcoidosis can do so as well.

8.3.1 Neuromyelitis Optica

Pathogenesis. NMO (earlier known as Devic disease) is a **severe demyelinating disease** of the CNS, characterized by optic neuritis and acute myelitis. It is much rarer than MS, affects **women** more often than men, and usually begins **at a later age** than MS. The autoimmune process underlying NMO is traceable to a disease-specific immunoglobulin G (IgG) antibody (NMO-IgG) directed against aquaporin-4. Necrotizing inflammation in the CNS is the pathologic hallmark of the disease.

Clinical features. The main clinical features appear either simultaneously or rapidly one after the other and include **myelitis**, uni- or bilateral **optic neuritis**, or both. The neurologic deficits are severe. When the deficits reach peak severity, the patients are generally **blind** and **unable to walk**, as well as being **incontinent of urine**. The course can be monophasic, but a relapsing and remitting course is more common. The cerebrum and cerebellum are sometimes affected, but usually only in the later course of the disease, rather than as its initial manifestation.

Diagnostic evaluation. Spinal MRI reveals centrally located spinal cord lesions of long vertical extent (the height of at least three contiguous vertebral bodies) (**Fig. 8.9**). **Head MRI** typically reveals uni- or bilateral optic neuritis, but no lesions in the cerebral hemispheres. **CSF** analysis reveals pleocytosis (> 50 leukocytes/mm^3 or at least 5 neutrophils), but no oligoclonal bands. The most useful diagnostic test is a **serologic study** for NMO-IgG antibodies.

The definitive diagnosis of NMO is made when the following three criteria are met:
- Optic neuritis.
- Acute myelitis.
- At least two of the following three features:
  - A **lesion** on **spinal MRI** that extends vertically over the height of at least three vertebral bodies.
  - No MS-specific signal abnormalities on head MRI.
  - Serologic demonstration of **NMO-IgG**.

The **differential diagnosis** depends on the main manifestation of the disease and corresponds to those of uni- or bilateral visual disturbances (see section 12.2.2) and of acute myelitis (see section 7.5.1).

Treatment. Episodes are treated with **corticosteroids**, for example, methylprednisolone 1,000 mg IV once a day for 5 days followed by long-term oral prednisone. Immunosuppressant drugs of first choice are **azathioprine** (2.5–3 mg/kg body weight/day) and **rituximab** (2 × 1,000 mg, given 2 weeks apart, every 6 months).

Prognosis. The prognosis is better when the disease has a monophasic rather than a relapsing–remitting course but is nonetheless unfavorable, unless intensive treatment is given. NMO-IgG antibodies are associated with a high risk of recurrence.

8

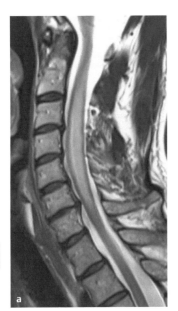 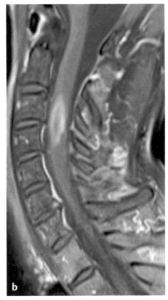 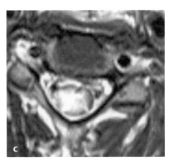

Fig. 8.9 **MRI of the cervical spinal cord in a 58-year-old man with neuromyelitis optica** and, clinically, a partial spinal cord transection syndrome. **(a)** The T2-weighted image reveals a signal abnormality extending from C2 to C7. **(b)** The contrast-enhanced T1-weighted image reveals uptake of contrast medium in the center of the inflammatory lesion. **(c)** Axial T2-weighted image: the lesion affects both the gray and the white matter of the spinal cord.

8.3.2 Acute Disseminated Encephalomyelitis

Pathogenesis and clinical features. ADEM is an **acute**, **monophasic**, autoimmune-inflammatory demyelinating disease that usually arises in the aftermath of an infection. It affects children more commonly than adults. There are **rapidly progressive** neurologic deficits that can become very severe; in the extreme case, the disease can cause **hemorrhagic encephalomyelitis** and death.

Diagnosis and treatment. **MRI** reveals extensive, multifocal, subcortical signal abnormalities, which are all of the same age, but of nonspecific type. **CSF examination** reveals pleocytosis, and oligoclonal bands may be (but are not necessarily) present. There is no specific diagnostic test. ADEM is treated with **steroids**, **immunosuppressive drugs**, and **plasmapheresis**.

Prognosis. If the patient survives, the brain lesions and the neurologic deficits can resolve to a greater or lesser extent. More than 90% of affected children recover completely.

8.3.3 Behçet Disease

This disease is a type of **systemic vasculitis** affecting both arteries and veins. It classically manifests itself with the clinical triad of **genital and oral aphthous sores** and **iritis**. Its cause is unknown. Most patients carry HLA-B51; along with this genetic component,

exogenous precipitating factors are presumed. The disease can affect the **CNS** as well as the eyes—both directly, through inflammation, and indirectly through vascular disturbances, for example, cerebral venous or venous sinus thrombosis.

The treatment is symptomatic, with **immunosuppressive drugs** (steroids, azathioprine, cyclosporine A, or cyclophosphamide).

8.3.4 Subacute Myelo-Optic Neuropathy

In 1970, Japanese authors described a subacute myelo-optic neuropathy that arose after the consumption of medications containing oxyquinoline. In **Japan**, 15 to 40% of MS patients have an **opticospinal relapsing–remitting inflammation** that differs in various ways from MS as it commonly appears in Europe, North America, and Australia and shares many features with NMO.

8.3.5 Other Autoimmune Diseases

There are several other autoimmune diseases that can involve the central and/or peripheral nervous system, including **sarcoidosis** and the **collagenoses** (see section 6.8.6), giant cell arteritis, systemic lupus erythematosus, antineutrophil cytoplasmic antibody–associated vasculitides (Wegener granulomatosis, Churg–Strauss syndrome), periarteritis nodosa, and granulomatous angiitis of the CNS.

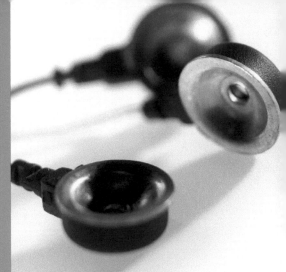

Chapter 9

Epilepsy and Its Differential Diagnosis

Blackout

The patient was 76 years old when his wife, returning home from a brief shopping trip, found him confused and disoriented. His trousers were wet, and a broken coffee cup lay on the floor. She phoned the family doctor. The patient returned to normal consciousness within half an hour; by the time the doctor arrived, he was fully alert and oriented, but he had no recollection of what had happened and spoke of a complete "blackout." The doctor examined him thoroughly and told him and his wife to call him at once if anything similar happened again. A few weeks later, while out walking with his wife, he suddenly fell. His eyes looked to one side, and, a few seconds later, the right corner of his mouth began to twitch, followed by his right arm and, finally, his entire body. Bloody froth came out of his mouth. A minute or two later, he was still lying motionless and unconscious on the ground. His wife called an ambulance. On arrival in the hospital he was awake again, but confused; half an hour later, he was fully alert and oriented.

The emergency medical team took a thorough history from the patient's wife, as he once again had no recollection of the event. He had always been healthy in the past, except for high blood pressure. About 6 months previously, however, he had had a transient "speech problem," and, at the same time, the right corner of his mouth had hung down, and his right arm had been weak. These problems had all resolved within a few days.

Clearly, the patient had had two epileptic seizures a few weeks apart. The initial disturbance, with disorientation, was a seizure of the "dyscognitive" type. The course of the second seizure, as observed by his wife, with twitching that successively spread from the right corner of the mouth to the right arm to the whole body, implied a focal onset of epileptic activity with secondary generalization. The epileptic focus was most likely to be in the left cerebral hemisphere. The focal onset and the patient's advanced age implied that the seizures, in this case, were probably symptomatic. Accordingly, his electroencephalogram (EEG) showed a focus with slow waves and periodic steep potentials in the left frontal lobe. A magnetic resonance imaging scan revealed scarring in the area of an old stroke, presumably reflecting the event of 6 months before, in which he had been transiently aphasic with a mainly brachiofacial hemiparesis.

Lamotrigine was given to prevent further seizures, and he remained seizure-free for 2 years thereafter. Lamotrigine was then slowly tapered to off. He is now 81 and has had no further seizures.

Stroke is the most common cause of symptomatic epilepsy in the elderly. This type of epilepsy generally takes a benign course; anticonvulsive treatment is usually needed only for a limited time.

9.1 Fundamentals

 Key Point

An epileptic seizure is produced by a tempo-rally limited, synchronous electric discharge of neurons in the brain. It involves a combination of suddenly arising motor, somatosensory, special sensory, autonomic, and/or behavioral disturbances that reproduces itself in charac-teristic fashion each time the patient has a seizure, but varies from patient to patient. On rare occasions, seizure activity persists for more than 20 minutes and may go on for hours, or even longer, without interruption (status epilepticus). The epileptic event may affect a circumscribed area of the brain (partial or focal seizures) or both cerebral hemispheres at the same time (generalized seizures). Some, but not all, seizures involve an impairment of consciousness.

In their differential diagnosis, epileptic seizures must be carefully distinguished from other episodic events involving neurologic deficits and disturbances of consciousness.

Epidemiology. One percent of all persons have epi-leptic seizures. The child of a parent with genetic epilepsy has a 4% likelihood of suffering from it.

Pathophysiology. Epileptic seizures are due to the uncoordinated activity of neurons in the brain, which expresses itself electrophysiologically as an abnormality of the fluctuations of electrical potential that are seen in an EEG (see section 4.3.2). (If the sur-face EEG is normal, such abnormalities can be revealed by recording with depth electrodes.) The underlying cause is an **imbalance of excitatory and inhibitory currents**, with predominance of excitatory neurotransmitters such as glutamate and aspartate, or diminished activity of inhibitory neurotransmit-ters such as gamma-aminobutyric acid. **Altered net-work structures** are responsible: these promote the generation and intermittent spread of uncoordinated neural activity. The uncoordinated discharge of neu-rons in a particular area of the brain is accompanied by a local increase in blood flow.

Etiology. In **structural epilepsy**, epileptic seizures are produced by structural lesions in the brain (so-called epileptogenic structural changes: scar, tumor, con-genital malformation). **Metabolic epilepsy** is due to metabolic disturbances (e.g., hypoglycemia) or toxic influences (e.g., alcohol). These are both types of **symptomatic epilepsy**. In contrast, the **genetic epi-lepsies** involve a genetic predisposition to epileptic seizures, in the absence of a structural lesion. The **epilepsies of unknown cause** are presumed to be of symptomatic origin, although their cause cannot (yet) be demonstrated. Molecular genetic techniques have made it possible to trace certain forms of focal epilepsy back to specific mutations in the genome.

This threefold classification, like all classifications, has its limits. There will always be cases whose clas-sification is ambiguous or uncertain; for example, there are some genetically based structural changes of the brain that are epileptogenic. Moreover, there is often more than one etiologic factor at work. Thus, diseases of the brain are more likely to produce epileptic seizures in persons with an inherited predisposition to seizures than in other, normal individuals.

Clinical features. General characteristics of epileptic seizures are as follows:

- Epileptic seizures are **events of sudden onset**.
- They occur with **variable frequency** (generally in the range of a few seizures per year to several per day).
- **Stereotypy**: epileptic seizures generally take a similar course each time they occur, with an iden-tical, "predetermined" sequence of manifesta-tions, and are of similar duration each time as well.
- They often present with **motor phenomena** (in particular, repetitive, clonic twitching or changes of muscle tone) and sometimes with **somatosen-sory**, **special sensory**, and/or **autonomic manifes-tations**.
- Depending on their type, they may involve an **impairment or loss of consciousness**, or con-sciousness may be preserved during the seizure.
- The seizure may be preceded by premonitory symptoms of various kinds (**auras**, e.g., nausea, a rising sensation of warmth, or a feeling of unreality).
- In some patients, seizures occur in response to specific **provocative** and **precipitating factors** (sleep deprivation, alcohol withdrawal, medica-tions, strobe lighting, hyperventilation, fever).

9.1.1 Classification of the Epilepsies

Epilepsy can be **classified** according to several crite-ria (**Table 9.1** and **Table 9.2**), including:

- **Etiology**, for example:
  - "Genuine/idiopathic" = genetic.
  - Symptomatic = structural or metabolic.
  - Cryptogenic = of unknown cause.
- **Age of onset**, for example:
  - Epilepsy of childhood or adolescence.
  - Epilepsy of adulthood.
  - Late epilepsy (age 30 and up; always consider a primary organic disease as the cause).
- **Setting in which seizures are most frequent**, for example:
  - Sleep epilepsy.

9

- Epilepsy on awakening.
- **EEG correlate** and corresponding topographic localization, for example:
  - Generalized epilepsy.
  - Focal (= partial) epilepsy.
- Finally, the **clinical features** of each seizure. The International League against Epilepsy has developed, and recently revised, a nomenclature for the different clinical types of epileptic seizure, which is reproduced in **Table 9.2**. For completeness, the table includes both the older and the newer nomenclature, because the older system is still in widespread use. **Table 9.1** (classification of the epilepsies) also includes the terminology of both systems of classification.

9.1.2 Practical Clinical Management of a Suspected Epileptic Seizure

History and physical examination. A **thorough history** is of the essence for the diagnosis of epilepsy and its differentiation from other, nonepileptic disorders (see later). A description of the seizures should

Table 9.1

Classification of the epilepsies

Previous terminology	New terminology
— Idiopathic	— **Genetic** According to current knowledge, the seizures are the direct result of one or more known or presumed genetic changes. The epileptic seizures are the main manifestation of the genetic disease
— Symptomatic	— **Structural or metabolic** The patient is suffering from an entirely different condition or disease that has been shown in conclusive scientific studies to be associated with a markedly elevated risk of developing epilepsy, or there are clearly recognizable structural changes in the brain of a type known to be epileptogenic
— Cryptogenic	— **Of unknown cause** "Of unknown cause" is a neutral designation of the fact that the nature of the underlying cause of the patient's epilepsy could not be determined up to the present time

Source: Adapted from Diener HC, Weimar C, Berlit P, et al. Leitlinien für Diagnostik und Therapie in der Neurologie. Stuttgart: Thieme; 2012.

Table 9.2

Classification of epileptic seizure types as proposed by the International League against Epilepsy

Previous terminology	New terminology
Localization-related (focal, partial) seizures	*Focal seizures*

— Simple focal (simple partial)
  • Focal motor
  • Aura
  • Automatisms
— Complex focal (complex partial), psychomotor
— Secondary generalized
	Characteristics of focal seizures relating to impairment during the seizure:
	— Without impairment of consciousness or attention:
	  • With observable motor or autonomic components (cf. section 9.3.1 and **Table 9.9**)
	  • With only subjective somatosensory, special sensory, or mental phenomena (cf. **Table 9.9**)
	— With impairment of consciousness or attention: dyscognitive type
	— With progression to a bilateral convulsive seizure (with tonic, clonic, or tonic–clonic elements)

Generalized seizures	*Generalized seizures*

— Tonic–clonic (grand mal)
— Absences
— Myoclonic
— Clonic
— Tonic
— Atonic (astatic)
	— Tonic–clonic (in any combination)
	— Absences
	  • Eyelid myoclonus with absence
	  • Typical
	  • Atypical
	  • With special features
	  • Myoclonic absence
	— Myoclonic
	  • Myoclonic
	  • Myoclonic–atonic
	  • Myoclonic–tonic
	— Clonic
	— Tonic
	— Atonic

Unclassifiable seizures	*Unknown*
–	Epileptic spasms

Source: Adapted from Diener HC, Weimar C, Berlit P, et al. Leitlinien für Diagnostik und Therapie in der Neurologie. Stuttgart: Thieme; 2012.

also be obtained from **someone who saw the patient having a seizure**, if possible, because patients usually suffer amnesia for the seizures. The questions to be asked are summarized in **Table 9.3**. A video clip of a seizure is also a helpful part of the history that can be very useful in differential diagnosis: nowadays, the patient's family can generally make one of these easily with a smartphone. The position of the eyes during the seizure is particularly significant (**Fig. 9.1**). When performing the **physical examination**, the examiner should pay special attention to the following:

— Any physical evidence that a seizure has occurred.

— Any signs of a neurologic or general medical disease that may have caused the seizure (**Table 9.4**).

General diagnostic aspects. If the clinical findings suggest that an epileptic seizure has occurred, a series of **laboratory studies and ancillary tests** should be performed. These are indicated as part of the initial evaluation of every case of suspected epilepsy and mainly serve to detect, or rule out, any possible symptomatic cause of the seizure (**Table 9.5**).

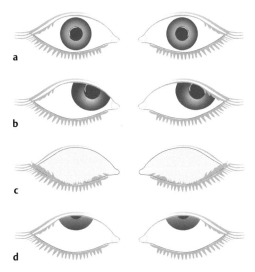

Fig. 9.1   Eye position in seizures and seizure-like disturbances. (a) Temporal lobe seizure, **(b)** extratemporal seizure, **(c)** psychogenic nonepileptic seizure, and **(d)** syncope. (Reproduced from Diener HC, Weimar C, Berlit P, et al. Leitlinien für Diagnostik und Therapie in der Neurologie. Stuttgart: Thieme; 2012.)

Table 9.3	
History	
Questions to be asked after a suspected epileptic seizure	
About the current seizure	— Premonitory signs?
	— Amnesia?
	— Loss of consciousness?
	— Eyes open or closed during the seizure?
	— Manner of waking up (rapidly or slowly)?
	— Postictal fatigue?
	— Injuries?
	— Tongue biting?
	— Urinary or fecal incontinence?
	— Possible provocative factors?
Past history	Family history of epilepsy?
	Past events possibly causing brain damage?
	— Perinatal injury (left handedness, strabismus, psychomotor retardation)?
	— Meningitis, encephalitis?
	— Head trauma?
	Prior episodes of impaired consciousness?
	— Febrile seizure(s) in childhood?
	— Unconsciousness?
	— Bedwetting (possibly due to nocturnal grand mal seizures)?
	— Twilight states? (Ask specifically about partial complex seizures and déjà vu)
	If epileptic seizures have occurred in the past:
	— When was the first one?
	— When was the most recent previous one?
	— Frequency?
	— Characteristics of each seizure?
	— EEG obtained? If so, with what result?
	— Antiepileptic drugs taken, if any: which ones? In what dose? Taken regularly as directed? Adequate effect on seizures? Any side effects?

Abbreviation: EEG, electroencephalogram.

Table 9.4

Physical examination

The physical examination of a patient after a suspected seizure

Evidence that an epileptic seizure has occurred	− Tongue bite − Incontinence of urine or stool − Conjunctival hemorrhage − External injury − Fractures − Shoulder dislocation
Evidence implicating an underlying illness as the cause of the seizure	− Neurologic deficits on physical examination, signs of intracranial hypertension (especially papilledema); these indicate an underlying organic disease of the brain − Abnormal mental status (indicating intoxication or the effect of licit or illicit drugs) − Evidence of general medical illness as the underlying condition (e.g., metabolic or endocrine disease, cardiovascular disease as a cause of a possible prior stroke)

Table 9.5

Laboratory tests and ancillary testing

Laboratory tests and ancillary testing after a suspected epileptic seizure

Evidence that an epileptic seizure has occurred	Laboratory tests	Elevated CK Elevated serum prolactin level (a few minutes after the seizure)
Evidence implicating an underlying illness as the cause of the seizure	EEG	If the routine EEG is normal, EEG with special provocative maneuvers may be indicated (e.g., sleep deprivation, hyperventilation); also long-term EEG, video-EEG, video telemetry
	Brain imaging (to detect or rule out a structural lesion)	− MRI: special MRI protocols may be used depending on the type of seizure − CT: only to detect skull fractures, or if MRI is contraindicated
	Lumbar puncture	If an inflammatory disease of the brain or meninges is suspected
	Further laboratory tests	Routine and specialized tests, depending on clinical suspicion and the questions to be asked in the particular case

Abbreviations: CK, creatine kinase; CT, computed tomography; EEG, electroencephalogram; MRI, magnetic resonance imaging.

General therapeutic aspects. If the diagnosis of epilepsy can be made securely on the basis of the clinical findings and further testing, an appropriate course of therapy must be decided upon. Any underlying cause of symptomatic epilepsy should be treated (**causally directed treatment**); moreover, the predisposition to seizures can be treated **symptomatically** with one or a combination of drugs (**antiepileptic drugs**, AEDs). Not every epileptic seizure implies a need for treatment. In many patients with a first seizure, it may be best to wait and see whether the event will repeat itself, as long as this presents no special danger and the patient agrees. The decision whether to treat with drugs must always be taken on an individual basis, with due consideration of the patient's personality, life situation, occupation, need to drive a car, and so forth.

NOTE

The following situations are generally considered **indications for treating epilepsy with drugs**:
− Two or more unprovoked epileptic seizures.
− One or more unprovoked epileptic seizures in the setting of a known disease of the brain (epileptogenic structural lesion, encephalitis, cerebral hemorrhage, tumor, etc.).
− Epilepsy-typical potentials on EEG.
− Initial status epilepticus.

The general principles of the treatment of epilepsy are as follows:
− Thorough **patient education**.
− **Avoidance of precipitating factors** (regular sleep habits, no excessive alcohol consumption, no illicit drugs, caution with prescription drugs, avoidance of strobe lights).
− Treatment of the **underlying disease**, if any (e.g., resection of a meningioma).
− If pharmacotherapy is indicated: choice of a suitable **drug** for the particular seizure type (**Table 9.6**).
− Gradual **increase of the dose** till seizure control is achieved or intolerable side effects arise. Beware of treatment failure through underdosing: the side effect threshold varies greatly from patient

Table 9.6

Antiepileptic drugs and their indications, by type of epilepsy. The drugs are listed in alphabetic order

	Focal seizures	Generalized seizures				Special epilepsy syndromes of childhood		
	Focal seizures with or without secondary generalization	Primary generalized tonic–clonic seizures	Absences	Myoclonic seizures	West syndrome (salaam spasms)	Lennox–Gastaut syndrome (myoclonic–astatic petit mal)	Rolandic epilepsy (benign epilepsy in childhood and adolescence with central spikes on EEG)
First choice	Carbamazepine	Lamotrigine	Valproate	Lamotrigine	Valproate	Valproate	Carbamazepine
	Lamotrigine	Levetiracetam		Valproate	Vigabatrin		Sultiame
	Levetiracetam	Topiramate					
	Oxcarbazepine	Valproate					
	Topiramate						
	Valproate						
Second choice	Clonazepam	Phenobarbital	Ethosuximide	Clonazepam	ACTH	ACTH	Valproate
	Gabapentin	Primidone	Clonazepam	Ethosuximide	Clonazepam	Carbamazepine	Phenytoin
	Phenobarbital		Lamotrigine	Levetiracetam		Clobazam	
	Phenytoin		Topiramate	Primidone		Felbamate	
	Primidone					Phenytoin	
	Tiagabine						
	Vigabatrin						
Third choice: combinations	Lamotrigine + valproate	Valproate + clonazepam	Valproate + ethosuximide	Valproate + clonazepine	Lamotrigine + levetiracetam	Valproate + lamotrigine	–
	Lamotrigine + levetiracetam	Valproate + topiramate	Lamotrigine + topiramate				

Abbreviations: ACTH, adrenocorticotropic hormone; EEG, electroencephalogram.

to patient and must be crossed, or nearly so, before a drug can be declared ineffective.
- Meticulous **follow-up** for possible side effects, with especially close observation in the initial phase of treatment.
- Checking for **compliance**, for example, with serum levels, if the drug seems to be ineffective.
- If treatment with the first drug tried is truly ineffective despite maximal dosing and adequate compliance, **switch** to another drug of first choice, in gradual and overlapping fashion.
- **Combination therapy** only if monotherapy fails.
- Determination of **serum levels** when:
  - Poor compliance is suspected.
  - Toxic drug effects are suspected.
  - Drug interactions are suspected, particularly those involving enzyme induction.
  - An already high dose is to be raised even further.
  - Medicolegal questions arise, particularly with respect to permission to drive.

- Rules of thumb for the **discontinuation of AEDs**: the patient should be free of seizures for at least 2 years; the EEG should be free of potentials that are typical for epilepsy; traditionally, the drug is slowly tapered to off over several months (although the need for this has not been demonstrated); the patient and family must be explicitly told that seizures may recur during or after the tapering phase.
- If a patient with focal seizures has not become seizure-free with two AEDs, the possibility of **epilepsy surgery** should be considered early.
- In patients with treatment-resistant focal or generalized seizures, the seizure frequency can be reduced with **vagus nerve stimulation**.

Table 9.6 contains an overview of the major AEDs that are currently available and the indications for each. A practical algorithm for the treatment of epilepsy is shown in **Fig. 9.2**.

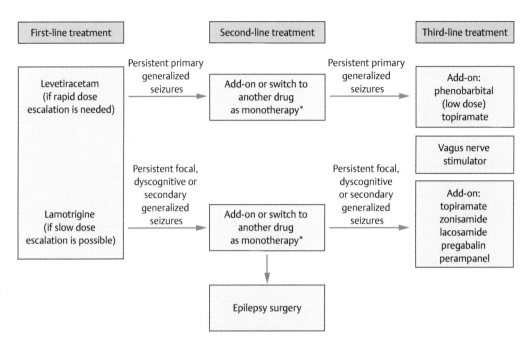

Fig. 9.2   Pragmatic treatment algorithm for adult patients with epilepsy. *Choice of drug as in **Table 9.6**.

Practical Tip
When the patient is a woman of child-bearing age, it is important to note that some AEDs (e.g., valproate) are teratogenic. Women who take AEDs should be informed of the need for concomitant effective contraception. Moreover, note should be taken of the possible interactions of some AEDs with hormonal contraceptive drugs.

9.2 Generalized Seizures

Key Point
Primary generalized seizures occur in both cerebral hemispheres simultaneously; that is, they spread from one hemisphere to the other so rapidly that the extracranially recorded EEG shows extensive bilateral epileptiform activity right from the beginning of the seizure. Focal seizures can also become secondarily generalized (see section 9.3). Generalized seizures are usually accompanied by an obvious impairment of consciousness. There are always changes of muscle tone, and there are often repetitive involuntary movements of both sides of the body (myoclonus or clonus, cf. Table 9.1). Consciousness may be preserved in seizures with generalized myoclonus (i.e., myoclonus in all four limbs at the same time)—for example, in frontal lobe seizures.

The most common clinical types of seizure are described in the following sections.

9.2.1 Tonic–Clonic Seizures (Earlier Term: "Grand Mal Epilepsy")

Pathogenesis and etiology. A generalized seizure may be of **genetic** (idiopathic) origin, or it may be due to a **structural** abnormality (a focal brain lesion; focal seizure with **secondary generalization**) or a **metabolic** disturbance. The cause in the individual case can usually be determined from the history, physical examination, imaging studies, laboratory findings, and EEG, but, in many cases, the cause remains unknown. It is now thought that all seizures are, in fact, of **focal onset**; so-called primary generalized seizures are those that spread from one hemisphere to the other so rapidly that the extracranially recorded EEG shows extensive bilateral epileptiform activity right from the beginning of the seizure.

Practical Tip
Despite the foregoing, the distinction between primary and secondary generalized seizures is clinically important, because some medications that are highly effective against secondary generalized seizures can make primary generalized seizures worse (e.g., phenytoin or gabapentin).

Clinical features. Epilepsy with generalized seizures is a visually impressive disturbance, statistically common and generally familiar to lay people. The

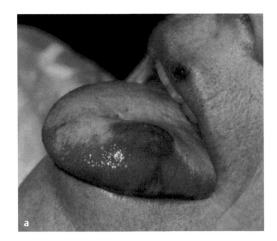

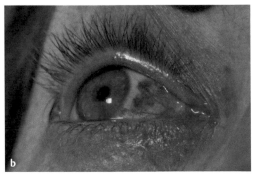

Fig. 9.3   Clinical signs in the aftermath of a generalized tonic–clonic seizure. (a) Tongue bite. **(b)** Subscleral hemorrhage.

seizures are often introduced by **auras** (see section 9.1) and by an **initial shout**; these are followed by **loss of consciousness** and, often, a **fall**. Simultaneously, there is **tonic spasm** of the skeletal muscles: the limbs are extended, the trunk and head overextended. The eyes are typically open, staring rigidly into the distance. After 10 to 20 seconds, **rhythmic, clonic, generalized twitching** appears in all of the patient's muscles. This is accompanied by cyanosis of the face, frothing at the mouth, and, possibly, tongue biting and involuntary loss of urine or stool. The twitching lasts about 1 minute (typically seeming longer to bystanders) and is followed by a phase of, at first, deep **unconsciousness**. There is then a transition over a few minutes to confusion and somnolence (the **postictal twilight state**) and, finally, normal consciousness is regained. In the postictal phase after a generalized epileptic seizure, there can also be marked cardiovascular depression, leading in some cases to total cardiovascular arrest.

The patient may remember an aura but is otherwise totally amnestic for the time of the seizure. After the seizure, the patient is tired and may complain of muscle pain. A lateral tongue bite and subscleral hemorrhages are sometimes seen (**Fig. 9.3**); further accompaniments of generalized seizures include urinary and fecal incontinence and fall-related injuries such as shoulder dislocation and spinal or other fractures.

Diagnostic evaluation. The **EEG** (even if recorded interictally, i.e., in the interval between seizures) may show the typical picture of synchronous generalized **spikes and waves** in all leads (**Fig. 9.4**).

Treatment. The drugs of first choice for generalized seizures are **lamotrigine**, **levetiracetam**, **topiramate**, and **valproate** (**Table 9.6**).

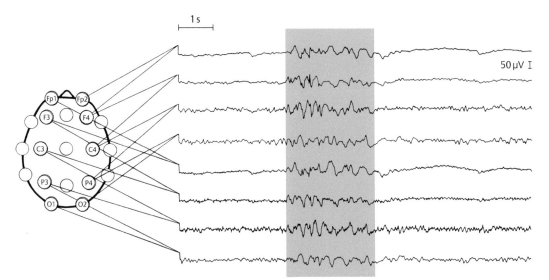

Fig. 9.4   Interictal EEG in a patient with primary generalized seizures. There is a sudden, simultaneous eruption of paroxysmal, generalized, partly atypical spikes and waves in all leads.

9.2.2 Absences (Earlier Term: "Petit Mal Epilepsy")

This term designates primary generalized seizures that involve a brief, transient impairment of consciousness without loss of consciousness. They are usually seen in children and adolescents.

Etiology. Absences, like many other kinds of childhood epilepsy, are of **genetic** origin.

Clinical features. Motor phenomena are not always seen; if present, they are only mild (blinking, automatisms, loss of muscle tone, brief clonus). In the simplest type of absence epilepsy, **petit mal epilepsy of school-aged children**, the seizures often seem to be no more than brief periods of **daydreaming**: the child stares fixedly with eyes turned upward, blinks, and may make movements of the tongue or mouth, or pick at his or her clothes. These types of movements are called petit mal automatisms. The entire event lasts no more than a few seconds. Absences usually occur multiple times per day. The examining physician may be able to provoke an absence by having the patient hyperventilate.

Diagnostic evaluation. The **EEG** reveals a pathognomonic pattern of bursts of synchronous, generalized spike-and-wave activity at a frequency of approximately 3 Hz. These can be provoked by **hyperventilation** (Fig. 9.5).

Treatment. The medications of first choice for the treatment of absences are **valproate** and **lamotrigine**. **Ethosuximide** is now considered a drug of **second choice**.

Prognosis. About one in four affected children becomes free of seizures during puberty; in the remainder, seizures persist. One-half of these patients with persistent absence seizures will go on to develop grand mal seizures as well.

9.2.3 Atypical Absences and Other Types of Epilepsy in Childhood

The other types of childhood epilepsy are summarized in **Table 9.7**.

9.3 Focal (Partial) Seizures

Key Point

Focal seizures are always due to a circumscribed lesion in the brain, which may or may not be detectable in imaging studies. The specific manifestations of the seizure correspond to the site of the lesion. Unlike primary generalized seizures, which always involve an impairment of consciousness, focal seizures may occur with the patient remaining fully conscious (earlier term, "simple partial seizures"). They can, however, involve an impairment of consciousness (earlier term, "complex partial seizures;" current term, "dyscognitive seizures"). The uncoordinated neural activity arising in the epileptic focus may spread to wider areas of the brain and thereby induce a secondarily generalized tonic–clonic seizure. In such patients, the initial focal phase may be very brief and is not always clinically recognizable.

Fig. 9.6 schematically represents the clinical manifestations that can be expected in focal seizures arising from various brain areas. The major types of focal seizure will be described in detail in the remainder of this section.

9.3.1 Focal Seizures without Altered Consciousness

Focal seizures without any alteration of consciousness (= simple partial seizures) can be purely motor, mixed sensory and motor, or purely sensory (either

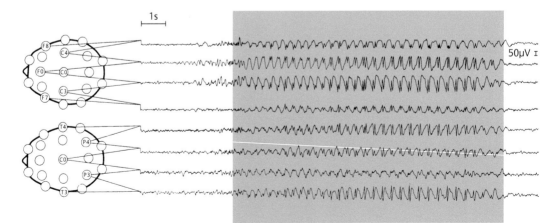
Fig. 9.5 EEG in a patient with absence seizures, showing generalized spikes and waves at 3–4 Hz induced by hyperventilation.

Table 9.7

Types of epilepsy mainly or exclusively affecting children

Designation	Age group	Features	Remarks
West syndrome (propulsive petit mal, infantile spasms, salaam spasms)	First year of life	Rocking and nodding movements, twitching of the trunk, forward thrusting of the arms	Often seen in brain-damaged, retarded children. Typical EEG finding: hypsarrhythmia (irregular high delta waves with interspersed desynchronized short-lasting spikes)
Febrile seizures	0–5 y	Generalized seizures during episodes of fever	Later development of true epilepsy is not uncommon
Myoclonic–astatic petit mal (Lennox–Gastaut syndrome)	0–8 y	Variable loss of muscle tone (ranging from nodding to collapse and falling), very brief unconsciousness	More common in boys; often associated with tonic seizures
Typical absences	1–13 y	Very brief period of unconsciousness, rare falls, occasional minor motor phenomena (picking at clothes), vacant stare; many times a day, can be precipitated by hyperventilation	Sometimes found in association with grand mal seizures (mixed epilepsy); EEG typically shows a 3-Hz spike-and-wave pattern (**Fig. 9.5**)
Myoclonic seizures (impulsive petit mal)	Second decade and onward into adulthood	Irregular rocking twitches, more frequent on awakening, no loss of consciousness	Later often combined with grand mal seizures
Benign focal epilepsy of childhood and adolescence	First and second decades	Focal twitching, usually during sleep; the patient is conscious during seizures that occur when he/she is awake; one-third also have generalized seizures	Multiple subtypes; typical EEG pattern with biphasic centro-temporal spikes; good prognosis for spontaneous recovery

Abbreviation: EEG, electroencephalogram.

somatosensory or special sensory). Consciousness is impaired only if the seizure undergoes secondary generalization.

There are various types of focal seizure without altered consciousness:

- There may be **focal motor twitching** on one side of the body, or sensory disturbances that suddenly arise in a circumscribed area of the body. Focal twitching confined to a very small area (e.g., a hand) and lasting for a very long time (hours or more) is called **epilepsia partialis continua** (of Kozhevnikov).
- In a **jacksonian seizure**, the motor (or sensory) phenomena rapidly spread over the entire ipsilateral half of the body ("**jacksonian march**").
- If the seizure focus lies in the precentral region or the supplementary motor area, the seizure will be of **adversive** type: the patient's head and eyes turn tonically to the opposite side, while the contralateral arm is abducted and elevated.
- If the seizure focus lies in the visual or auditory cortex or the neighboring association areas, the seizure may consist of, or begin with, auditory or visual sensations, or even scenic images.

Diagnostic evaluation. The focal nature of the seizure, or its focal origin (in the case of secondarily generalized seizures), is demonstrated not only by its clinical features, but also by the **EEG**, which reveals localized epileptic activity over the seizure focus (**Fig. 9.7**).

Treatment. The drugs of first choice for focal seizures are **lamotrigine** and **levetiracetam**. The latter is preferred if **rapid dose escalation** is needed.

9.3.2 Focal Seizures with Altered Consciousness (Earlier Term, "Complex Partial Seizures;" Current Term, "Dyscognitive Seizures")

This type of seizure is typically (but not exclusively) seen in **temporal lobe epilepsy**. As these seizures involve altered consciousness and, often, motor automatisms, they were also called "psychomotor seizures" in the earlier literature.

Etiology. The most common cause of focal seizures with altered consciousness is a **perinatal lesion** of anoxic or inflammatory origin (mesial temporal sclerosis or hippocampal sclerosis). Other causes include **congenital developmental anomalies** (e.g., cavernomas and neuroblast migration disorders).

Clinical features. Focal dyscognitive seizures have **sensory, behavioral**, and **autonomic manifestations**, accompanied by **altered attention** or **impaired consciousness**. These manifestations are described in **Table 9.8**.

Which of these manifestations will be present in the individual patient depends on the precise location of the epileptic focus and the pattern of spread of seizure activity. Patients whose seizure focus lies in the uncinate gyrus also have **olfactory and gustatory hallucinations**, or, as they are called, **uncinate fits**. These are often caused by a mass in the temporal lobe.

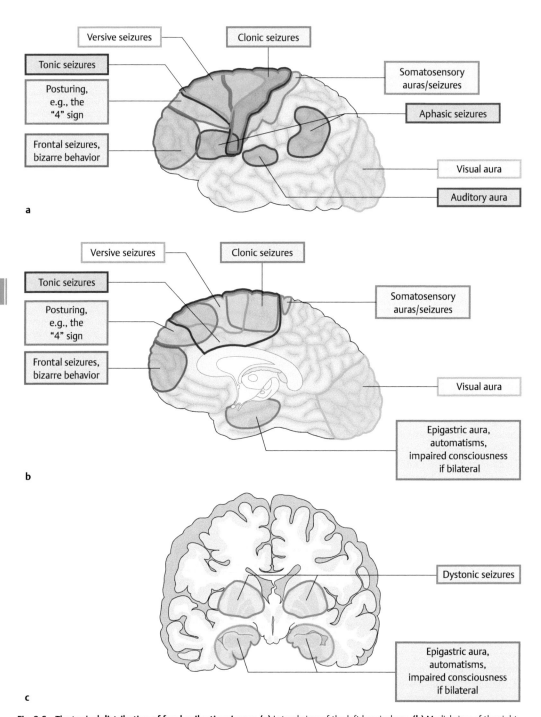

Fig. 9.6   The topical distribution of focal epileptic seizures. (a) Lateral view of the left hemisphere. **(b)** Medial view of the right hemisphere. **(c)** Coronal section through both hemispheres.

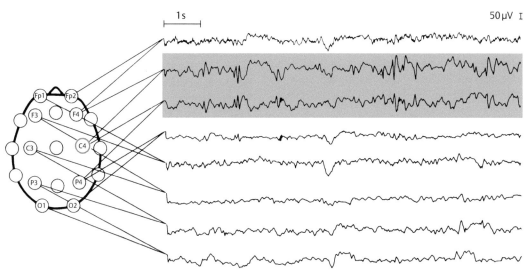

Fig. 9.7   EEG during a focal epileptic seizure. Epileptiform signals are seen in the central leads on the right, with spikes and sharp and slow waves. Phase reversal (= location of maximal surface negativity) at lead C4.

Table 9.8

Clinical features of focal seizures with or without impairment of consciousness and/or altered attention

Category	Clinical features	Remarks
Sensory disturbances	Dizziness, somatosensory phenomena (numbness, tingling), visual phenomena (lightning, bright dots or shapes, metamorphopsia,[a] auditory phenomena (noises, tones, voices), gustatory sensations, unpleasant olfactory sensations	Uncinate fits (= predominantly olfactory or gustatory sensations)
Autonomic disturbances	Dilated pupil (mydriasis), shortness of breath, palpitations, diaphoresis, blushing, goosebumps, nausea, salivation, dry mouth, hunger, urge to urinate, abdominal sensations	Often, ascending sensation from stomach to throat (the patient typically demonstrates this to the doctor with an upward hand movement)
Behavioral and psycho-motor manifestations	Traumatic experience, feeling of unreality or alienation, obsessive thoughts, déjà vu (factually incorrect feeling of having experienced present experiences before) and jamais vu (the opposite incorrect feeling of never having experienced present experiences before), affective disturbances (unfounded anxiety or rage), structured hallucinations, altered perception of time	-
Twilight states	Automatic, semiorganized, but inappropriate behavior, e.g., picking at clothes, senseless moving around of objects, etc. (twilight attacks); long-lasting, semiorganized complex behaviors that may even involve travel over a long distance (twilight state, fugue épileptique)	Amnesia for these states
Temporal syncope	Collapse, usually immediately following one of the above phenomena, typically with only brief unconsciousness	No sudden falling
Psychomotor status epilepticus	Very long persistence of the above phenomena, or repeated occurrence with incomplete recovery in between	Rare

[a]Metamorphopsia is a distorted visual perception of the environment; types include micropsia (things seem small), macropsia (things seem large), dysmorphopsia (things seem to be out of shape), and teleopsia (things seem far away).

Illustrative Case

A patient suddenly experiences a peculiar feeling of **distance** from his surroundings. Everything seems to be far away, unreal, like a dream. At the same time, he notices a strange **sensation in the pit of his stomach, ascending into his throat.** He sometimes has palpitations or shortness of breath as well. Often, he experiences **anxiety**, which can be vague or very intense. On some occasions, his **consciousness** is more severely **affected**: he stares blankly ahead, makes chewing and swallowing movements, produces gagging noises, and fails to answer questions. He picks at his clothes, makes **purposeless hand movements**, and sometimes **falls over**. The entire episode usually lasts 1 or a few minutes, but is sometimes longer.

Diagnostic evaluation. This type of seizure can generally be diagnosed from its typical clinical picture. The **EEG** reveals temporal slow waves or spikes. In the interictal period, however, it is usually normal.
Treatment. The drugs of first choice for focal seizures with altered consciousness are **carbamazepine**, **oxcarbazepine**, **lamotrigine**, **levetiracetam**, **topiramate**, and **valproate**.

9.4 Status Epilepticus

Key Point
The term "status epilepticus" refers to a prolonged, uninterrupted epileptic seizure or to multiple seizures occurring in rapid succession without full recovery in between. Generalized status epilepticus, in which the patient does not regain consciousness between seizures, is a life-threatening emergency because of the danger of respiratory complications (aspiration) and ensuing hypoxic brain damage.

The current definition of status epilepticus is as follows:
— A generalized tonic–clonic seizure lasting at least **5 minutes**, or
— A focal seizure or absence lasting at least **20 to 30 minutes**.
In **absence status**, the patient is not unconscious, but rather confused or mildly dazed, with inappropriate behavior. The EEG is diagnostic.
Hypoglycemia can present clinically as status epilepticus.
Focal status epilepticus with altered consciousness and attention, **that is, dyscognitive (complex partial) status epilepticus**, can be mistaken for an acute psychotic episode.
Treatment. Grand mal status epilepticus with secondarily generalized seizures should be treated initially

with thiamine and glucose IV, followed by a bolus dose of a **benzodiazepine** (e.g., lorazepam, clonazepam, or diazepam IV) and then intravenous **phenytoin, valproate, or levetiracetam**. If the seizure activity does not stop within 30 minutes, the patient must be **intubated and ventilated** and put in artificial coma with a barbiturate such as **thiopental** or **propofol** (**Table 9.9**). Petit mal status epilepticus and psychomotor status epilepticus respond to **clonazepam** 2 to 4 mg IV.

9.5 Episodic Neurologic Disturbances of Nonepileptic Origin

Key Point
Because the clinical presentations of epileptic seizures are so highly varied, their differential diagnosis necessarily includes a wide variety of conditions. Any episodic loss of consciousness, impairment of motor function, or fall might be due either to an epileptic seizure or to a nonepileptic event of another etiology, as will be discussed in this section.

Episodic neurologic disturbances of nonepileptic origin can be classified into the following major categories:
— Nonepileptic psychogenic seizures.
— Episodic disturbances with brief impairment of consciousness and falling.
— Episodic falling without impairment of consciousness.
— Episodic impairment of consciousness without falling.
— Episodic movement disorders.
— Episodic impairment of memory and confusion.

9.5.1 Nonepileptic Psychogenic Seizures
Ten to twenty percent of adults evaluated for refractory seizures have **dissociative disorders** or (to use an alternative term) **pseudoseizures**. Their episodes are of a demonstrative, appellative character and usually occur when there is someone present to observe them. The phenomenology of psychogenic seizures differs markedly from that of the usual types of epileptic seizure.

NOTE

Unlike true epileptic seizures, nonepileptic psychogenic seizures are not stereotypic. Their symptoms and signs do not occur in a characteristic sequence, but rather **without any clear pattern**. The **spasms** are alternating and **asymmetric**, the patient's **mouth** usually stays **open**, and the **eyes** are **closed** (**Fig. 9.1**); the patient resists passive opening of the eyelids.

The patient's movements tend to be tremor-like ("sinusoidal"), instead of possessing a rapid phase

Table 9.9

Treatment algorithm for generalized status epilepticus

Treatment step	Drug/treatment measure	Dose, administration, remarks
Step 1	Thiamine	100 mg IV
	Glucose	40% 60 mL IV
Step 2	Initial treatment with a benzodiazepine:	
	Lorazepam (Tavor)	2–4 mg IV
	Diazepam (Valium)	10–20 mg IV
	Clonazepam (Rivotril)	1–2 mg IV
Step 3	If seizure activity persists, repeat benzodiazepine injection in 3–5 min	
Step 4	Phenytoin (Epanutin, Phenhydan)	750 mg over 15–30 min as a rapid infusion Then 250–750 mg as an infusion over the next 24 h Then maintenance therapy with 300–400 mg/d
	Valproate	900 mg over 30 min as a rapid infusion Then 1,500 mg as an infusion over the next 12 h Then maintenance therapy with 1,200–1,500 mg/d
	Levetiracetam (Keppra)	1,500–3,000 mg as a rapid infusion
Step 5	If seizure activity persists 30 min after the administration of phenytoin or valproate:	
	Intubation and ventilation	(If not already performed)
	Thiopental (Trapanal)[a]	100–200 mg IV Then 50 mg IV bolus with EEG monitoring until a burst-suppression pattern[b] appears Then 3–5 mg/kg body weight/h (ca. 300 mg/h) for at least 12 h Attempt to lower the dose after 12 h or longer
	Propofol (Disoprivan)[a]	1–2 mg/kg body weight as an IV bolus then 2–10 mg/kg body weight/h

Abbreviation: EEG, electroencephalogram.
[a]During treatment with thiopental or propofol, phenytoin, valproate, or levetiracetam should continue to be given.
[b]Burst-suppression pattern: The EEG shows high-amplitude waves in between flat segments of the tracing.

and a slow phase. Proximal muscle groups are activated that do not have a large cortical representation. **The EEG is normal.** Nonepileptic psychogenic seizures are an expression of mental illness with subjective suffering but without any organic correlate. The affected patients need behaviorally oriented **psychotherapy**.

9.5.2 Episodic Disturbances with Brief Impairment of Consciousness and Falling

A concise overview of such disturbances, including, for completeness, types of epilepsy that involve impaired consciousness, is provided in **Table 9.10**. The main diseases listed are described in the following sections in greater detail.

Syncope

Syncope is defined as a very brief loss of consciousness during which the affected person falls to the ground. It is due to a very brief loss of function of the brainstem reticular formation, which, in turn, is usually caused by temporary ischemia and tissue hypoxia. Syncope can be associated with motor phenomena, but these are generally less pronounced and of shorter duration than those seen in

epilepsy. The eyelids are closed or half-closed, and the eyes are directed upward (**Fig. 9.1**). Syncope can be of orthostatic, vasomotor, or cardiogenic origin.

Orthostatic Syncope

Orthostatic syncope occurs when the patient stands up from the lying or sitting position. Venous blood pools in the lower half of the body, and the blood pressure falls (hypotension). Normally, the autonomic nervous system counteracts the drop in blood pressure. When circulatory regulation is defective, however, hypoperfusion of the brain may arise and lead to syncope. The etiologic subtypes of orthostatic syncope include **idiopathic vasomotor collapse of adolescence**, orthostatic hypotension due to **inadequate sinus tachycardia**, and the **postural orthostatic tachycardia syndrome**. Moreover, orthostatic syncope is an accompaniment of many **neurologic** and **general medical conditions**, including multisystem atrophy, autonomic polyneuropathy, hypovolemia, and sodium deficiency.

Reflex Circulatory Syncope

This is the commonest kind of syncope, also called vasovagal or neurocardiogenic syncope. It is caused

Table 9.10

Clinical features of various conditions causing brief loss of consciousness and falls

	"Falling sicknesses"	Found in:	Precipitating factors	Prodromal phenomena
Syncopal	*Orthostatic hypotension (vasomotor collapse)*			
	– Chronic sympathetic defect	– Multisystem atrophy – Tabes dorsalis	– Prolonged standing – Rapidly standing up from a lying position	– Yawning – Tinnitus – Seeing black – Feeling of heat – Epigastric pressure
	– Drugs	– β-blockers, diuretics, antihypertensive drugs – L-dopa		
	– Adolescents – POTS	– May be due to anemia – Poor general condition – Sympathetic dysregulation		
	Reflex circulatory syncope (vagal inhibition)			
	– Vasovagal syncope	– Hyperventilation – Heat, fright, etc.	– Intense emotion – Pain	– Like orthostatic hypotension (see above)
	– Swallowing syncope	– Glossopharyngeal neuralgia	– Paroxysms – Cold drinks, chewing	
	– Carotid sinus syndrome	– Elderly men	– Pressure on carotid sinus	
	– Micturition syncope	– Men – Alcohol consumption	– Urinating while standing	
	– Extension syncope/squatting	– Children – May be deliberate	– Hyperextension – Squatting and pressing	
	Pressor syncope (inadequate venous return)			
	– Coughing/laughing syncope	– Persons with emphysema	– Coughing fit or laughing fit (Valsalva maneuver)	–
	Primary cardiovascular syncope			
	– Cerebrovascular syncope	– Subclavian steal syndrome	– Physical exertion (arm)	– Fright/anxiety – Usually without warning
	– Cardiac syncope	– Congenital malformations of the heart – Heart failure – Arrhythmia[a] (Stokes–Adams attack)	– Possibly precipitated by emotion – Independent of position	
	Respiratory affect seizure			
	– Cyanotic affect seizure	– Infants	– Anger/spite	–
	– "White" affect seizure	– School-aged children	– Fright – Pain	
Falling attacks	True reflex "vestibular" syncope or falling (Tumarkin syndrome)	– Ménière disease – Paroxysmal positioning vertigo	– Bending the head forward – Craning the neck – Lying down	– Vertigo – Nausea (sometimes)
	Intermittent vertebro-basilar ischemia	– Elderly patients – Vascular risk factors – Stenosis and occlusion of the vertebral and basilar arteries	– Head turning (sometimes)	– Nausea/dizziness – Visual disturbances, etc.
	Cryptogenic falling attacks in women	– Middle-aged women	– Only while walking	– No prodromal phenomena
	Cataplectic falling	– Isolated – In a patient with narcolepsy	– Intense emotion – Laughing – Fright	– Without warning
Epilepsy	"Temporal lobe syncope"	– Psychomotor epilepsy	– Intense emotion (sometimes)	– Psychomotor aura possible
	Generalized seizure	– Possibly several times per day – Any age	– Sleep deprivation – Alcohol	– Psychomotor aura (sometimes)
	Drop attacks (myoclonic–astatic)	– Lennox–Gastaut syndrome (children)	–	–
Acute confusion	– TGA – Other acute amnesias	– Older persons – Temporal or frontal epilepsy – Traumatic brain injury – Licit or illicit drugs	–	–

Table 9.10

Clinical features of various conditions causing brief loss of consciousness and falls (continued)

	"Falling sicknesses"	Found in:	Precipitating factors	Prodromal phenomena
Psycho-genic	— Hysterical falling (with pseudoimpairment of consciousness)	— Neurotic disorders — psychological gain	— Other persons present	–
	— Factitious seizures	— May occur in patients who also have true epileptic seizures — "Compensation neurosis"		

Abbreviations: POTS, postural orthostatic tachycardia syndrome; TGA, transient global amnesia.
[a]Bradyarrhythmias (e.g., third-degree atrioventricular block), tachyarrhythmias, special type: sick sinus syndrome (sinus node syndrome).

by **reflex vasodilatation and bradycardia** and can be precipitated by intense emotion (e.g., the sight of blood, anticipatory anxiety), heat, prolonged standing, or physical pain.

NOTE

Reflex circulatory syncope is typically preceded by certain **prodromal symptoms**: the affected person becomes dizzy, sees black, turns pale, breaks out in a sweat, and then collapses to the ground.

Most patients regain wakefulness and **full orientation** at once.

The subtypes of reflex circulatory syncope include **micturition syncope**, **swallowing syncope**, and **extension syncope** (mainly seen in younger patients who stand up too quickly from a squatting position). **Carotid sinus syncope** is rarer than once thought.

Pressor Syncope

Pressor syncope, precipitated (for example) by prolonged **coughing or laughing**, is due to **elevated intrathoracic pressure** that is transmitted by way of the spinal venous system to the intraspinal and intracranial compartments, raising the intracranial pressure. If the intracranial pressure exceeds the arterial pressure, the **cerebral circulation** comes to a **standstill**; if this situation persists for a few seconds, the patient loses consciousness, collapses, goes limp, and thereby ceases to cough or laugh. The circulation then rapidly recovers, and consciousness is regained.

Cardiogenic Syncope

Syncope of cardiac origin is especially common in older patients. Its causes include **cardiac arrhythmias** (third-degree atrioventricular block, sick sinus syndrome, tachycardias) and other types of **heart disease** (e.g., valvular aortic stenosis, atrial myxoma, and chronic pulmonary hypertension with cor pulmonale). **Pulmonary embolism** can also cause syncope.

"Convulsive Syncope"

Prolonged syncopal episodes are sometimes accompanied by brief, clonic muscle twitching. This may make a syncopal episode even harder to distinguish from an epileptic seizure.

9.5.3 Episodic Falling without Impairment of Consciousness

In a so-called **drop attack**, the patient suddenly falls to the ground without braking the fall. Consciousness is apparently preserved during the event; in some patients, however, the patient may, in fact, lose consciousness without realizing it afterward, and too briefly for others to observe. Some drop attacks are due to **atonic epilepsy**, others to **basilar ischemia**. **Cryptogenic drop attacks** have been described in older women ("climacteric drop syncope"). Drop attacks can also be caused by basilar impression and other structural abnormalities of the craniocervical junction. Acute labyrinthic disturbances can also cause **falls of vestibular origin**, for example, in acute paroxysmal positioning vertigo and Ménière disease.

9.5.4 Episodic Impairment of Consciousness without Falling

Certain **metabolic disturbances** (e.g., hypoglycemia) and **electrolyte disturbances** (especially hyponatremia), as well as **endocrine diseases** (hypothyroidism, hypoparathyroidism), can episodically impair consciousness. Loss of consciousness can also be the main manifestation of **tetany**, for example, in hyperventilation. Further clinical features include a positive Chvostek sign, digital and perioral paresthesiae, and tonic muscle contraction (claw hand).

9.5.5 Episodic Movement Disorders without Impairment of Consciousness

The following types of abnormal movement must be distinguished from focal motor epilepsy:
— **Focal repetitive twitching**: this can be seen in, for example, hemifacial spasm, in which all of the muscles innervated by the facial nerve contract synchronously at irregular intervals. Tics and blepharospasm are usually unilateral. Palatal nystagmus is due to a lesion of the inferior olive or the central tegmental tract. Myoclonus and myorhythmia are usually of inconstant localization.

9

— **Episodic generalized motor dysfunction**: this can be seen in, for example, the (usually familial) episodic ataxias, paroxysmal choreoathetoses and dyskinesias, hyperekplexia ("startle disease"), and the so-called tonic brain stem seizures seen in multiple sclerosis (see section 8.2).

9.5.6 Episodic Impairment of Memory and Confusion

Any impairment of immediate and recent memory causes confusion: the patient's behavior and reactions become inappropriate, and he or she can no longer act logically and correctly.

Transient global amnesia (TGA) usually affects elderly persons. For a period of several hours, they cannot store new memories; they ask the same questions over and over, but still have normal motor function and reactions. TGA leaves an amnestic gap behind. It is due to a transient, bilateral dysfunction of the hippocampus or the limbic system whose cause is currently unknown.

Acute confusional episodes can also be caused by temporal or frontal **epileptic seizures**, mesiotemporal **ischemia**, the use of **prescription drugs** (e.g., benzodiazepines) or illicit drugs, and **traumatic brain injury**.

9

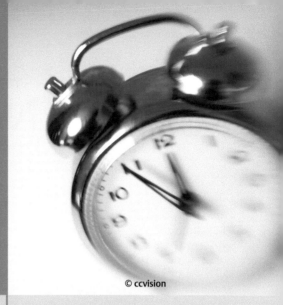
© ccvision

Chapter 10

Sleep and Its Abnormalities

Restful? Not Quite

The patient, a 50-year-old chef and restaurateur, proprietor of a popular establishment amid the old-town arcades of the Swiss capital, often worked from early in the morning till late at night. His heavy workload and the constant temptations around him had led to steadily increasing alcohol consumption over the last few years. Though already obese, he had put on a good deal more weight. His employees respected him and liked him for his jovial, enthusiastic manner, but they noticed that he had become irritable and impatient in recent months. He had also become slower and less concentrated in his work; ever more frequently, a meal emerged burnt from the oven or a soup was spoiled with too much salt. One afternoon, the staff even caught him taking a nap on a chair in the kitchen. This began to happen with increasing regularity.

The patient himself was very worried and consulted his family physician, telling him about the embarrassing happenings in the restaurant. Asked about his sleep habits, he said he had often, in recent months, woken up from sleep with a start and found himself covered in sweat. He had the feeling of having woken up from a nightmare but could not remember dreaming. He was now getting up with a headache and a dry mouth every morning, and he felt exhausted all day long.

Sleep can be disturbed in many different ways. Difficulty falling asleep and difficulty staying asleep are very common; abnormal behavior during sleep and daytime somnolence can occur as well. Thorough history-taking with specific questioning, not just of the patient, but also of his or her bedmate and other family members, often brings the underlying cause to light. Sometimes, however, the diagnosis can only be established by further evaluation, including polysomnography (PSG; a "sleep study"), nocturnal oximetry, and video observation of the sleeping patient with an infrared camera.

He was obviously suffering from a marked sleep disturbance with excessive daytime somnolence. The family physician called his wife in to ask her a few questions and clarify the situation. She said her husband had always been a snorer, but his snoring had gotten louder over the past 2 years or so. Lately, he had often temporarily stopped breathing during sleep; this worried her very much. The pauses in breathing usually lasted several seconds and were then followed by a deep sigh, as if he were gasping for air. On a few occasions, he had stopped breathing for such a long time that she panicked and shook him awake, because she was afraid he might die.

This patient's symptoms and the clear history given by his wife led to the diagnosis of sleep apnea syndrome. Nocturnal oximetry revealed as many as 25 desaturations per hour, sometimes to values below 80%. The doctor urgently advised him to lose weight and to give up alcohol entirely, because overweight and alcohol both contribute to the pathogenesis of the syndrome. He also told him to avoid sleeping on his back. Because of daytime somnolence in particular, the patient was given a biphasic positive airway pressure (BIPAP) device. He tolerated it poorly at first, but his symptoms then improved so much that he became a devoted user. After the first night of successful BIPAP therapy, he was no longer sleepy during the day. He lost 8 kg of weight over the next 3 months.

Photo: Kirsten Oborny/Thieme Verlagsgruppe

Key Point
The individual sleep requirement is genetically determined: it varies from 4 to 11 hours per night, with an average of 7 to 8 hours. The body's "internal clock" has an intrinsic "day" lasting somewhat longer than 24 hours and needs to be continually reset by external stimuli to keep pace with the environmental day/night cycle. This sensitive process can be impaired by various exogenous factors and diseases. The resulting disturbances are best classified by their main clinical features: disturbances of sleep duration and the sleep–wake rhythm, insomnia, hypersomnia, excessive daytime somnolence, and special abnormal phenomena occurring during sleep (parasomnias).

10.1 Shortened Sleep Duration and Abnormal Sleep–Wake Rhythm

> **NOTE**
>
> The patient sleeps **too little**, falls asleep **too late**, or wakes up **too early**. Often, the problem is an organic or psychological disturbance affecting the ability to fall asleep and/or stay asleep, or an abnormal setting of the internal clock.

If the patient sleeps **too little at night**, the most common cause is simply that the patient's social environment prevents adequate sleep. Pathologic causes include somatic conditions (e.g., pain), internal medical illnesses, psychosocial problems or conflicts, and endogenous depression. These usually lead to difficulty falling asleep, staying asleep, or both.

If the patient falls asleep much **too late** and tends to sleep for a long time in the morning, the internal clock is incorrectly set. This is called the **delayed sleep phase syndrome** and is most common among adolescents.

10.2 Insomnia

 Key Point
Insomnia is now defined as a condition in which the patient finds that he or she does not get enough sleep and that the normal restorative benefit of sleep is lacking. Insomnia can occur as a primary disorder or as a consequence of many different environmental situations and physical and mental illnesses. Patients with restless legs syndrome (RLS) complain of abnormal sensations in the limbs and an abnormal urge to move them, often in combination with difficulty falling asleep.

10.2.1 General Principles

Insomnia can be divided into **difficulty falling asleep**, **difficulty staying asleep** (often called "sleep continuity disturbance" in the specialized literature), and **early morning awakening**. Sleep can also be **subjectively inadequate**, even if its quality and duration seem adequate when objectively assessed. Insufficient nighttime sleep can lead to daytime somnolence, exhaustion, and depression. The evaluation of insomnia should include a search for contributory extrinsic factors (noise, shift work, jet lag, etc.), physical and mental illnesses, and substances that can impair sleep, such as alcohol, caffeine, steroids, and stimulant drugs (both licit and illicit).

Treatment. If an underlying disease is found, the treatment of insomnia begins with the treatment of the disease. **Behavior changes**, such as proper sleep hygiene, the elimination of exogenous disturbances, getting to bed on time, and the use of relaxation techniques, are a further major component of treatment. **Sedatives** can be used as well; the choice of drug depends on the underlying problem. Benzodiazepines should be used only to treat acute insomnia, and for no more than a few weeks' time, for example, for a student who cannot sleep because of impending examinations.

10.2.2 Restless Legs Syndrome

About 20% of patients with insomnia suffer from RLS. They complain mainly of **difficulty falling asleep**.

> **NOTE**
>
> Patients with RLS suffer from a distressing **urge to move the legs** that is worst toward the evening when they sit in a relaxed position or lie in bed and that improves with mental or physical activity. Most patients actually do move their legs whenever they sit or lie down. To gain relief, they sometimes need to get up and walk around.

Epidemiology. The prevalence of RLS increases with age; it is 5 to 10% overall. Women are twice as commonly affected as men.

Etiology and pathogenesis. **Primary** RLS is usually **idiopathic**; in other words no specific cause can be found. One-third of patients, particularly those who develop the syndrome when young, have this disorder as a familial condition with autosomal dominant inheritance. Mutations are found at various genetic loci.

Secondary RLS can be due to iron deficiency, renal insufficiency, hypothyroidism, spinal cord lesions, polyneuropathy, pregnancy, or drugs (licit and illicit) such as neuroleptic drugs, antiemetic drugs (exception: domperidone), tricyclic antidepressants, selective serotonin reuptake inhibitors, and ecstasy.

10

10

The pathogenesis of RLS is not fully clear. The dopaminergic and endogenous opioid systems and the body's iron metabolism all appear to be involved.

Definition, clinical features, and diagnostic evaluation. RLS is defined by the following criteria:

- Urge to move the limbs and abnormal sensations (such as burning or tingling) in the limbs; symptoms mainly but not exclusively in the lower limbs.
- Worsening of symptoms at rest (lying down, sitting).
- Improvement of symptoms with mental or motor activity (concentration, walking around).
- Worst symptoms in the evening or at night.

Confirmatory criteria include a positive family history, periodic leg movements in the night (particularly in the superficial stages of sleep), and response to treatment with dopaminergic drugs. RLS may cause daytime fatigue and irritability because of the lack of sleep. The neurologic examination is normal in patients with idiopathic RLS.

The diagnosis is usually made **on clinical grounds alone**. **L-dopa** can be given to test responsiveness to dopaminergic treatment. The additional diagnostic evaluation, serving mainly to exclude the possible causes of RLS, includes the following:

- **Laboratory testing**, for example, to exclude iron deficiency, renal insufficiency, or hypothyroidism.
- **Electromyography and electroneurography** to detect or rule out polyneuropathy.
- **PSG**, for example, in children with pronounced RLS, or if respiratory problems during sleep are suspected.

The **differential diagnosis** includes polyneuropathy, hypnagogic myoclonus, akathisia, and the so-called painful legs and moving toes syndrome.

Treatment. The treatment usually consists of **non-pharmacologic** measures, for example, mental activity (distraction), light exercise, abstinence from coffee and alcohol, and sleep hygiene. If RLS is secondary to another disorder, the **underlying disease** should be treated, for example, with iron supplementation or the discontinuation of the drugs that are causing the problem. Only one-third of patients need drugs to treat the syndrome; the agents of choice are **dopamine agonists** such as ropinirole, pramipexole, and rotigotine, initially in combination with domperidone to prevent nausea (if necessary). Sometimes these treatments worsen the condition instead of improving it ("symptom augmentation"). In such cases, an **anticonvulsant** such as gabapentin or pregabalin or an **opioid** such as codeine or tramadol can be given. **L-dopa, with or without** a decarboxylase inhibitor, leads to symptom augmentation more commonly than the dopamine agonists do and is thus only rarely given to treat RLS.

10.3 Hypersomnia and Excessive Daytime Somnolence

 Key Point

Among the disorders that cause excessive daytime somnolence, sleep apnea syndrome is the most common, and narcolepsy–cataplexy syndrome is probably the most impressive. A commonly overlooked cause is hypersomnia due to depression or an anxiety disorder. If a patient with hypersomnia is found to be cognitively impaired, a previously unrecognized dementia may be the cause of both problems.

10.3.1 Sleep Apnea Syndrome

Clinical features. When sleeping in the supine position, the patient snores very intensively and has **respiratory pauses** occurring more than 10 times per hour and lasting at least 10 seconds each; they are sometimes frighteningly long (1 minute or even longer). Patients do not always realize that they have a problem relating to sleep, although their bedmates usually do. They feel inadequately rested in the morning and often fall asleep during the day. This tends to happen in situations that ordinarily promote sleep, but it can also happen while the patient is at work, causing frequent embarrassment and stress. Such involuntary daytime naps generally have no restorative benefit. Patients often complain of **morning headaches**, seem depressed, tend to be in a bad mood, and suffer from diminished libido. As the years go by, psycho-organic changes can appear as well.

Men are more commonly affected than women. Most patients are **obese**, and many have **arterial hypertension**.

Diagnostic evaluation. The evaluation begins with **respiratory polygraphy** with any of the various commercially available devices for this purpose (e.g., ApneaLink). A simple **audio recording** of the patient's snoring, breathing, and respiratory pauses during sleep, for example, with a smartphone, is a useful screening test. **Transcutaneous oximetry** during sleep is not sensitive enough as an isolated test, because the oxygen saturation does not necessarily drop during each respiratory pause.

PSG (**Fig. 10.1**) with video, electroencephalogram (EEG), electrocardiogram, and respiratory recording enables a thorough analysis of sleep and of individual physiologic variables, as well as of behavioral abnormalities, movements, and body posture during sleep. It is performed in a sleep laboratory. PSG can be used to distinguish sleep apnea syndrome from other sleep disturbances such as parasomnias or epileptic seizures.

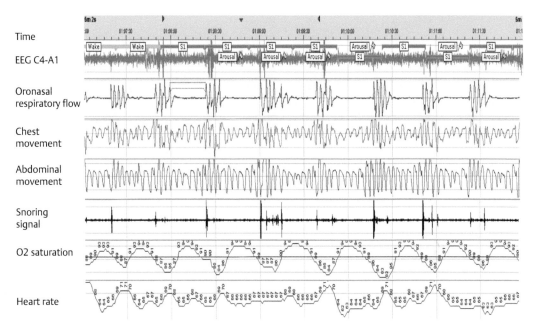

Fig. 10.1   Obstructive sleep apnea syndrome. Polysomnography.

Treatment. The treatment is directed against the pathogenic factors that are operative in the individual case. In some patients, simple measures such as **avoidance of the supine position** during sleep (by strapping a bulky object to the patient's back) effectively eliminate the problem. At the other end of the therapeutic spectrum, **positive-pressure mask ventilation** can be provided at night and often markedly improves the symptoms. Its variations include continuous positive airway pressure, ventilation with different pressures in the inspiratory and expiratory phases (**BIPAP**), and ventilation with automatically adjusted pressures (automatic positive airway pressure).

Obesity-hypoventilation syndrome. Patients with this syndrome also suffer from **daytime somnolence**. The syndrome is characterized by **obesity** (body mass index > 30 kg/m^2), **hypoxia** during sleep, and **hypercapnia** in the daytime. It can appear in combination with sleep apnea syndrome.

Obesity-hypoventilation syndrome used to be known in the English-speaking world as the pick-wickian syndrome, after a character in the Dickens novel *The Pickwick Papers* (not Samuel Pickwick himself, but Joe, the "fat boy").

10.3.2 Narcolepsy–Cataplexy Syndrome

Epidemiology. The estimated overall prevalence of narcolepsy–cataplexy syndrome is 0.6%.

Pathogenesis. Narcolepsy–cataplexy syndrome is thought to be caused by loss of the hypocretin-

binding cells in the hypothalamus. This loss, in turn, is thought to be due to immune mechanisms that become clinically manifest because of a genetic predisposition.

Clinical features. Typically, extreme daytime somnolence is combined with diverse phenomena that occur in REM sleep, and with a paradoxical sleep disturbance. **During the daytime**, patients have the following problems:

- **Excessive daytime somnolence** leads to **sleep attacks** that are often irresistible. In sleep-promoting situations, the patient cannot help falling asleep and then wakes up again a short time later, feeling rested.
- Patients who cannot take naps in the daytime have **twilight states** and **automatic behaviors**.
- Sudden emotional excitement—laughter, startle, other emotions—leads to a sudden loss of muscle tone (**affective loss of tone**), causing a fall, that is, **cataplexy**. Cataplectic attacks often give the initial impression of an unexplained atonic fall. The loss of tone may be generalized, or else only a few muscle groups may be affected with brief, focal atonia.

At night, patients have the following problems:

- **Hypnagogic hallucinations**, that is, hallucinations that are experienced just as the patient is falling asleep (less commonly, just as the patient is waking up).
- **Nightmares**, that is, intense, frightening, oppressive dreams during sleep.

Normal sleep profile

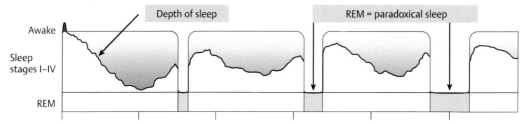

Sleep profile in narcolepsy–cataplexy syndrome

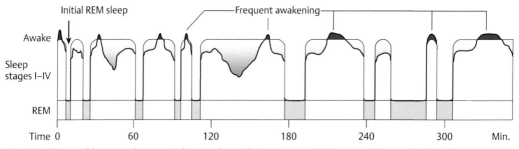

Fig. 10.2   **Sleep profile in narcolepsy–cataplexy syndrome** (below) compared with a normal sleep profile (above).

— **Sleep paralysis**, that is, the inability to move for a short time after waking up; this may be only partial (e.g., inability to open the eyes).

In the **monosymptomatic type** of narcolepsy—approximately 10% of cases—the sole abnormality is excessive daytime somnolence with irresistible sleep attacks. On the other hand, cataplexy can also be the main symptom leading to the diagnosis of the narcolepsy–cataplexy syndrome; in such cases, patients do not complain of daytime somnolence as a major problem and will only say they suffer from it if directly asked.

Diagnostic evaluation. The monosymptomatic type can be diagnosed only with the aid of ancillary tests—in particular, a **multiple sleep latency test** and **PSG**. The EEG abnormalities are characteristic: very short sleep latency (the official threshold is 8 minutes, but actual latencies are usually less than 5 minutes), the appearance of early REM sleep stages only a few minutes after falling asleep (SOREM = sleep-onset REM), and the frequent alternation of REM sleep with non-REM sleep and wakefulness (**Fig. 10.2**). Moreover, more than 95% of patients with narcolepsy have the **histocompatibility antigen** HLA DQB1*0602. Patients who have narcolepsy and cataplexy have a low **cerebrospinal fluid** concentration of hypocretin (=orexin).

Differential diagnosis. The key distinguishing features of the narcolepsy–cataplexy and sleep apnea syndromes are listed in **Table 10.1**.

Treatment. Narcolepsy is treated with **nonpharmacologic** measures such as sleep hygiene and coping strategies. Daytime somnolence can be alleviated with **drugs** such as modafinil (Vigil). Cataplexy can be treated with various drugs, including sodium oxybate and certain antidepressants.

10.3.3 Kleine–Levin–Critchley Syndrome

This syndrome is characterized by **periodic bouts of sleep for several hours** in the daytime, combined with disturbances of **perception** and **behavior** (food craving attacks, dysfunctional sexual behavior, sometimes other vegetative disturbances and abnormal emotional behavior). It affects male adolescents almost exclusively.

10.3.4 Other Causes of Daytime Fatigue and Somnolence

Persons suffering from temporary sleep deprivation can usually correct the problem by sleeping longer. If not, their lack of sleep causes daytime fatigue, impaired concentration, and somnolence. External circumstances, either job-related or social, are the usual causes of the inability to make up for a lack of sleep. Such situations need to be recognized and remedied, as long-term sleep deprivation can lead to **altered metabolism**, **weight gain**, and further sequelae.

Daytime fatigue and somnolence often have a nonorganic, mental or emotional cause. **Depression** and **anxiety disorders** are often associated with a subjective lack of sleep, a feeling of being poorly rested, fatigue, and a lack of drive, even if the patient in fact sleeps more than enough in each 24-hour period.

Table 10.1

Distinguishing features of the narcolepsy–cataplexy and sleep apnea syndromes

Aspect		Narcolepsy–cataplexy	Sleep apnea syndrome
History		— Onset usually in second or third decade	— Onset usually in middle or old age
Daytime sleep		— Overwhelming, even in active situations — Patient feels rested afterward — There are also hypovigilant states and twilight states with automatic behaviors	— Mainly in sleep-promoting situations — Patient does not feel rested afterward
Nighttime sleep		— Often interrupted by periods of wakefulness — Nightmares — Sometimes, sleep paralysis — Patients usually feel rested in the morning — No headache — Often, REM sleep behavioral disturbances — Often, difficulty staying asleep	— Loud snoring — Respiratory pauses lasting more than 10 s (hallmark) — Low O_2 saturation of the blood — Sometimes, angina pectoris during sleep — Patients usually do not feel rested in the morning — Headache
Other features		— Cataplectic states, e.g., loss of affective tone — Hypnagogic hallucinations — No dementia	— No cataplexy — Sometimes, hypnagogic hallucinations and automatic behaviors — In some cases, (reversible) dementia
Clinical findings		— Often mildly overweight	— Usually men — Almost always obese — Often hypertensive — Occasional anomaly of nasopharynx
Ancillary tests:	EEG, PSG	— Marked evidence of somnolence — Short sleep latency — Early REM sleep stages — Frequent alternation with non-REM sleep and wakefulness —	— Often, somnolence
	Other	— HLA-DQB1*0602 constellation — In narcolepsy with cataplexy: low CSF hypocretin (=orexin) level	— No specific HLA type

Abbreviation: CSF, cerebrospinal fluid.

10

10.4 Abnormal Movements in Sleep (Parasomnias)

 Key Point

Abnormal movements in sleep, also called parasomnias, are relatively common. They cover a broad spectrum, ranging from physiologic phenomena such as isolated twitching to complex behaviors and serious disease (Table 10.2).

Sudden jerking of the arms or legs ("sleeping jerks") constitutes **hypnagogic myoclonus**, a common and harmless phenomenon.

Nocturnal epileptic seizures should be suspected if rhythmic, clonic movements occur in sleep and the affected person cannot be awakened afterward; if tongue-biting occurs in sleep (manifested, perhaps, by blood on the pillow); if bedwetting appears and was not previously a problem; or if the patient has pain in the limbs and/or headache in the morning.

Periodic limb movements in sleep, previously known as **nocturnal myoclonus**, consists of repetitive twitching of the feet, the toes (resembling the Babinski response), or even both legs during sleep. Such movements are seen in 80% of patients with RLS and

are also common in Parkinson disease and narcolepsy. They can occur in healthy elderly persons as well.

Jactatio capitis is rhythmic head movement before falling asleep and during sleep. It is usually seen in mentally retarded children, less commonly in adults. Jactatio capitis must be included in the differential diagnosis of nocturnal epilepsy.

Bedwetting (enuresis) usually reflects the delayed development of nighttime continence in children and adolescents and resolves spontaneously. It is only rarely due to an organic disorder that needs to be treated.

Bedwetting sometimes appears together with **sleepwalking** (somnambulism).

Sleepwalking, pavor nocturnus (night terror) and confused awakening all occur as the sufferer is awakening from a deep sleep. They are thought to be due to a dissociated brain state in which the motor centers are already awake and active, but the brain areas subserving memory and control are still asleep. In **sleepwalking**, the individual actually gets out of bed; in **confused awakening**, he or she briefly sits up and seems confused. **Pavor nocturnus** (night terror) consists of expressions of intense fear, including crying

Table 10.2

Parasomnias

Sleep stage	Parasomnia
Wakefulness, falling asleep	– Restless legs syndrome
Falling asleep and early sleep stages (Stages I and II)	– Hypnagogic myoclonus, sensory paroxysms (EHS) – Hypnagogic hallucinations – Periodic leg movements – Bruxism (grinding the teeth) – Jactatio capitis (rhythmic head movements) – Somniloquy (sleep talking)
Mainly in the first half of the night (deep sleep and arousal; arousal disorders and awakening disorders)	– Sleepwalking – Pavor nocturnus – Confused awakening
Mainly in the second half of the night (REM sleep)	– Nightmares – RBD – Cluster headaches and hypnic headache – Painful erections
Toward morning (neither REM nor non-REM sleep)	– Cardiovascular symptoms – Asthma
Awakening phase	– Epilepsy in the awakening phase – Hypnopompic hallucinations (REM sleep) – Sleep inertia – Sleep paralysis (REM sleep, also in the stage of falling asleep) – Nocturnal paroxysmal dystonia
Entire night	– Psychomotor seizures, frontal lobe seizures – Bedwetting (enuresis) – Calf cramps

Abbreviations: EHS, exploding head syndrome; RBD, REM sleep behavior disorder.

and screaming, that last about ten minutes. It is mainly seen in children. During night terrors, the eyes are open, but the individual does not respond in the normal way to external stimuli. These disturbances of the awakening phase can be alleviated by benzodiazepines such as clonazepam if they are very severe.

REM sleep behavior disorders (RBD), in which muscle tone is preserved (i.e., the normal atonia of REM sleep is lacking), generally occur in the second half of the night. Most of the affected persons are elderly men. These disorders are characterized by complex behaviors, often of an aggressive or auto-aggressive nature, e.g., wild thrashing of the limbs, as if the patient were acting out a dream. The diagnosis is established by video-polysomnography. RBD are often an early sign of Parkinson disease, multisystem atrophy, or another **neurodegenerative disease**; anti-neuronal antibodies have been found in a few cases. **Fatal familial insomnia** is a rare prion disease (cf. section 6.7.9) whose sufferers have progressive autonomic dysfunction and, in many cases, ataxia, dysarthria, myoclonus, and pyramidal tract signs.

 Practical Tip

The differential diagnosis of abnormal movements in sleep (parasomnias) should always include nocturnal twilight states with behavioral automatisms as a manifestation of temporal or frontal lobe epilepsy, particularly when similar disturbances occur during the day or a temporal or frontal brain lesion is present.

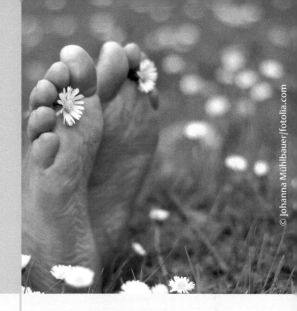

Chapter 11

Polyradiculopathy and Polyneuropathy

Suddenly Paralyzed

A few days after his return from a Caribbean holiday, a 23-year-old man developed mild flulike symptoms, including a sore throat and low-grade fever. He recovered from this illness completely. Several days later, however, he felt a mild tingling in his toes, and it seemed to him that his legs were weak. The next day, the weakness was so pronounced that he could only stand up from a sitting position by pushing himself up from the chair with his arms, and he had trouble walking as well. At first, he thought this weakness had something to do with his cold. A little while later, when he began to notice weakness in his arms as well; he panicked and presented himself to the emergency room of a nearby hospital.

The admitting physician examined him thoroughly, finding mainly proximal weakness of all four limbs. The intrinsic muscle reflexes were weakly elicitable. Sensation was intact, except for impaired vibration sense on the feet and calves. The patient had no difficulty urinating.

The rapid development of mainly proximal, flaccid weakness of all four limbs (quadriparesis) with only mild sensory impairment and intact micturition is characteristic of Guillain–Barré syndrome (GBS). This disease is often associated with a prior upper respiratory or gastrointestinal infection; autoimmune processes play a role its pathogenesis. The cause of GBS remains unclear in most cases (idiopathic GBS). Treatment with immunoglobulins or plasmapheresis lessens the severity of the disease and accelerates the resolution of weakness.

This patient had had a mild cold before the neurologic deficits set in. As he had always been healthy up to that point, the doctors presumed he had idiopathic GBS. They nonetheless tested him for HIV, for the sake of completeness.

Three days after admission, the doctors were surprised by a laboratory report of a positive HIV test. There had been nothing in the history or the physical findings to arouse suspicion of an HIV infection. On repeated questioning, the patient said he had, in fact, had unprotected sexual intercourse on multiple occasions.

HIV infection rarely presents with acute polyradiculitis, as in this case. Thus, this patient had a type of symptomatic rather than idiopathic GBS. Like idiopathic GBS, this form of the disease is treated with immunoglobulins; antiretroviral drugs are given at the same time. The prognosis of HIV-associated GBS, like that of other forms of the disease, is favorable.

On discharge to a rehabilitation hospital 2 weeks later, the patient's muscular strength had already markedly improved. He regained full strength during a brief rehabilitation period. He tolerated antiretroviral therapy without any further problems.

11.1 Fundamentals

 Key Point
In this chapter, we will describe the characteristic syndromes produced by lesions that affect multiple nerve roots or peripheral nerves simultaneously (polyradiculopathy and polyneuropathy, respectively). If nerve roots and peripheral nerves are affected, the disorder is termed polyradiculoneuropathy.

Classification. These very heterogeneous syndromes can be classified in various ways. Today, they are most commonly classified by the following criteria:
- Temporal course: polyradiculoneuropathy may present acutely with complete or partial remission, or it may take a chronically recurrent or chronically progressive course.
- Localization: symmetric versus asymmetric, distal versus proximal, lower or upper limbs affected versus lower and upper limbs affected, involvement of a few individual nerves (mononeuropathy multiplex).
- Etiology: polyradiculoneuropathy may be of metabolic, endocrine, toxic, genetic/hereditary, infectious, inflammatory, autoimmune, or paraneoplastic origin.
- Pathology: the functioning of the nerve roots and/or peripheral nerves may be impaired either by demyelination or by axon degeneration. Different types of nerve fibers may be affected (e.g., motor vs. sensory, large fibers vs. small fibers). Slowing of nerve conduction (or conduction block) early in the course of the illness is a distinguishing feature of demyelinating polyradiculoneuropathy, as opposed to diseases that involve axon degeneration.

General clinical features. Polyradiculopathy and polyneuropathy are characterized by:
- Paresis.
- Weak or absent reflexes.
- Muscle atrophy.
- Sensory deficits and positive sensory phenomena (paresthesia, dysesthesia), with or without pain.
- Mainly distal manifestations in a symmetric distribution (rarely, asymmetric).
- Usually beginning in the lower limbs.
- With more or less rapid progression.
- With variable involvement of the autonomic nervous system.

The extent, severity, and distribution of these manifestations vary from patient to patient. In particular, mainly radiculopathic processes are clinically distinguishable from exclusively neuropathic processes. These two types of process are, therefore, presented separately in what follows.

11.2 Polyradiculitis

 Key Point
This term refers to an inflammatory process that affects many spinal nerve roots (most commonly the anterior ones), usually with simultaneous involvement of the proximal segments of the peripheral nerves. The cause of the inflammation is sometimes a direct infection, but more often an autoimmune reaction. Clinical variants of polyradiculitis are distinguished from one another by the temporal course and predominant localization of the inflammation. The acute form, GBS, is more common; the chronic form (chronic inflammatory demyelinating polyradiculoneuropathy [CIDP]) is rarer.

Another rare form is localized polyradiculoneuritis exclusively affecting either the cranial nerves or the cauda equina.

In most cases, the inflammation is not directly due to an infection, but rather due to an autoimmune-mediated process, that is, an autoallergic radiculitis/neuritis following a viral or bacterial infection (which may be subclinical).

Demyelination is the main pathophysiologic mechanism of autoimmune polyradiculitis. Axon degeneration is also present, to a varying degree, in CIDP, which explains its protracted course.

11.2.1 Guillain–Barré Syndrome
GBS (also called Landry–Guillain–Barré syndrome) is the classic example of a polyradiculitis.

NOTE

Acute polyradiculitis is characterized by **rapidly ascending paresis** and only **mild sensory disturbances**. In severe cases, the cranial nerves and autonomic system can be involved. Weakness usually improves spontaneously in all involved muscles; those that became weak first recover last. The prognosis is favorable.

Epidemiology. GBS can strike at any age. Its incidence is from 0.5 to 2 cases per 100,000 persons per year. It tends to appear in the spring or fall.

Etiology and pathogenesis. This syndrome has more than one cause, and the etiology often remains unclear. In some patients, the illness is preceded by Mycoplasma pneumonia or by infection with varicella zoster virus (chickenpox), paramyxovirus (mumps), HIV, Epstein–Barr virus (infectious mononucleosis), or *Campylobacter jejuni*. The last-named organism often produces axonal lesions and is associated with a particularly severe form of the illness. Immunologic processes play an important role in

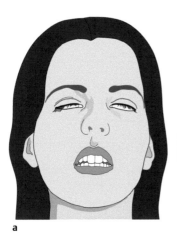
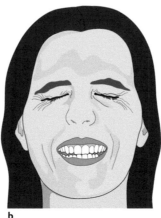

a   b

Fig. 11.1   Bilateral peripheral facial nerve palsy in Guillain–Barré polyradiculitis.
a Acute phase. **b** After recovery.

pathogenesis; in particular, antimyelin antibodies are often found. Anti-GD1a antibodies are sometimes found in the rarer forms of the illness that involve axon degeneration, but not in the more common, demyelinating forms (see earlier).

Clinical features. The first sign is weakness of the lower limbs, beginning distally, occasionally in the aftermath of an upper respiratory or gastrointestinal infection. There is no fever. Weakness ascends within a few hours or days, and the patient may become unable to walk. Distal paresthesiae and sensory disturbances are usually present, but much less disturbing to the patient than the weakness. Though the weakness ascends rapidly, its ultimate extent is variable. In very severe cases, the upper limbs, diaphragm, and accessory muscles of respiration are affected within a few days of onset, as well as the muscles of the head and neck that are supplied by the cranial nerves. Inability to swallow and bilateral facial palsy ensue (**Fig. 11.1**). Life-threatening respiratory failure often develops very rapidly. In addition, possible involvement of the autonomic nervous system can cause life-threatening abnormalities of blood pressure regulation, cardiac rhythm, central respiratory drive, and, less commonly, bladder function.

Diagnostic evaluation. The diagnosis is generally made from the clinical findings and confirmed by the characteristic finding of albuminocytologic dissociation in the cerebrospinal fluid (CSF), classically described in 1916 by Guillain, Barré, and Strohl: the CSF protein concentration is elevated, without any accompanying elevation of the cell count. This finding may not be present, however, until 2 or 3 weeks after the onset of illness. Electrophysiologic testing usually reveals focal demyelination with conduction block, or, less commonly, axonal lesions.

Treatment. In mild cases, general supportive care is all that is needed, with close monitoring of muscle strength and vital capacity. In severe cases, with profound weakness and rapidly progressive respiratory dysfunction, the intravenous infusion of immunoglobulins is indicated (0.4 g/kg body weight daily for 5 consecutive days). A second course of treatment can be given 4 weeks later if necessary. Plasmapheresis is an effective alternative, for example, for patients with contraindications to immunoglobulin therapy. Patients with rapidly ascending paresis and impending respiratory failure must be hospitalized in an intensive care unit, so that their circulatory and respiratory functions can be closely monitored and they can be intubated without delay, if necessary. Cardiac complications and pain are treated symptomatically. Patients with dysphagia are fed through a nasogastric or gastrostomy tube. Other important elements of care are: prophylaxis against deep venous thrombosis (and pulmonary embolism), urinary catheterization if needed, and, later, physical therapy.

Prognosis. The prognosis is generally favorable. Intensive care may be needed in the acute phase, but, once this is past, the weakness usually resolves in all affected muscles. The muscles that were weak first recover last. Recovery may take several months, however, or even up to 2 years in very severe cases. Permanent, mainly distal muscle atrophy is not uncommon. Most of the deaths caused by GBS are attributable to prolonged immobility (pneumonia, pulmonary embolism) or autonomic dysfunction (respiratory failure, sudden cardiac death). Death from this disease is rare in the current era of intensive care and complication prevention.

11.2.2 Chronic Inflammatory Demyelinating (Recurrent) Polyneuropathy

NOTE

CIDP, the **chronic** variant of **polyradiculitis**, is pathophysiologically similar to the acute variant (GBS, see section 11.2.1). It develops over a period of 8 weeks or more. The weakness and autonomic dysfunction are usually **less severe** than in GBS, but they last **longer.**

Pathogenesis. The idiopathic form of this condition is presumed to have an autoimmune basis. Immunoglobulins are found in the CSF, and immunoglobulin deposits are seen in biopsy specimens of the sural nerve. There are also forms of CIDP associated with HIV and systemic lupus erythematosus.

Clinical features. CIDP differs most obviously from classic, benign Guillain–Barré polyradiculitis in its slower course. Its main clinical features are:

- Chronic or relapsing–remitting course (at least 8 weeks).
- (Possibly) subacute course.
- (Often) pain.
- Symmetric or asymmetric distribution of neurologic deficits.
- Recurrent cranial nerve involvement.
- Central nervous manifestations are more common than in GBS.
- Electroneurography (ENG) reveals evidence of focal demyelination or axonal involvement.
- Marked elevation of CSF protein concentration, often combined with an elevated immunoglobulin G index, while the cell count is normal.

Fluctuation of the signs and symptoms is also typical: there may be phases of complete remission followed by relapse, or else the manifestations may progress slowly over a long period of time.

Diagnostic evaluation. ENG reveals slowed nerve conduction, partial conduction blocks, and a delayed or absent F wave. In cases with axonal involvement, electromyography (EMG) reveals low-amplitude summed muscle potentials and abnormal spontaneous muscle activity.

Treatment. CIDP can be treated effectively with corticosteroids and immunoglobulins and with plasmapheresis. Depending on the response, long-term treatment may be needed, either with immunoglobulins or with immunosuppressive drugs (corticosteroids, azathioprine, cyclophosphamide).

Practical Tip

Corticosteroids are indicated to treat CIDP, but not GBS.

Prognosis. CIDP takes either a relapsing–remitting or a chronic progressive course; the former carries a better prognosis. More than half of all patients need long-term treatment.

Multifocal Motor Neuropathy

NOTE

Multifocal motor neuropathy (MMN) is a special variant of CIDP.

Clinical features. MMN is characterized by asymmetric, slowly or rapidly progressive weakness with muscle atrophy and, sometimes, fasciculations (which may make MMN hard to distinguish from amyotrophic lateral sclerosis). There may also be dysarthria and sensory deficits. Some reflexes are lost.

Diagnostic evaluation. The key diagnostic finding in ENG is that of sporadic, circumscribed nerve conduction blocks. Laboratory testing often reveals elevated anti-GM1 titers.

Treatment. MMN is treated like other forms of CIDP.

11.2.3 Cranial Polyradiculitis

Polyradiculitis of the cranial nerves may be a component of ascending polyradiculitis, in which case it generally arises only after the limbs have become paretic. Sometimes, however, it is the first, main, or only clinical manifestation of polyradiculitis.

Practical Tip

The differential diagnosis of patients with cranial polyradiculitis must always include borreliosis and chronic meningitis (see section 6.7.4).

Miller Fisher Syndrome

Miller Fisher syndrome is a variant of cranial polyradiculitis that mainly affects young men. It is presumed to share a pathogenesis with Bickerstaff encephalitis, in which brain stem involvement predominates.

Clinical features. Miller Fisher syndrome is characterized by the following:

- Ophthalmoplegia.
- Somatosensory ataxia.
- Areflexia.
- (Sometimes) pupillary involvement—an Adie pupil (see section 12.3.6 and **Fig. 12.16**),
- (Sometimes) facial nerve palsy (**Fig. 11.1**).
- (sometimes) accompanying brainstem signs.
- Electrophysiologic evidence of a sensory axonal neuropathy.

Diagnostic evaluation. The diagnosis rests on the typical clinical features and the serologic demonstration of antiganglioside antibodies GQ1a and b. The CSF protein concentration is elevated.

11

Treatment. Miller Fisher syndrome has a favorable prognosis and generally needs no specific treatment.

11.2.4 Polyradiculitis of the Cauda Equina
This rare type of polyradiculitis, also called Elsberg syndrome, is characterized by isolated involvement of the sacral roots, producing distal weakness, areflexia of the lower limbs, and sphincter dysfunction. Many cases are presumably due to borreliosis or a type 2 herpes virus infection.

11.3 Polyneuropathy

    Key Point
Polyneuropathy is a condition that affects multiple peripheral nerves, usually simultaneously, though sometimes sequentially (with a more or less rapid switch from one nerve to the next). The clinical features are nearly always symmetrically distributed and slowly progressive. The first signs of the condition are nearly always in the lower limbs. Its causes are many.

Etiology. The common causes of polyneuropathy are listed and classified in **Table 11.1**.

Pathogenesis. Various harmful influences can affect peripheral nerves in different ways to produce different types of histopathologic lesion. Initial damage of the neuronal nuclei leads to secondary, distal, retrograde axon degeneration. On the other hand, primary damage to axons leads to wallerian degeneration of the distal axon segments, as in many types of toxic polyneuropathy. The Schwann cells are another possible target of pathogenic influences, for example, autoimmune processes such as dysproteinemia. Loss of Schwann cells leads to demyelination.

General clinical features. Polyneuropathy is characterized by:
- First signs appearing distally in the lower limbs.
- Paresthesiae in the toes or soles of the feet, mainly at night.
- Tingling.
- Muffled sensation on the soles, "as if I had socks on."
- Loss of the Achilles reflexes.
- Diminution or loss of vibration sense, beginning distally.
- As the condition progresses, there is paresis of the short toe extensors on the dorsum of the foot and of the interossei (the patient can no longer spread his or her toes), and, later, paresis of the long toe extensors and foot extensors.
- This produces a bilateral foot drop, for which the patient compensates with a steppage gait.

- Finally, sensory disturbances and weakness spread to the upper limbs as well (**Fig. 11.2**, see also **Fig. 5.3**c).

Diagnostic evaluation. When the typical clinical findings imply a polyneuropathy, a series of laboratory tests is performed to determine its etiology (**Table 11.2**).

If a paraneoplastic cause is suspected, a primary tumor should be sought, for example, with imaging studies.

> **NOTE**
> **ENG** reveals a variable degree of impairment of impulse conduction, depending on the etiology. In **demyelinating** polyneuropathies, the nerve conduction velocity is slow. In **axonal** polyneuropathies, it is normal or only mildly slowed, but **EMG** reveals evidence of denervation or neurogenically altered potentials.

The CSF protein concentration is elevated in many types of polyneuropathy (e.g., diabetic polyneuropathy); in rare cases, CSF examination may yield evidence of an infectious process. Sural nerve biopsy is an additional means of distinguishing axonal from demyelinating forms of polyneuropathy, if the findings of ENG and EMG are inconclusive; it may also provide direct evidence for certain etiologies (e.g., vasculitis). Sural nerve biopsy is an invasive and hence uncommon procedure that should only be performed in specialized centers. Skin biopsy is less invasive and enables a quantitative assessment of the thin, unmyelinated fibers that are lost in small-fiber neuropathies (see later) (**Fig. 11.5**).

11.3.1 Particular Etiologic Types of Polyneuropathy
The types of polyneuropathy that are clinically most important, either because they are common or for other reasons, are described in the following sections.

Hereditary Motor and Sensory Neuropathies (HMSN)
The current classification of hereditary polyneuropathies is shown in **Table 11.3**.

HMSN Type I (Charcot–Marie–Tooth disease)
This is the most common hereditary polyneuropathy, with a prevalence of 2 per 100,000 persons. It is of autosomal dominant inheritance; at least five causative genetic mutations have been identified. About 70 to 80% of cases are due to duplication of the PMP22 (peripheral myelin protein 22) gene on chromosome 17 (type 1a CMT).

11

Table 11.1

Causes of common polyneuropathies

Type of polyneuropathy	Underlying disease
Polyneuropathies of genetic origin	— Hereditary motor and sensory neuropathies — Neuropathy with tendency to pressure palsy — Porphyria — Primary amyloidosis
Inflammatory, autoimmune polyneuropathies	— Acute polyradiculitis (Guillain–Barré syndrome) — CIDP — Cranial polyradiculitis — Polyradiculitis of the cauda equina
Metabolic polyneuropathies	— Diabetic neuropathy: • Symmetric, mainly distal type • Asymmetric, mainly proximal type • "Mononeuropathy" • Amyotrophy or myelopathy — Uremia — Cirrhosis — Gout — Hypothyroidism
Polyneuropathies due to undernutrition or malnutrition	— Vegan or strict vegetarian diet
Polyneuropathies due to vitamin B_{12} deficiency and other malabsorptive disorders	— Chronic gastritis — Status post gastrectomy — gluten-sensitive enteropathy (celiac sprue)
Polyneuropathies due to dysproteinemia or paraproteinemia	— Multiple myeloma — Waldenström disease — Other
Polyneuropathies due to infectious disease	— Leprosy — Mumps — Infectious mononucleosis — Typhoid and paratyphoid fever — Spotted fever — HIV infection — Diphtheria — Botulism — Borreliosis — Hepatitis C
Polyneuropathies due to arterial disease	— Atherosclerosis, ischemic neuropathy — Polyarteritis nodosa — Other collagenoses
Polyneuropathies due to exogenous toxic substances	— Ethanol — Lead — Arsenic — Thallium — Triaryl phosphate — Solvents (e.g., carbon disulfide) — Drugs (isoniazid, thalidomide, nitrofurantoin, antiretroviral drugs, antineo-plastic drugs, etc.)
Polyneuropathies of other causes	— Serogenic (after vaccination) — Sarcoidosis — Neoplasia — Paraneoplastic — Critical illness neuropathy

Abbreviations: CIDP, chronic inflammatory demyelinating polyneuropathy; HIV, human immunodeficiency virus.

Clinically, an early manifestation is pes cavus, later followed by atrophy of the calf muscles, while the thigh muscles retain their normal bulk ("stork legs," "inverted champagne-bottle sign," **Fig. 11.3**). As the disease progresses, predominantly distal muscle atrophy is seen in the upper limbs as well. Distal sensory impairment may not arise until much later and even then is usually only mild. ENG reveals marked slowing of nerve conduction; histopathologic examination of a sural nerve specimen reveals axon degeneration, myelin changes, and onion-skin-like Schwann cells.

The course of HMSN type I is characterized by very slow progression. Patients can often keep working until the normal retirement age or beyond.

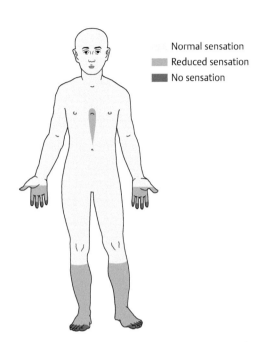

Normal sensation
Reduced sensation
No sensation

Fig. 11.2　Sensory disturbances in symmetric polyneuropathy.

Hereditary Neuropathy with Predisposition to Pressure Palsies (HNPP)

This autosomal dominant disorder is also due to a point mutation in chromosome 17p11.2–12. Clinically, patients develop recurrent pressure palsies of individual peripheral nerves, even after very light pressure. The histopathologic substrate of the disorder is an abnormality of the myelin sheaths of peripheral nerves. Microscopy reveals sausage-like, segmental swelling of the sheaths ("tomaculous neuropathy").

Diabetic Polyneuropathy
Epidemiology.

> **NOTE**
>
> **Diabetic polyneuropathy** is the second **most common** type of polyneuropathy. Only the **alcohol-induced** type is more common.

About 20 to 40% of diabetics have some degree of diabetic polyneuropathy, which typically afflicts persons aged 60 to 70 who have suffered from diabetes for 5 to 10 years or more. In 10% of patients with

11

Table 11.2

Laboratory testing in polyneuropathy

Step of diagnostic evaluation	Tests
Basic testing	— ESR or CRP
	— Complete blood count
	— Na$^+$, K$^+$, creatinine, blood urea nitrogen
	— ALT (GPT), AST (GOT), γ-GT
	— Glucose, HBA$_{1c}$, glucose tolerance test if indicated
	— TSH; T3 and fT4 if indicated
	— Vitamin B$_{12}$; inconclusive test → homocysteine; if still unclear, methylmalonic acid
	— Vasculitis battery: ANA, anti-dsDNA antibodies, rheumatoid factor, anticardiolipin antibodies, c-ANCA, p-ANCA, SS-A, SS-B, C3, C4
	— CDT
	— Serologic examination for borreliosis, syphilis, HIV
	— Serum electrophoresis and immune fixation
Specific testing	— CSF examination
	— Erythrocyte transketolase (vitamin B$_1$)
	— Erythrocyte AST (vitamin B$_6$)
	— Vitamin E
	— Serologic examination for *Campylobacter jejuni*, HSV, hepatitis B and C
	— Antiganglioside antibodies (GM1, GQ1b)
	— Anti-glycoprotein antibodies (MAG)
	— Paraneoplastic antibodies (Hu, CV2, VGKC)
	— Urinary δ-aminolevulinic acid and porphobilinogen
	— Heavy metals (arsenic, lead, thallium, mercury)
	— Phytanic acid
	— Genetic testing
	— Nerve biopsy
	— Skin biopsy
	— Detection of amyloid in abdominal fatty tissue, rectal mucosa, etc.

Abbreviations: ALT, alanine aminotransferase; ANA, anti-nuclear antibodies; ANCA, anti-neutrophil cytoplasmic antibodies; AST, aspartate aminotransferase; CDT, carbohydrate-deficient transferrin; CRP, C-reactive protein; CSF, cerebrospinal fluid; ESR, erythrocyte sedimentation rate; γ-GT, γ-glutamyl transferase; HBA$_{1c}$, glycated hemoglobin; HIV, human immunodeficiency virus; HSV, herpes simplex virus; T3, triiodothyronine; fT4, free thyroxine; TSH, thyroid-stimulating hormone.

| Table 11.3 |

Hereditary motor and sensory neuropathies

Type of HMSN	Inheritance pattern	Age at onset	Muscle weakness and atrophy	Sensory deficit	Nerve conduction velocity	Other remarks
Type I Charcot–Marie–Tooth disease	Autosomal dominant	Second to fourth decade	– Mainly distal, beginning in the feet and calves – Later in the hands and forearms – Pes cavus	None or mild, mainly acral	Markedly slowed	– Peripheral nerves thickened – Sural nerve biopsy reveals axon degeneration, de- and remyelination, onion-skin structures
Type II Neuronal type of peroneal muscle atrophy	Autosomal dominant	Second to fourth decade	– Distal atrophy, mainly in the feet and calves – Pes cavus	Mild, mainly acral	Mildly slowed	– Peripheral nerves not thickened – Sural nerve biopsy reveals axon degeneration, no onion-skin structures
Type III Déjerine–Sottas Hypertrophic neuropathy	Autosomal dominant	First decade	Rapidly progressive weakness of legs and hands	Marked, mainly acral	Severely slowed	– Peripheral nerves thickened – Sural nerve biopsy reveals hypo-, de-, and remyelination, onion-skin structures, only thin myelinated fibers
Type IV Hypertrophic neuropathy in Refsum disease	Autosomal recessive	First to third decade	Mainly distal	Marked, mainly distal	Markedly slowed	– Sensorineural hearing loss – Possibly, retinitis pigmentosa – Thickened peripheral nerves – Sural nerve biopsy reveals axon degeneration, de- and remyelination, onion-skin structures – Phytanic acid accumulation in various tissues
Type V HMSN with spastic paraparesis	Autosomal dominant	Second decade or later	Mainly distal muscle atrophy and spastic paraparesis	None or mild	Normal or mildly slowed	– Sural nerve biopsy may reveal reduced number of myelinated fibers
Type VI HMSN with optic nerve atrophy	Autosomal dominant or recessive	Highly variable	Mainly distal	None or mild	Normal or mildly slowed	– Visual loss, progressive blindness – Thickened nerves in rare cases
Type VII HMSN with retinitis pigmentosa	Autosomal recessive	Variable	Mainly distal	Mild	Slowed	– Retinitis pigmentosa

Abbreviations: HMSN, hereditary motor and sensory neuropathies.
Source: Dyck PJ, Thomas PK. Peripheral Neuropathy, 4th ed. Philadelphia: Saunders; 2005.

diabetic neuropathy, it is only the diagnostic evaluation of neuropathy that brings the underlying diabetes to light.

Pathogenesis. Polyneuropathy is caused both by diabetic angiopathy and by the direct effect of elevated blood sugar. Axon degeneration is usually the most prominent histologic finding, though segmental demyelination is sometimes marked as well.

Clinical features. Irritative sensory symptoms are most prominent at first, including paresthesia and, often, burning dysesthesia of the feet. The latter is particularly disturbing when the feet are warm, for example, at night under a blanket. Typically,

Achilles reflexes are absent, and there is a mainly distal impairment of touch and vibration sense. It is only later that about half of the affected patients develop motor deficits. The neurologic deficit may be asymmetric, or there may be isolated disease of an individual nerve, such as cranial nerves III, IV, or VI or the femoral nerve. Disturbances of autonomic innervation are also typical: dry, often reddened skin, bladder dysfunction, orthostatic hypotension, tachycardia, diarrhea, and erectile dysfunction in young male diabetics. The effects of diabetes on the nervous system are listed in **Table 11.4**.

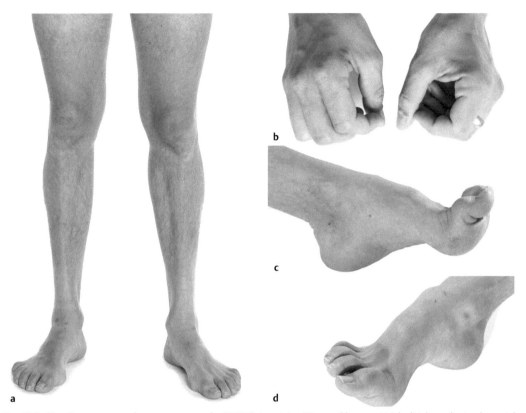

Fig. 11.3 Hereditary motor and sensory neuropathy (HMSN), type I, in a 30-year-old man. **a** Mainly distal muscle atrophy, mainly visible in the calves and feet. **b** Atrophy of the intrinsic hand muscles. **c, d** Pes cavus, with claw-like toes because of atrophy and loss of the intrinsic muscles of the feet, so that the action of the long toe flexors predominates.

Treatment. Optimal glycemic control is of paramount importance. The neuropathic pain of diabetic neuropathy, which is often very disturbing, is primarily treated with anticonvulsant drugs such as pregabalin and gabapentin. It can be treated alternatively, or additionally, with tricyclic antidepressants such as amitriptyline. Opioids may be necessary in otherwise intractable cases.

If the pain of diabetic neuropathy is locally circumscribed, it can be treated topically with a capsaicin or lidocaine ointment.

Toxic Polyneuropathies

The numerous substances that can cause a toxic polyneuropathy will not all be listed here. We will merely indicate the broad clinical spectrum of toxic polyneuropathy by describing two very different, highly characteristic syndromes.

Alcoholic Polyneuropathy

Alcoholic polyneuropathy is very common, but its pathogenesis is not fully understood. In addition to the direct effects of ethanol and acetaldehyde, the nutritional deficiencies that are common in

alcoholics play a role as well. Further contributing factors include possible defects of the enzymes alcohol dehydrogenase and acetaldehyde dehydrogenase. Clinically, intense pain in the legs is often the most prominent symptom. Many patients also suffer from muscle cramps. The intrinsic muscle reflexes are weak; the Achilles reflexes are usually absent. Proprioception is impaired, and touch and vibration sense are diminished distally. The calves are often tender to deep pressure. The foot dorsiflexors are weak. Sural nerve biopsy reveals axon degeneration.

Triaryl Phosphate Poisoning

This entity will serve here as an example of an acute toxic neuropathy whose manifestations can persist, either fully or in part. Triaryl phosphate is found in certain mineral oil derivatives used in industry. Their erroneous use as cooking oil leads to a clinical syndrome that manifests itself initially with diarrhea, followed 1 to 5 weeks later by fever and other constitutional symptoms. The neuropathy only becomes evident several weeks after the exposure: flaccid paresis affects the feet at first, spreading to all four

Table 11.4

Effects of diabetes mellitus on the nervous system

Site	Manifestation	Special features
Central nervous system	▬ Stroke ▬ Spinal cord ischemia	
Peripheral nervous system	**Polyneuropathies**	
	▬ Sensorimotor	Distal, sometimes painful, symmetric, gradually worsening paresthesiae or burning pain in the feet, absent Achilles reflexes, diminished vibration sense, hypesthesia in a stocking distribution, sometimes dorsiflexor weakness (with steppage gait), sometimes toe ulcers and toe joint destruction
	▬ Proximal asymmetric	Mainly affects the lumbar plexus or femoral nerve, unilateral, acute, painful, weakness of hip flexors and quadriceps muscle, diminished knee-jerk reflexes, positive reverse Lasègue sign, hypesthesia in femoral nerve distribution, sometimes similar findings in upper limbs, spontaneous improvement possible (as in mononeuropathy, see below)
	Mononeuropathies	
	▬ CN III (most common)	Painful, spares the intraocular muscles, regresses within a few months (**Fig. 12.10**)
	▬ Other peripheral nerve	For example, thoracic nerves with abdominal muscle weakness (**Fig. 13.50**)
Autonomic nervous system	▬ Bladder dysfunction	Sphincter disturbance, atonic flaccid bladder
	▬ Erectile dysfunction	In younger male patients
	▬ Diarrhea	Chiefly at night
	▬ Necrobiosis lipoidica	Polycyclic cutaneous atrophy in women
	▬ Osteoarthropathy	Particularly in the toes
	▬ Ulcers	Particularly on the soles of the feet

limbs within a few days. Sensation is also impaired. Many patients' deficits resolve only in part, or not at all, and spasticity of central origin frequently develops in the ensuing years. Histopathologic examination reveals axonal lesions both in the peripheral nerves and in the central nervous system.

Mononeuropathies and Mononeuritis Multiplex

This term subsumes the types of polyneuropathy that affect individual peripheral nerves one after another, in highly variable temporal sequence (**Fig. 11.4**). Individual mononeuropathies summate to create a polyneuropathy.

As for their pathogenesis, most cases of these two entities are due to a vasculopathy, such as diabetic microangiopathy, polyarteritis nodosa, systemic lupus erythematosus, Sjögren syndrome, Wegener granulomatosis, or atherosclerosis. Clinically, they are characterized by asymmetrically distributed weakness, sensory deficits, or autonomic dysfunction in the distribution of a single peripheral nerve or (in later stages of mononeuritis multiplex) multiple peripheral nerves. Other manifestations of the

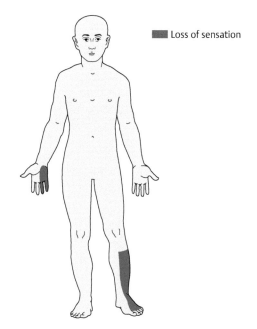

Loss of sensation

Fig. 11.4   Mononeuropathy multiplex.

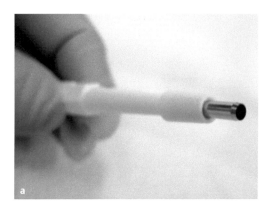

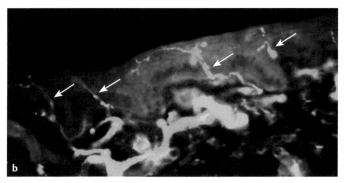

Fig. 11.5   The technique of skin biopsy.
a A skin biopsy punch, diameter 3 mm.
b Immunohistochemical staining (arrows: intraepidermal nerve fibers).

underlying illness are usually present as well, for example, constitutional symptoms such as fever, night sweats, and weight loss, an elevated erythrocyte sedimentation rate, and symptoms referable to the internal organs.

Small-Fiber Neuropathy

Small-fiber neuropathies affect unmyelinated and thin myelinated fibers, but not thicker myelinated ones.

> **NOTE**
>
> Small-fiber neuropathies manifest themselves clinically with **burning feet** or generalized, mainly **distal**, painful or **burning dysesthesia**. Pain and temperature sensation are reduced, while touch, vibration, and position sense are intact, and the intrinsic muscle reflexes are elicitable.

Further manifestations may include orthostatic hypotension and other types of autonomic dysfunction (see chapter 16).

The conventional electrophysiologic studies reveal no abnormality. The key diagnostic procedure is skin biopsy, which reveals reduced nerve fiber density (**Fig. 11.5**). Small-fiber neuropathy is often the presenting manifestation of a hereditary or acquired polyneuropathy, for example, diabetic or alcohol-induced polyneuropathy (which are the most common and second most common causes of small-fiber neuropathy, respectively). The differential diagnosis of small-fiber neuropathy includes most of the same entities that can cause large-fiber neuropathy, and the diagnostic evaluation therefore follows similar lines (see earlier).

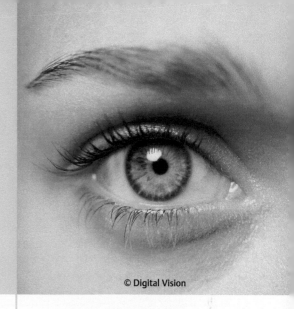

© Digital Vision

Chapter 12

Diseases of the Cranial Nerves

Better Than the Alternative

The patient, a law student, was 24 years old when she was bitten by a tick in the autumn of 2013. An expanding ring of erythema developed around the site of the bite. She was given oral doxycycline and the rash subsided.

In the summer of 2014, she woke up with a stabbing pain behind the right ear. By midday, she had difficulty drinking; whenever she tried, the beverage dribbled out of the right corner of her mouth, which she noticed was no longer straight. She immediately went to see a general practitioner, who examined her and found marked weakness of all muscles supplied by the right facial nerve, including the muscles of the forehead. Eye closure was incomplete on the right.

Here, as in all problems of neurologic diagnosis, the first task is to localize the lesion. The most common cause of facial weakness is damage to the facial nerve in the petrous canal: inflammatory swelling of the nerve, probably caused by a viral infection, leads to pressure on the nerve in the canal, with ensuing ischemia. In this disorder, called idiopathic or crypto-genic facial nerve palsy (also known by the eponym Bell palsy), lacrimation and taste are typically affected as well—a fact that can be useful in differential diagnosis. Weakness predominates, while lacrimation and taste are intact, if the facial nerve is affected more distally after its exit from the skull base via the stylomastoid foramen, or more proximally within the brainstem, either in its intramedullary fascicle (fascicular lesion) or in the facial nerve nucleus itself (nuclear lesion). Finally, the lesion may also lie above the facial nerve nucleus within the central nervous system (central facial palsy). The cells in the facial nerve nucleus that project to the forehead muscles receive afferent input from higher centers on both sides of the brain; thus, in central facial palsy, the forehead muscles are spared, and full eye closure is possible.

The doctor was able to exclude central facial palsy on the basis of his findings, but was nonetheless very concerned, fearing that the tick-borne borreliosis of the year before had not been fully eradicated and was now affecting the nervous system.

Nonidiopathic facial nerve palsy is often due to an infection with *Borrelia burgdorferi* (Lyme disease) or the varicella-zoster virus. Borreliosis, however, generally causes polyneuritic or polyradiculopathic weakness, rather than facial nerve mononeuropathy.

The doctor tested the patient's sense of taste with various aqueous solutions: taste was impaired on the right side in the anterior two-thirds of the tongue. Moreover, he found by a Schirmer test that lacrimation was also diminished on the right. These findings are typical of idiopathic facial nerve palsy. Borreliosis serology revealed no evidence of a florid infection. There were no cutaneous vesicles indicating a reactivated varicella infection. Therefore, the doctor diagnosed idiopathic facial nerve palsy and prescribed a 5-day course of prednisone by mouth, as well as an ophthalmic ointment to prevent drying and damage of the cornea at night. The patient's symptoms regressed completely within a few weeks.

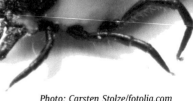

Photo: Carsten Stolze/fotolia.com

12.1 Disturbances of Smell (Olfactory Nerve)

Key Point

Neurologic disturbances of smell are usually due to traumatic or mechanical damage to the fila olfactoria or the olfactory bulb.

Anatomy. The peripheral olfactory receptors can only be excited by substances dissolved in liquid. The receptors of the olfactory mucosa project their axons through the cribriform plate to the olfactory bulb (see **Fig. 3.3**), which lies on the floor of the anterior cranial fossa, beneath the frontal lobe. These axons make up the fila olfactoria, which collectively constitute the olfactory nerve. After a synapse onto the second neuron of the pathway in the olfactory bulb, olfactory fibers travel onward through the lateral olfactory striae to the amygdala and other areas of the temporal lobe. Olfactory fibers also travel by way of the medial olfactory striae to the subcallosal area and the limbic system (see section 5.5.4).

Clinical features. Techniques for examining the sense of smell are discussed in section 3.3.2. Only the following types of olfactory disturbances are relevant to neurologic diagnosis:

- **Anosmia**. A more or less complete loss of the sense of smell is most often due to a disorder of the nose, particularly rhinitis sicca. The most common neurologic cause of anosmia is a traumatically induced brain contusion and/or avulsion of the fila olfactoria as they traverse the cribriform plate. Anosmia regresses in one-third of patients, but distortions of olfactory perception, so-called **parosmias**, often persist, sometimes in the form of unpleasant **kakosmia**. Anosmia is the characteristic symptom of an olfactory groove meningioma and is often its initial manifestation. Rarer causes of hyposmia include Paget disease, Parkinson disease, prior laryngectomy, diabetes mellitus, and Kallmann syndrome (hyposmia or anosmia with hypogonadotropic hypogonadism, of genetic origin). Medications often alter or impair the sense of smell.
- Anosmia always carries with it an impairment of the sense of taste (**ageusia**). The differential perception of gustatory stimuli requires not only an intact sense of taste but also an intact sense of smell.
- **Olfactory hallucinations**—usually in the form of spontaneous kakosmia—are produced by epileptic discharges from a focus in the anteromedial portion of the temporal lobe. Such hallucinations are called uncinate fits (see "Temporal Lobe Syndrome" in section 5.5.1).

12.2 Neurologic Disturbances of Vision (Optic Nerve)

Key Point

Visual disturbances can be caused by lesions of the retina or of its connections with the visual cortex, or of the cortex itself. Depending on the etiology, the clinical manifestation may be either impaired visual acuity (ranging to total blindness) or a visual field defect. The site of the lesion determines the type of visual abnormality that will be present and whether it will affect only one eye or both. As a rule, lesions of the retina and optic nerve cause monocular impairment of visual acuity and of the visual field; chiasmatic lesions impair visual acuity and the visual fields in both eyes; and retrochiasmatic lesions (from the optic tract to the visual cortex) cause visual field defects but spare visual acuity, unless there is more than one lesion and the lesions are located on both sides.

12.2.1 Visual Field Defects

NOTE

A visual field defect is defined as the absence of some part of the normal visual field. The diagnostic assessment of a visual field defect involves, first, localization of the underlying lesion to a particular part of the visual pathway, and, second, determination of the etiology on the basis of the history, neurologic examination, and ancillary test findings.

Types of Visual Field Defect and Their Localization

The manual confrontation technique for examining the visual fields is described in section 3.3.2, and the use of special instrumentation for this purpose is described in section 4.5.3. Visual field defects may be either monocular or binocular.

NOTE

Monocular visual field defects are caused by lesions of the retina and optic nerve; **binocular** visual field defects are caused by lesions in or behind the optic chiasm.

As shown in **Fig. 12.1** and **Table 12.1**, different kinds of visual field defect are characterized by their **spatial configuration**:

Homonymous visual field defects. If a binocular visual field defect involves a corresponding area of the visual field in both eyes (e.g., the right half of the visual field in both eyes), it is called a **homonymous** visual field defect.

12

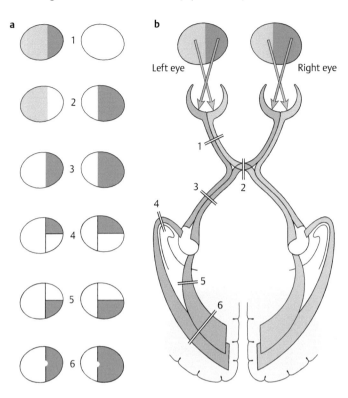

Fig. 12.1   Sites of lesions in the visual pathway and the visual field defects that they produce. 1 Left amaurosis due to a left optic nerve lesion. **2** Bitemporal hemianopsia due to a chiasmatic lesion. **3** Right homonymous hemianopsia due to a left optic tract lesion. **4–6** Lesions along the left optic radiation. **4** Right upper temporal quadrantanopsia. **5** Right lower temporal quadrantanopsia. **6** Right homonymous hemianopsia sparing central (macular) vision.

| Table 12.1 |

Classification of visual field defects

Term	Definition
Amaurosis	Blindness in one or both eyes, either congenital or acquired
Hemianopsia	A defect occupying one half of the visual field (right or left)
Quadrantanopsia	A defect occupying one quarter of the visual field
Scotoma	A defect occupying a small spot or patch within the visual field (a central scotoma is an impairment of central vision—and therefore a reduction of visual acuity—due to a lesion of the macula lutea or its efferent nerve fibers)
Temporal crescent	A near-hemianopic visual field defect sparing far lateral vision, caused by a contralateral occipital lesion that spares the rostral portion of the visual cortex on the banks of the calcarine fissure
Homonymous visual field defect	The same area of the visual field is affected in each eye (e.g., the right visual field of each eye)
Heteronymous visual field defect	**Different areas** of the visual field are affected in the two eyes (e.g., bitemporal hemianopsia)

— A lesion of the **right** optic tract, lateral geniculate body, optic radiation, or visual cortex produces a **left homonymous hemianopsia**, while a lesion of any of these structures on the left produces a right homonymous hemianopsia (**Fig. 12.1**).

— A lesion along the course of the optic radiation or in the visual cortex may affect only part of these structures, causing a homonymous visual field defect that is less than a complete hemianopsia: thus, depending on the site and extent of the lesion, there may be a homonymous quadrantanopsia or a homonymous scotoma.

Heteronymous visual field defects. These are defects involving noncorresponding areas of the visual field in the two eyes:

— Most lesions of the **optic chiasm** affect the decussating fibers derived from the nasal half of each retina to produce a bitemporal hemianopsia or bitemporal quadrantanopsia (**Fig. 12.1**). The defect lies in the temporal half of each visual field, that is, in the right half of the visual field of the right eye and the left half of the visual field of the left eye.

— If a tumor, such as a pituitary adenoma, compresses the optic chiasm from *below*, there is initially an *upper* bitemporal quadrantanopsia only later followed by bitemporal hemianopsia. If a tumor compresses the optic chiasm from *above* (e.g., a craniopharyngioma), there is initially a *lower* bitemporal quadrantanopsia, and later a bitemporal hemianopsia.

— If a tumor compresses the optic chiasm from one side, it will affect not only the decussating medial fibers but also the uncrossed fibers from the retina on that side. The resulting visual field defect involves the entire visual field on the side of the lesion and the temporal hemifield on the opposite side.

The Localization of Lesions That Impair Visual Acuity

Half of the efferent neurons of the macula project to the ipsilateral cerebral hemisphere, and the other half to the contralateral hemisphere. An eye can see with full acuity if at least half of the neural output from the macula is intact. Thus, lesions of the retina, optic nerve, or chiasm affecting more than half of the fibers from one eye impair visual acuity, but unilateral retrochiasmatic lesions do not.

NOTE

Lesions of the retina, optic nerve, or optic chiasm impair visual acuity, while unilateral retrochiasmatic lesions do not.

Etiologic Classification of Visual Field Defects

A visual field defect that arises suddenly is generally due to either **ischemia** or **trauma**. The shape of the visual field defect sometimes provides a clue to its etiology; thus, a temporal crescent is highly characteristic of a **vascular lesion**. A slowly progressive visual field defect suggests the presence of a **brain tumor.** In such patients, the patient may fail to notice the visual field defect, particularly if the tumor lies in the right parietal lobe. There may be **visual hemineglect** accompanying, or instead of, a "true" visual field defect. The patient ignores visual stimuli in the affected hemifield, even though he or she may still be able to see them, and is unaware of the deficit. Neuroimaging generally reveals the site and nature of the underlying lesion (**Fig. 12.2**).

Special Types of Visual Field Defect

In the **Riddoch phenomenon**, the patient cannot see stationary objects in the affected area of the visual field, though movement can be perceived. In **palinopsia**, the perception outlasts the stimulus: the patient continues to "see" the presented image long after it has been removed. This phenomenon is produced by right temporo-occipital lesions.

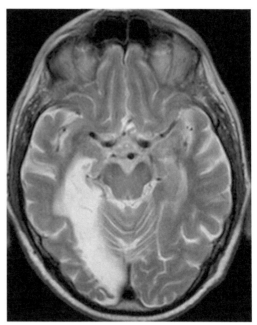

Fig. 12.2   Infarct in the territory of the right posterior cerebral artery in a patient with left homonymous hemianopsia.

12.2.2   Impairment of Visual Acuity

NOTE

Impairment of visual acuity can be partial or total (blindness); it can arise suddenly or progress slowly, and it can affect one or both eyes. All of these distinctions, along with the ocular and retrobulbar findings, are relevant to the localization of the lesion and the determination of its etiology. To evaluate such problems, neurologists often collaborate with ophthalmologists.

Sudden Unilateral Loss of Vision

Sudden unilateral loss of vision, as long as its cause does not lie in the eye itself, is usually due to a **lesion of the optic nerve**. Sudden onset implicates ischemia as the cause. A defect of this type may be permanent, for example, in occlusion of the central retinal artery due to temporal arteritis or embolization from an atheromatous plaque in the carotid artery, or it may be temporary, in which case it is called amaurosis fugax (transient monocular blindness). Rarely, transient visual loss can be produced by a functional neurologic disturbance such as migraine (retinal migraine). **Papilledema**, too, can be accompanied by episodes of sudden visual loss (amblyopic attacks). The differential diagnosis includes trauma and **ocular causes** such as retinal detachment, preretinal hemorrhage, and central vein thrombosis. Correct diagnosis requires precise history-taking and meticulous examination of the optic disc and fundus.

Sudden Bilateral Loss of Vision

Bilateral visual loss of more or less sudden onset is usually due to **simultaneous ischemia of both occipital lobes**. Such events are often preceded by hemianopic episodes and loss of color vision as prodromal manifestations. The possible causes include embolization into the territory of the posterior cerebral arteries on both sides simultaneously, basilar artery thrombosis, and compressive occlusion of both posterior cerebral arteries by an intracranial mass. Patients often deny that they cannot see (anosognosia). Despite the severe visual loss, the pupillary light reflex is still present, because the pathway for visual impulses to the lateral geniculate body, where the fibers for the reflex branch off, remains intact. The visual evoked potentials (see section 4.3.3 and **Fig. 4.26**), however, are pathologic. In rare cases, sudden bilateral loss of vision is due to **bilateral retinal ischemia**, for example, on standing up in a patient with stenosis or occlusion of the cerebral vessels that arise from the aorta (aortic arch syndrome). Certain types of **intoxication** can also rapidly produce bilateral optic nerve lesions, for example, methanol poisoning, which causes blindness within hours.

Progressive Impairment of Visual Acuity in One or Both Eyes

Unilateral impairment is due to a process causing more or less rapid, progressive damage to the optic nerve or chiasm. **Retrobulbar neuritis** (see "Clinical features and neurologic findings" in section 8.2), that is, inflammation of the optic nerve between the retina and the chiasm, and **optic papillitis**, that is,

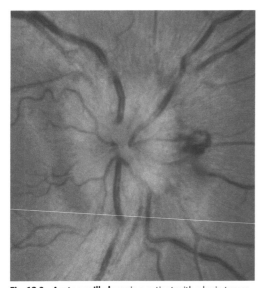

Fig. 12.3   Acute papilledema in a patient with a brain tumor. The optic disc is swollen, with blurred margins and a small hemorrhage at 3 o'clock.

inflammation of the optic nerve at the level of the optic disc, cause unilateral visual loss within a few days. Progressive, unilateral visual loss should also always prompt suspicion of a **mass**: optic glioma, for example, is a primary tumor within the optic nerve that is more common in children, while an optic sheath meningioma can compress the nerve from outside. Retrobulbar neuritis rarely occurs *bilaterally*, sometimes in combination with myelitis (cf. neuromyelitis optica, section 8.3.1). Further causes of bilateral loss of visual acuity are *Leber hereditary optic neuropathy* (LHON, a hereditary mitochondrial disease seen in men), and *tobacco–alcohol amblyopia*. In the latter condition, the most prominent initial finding is an inability to distinguish red from green. *Vitamin B_{12} deficiency* can cause progressive optic nerve atrophy in combination with polyneuropathy. Infections (syphilis, sarcoidosis) can also cause uni- or bilateral optic neuritis with impaired visual acuity.

Pathologic Findings of the Optic Disc

This is an area requiring close collaboration between the neurologist and the ophthalmologist.

Papilledema generally reflects intracranial hypertension but can also be seen in infectious or inflammatory disorders (e.g., syphilis). The typical findings include a somewhat enlarged, hyperemic optic disc with blurred margins, enlarged veins, and usually hemorrhages (**Fig. 12.3**). Inexperienced clinicians often have difficulty distinguishing papilledema from other changes of the optic disc.

Optic nerve atrophy is a permanent residual finding in the aftermath of an optic nerve lesion. The degree of visible atrophy does not necessarily correspond to the extent of visual loss. The optic disc is pale all the way to its margin, which remains sharp. These findings are typically seen after retrobulbar neuritis (see **Fig. 3.4**), but also after optic nerve compression (whether from outside, as by a meningioma, or from inside, as by an optic glioma). Further causes of optic nerve atrophy include chronic papilledema, syphilis, LHON, many types of spinocerebellar degeneration, ischemia, and exogenous intoxication.

12.3 Disturbances of Ocular and Pupillary Motility

   Key Point

Eye movements enable the centering of objects in the visual field and the ocular pursuit of moving objects. They are anatomically subserved by multiple neural structures, as discussed later. *Lesions of the supranuclear structures* (certain cortical areas, the brainstem gaze centers, and their connections to the brainstem nuclei that control eye movement)

cause horizontal or vertical gaze palsy, or inter-nuclear ophthalmoplegia. Such lesions must be distinguished from *nuclear and infranuclear lesions of the third, fourth, and sixth cranial nerves*. Lesions of all of these types can have a wide variety of causes. Moreover, abnormal eye movements and diplopia can also be due to *diseases of neuromuscular transmission* (e.g., myasthenia gravis), *diseases of the extraocular muscles themselves*, and orbital processes. Impaired pupillary motility has many different causes as well.

12.3.1 The General Principles of Eye Movements

> **NOTE**
>
> Saccades, slow pursuit, and convergence are physiologic types of eye movement. Multiple anatomic structures are involved in their coordination and control: the extraocular muscles, the three cranial nerves that innervate them (the oculomotor, trochlear, and abducens nerves), and the corresponding brainstem nuclei. These nuclei, in turn, are under the influence of central impulses that originate in certain areas of the cerebral cortex and are transmitted to the brainstem nuclei via the brainstem gaze centers or the vestibular system. The brainstem nuclei that control eye movement are also linked to each other by the medial longitudinal fasciculus.

The Anatomic Substrate of Eye Movements

The anatomic substrate of eye movements consists of the following structures:

- **Cortical areas** in the frontal, occipital, and temporal lobes, in which the impulses for voluntary conjugate eye movements and ocular pursuit are generated.
- Several important **gaze centers in the brainstem** (particularly the paramedian pontine reticular formation [PPRF] and midbrain nuclei) that relay the cortical impulses onward to the motor nuclei innervating the extraocular muscles, which, in turn, effect coordinated movement around the three major axes (horizontal, vertical, and rotatory eye movements). Special white matter tracts play an important role in this process, particularly the medial longitudinal fasciculus (MLF, **Fig. 12.4**).
- Finally, the **motor nuclei** and cranial nerves that innervate the **extraocular muscles**, and these **muscles** themselves (see **Fig. 3.8**).
- The entire process is also affected by cerebellar impulses and by **vestibular impulses** that enter the central nervous system through the eighth cranial nerve.

Types of Eye Movement

Eye movements can be divided into the following types:

- **Saccades** are rapid conjugate movements that are executed voluntarily or in reflex fashion in response to stimuli of various kinds. They serve to fix a newly selected object in the center of vision. Small microsaccades have an angular velocity of 20 degree/s, larger ones up to 700 degree/s. Saccades are the elementary type of rapid eye movement.
- Once the gaze has been fixated on a given object, **slow pursuit movements** serve to keep it in view if it is moving. The pursuit system is responsible for executing these conjugate eye movements: from the visual cortex in the occipital lobe, impulses travel to the eye fields of the temporal lobe ("medial superior temporal visual area") and the neighboring parietal cortex. These areas are interconnected with the PPRF and the cerebellum. Impulses from the PPRF control the nuclei of the eye muscles either directly or by way of interneurons.
- Disturbances of the pursuit system result in saccadic (jumpy) pursuit movements. If the saccade system is damaged as well, gaze palsy results (see later).
- **Convergence** enables fixation on a near object and is accomplished by simultaneous adduction of both eyes.

12.3.2 Nystagmus

> **NOTE**
>
> In purely descriptive terms, nystagmus is an involuntary, repetitive, rhythmic movement of the eyes. Nystagmus is often, but not always, pathologic.

Examples of physiologic nystagmus include optokinetic nystagmus (see "Physiologic Nystagmus") and the type of vestibular nystagmus that is induced by rotation in a swivel chair. End-gaze nystagmus (see "Vestibular Function" in section 3.3.2) is also physiologic, as long as it is symmetric in both directions. Pathologic nystagmus, on the other hand, indicates the presence of a lesion in the anatomic structures that subserve eye movements. Many components in this system can be damaged, and thus nystagmus has a wide spectrum of possible causes (see later).

Phenomenologic Classification of Nystagmus

As already discussed to some extent in section 3.3.2, nystagmus can be classified by various criteria:

- **Saltatory versus pendular nystagmus**: most types of nystagmus are either of the salutatory (jerking) type, that is, with a fast and a slow phase, or pendular (back-and-forth).

12

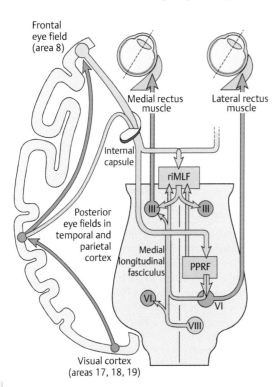

Frontal eye field (area 8)

Medial rectus muscle

Lateral rectus muscle

Internal capsule

riMLF

III   III

Posterior eye fields in temporal and parietal cortex

Medial longitudinal fasciculus

PPRF

VI   VI

VIII

Visual cortex (areas 17, 18, 19)

Fig. 12.4   Anatomic substrate of conjugate eye movements. The diagram shows the anatomic pathways for a conjugate movement to the right: neural impulses flow from the cortical eye fields of the left hemisphere to the right PPRF and onward to the nucleus of the right abducens nerve. Impulses in the abducens nerve induce contraction of the lateral rectus muscle of the right eye. Meanwhile, cortical impulses also travel by way of the medial longitudinal fasciculus to the nucleus of the left oculomotor nerve, and impulses in this nerve induce contraction of the medial rectus muscle of the left eye. Thus, lesions of the hemispheres or of the PPRF result in a palsy of conjugate horizontal gaze (hemispheric lesion: contralateral gaze palsy, PPRF lesion: ipsilateral gaze palsy). On the other hand, lesions of the medial longitudinal fasciculus cause an isolated loss of adduction of one eye during horizontal eye movement (internuclear ophthalmoplegia). Vertical eye movements are generated by the midbrain reticular formation (riMLF = rostral interstitial nucleus of the medial longitudinal fasciculus, see "Internuclear Ophthalmoplegia" in section 12.3.3), which receives input from both the cerebral cortex and the PPRF.

— **Direction of beat in relation to the three major axes of eye movement**: one speaks of horizontal, vertical, or rotatory nystagmus.
— **Direction of beat in relation to the midline of the eye**: nystagmus may beat to the left, to the right, upward, downward, or diagonally.
— In saltatory nystagmus, the **direction of beat is defined, by convention, as that of the rapid phase**, even though the slow phase is actually the pathologic component. The rapid phase is a physiologic correction that returns the eyes to their original position.
— Nystagmus can be **spontaneous** (see "Vestibular Function" in section 3.3.2) or else present only in response to **specific precipitating stimuli** (e.g., position, change of position, a rotatory or thermal stimulus to the vestibular system, or a particular direction of gaze [see discussion on gaze-evoked nystagmus later]).
— The examiner must also determine whether nystagmus is equally severe in both eyes, or whether it is weaker or perhaps absent in one eye. Nystagmus that is unequal in the two eyes is also called **dissociated nystagmus**.

A mainly phenomenologically oriented listing and illustration of the important types of nystagmus and their causes is found in **Table 12.2** and **Fig. 12.5**.
There are a few rarer types of nystagmus whose phenomenology is quite complex and not easily

described by the criteria listed earlier. These types of nystagmus are summarized in **Table 12.3**.

Topical Classification of Pathologic Nystagmus
Often, the type of nystagmus that is present provides a clue to the site of the lesion:
— **Gaze-paretic nystagmus** may be due to disease of the eye muscles themselves or a lesion of the cranial nerves innervating them or the corresponding brainstem nuclei. It is usually slow, coarse, and in the direction of the impairment of gaze.
— **Vestibular nystagmus** is due to a lesion of the vestibular organ itself or of the vestibular nerve or its brainstem nuclei. It is typically a spontaneous nystagmus that beats away from the side of the lesion, regardless of the direction of gaze (nystagmus in a fixed direction, cf. **Table 12.2**). It is typically inhibited by fixation; often, it can be observed only when the patient wears Frenzel goggles or shakes the head rapidly.
— **Gaze-evoked nystagmus** beats in the direction of gaze and indicates a lesion in the brainstem or its afferent or efferent connections with the cerebellum. If caused by a unilateral cerebellar lesion, it can be highly asymmetric or even beat only to the side of the lesion. If so, it may be hard to distinguish from vestibular nystagmus.
— **Nystagmus due to brainstem lesions.** Vestibular spontaneous nystagmus, gaze-evoked nystagmus, upbeat or downbeat vertical nystagmus, and

Table 12.2

Important physiologic and pathologic types of nystagmus

Type of nystagmus	Physiologic	Pathologic	Remarks
Optokinetic nystagmus	Must be symmetrically present	If asymmetric, dissociated, slowed, or absent	− Can be seen and tested by having the patient fixate on the pattern on a rotating drum
Vestibular nystagmus	Must be symmetrically present	If asymmetric, dissociated, or absent	− Elicited by lavage of the external auditory canal with cold or warm water (always after otoscopy to exclude a tympanic defect) − Also elicitable by rotating the patient in a swivel chair, if Frenzel goggles are worn to prevent fixation
Spontaneous nystagmus	Up to 5 degrees/s is normal in the dark	If present in the light	− Unidirectional: the nystagmus always beats in the same direction, independent of the direction of gaze − Can be inhibited by visual fixation − May be due to a central or peripheral vestibular lesion − **Grade III**: present in all directions of gaze − **Grade II**: visible with gaze straight ahead or in the direction of nystagmus − **Grade I**: visible only with gaze in the direction of nystagmus − **Head-shaking nystagmus**: inducible only by vigorous shaking of the head
Gaze-evoked nystagmus	Never	Always	− Beats in the direction of gaze − Defined as nystagmus in binocular visual field − Always due to a central lesion
End-gaze nystagmus	If symmetric	If asymmetric or dissociated	− Defined as nystagmus in monocular visual field
Positional nystagmus		Always pathologic	− Elicited by rapidly placing the patient supine with the head hanging down 30 degrees and to one side (Hallpike maneuver, **Fig. 12.28**) − Latency of 1 to several seconds, with increasing intensity for a few seconds followed by an equally rapid decline − Accompanied by a strong sensation of rotation and dizziness − Mainly rotatory; clockwise when the head hangs down and to the left, counterclockwise when it hangs down and to the right − Diminishes (habituates) on repeated elicitation
Pendular nystagmus		Always pathologic, but need not indicate active disease	− Sinusoidal back-and-forth movement − Increasing with attention or monocular fixation − Usually congenital, rarely acquired
Nystagmus induced by the vestibulo-ocular reflex suppression test (cf. VOR suppression test; nystagmus suppression test, **Fig. 12.6**)		Always pathologic	− When the patient is passively rotated en bloc while extending the arms in front and staring at the thumbs, visual fixation normally completely suppresses vestibular nystagmus − If nystagmus nonetheless appears, this indicates a lesion of the vestibulocerebellum or of its afferent or efferent connections − This test can be falsely positive with inadequate fixation

Source: Henn V. Nystagmus: Klinische Prüfung und Pathophysiologie. Akt Neurologie 1978;5:237–244.

positional and/or positioning nystagmus can all indicate the presence of a brainstem lesion. These types of nystagmus are often rotatory or dissociated (as in internuclear ophthalmoplegia [INO]).

− **Positioning nystagmus** is a mainly rotatory nystagmus that lasts several seconds after changes of position of a particular type; it is found in benign paroxysmal positioning vertigo, a disorder of the peripheral portion of the vestibular system (see section 12.6.2).

− **Congenital pendular nystagmus** is characterized by conjugate, pendular eye movements that increase with attention or monocular fixation. It is normally well compensated. There is no underlying, pathologic structural lesion.

Physiologic Nystagmus

The most important example is optokinetic nystagmus. This normal phenomenon serves to stabilize the visual image of a moving object on the retina and thus has the same purpose as the vestibulo-ocular reflex (VOR).

Optokinetic nystagmus consists of slow pursuit movements alternating with rapid return movements (saccades). The return movements occur whenever the moving object "threatens" to leave the visual field. If the object is moving very rapidly, optokinetic nystagmus can be voluntarily suppressed. Absent, asymmetric, or dissociated optokinetic nystagmus is pathologic.

12

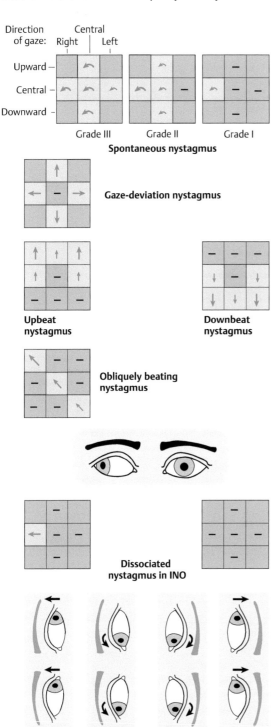

Fig. 12.5   The main types of nystagmus. For each type of nystagmus, the figure shows the intensity and direction of beating, depending on the direction of gaze. Positioning nystagmus is rotatory when the patient looks toward the lower ear (an exceptional case).

Table 12.3

Rare types of nystagmus

Type	Characteristics	Localization	Cause (examples)
Seesaw nystagmus	– Alternating movement of one eye upward and the other eye downward, accompanied by rotation – Various other kinds of eye movement can resemble this type of nystagmus	Oral brainstem and diencephalon	– Tumor – Multiple sclerosis – Vascular – Syringobulbia
Downbeat nystagmus	– Vertical nystagmus with rapid downward component	Caudal medullary lesion, floccular lesion, vitamin B_{12} deficiency	– As above – Phenytoin intoxication – Drugs of abuse
Convergence nystagmus	– Slow abduction followed by rapid adduction of both eyes	(Rostral) midbrain tegmentum	As above
Retraction nystagmus	– Jerking movements of both eyes back into their sockets – Usually accompanied by other oculomotor disturbances	Midbrain tegmentum	– Rare – Tumor – Multiple sclerosis – Vascular
Nystagmus with eyelid retraction	– Vertical nystagmus with upward rapid component – Accompanied by simultaneous rapid raising of upper lid	Pons and periaqueductal region	– Often vascular
Monocular nystagmus	– In internuclear ophthalmoplegia – As an ictal phenomenon in epilepsy	Medial longitudinal fasciculus	– Very rarely ictal – Multiple sclerosis – Vascular –
Opsoclonus (gaze myoclonus, dancing eyes)	– Spontaneous, grouped, variably rapid, nonrhythmic conjugate eye movements – Irregularly "dancing" back and forth	Brainstem and cerebellum	– Paraneoplastic – Neuroblastoma – Multiple sclerosis – Encephalitis
Ocular bobbing	– Rapid, nonrhythmic downward beating of the eyes, which stay down for a few seconds, then slowly return to the central position – Unilateral; the other side is usually blocked by oculomotor nerve palsy – May also be accompanied by synchronous palatal nystagmus	Pons, compression by cerebellar hemorrhage (lesion of central tegmental tract)	– Tumor – Ischemia – Hemorrhage
Gaze dysmetria	– Overshooting movements when redirecting gaze to a new target, followed by compensatory corrections (ocular apraxia)	Cerebellar	– For example, multiple sclerosis
Ocular flutter (ocular myoclonus)	– Rapid, irregular back-and-forth movements around the point of fixation	As for opsoclonus and gaze dysmetria	

The **vestibulo-ocular reflex** is a function of the labyrinth that serves to stabilize gaze fixation during rapid movements of the head: it produces a compensatory eye movement in the direction opposite to the head movement. Slower head movements do not need to be compensated for by the vestibular system, as the ocular pursuit system suffices to keep gaze fixated in this case (see section 12.3.1, The Anatomic Substrate of Eye Movements). Vestibular nystagmus can be suppressed by fixation on an object moving in tandem with the head (nystagmus or VOR suppression test, see later). An inability to suppress the VOR by fixation is pathologic.

– **Nystagmus suppression** test (= VOR suppression test). In this test, the person stretches both arms forward, holds his or her thumbs up, and fixates gaze on them. When the person is rapidly rotated around the long axis of the body, there is normally no nystagmus, because vestibular nystagmus can be suppressed by visual fixation (**Fig. 12.6**). If nystagmus does appear, this indicates a lesion in the cerebellum or its connections with the vestibular apparatus of the brainstem.

12.3.3 Supranuclear Oculomotor Disturbances

NOTE

These disturbances are characterized by the simultaneous impairment of the voluntary movements and involuntary pursuit movements of both eyes. The eyes generally remain parallel to each other ("conjugated") but cannot be moved together in the horizontal or

12

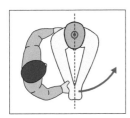
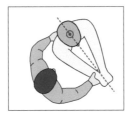

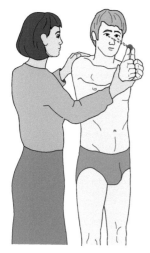
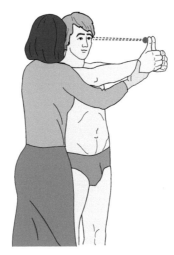

Fig. 12.6 Nystagmus suppression test. The patient extends the arms, fixates gaze on his or her own thumbs, and is then rapidly rotated "en bloc" by the examiner. In a normal individual, gaze fixation on the thumbs prevents the appearance of nystagmus. Failure to suppress nystagmus indicates a central lesion, usually in the cerebellum.

vertical plane. The lesion lies above the level of the cranial nerve nuclei, that is, "supranuclear." In disorders of the brainstem, supranuclear lesions may coexist with nuclear lesions so that the eyes can be disconjugate. Only in this case will there be diplopia.

Horizontal Gaze Palsy

A patient with horizontal gaze palsy cannot make a conjugate movement of the eyes to the right, to the left, or (rarely) in either of the two directions. The causative lesion may be at any of several sites in the central nervous system:

- **Cortical centers** that generate the impulses for horizontal gaze movements, particularly the frontal eye field of the frontal lobe.
- The **paramedian pontine reticular formation**, which receives the impulses from the higher cortical centers and relays them to the ipsilateral abducens nerve nucleus (innervation of the lateral rectus muscle) and simultaneously, by way of interneurons, to the contralateral oculomotor nerve nucleus (innervation of the medial rectus muscle). The latter connection is by way of the MLF (see **Fig. 12.4**). The result is an ipsilateral, conjugate, horizontal gaze movement (i.e., to the left on activation of the left PPRF and to the right on activation of the right PPRF).
- **A lesion of the abducens nucleus** has the same effect as a PPRF lesion, that is, a conjugate horizontal gaze palsy to the side of the lesion.

Lesions of the Frontal Eye Field

This field is in area 8 in the middle frontal gyrus. The right eye field generates conjugate gaze movements to the left, and vice versa. When the frontal eye field is affected by an acute lesion, the influence of the contralateral field predominates for a few hours (or, rarely, days), so that the eyes (and the head) deviate to the side of the lesion: **déviation conjuguée** (**Fig. 12.7**), the patient "looks at the lesion." Déviation conjuguée is usually accompanied by contralateral hemiparesis.

Active gaze movements toward the midline rapidly become possible again; so, later, do movements to the opposite side. As contralateral movements begin to reemerge, they are accompanied by *gaze-paretic nystagmus*, whose rapid component beats away from the side of the lesion.

Lesions of the Posterior Hemispheric Cortex

Horizontal gaze palsy due to an occipital lesion is often accompanied by hemianopsia. The gaze palsy is characterized by saccadic ocular pursuit. Optokinetic nystagmus (see "Physiologic Nystagmus" in section 12.3.2) is also impaired.

Lesions of the Paramedian Pontine Reticular Formation

These affect the last supranuclear relay station for horizontal gaze movements. They usually cause long-lasting or permanent *gaze palsy to the side of the lesion*.

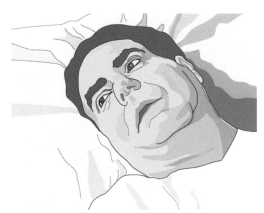

Fig. 12.7   Déviation conjuguée of the head and eyes (to the right). This 65-year-old man has sustained an acute ischemic stroke in the territory of the right middle cerebral artery and is hemiplegic on the left.

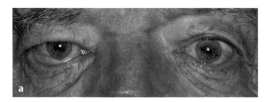

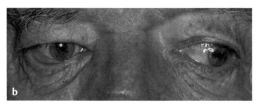

Fig. 12.9   Right internuclear ophthalmoplegia in a patient with a lacunar brainstem infarct. **a** When the patient looks straight ahead, the eyes are parallel. **b** On attempted leftward gaze, right eye adduction is impaired (weakness of the medial rectus muscle).

Lesions of the Abducens Nucleus

These affect not only the neurons whose axons constitute the sixth cranial nerve but also interneurons that connect the nucleus by way of the adjacent MLF to the contralateral oculomotor nucleus, which innervates the contralateral medial rectus muscle. *The clinical picture is initially very similar to that of a PPRF lesion.* PPRF lesions, however, spare the vestibulo-ocular connections in the MLF and do not directly involve the cranial nerve nuclei subserving eye movement; thus, in PPRF lesions, the gaze palsy can be overcome by a vestibular stimulus. Gaze palsy due to a lesion of the abducens nerve nucleus cannot be overcome either voluntarily or through any kind of reflex.

Vertical Gaze Palsy

Impairment of upward or downward conjugate gaze is always due to a **midbrain lesion** involving either

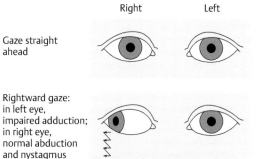

Fig. 12.8   Internuclear ophthalmoplegia (INO), left. When the patient looks straight ahead, the eyes are parallel. On attempted rightward gaze, the left medial rectus muscle fails to contract (no adduction of the left eye) and there is nystagmus of the abducted right eye.

the *rostral interstitial nucleus* of the MLF (the Büttner–Ennever nucleus) or its *efferent fibers* (**Fig. 12.4**). In most patients, both upward and downward gaze are impaired, but pretectal lesions can cause isolated upward gaze palsy. Vertical gaze palsy is one of the clinical features of progressive supranuclear palsy (see section 6.9.4).

Internuclear Ophthalmoplegia

This condition is caused by a **lesion of the MLF.** When the patient attempts to look away from the side of the lesion, the ipsilateral (adducting) eye cannot fully adduct, and the contralateral (abducting) eye exhibits end-gaze nystagmus. The inability of the ipsilateral eye to adduct is not due to a lesion of the oculomotor nerve nucleus, as is demonstrated by a preserved ability to adduct (converge) in the near reflex. INO can also be bilateral if the MLF is damaged on both sides. **Fig. 12.8** illustrates the clinical findings in INO with total loss of adduction of the left eye. **Fig. 12.9** shows a more common type of INO, in which the inward movement of the adducting eye is merely delayed and eventually takes place with slow, horizontal saccades. This type of INO is particularly common in multiple sclerosis.

One-and-a-Half Syndrome

This name is given to the combination of horizontal gaze paresis to one side ("one") with INO on attempted gaze to the other side ("… and a half"). As one might expect, it is due to **combined lesions of the PPRF or abducens nerve nucleus** on one side and of the **ipsilateral MLF.** The sole horizontal eye movement that remains possible is abduction of the contralateral eye on attempted contralateral gaze.

Skew Deviation

Skew deviation, also called Hertwig-Magendie syndrome or Hertwig-Magendie strabismus, is a vertical strabismus in which one eye is higher than the other, usually with cycloversion of both eyes in the same direction. The subjective vertical axis is displaced. Skew deviation can be detected with a cover test; cycloversion is best demonstrated by photography of the fundi. The underlying lesion is in the brainstem, usually in the dorsal part of the mesencephalon.

Oculomotor Disturbances of Cerebellar Origin

Cerebellar lesions can cause the following disturbances of eye movement:
- Gaze-deviation nystagmus.
- Inability to suppress the oculovestibular reflex by fixation.
- Saccadic pursuit.
- Diminished optokinetic nystagmus.
- Dysmetric saccades (under- and overshoot).
- Overshooting VOR.
- Special types of nystagmus, such as upbeat nystagmus, downbeat nystagmus, rebound nystagmus, periodically alternating nystagmus, acquired pendular nystagmus, central positional nystagmus, other types.
- Unilateral cerebellar lesions produce ipsilateral nystagmus (as in spontaneous vestibular nystagmus).

Other Supranuclear Disturbances of Eye Movement

Another disturbance worth mentioning here is **oculomotor apraxia**. In the congenital form (**Cogan syndrome**), the patient is unable to direct his or her gaze voluntarily to the beginning of a line of text while reading. Instead, the entire head must be moved into position so that the beginning of the line lands in the center of the visual field. Once this is done, the head can be moved back to its original position without loss of fixation on the text.

12.3.4 Lesions of the Nerves to the Eye Muscles and Their Brainstem Nuclei

> **NOTE**
>
> Lesions of this type, like lesions of the eye muscles themselves, cause deviation of the axis of one eye, that is, paralytic strabismus. The patient reports seeing double (diplopia).

Oculomotor Nerve Palsy

An infranuclear lesion of the third cranial nerve causes paralysis of the medial, superior, and inferior rectus muscles; the inferior oblique muscles (cf. **Fig. 3.8**); and the levator palpebrae muscle (**external ophthalmoplegia**). In addition, the smooth muscle of the pupillary sphincter is paralyzed: the pupil is "fixed and dilated," that is, it is enlarged and responds neither to light nor to convergence (**internal ophthalmoplegia, Fig. 12.16**). The typical clinical appearance of oculomotor nerve palsy is thus immediately recognizable when the patient looks straight ahead (**Fig. 12.10**). **Fig. 12.11** illustrates the typical findings in primary position and in the position of greatest deviation, as well as the positions of the two visual images depending on the patient's direction of gaze.

The third cranial nerve can be affected by a lesion at its nucleus in the brainstem (**nuclear lesion**), at various points along its course within the brainstem (**fascicular lesion**), or in the periphery (**peripheral nerve lesion**). There are many possible causes and the resulting neurologic deficits are correspondingly varied. Typical symptom constellations involving oculomotor nerve palsy and various other findings, depending on the site and etiology of the lesion, are presented in **Table 12.4**. Lesions of the oculomotor nucleus also cause bilateral ptosis and upward gaze paresis.

Trochlear Nerve Palsy

Lesions of the fourth cranial nerve cause **paralysis of the superior oblique muscle** (cf. **Fig. 3.8**). The affected eye cannot be depressed in adduction, or rotated in abduction. Diplopia arises when the patient looks down; the images are vertically displaced and slightly tilted. The typical clinical situation is shown schematically in **Fig. 12.12**. The two images can be brought together again by tilting the head to the normal side; the distance between the images increases if the head is tilted to the affected side (**Bielschowsky phenomenon**).

Causes. The more common causes of trochlear nerve palsy are as follows:
- Congenital aplasia.
- Trauma.
- Midbrain hemorrhage.
- Multiple sclerosis.
- Ischemic neuropathy of the nerve, for example, in diabetes mellitus.
- Pathologic processes in the cavernous sinus.
- Pathologic processes in the orbit.

Differential diagnosis (pathologic processes affecting the superior oblique muscle). The tendon of the superior oblique muscle changes direction in the trochlea, sliding within it like a pulley. The tendon can sometimes be caught in the ring of the trochlea, thus becoming "stuck" in the middle of a movement. This causes intermittent vertical diplopia, typically when the patient looks up just after looking down, and typically only lasting for a very short time (Brown syndrome). Myokymia of the superior oblique muscle can arise in the aftermath of a trochlear nerve palsy, or independently. Its typical clinical sign is monocular, high-frequency nystagmus with oscillopsia and diplopia.

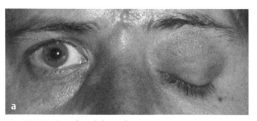
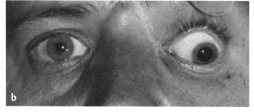

Fig. 12.10   Complete left oculomotor nerve palsy. a Complete ptosis of the left eye. **b** The examiner lifts the ptotic eyelid to reveal the mydriatic, fixed (i.e., unreactive) pupil. The eye is also mildly abducted through the predominant effect of the lateral rectus and superior oblique muscles, which are innervated by the abducens and trochlear nerves (cf. also **Fig. 3.8**).

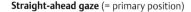

Straight-ahead gaze (= primary position)

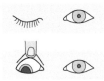

Greatest disparity of images

Fig. 12.11   Right oculomotor nerve palsy. Note the position of the eyes and the position of the two visual images (diplopia) in different directions of gaze.

Fixed, dilated pupil in total CN III palsy

Compensatory head position:

none if ptosis is present, because there is no diplopia

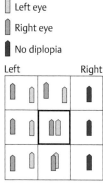

Weakness mainly of the medial rectus muscle

Table 12.4

Localization and etiology of oculomotor nerve palsy

Site of lesion	Clinical features	Causes
Nuclear	Oculomotor nerve palsy, bilateral vertical gaze palsy, bilateral ptosis	Infarct, hemorrhage, trauma, tumor, multiple sclerosis, inflammation, congenital hypoplasia
Fascicular (oculomotor nerve fascicle within the brainstem)	Oculomotor nerve palsy, contralateral hemiparesis, ataxia or rubral tremor (differential diagnosis: transtentorial herniation)	Infarct, hemorrhage, multiple sclerosis
Subarachnoid space	Isolated oculomotor nerve palsy	Aneurysm (posterior communicating artery, rarely other arteries such as the basilar artery), basilar meningitis, cranial polyradiculitis, intracranial hypertension, trauma, neurosurgical complication, tumor of the oculomotor nerve, transtentorial herniation
Cavernous sinus, superior orbital fissure, or orbit	Oculomotor nerve palsy accompanied by dysfunction of the trochlear, ophthalmic, and/or abducens nerves, in varying combinations	Aneurysm (internal carotid artery), carotid–cavernous fistula, cavernous sinus thrombosis, parasellar tumor or pituitary tumor with parasellar extension, sphenoid sinusitis, Tolosa–Hunt syndrome, herpes zoster
Orbital apex	Oculomotor nerve palsy accompanied by dysfunction of the optic, trochlear, ophthalmic, and/or abducens nerves, in varying combinations	See lists of causes above and below (cavernous sinus, orbit)
Orbit (superior branch of oculomotor nerve)	Ptosis and superior rectus palsy	Trauma, orbital tumor, orbital pseudotumor, infection, mucocele
Orbit (inferior branch of oculomotor nerve)	Palsy of inferior and medial recti and inferior oblique muscles	Trauma, orbital tumor, orbital pseudotumor, infection, mucocele
No localizing significance	Isolated external oculomotor nerve palsy (i.e., pupillary sparing)	Diabetes, hypertension, arteritis, migraine

12

Straight-ahead gaze (= primary position)

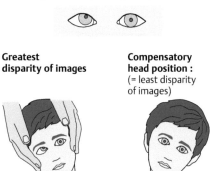

Greatest disparity of images

Compensatory head position : (= least disparity of images)

Head tilt to side of paretic muscle (Bielschowsky phenomenon)

Head tilt away from side of paretic muscle

☐ Left eye
☐ Right eye
■ No diplopia

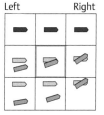

Weakness of the superior oblique muscle

Fig. 12.12 Right trochlear nerve palsy. Note the position of the eyes, the compensatory head tilt, and the position of the two visual images depending on the direction of gaze.

Abducens Nerve Palsy

Paralysis of the lateral rectus muscle (cf. **Fig. 3.8**) due to a lesion of the sixth cranial nerve causes weakness of abduction and, sometimes, inward strabismus of the affected eye. Horizontal diplopia is sometimes present even in the primary position of gaze and worsens when the patient looks toward the affected side. The findings are presented schematically in **Fig. 12.13. Fig. 12.14** shows the clinical findings in a patient with an incomplete right abducens palsy. The more common causes are listed in **Table 12.5**.

Combined Lesions of Multiple Cranial Nerves Innervating the Muscles of Eye Movement, and Other Disorders in the Differential Diagnosis of Diplopia

If multiple cranial nerves innervating the muscles of eye movement **on one side** are affected, the lesion usually lies in the cavernous sinus, at the orbital apex, or in the orbit itself.

Bilateral, multiple palsies of the muscles of eye movement are often due to brainstem processes; the differential diagnosis includes the entire spectrum of supranuclear oculomotor disturbances, brainstem lesions, and peripheral lesions such as cranial polyradiculitis, basilar meningitis (see section 6.7.4), carcinomatous meningitis, and skull base tumors. In addition, disorders of neuromuscular transmission, such as myasthenia gravis (see section 15.8.1), and diseases of the eye muscles themselves must be considered, including myositis of the eye muscles (rare), mitochondrial myopathy (Kearns–Sayre syndrome), or endocrine ophthalmopathy in hyperthyroidism (Graves disease).

12.3.5 Ptosis

> **NOTE**
>
> A common cause of ptosis is Horner syndrome. The narrower gap between the eyelids on the side of the Horner syndrome is best seen when the patient looks slightly downward.

Ptosis is present when the upper lid covers the upper border of the pupil. The cause of ptosis can be **myogenic**, **neurogenic**, or **mechanical** (e.g., dehiscence of the levator aponeurosis).

The eyelid is actively elevated mainly by the striated **levator palpebrae muscle**, which is innervated by the oculomotor nerve. Paralysis of this muscle causes ptosis that is most evident when the patient looks upward. The eyelid is also elevated, however, by the sympathetically innervated, smooth **superior tarsal muscle**. It follows that ptosis can be produced by lesions either of the oculomotor nerve or of the sympathetic innervation of the eye. The causes of ptosis are listed in **Table 12.6**.

Horner Syndrome

Horner syndrome is caused by loss of the sympathetic innervation of the eye and consists of the following:

- **Ptosis** (paralysis of the sympathetically innervated superior tarsal muscle), most evident when the patient looks slightly downward.
- **Miosis** (paralysis of the sympathetically innervated dilator pupillae muscle).
- Mild **enophthalmos** (paralysis of Müller's muscle, a smooth muscle in the orbit).
- **Conjunctival hyperemia** (loss of the constrictive effect of the sympathetic nervous system on the conjunctival vessels).

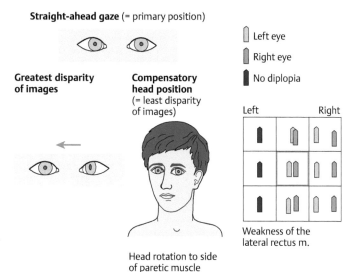

Straight-ahead gaze (= primary position)

Left eye

Right eye

No diplopia

Greatest disparity of images

Compensatory head position (= least disparity of images)

Weakness of the lateral rectus m.

Fig. 12.13   Right abducens nerve palsy. Note the position of the eyes, the compensatory rotation of the head, and the position of the two visual images depending on the direction of gaze.

Head rotation to side of paretic muscle

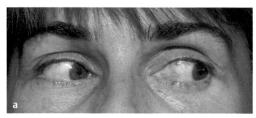
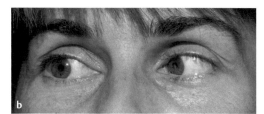

Fig. 12.14   Partial right abducens nerve palsy. a On leftward gaze, the eyes are parallel; **b** on rightward gaze, the right eye fails to abduct to the full extent.

The clinical findings in Horner syndrome are shown in **Fig. 12.15**.

Localization of the lesion.

- If Horner syndrome is not accompanied by a loss of sweating in one-half of the face, then the underlying lesion is located in the (ventral) roots of C8 through T2 proximal to their joining the sympathetic chain.
- If it is accompanied by a loss of sweating in the face, neck, and arm on one side, then the lesion is at the stellate ganglion, or at a more cranial level of the sympathetic plexus in the neck.
- A lesion of the sympathetic chain immediately below the stellate ganglion impairs sweating in the ipsilateral upper quarter of the body but does not produce Horner syndrome. (This is why thoracic sympathectomy is sometimes performed at this site to treat hyperhidrosis.)

12.3.6 Pupillary Disturbances

| NOTE

Disturbances of pupillary motility have many different causes. Lesions of the retina and optic nerve affect the afferent arm of the pupillary light reflex, while oculomotor nerve lesions affect its efferent arm. In the former case, the pupil constricts only when the contralateral eye is illuminated (consensual response); in the latter case, it does not constrict at all, either directly or consensually.

Pupillary motility is controlled by the parasympathetic portion of the oculomotor nerve (sphincter pupillae muscle) and by the sympathetic nervous system (ciliary muscle = dilator pupillae muscle). The constrictor and dilator muscles of the pupil are both smooth muscles; **the parasympathetic nervous system constricts the pupil and the sympathetic nervous system dilates it**.

| NOTE

A lesion of the oculomotor nerve thus produces a wide pupil, while a lesion of the sympathetic supply produces a narrow pupil.

Abnormalities of the Size and Shape of the Pupil

In **pupillary ectopia**, the pupil is eccentrically positioned in the iris. This may be due to a congenital malformation, prior inflammation of the iris, or

Table 12.5

Localization and etiology of abducens nerve palsy

Site of lesion	Clinical features	Etiology
Nuclear, pontine paramedian reticular formation	Gaze palsy, often combined with peripheral or nuclear facial nerve palsy	Infarct, hemorrhage, tumor, multiple sclerosis, inflammation, trauma, congenital aplasia
Fascicular	Abducens palsy with contralateral hemiparesis, occasionally also trigeminal deficit	Infarct, hemorrhage, multiple sclerosis
Subarachnoid space	Isolated abducens nerve palsy	Intracranial hypertension, intracranial hypotension, aneurysm (anterior inferior or posterior inferior cerebellar artery, basilar artery), subarachnoid hemorrhage, basilar meningitis, cranial polyradiculitis, trauma, neurosurgical complication, tumor of the abducens nerve, clivus tumor
Petrous apex, petrous bone	Deficits of trigeminal and abducens nerves, sometimes also facial and vestibulocochlear nerves	Extradural infection in otitis media
Cavernous sinus, superior orbital fissure	Abducens nerve palsy accompanied by dysfunction of the oculomotor, trochlear, and/or ophthalmic nerves, in varying combinations	Aneurysm (internal carotid artery), carotid–cavernous fistula, cavernous sinus thrombosis, parasellar tumor or pituitary tumor with parasellar extension, sphenoid sinusitis, Tolosa–Hunt syndrome, herpes zoster
Orbital apex	Abducens palsy accompanied by dysfunction of the oculomotor, trochlear, and/or ophthalmic nerves, in varying combinations	See lists of causes above and below (cavernous sinus, orbit)
Orbit	Lateral rectus palsy, either in isolation or combined with other deficits	Trauma, orbital tumor, orbital pseudotumor, endocrine ophthalmopathy, infection, mucocele
No localizing significance	Isolated lateral rectus (abducens nerve) palsy	Diabetes, hypertension, arteritis, migraine

Table 12.6

Causes of ptosis

Pathogenesis	Causes (examples)
Mechanical factors	— Connective tissue defect (e.g., dehiscence of levator aponeurosis) — Local orbital change — Microphthalmia
Muscle disease	— Progressive external ophthalmoplegia — Steinert myotonic dystrophy
Neuromuscular transmission disorder	— Myasthenia gravis — Botulism
Neurogenic: loss of innervation	— Oculomotor nerve lesion — Midbrain infarction — Cortical lesion — Sympathetic lesion (central or peripheral)
Neurogenic: excessively strong innervation	— Blepharospasm — Faulty regeneration after facial nerve palsy — Hemifacial spasm

incomplete nerve regeneration after a prior oculomotor nerve palsy. **Abnormally shaped pupils** are usually congenital. Mild inequality of pupillary size is a common, normal finding, but marked asymmetry is generally pathologic. Inequality of the pupils is called **anisocoria**; its causes include Horner syndrome and Adie syndrome (see later) and others.

Abnormalities of the Pupillary Reflexes

The direct and consensual pupillary light reflexes (see "Pupils" in section 3.3.2) can be impaired by any of the following:

- **Local affections of the eye**, such as glaucoma or posterior synechiae.
- **The Marcus Gunn phenomenon** is an impairment of the direct pupillary response to light on the

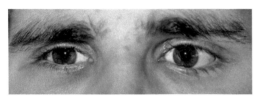

Fig. 12.15   Right Horner syndrome in a patient with right carotid artery dissection. The right pupil and eyelid gap are markedly narrower than on the left.

side of an acute or prior episode of retrobulbar neuritis.

- **Adie pupil** (pupillotonia) is usually unilateral, at least at first. The pupil is wider on the affected side and constricts very slowly in response to light, but more rapidly and completely on convergence. The subsequent widening of the pupil is slow (tonic). Women are more commonly affected than men; often, but not always, individual intrinsic muscle reflexes are absent. The underlying lesion is thought to lie either in the midbrain or in the ciliary ganglion.
- **Acute ciliary ganglionitis** (due to infection or trauma) renders the pupil unresponsive to light or convergence.
- **Reflex pupillary rigidity** (Argyll Robertson pupil) is a typical finding in late neurosyphilis. The pupils are generally narrow, usually oblong, and unresponsive to light (either directly or indirectly), but they constrict on convergence. It should be emphasized, however, that fixed and dilated pupils can also be seen in neurosyphilis.
- **A normal pupillary light reflex in a patient who is totally blind** implies bilateral damage to the visual pathway at some point between the lateral geniculate body and the visual cortex. The usual cause is bilateral infarction of the visual cortex. The direct and consensual light reflexes are preserved because the nerve fibers subserving them branch off the visual pathway proximal to the lateral geniculate body and then travel to the pretectal area to innervate their target nuclei.
- **Hippus**, a rhythmic fluctuation of pupillary width, is usually physiologic.
- The major abnormalities of pupillary size and responsiveness are summarized in **Fig. 12.16**.

12.4 Lesions of the Trigeminal Nerve

  Key Point

The trigeminal nerve is responsible for the somatosensory innervation of the skin of the face and forehead and of the mucous membranes of the nose, paranasal sinuses, and

mouth. It also carries motor fibers that innervate the muscles of mastication. Lesions of this nerve thus produce sensory deficits and weakness of the muscles of mastication.

The anatomic course and distribution of the **trigeminal nerve** are shown in **Fig. 3.10**, and the technique of clinical examination is presented in section 3.3.2.
Clinical features. Trigeminal lesions produce **sensory deficits in the face and head**. The somatosensory distribution of the three branches of the trigeminal nerve is shown in **Fig. 12.17**. Lesions of the trigeminal nuclei in the brainstem cause a sensory deficit that is centered on the upper lip and extends over the entire face in an onion-skin pattern (Lähr-Solder lines, **Fig. 12.17**). Lesions of the motor portion of the third branch cause **paralysis of the muscles of mastication**. The examiner can usually easily feel the diminished contraction of the masseter muscle on one side. When the mouth is opened, the jaw deviates toward the paralyzed side because of weakness of the pterygoid muscles (**Fig. 12.18**).
Causes. Nuclear lesions of the trigeminal nerve are located in the pons or medulla and are usually due to vascular processes, encephalitis, multiple sclerosis plaques, or a space-occupying lesion (glioma, syringobulbia). The nerve can also be affected in its **peripheral** course by mass lesions, toxic influences, or mechanical (iatrogenic) factors. The trigeminal nerve can also be affected in cranial polyradiculitis. Occasionally, no clear cause can be found (idiopathic trigeminal neuropathy, which is usually unilateral). Trigeminal neuralgia, a syndrome characterized by brief, intense, lightning-like, lancinating facial pain, is discussed in section 14.3.1.

12.5 Lesions of the Facial Nerve

  Key Point

This mainly motor cranial nerve innervates the muscles of facial expression. It also supplies taste to the anterior two-thirds of the tongue and innervates the lacrimal and salivatory glands. Lesions of the facial nerve usually lie in the peripheral nerve trunk and are clinically evident mainly as facial palsy. Peripheral facial nerve palsy often arises without any apparent cause, that is, it is often cryptogenic. Cryptogenic weakness must be carefully differentiated from symptomatic weakness of central or peripheral origin.

The anatomic course of the seventh cranial nerve is depicted in **Fig. 12.19**.

12

12.5.1 Topical Classification of Facial Palsy

The clinical picture of a (complete) facial nerve palsy varies depending on the site of the lesion (**Fig. 12.20**):

— **Lesions distal to the sternomastoid foramen** typically cause a purely motor paralysis of all the muscles of facial expression on one half of the face. The eye cannot be closed (lagophthalmos) and the forehead cannot be wrinkled. No other deficit is present.

— **Lesions in the petrous bone or the facial (Fallopian) canal** (the most common site) cause

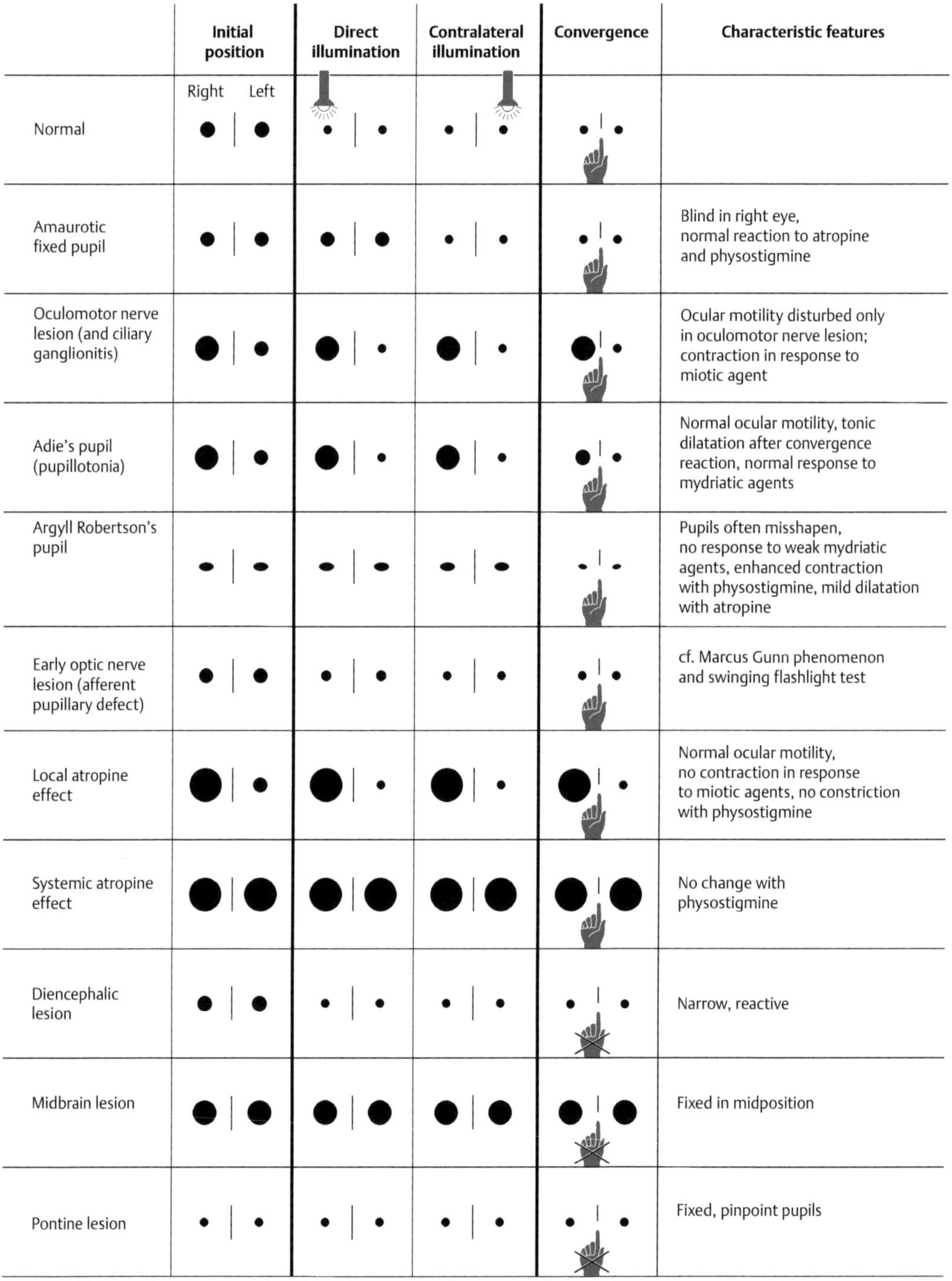

	Initial position		Direct illumination	Contralateral illumination	Convergence	Characteristic features
	Right	Left				
Normal	●	●	• | •	• | •	• | •	
Amaurotic fixed pupil	●	●	● | ●	• | •	• | •	Blind in right eye, normal reaction to atropine and physostigmine
Oculomotor nerve lesion (and ciliary ganglionitis)	● | •	● | •	● | •	● | •	Ocular motility disturbed only in oculomotor nerve lesion; contraction in response to miotic agent
Adie's pupil (pupillotonia)	● | •	● | •	● | •	• | •	Normal ocular motility, tonic dilatation after convergence reaction, normal response to mydriatic agents
Argyll Robertson's pupil	• | •	• | •	• | •	· | ·	Pupils often misshapen, no response to weak mydriatic agents, enhanced contraction with physostigmine, mild dilatation with atropine
Early optic nerve lesion (afferent pupillary defect)	• | •	• | •	• | •	• | •	cf. Marcus Gunn phenomenon and swinging flashlight test
Local atropine effect	● | •	● | •	● | •	● | •	Normal ocular motility, no contraction in response to miotic agents, no constriction with physostigmine
Systemic atropine effect	● | ●	● | ●	● | ●	● | ●	No change with physostigmine
Diencephalic lesion	• | •	• | •	• | •	• | •	Narrow, reactive
Midbrain lesion	● | ●	● | ●	● | ●	● | ●	Fixed in midposition
Pontine lesion	• | •	• | •	• | •	• | •	Fixed, pinpoint pupils

Fig. 12.16 Abnormalities of the pupillary reflexes (right side abnormal). (Reproduced from Mattle H, Mumenthaler M. Neurologie. Stuttgart: Thieme; 2013.)

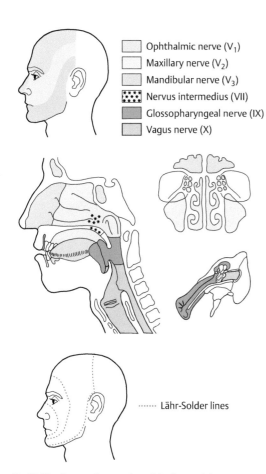

Ophthalmic nerve (V₁)
Maxillary nerve (V₂)
Mandibular nerve (V₃)
Nervus intermedius (VII)
Glossopharyngeal nerve (IX)
Vagus nerve (X)

········ Lähr-Solder lines

Fig. 12.17 Sensory innervation of the face and the mucous membranes of the head.

disturbances of lacrimation and salivation, impairment of taste, and/or hyperacusis in addition to the motor weakness of the face. All of these manifestations occur to varying extents depending on the precise location of the lesion.

— **Lesions of the facial nerve nucleus** or of its nerve fascicle within the brainstem are rarer and are mainly evident as a motor deficit including lagophthalmos and an inability to wrinkle the forehead. Lacrimation, salivation, and taste are normal, because the parasympathetic and gustatory fibers of the facial nerve are derived from (or travel to) other brainstem nuclei.

— **Lesions above the facial nerve nucleus** (central facial palsy). The typical finding in such cases is perioral weakness. The eye can still be closed on the affected side, and the forehead can be symmetrically wrinkled, because these muscles (like the respiratory muscles) derive their innervation from both cerebral hemispheres.

12.5.2 Etiologic Classification of Facial Palsy

Cryptogenic facial palsy is the most common type and must be distinguished from other, symptomatic varieties. Its cause is unknown and is thought to be either a viral infection (e.g., by a herpesvirus) or a parainfectious process (see later).

In **symptomatic forms**, an anatomic cause for the facial palsy can be found:

— **A basilar skull fracture** can damage the facial nerve. Transverse fractures of the petrous bone cause immediate and often irreversible facial palsy. Longitudinal fractures frequently give rise to facial palsy only after a delay, usually because of a slowly expanding hematoma in the wall of the facial canal; the prognosis in such cases is better than in transverse fractures.

— **Middle ear processes** (e.g., cholesteatoma) can cause facial nerve palsy.

12

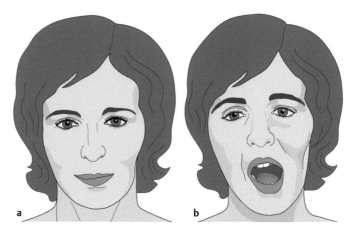

Fig. 12.18 Lesion of the motor portion of the left trigeminal nerve. a Atrophy of the left temporalis and masseter muscles.
b Deviation of the jaw to the left on opening.

a   b

Neural pathways of:
Lacrimation and salivation
Preganglionic ▬▬▬
Postganglionic ▪▪▪▪▪▪▪▪▪▪▪

Mucosal sensation
Taste
Cranial part
Caudal part

* Chorda tympani
** Stapedius muscle

Motor

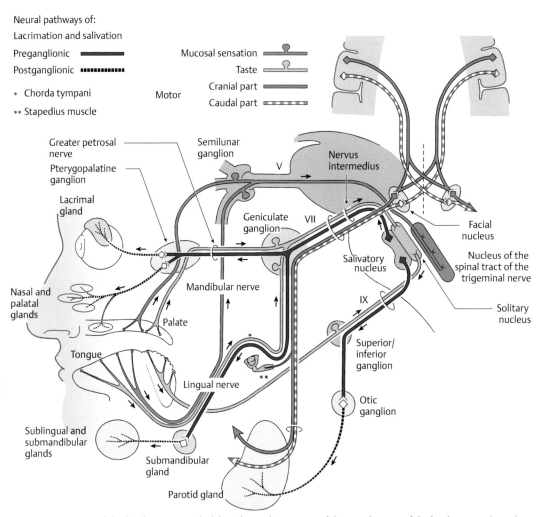

Fig. 12.19 Anatomy of the facial nerve. Note the bilateral central innervation of the cranial portion of the facial nerve nucleus. The caudal portion is innervated only by the contralateral hemisphere.

- **Tumors** of the skull base or the parotid gland can do so as well.
- **Viral infections**, particularly herpes zoster oticus, and borreliosis (Lyme disease) can affect the facial nerve to produce a facial palsy.
- **Nuclear facial palsy** arises if the facial nerve nucleus in the pons is damaged by ischemia or by a tumor (brainstem glioma).
- **Bilateral facial palsy** can be caused by (cranial) polyradiculitis, borreliosis, sarcoidosis, a meningeal tumor, or a brain tumor (see **Fig. 11.1**).

Cryptogenic Peripheral Facial Nerve Palsy
Epidemiology. This condition ("Bell palsy") accounts for three-quarters of all cases of facial palsy and has an annual incidence of approximately 25 per 100,000 individuals.
Etiology. The ultimate cause is unknown, but it is probably a viral infection. Swelling of the facial nerve

trunk in the narrow confines of the facial canal impairs nerve conduction and can cause axonotmesis in severe cases. The pathologic mechanism is thought to be compressive ischemia.
Clinical features. The most prominent finding is **weakness of the muscles of facial expression**, which can be of variable extent but is often complete; see **Fig. 12.21**. There is also an impairment of taste on the anterior two-thirds of the tongue on the affected side (for the technique of examination, cf. "Taste, Lacrimation, and Salivation" in section 3.3.2). Bitter tastes can usually still be perceived, because the receptors for this modality lie in the mucosa of the posterior third of the tongue, which is innervated by the glossopharyngeal nerve. **Lacrimation and salivation** are also ipsilaterally impaired. Dysacusis or hyperacusis, due to denervation of the stapedius muscle, is hardly ever clinically evident.
Treatment. Corticosteroids improve the outcome (e.g., prednisone 60 mg orally daily for 4 days, then

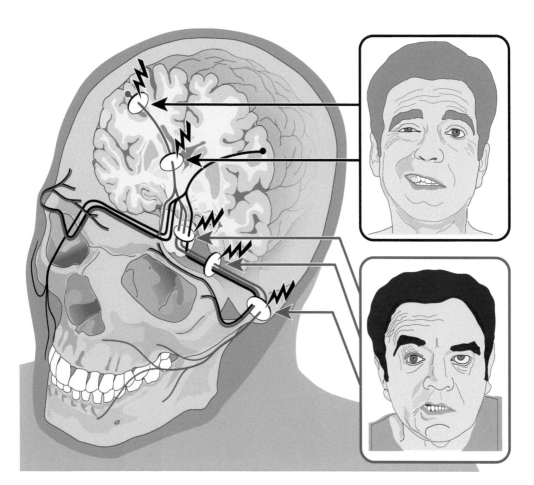

Fig. 12.20 Bilateral corticobulbar innervation of the facial nerve nucleus. A lesion of the cerebral cortex or internal capsule causes contralateral weakness of the perioral muscles, while eye closure and forehead wrinkling remain intact. A nuclear or peripheral lesion causes ipsilateral weakness of the perioral muscles as well as of eye closure and forehead wrinkling.

taper to off, lowering the dose by 5 mg every other day). Virostatic agents (e.g., valacyclovir 1,000 mg orally daily for 10 days) can yield an additional benefit. The benefit of surgical decompression of the facial nerve is questionable. An eye that cannot be closed must be protected from drying out and from trauma with ointment, artificial tears, and a moisture-chamber dressing.

Prognosis. The prognosis is generally favorable: in 80% of patients, the facial weakness resolves completely in 4 to 6 weeks. For the remaining 20%, whose facial musculature has been completely denervated, the recovery can take much longer (up to 6 months). **Residual manifestations** often include partial facial weakness or pathologic accessory movements due to misdirection of regenerating axons. In such cases, voluntary contraction of one part of the face is accompanied by simultaneous, involuntary contraction of another: thus, the eye on the affected side may close involuntarily when the patient whistles (synkinesia, **Fig. 12.22**).

Differential diagnosis. Facial weakness of central origin must be distinguished from peripheral facial nerve palsy. In central weakness, the lesion lies above the level of the facial nerve nucleus, that is, in the portion of the motor cortex subserving facial movements, or along the course of the corticobulbar efferent fibers. With meticulous clinical examination, one can always distinguish central from peripheral facial weakness; the criteria for this distinction are summarized in **Table 12.7**. The most important one is that **central facial palsy tends to spare the forehead and periocular muscles** (**Fig. 12.23**). The reason for this is that the neurons in the superior portion of the facial nerve nucleus in the pons receive impulses from both cerebral hemispheres; therefore, a unilateral lesion of the motor cortex or corticobulbar tract can usually be compensated for by the corresponding, intact pathway on the opposite side (**Fig. 12.19**). The caudal portion of the facial

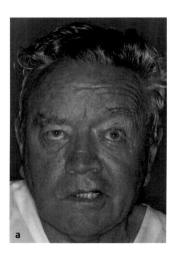
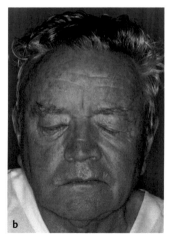

Fig. 12.21   Partial right peripheral facial nerve palsy. a The right corner of the mouth hangs limply downward and the right side of the forehead cannot be wrinkled. **b** The right eye cannot be completely closed.

nerve nucleus, on the other hand, is controlled only by the contralateral hemisphere.

> **NOTE**
>
> Central facial palsy is also often accompanied by weakness elsewhere in the body in areas not innervated by the facial nerve, for example, the tongue.

Hemifacial Spasm

This condition is characterized by synchronous, irregular, rapid, brief contractions of all of the muscles of facial expression supplied by the facial nerve on one side of the face, including the platysma. On close observation, it is readily distinguishable from a facial tic (**Fig. 12.24**). It rarely arises in the aftermath of a peripheral facial nerve palsy. The usual cause is **irritation of the facial nerve root by a looping blood vessel just distal to its point of exit from the pons**; this explains why neurosurgical intervention ("microvascular decompression") is usually successful. It is very rare for hemifacial spasm to be caused by a brainstem glioma. The condition can be treated symptomatically with anticonvulsants such as carbamazepine, or with injections of botulinus toxin.

12.6 Disturbances of Hearing and Balance: Vertigo

 Key Point

Lesions of the vestibulocochlear nerve can impair hearing, balance, or both. A lesion of its cochlear portion produces sensorineural hearing loss (impairment of sound perception), which must always be differentiated from conductive hearing loss (impairment of sound conduction, usually due to blockage of the external auditory canal by cerumen, or to a disease process in the middle ear). A lesion of the vestibular portion causes disequilibrium and vertigo.

The eighth cranial nerve (vestibulocochlear nerve, **Fig. 12.25**) conducts auditory and vestibular information to the central nervous system.

— **Auditory impulses** arise in the organ of Corti in the cochlea and travel by way of the cochlear nerve to the cochlear nuclei of the brainstem, and then onward in the auditory pathway (bilaterally) to the auditory cortex in the temporal lobe.

— **Vestibular impulses** arise in the ampullae and macula statica of the saccule and utricle, the organ of equilibrium; they then travel by way of the vestibular nerve to the vestibular nuclei, and then onward to multiple areas of the brain, including the cerebellum.

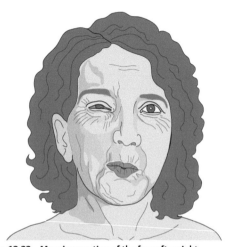

Fig. 12.22   Mass innervation of the face after right peripheral facial nerve palsy. Because of a misdirection of regenerating motor axons to their muscular targets, voluntary contraction of one muscle group in the face may be accompanied by involuntary contraction of other muscle groups. In the patient shown, whistling is accompanied by involuntary eye closure (a type of synkinesis).

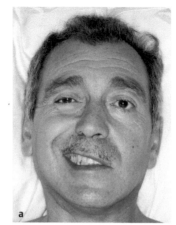 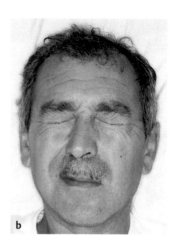

Fig. 12.23 Left central facial palsy. This 54-year-old man sustained an ischemic stroke in the right middle cerebral artery territory because of a right carotid artery dissection. Marked weakness of the perioral musculature on the left side (**a**). The forehead (**a,b**) is symmetrically innervated, and eye closure is symmetric (**b**).

Table 12.7

Differentiation of central and peripheral facial palsy

	Central facial palsy	Peripheral facial palsy
History	— Usually in the elderly — A sudden, acute event — Usually accompanied by hemiparesis that mainly affects the upper limb	— Any age — Often accompanied by retroauricular pain — Weakness develops over the course of one or two days, not suddenly
Facial appearance at rest	— Usually normal	— Often normal — Blinking may be less frequent — The affected side of the face is flaccid in long-standing, complete peripheral facial palsy
Muscles of facial expression	— The globe is always completely covered when the patient closes the eyes — The forehead is hardly affected	— If the palsy is complete, the patient cannot fully close the affected eye (possible in partial lesions) — The forehead is affected (**Fig. 12.21**)
Accompanying findings	— there may be ipsilateral tongue weakness (**Fig. 3.17**) or hemiparesis	— In the cryptogenic form, the sense of taste is lost on the ipsilateral side of the anterior two-thirds of the tongue — Diminished lacrimation and salivation — electromyography reveals denervation

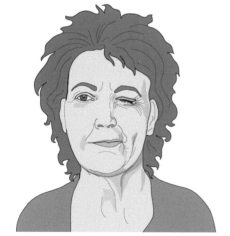

Fig. 12.24 Left hemifacial spasm. All of the muscles innervated by the facial nerve, including the platysma, contract repeatedly, synchronously, and involuntarily.

These anatomic relations are depicted in **Fig. 3.11** and discussed in an earlier chapter (section 3.3.2, "Vestibular Function").

12.6.1 Neurologic Disturbances of Hearing

NOTE

Most hearing problems are due to an abnormality of the ear rather than a neurologic condition, but many neurologic diseases can affect hearing. The neurologist's task is to distinguish conductive from (uni- or bilateral) sensorineural hearing loss and, if the latter is present, to determine the neurologic condition that is causing it.

The Differentiation of Sensorineural from Conductive Hearing Loss

On the basis of this distinction, one can determine whether the underlying cause is located in the

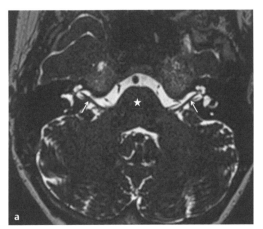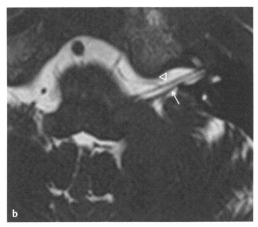

Fig. 12.25   MRI of the eighth cranial nerve: CISS sequences. **a** Axial section at the level of the pons (marked with an asterisk): the internal auditory canal and the eighth nerve are well seen on both sides (arrows). **b** The reconstructed image along the left internal auditory canal reveals the facial nerve (hollow arrowhead) and the vestibular part of the vestibulocochlear nerve (arrow).

middle ear or external auditory canal (conductive hearing loss, the more common kind) or in the sensory cells of the inner ear or the neural apparatus of hearing (sensorineural hearing loss, the less common kind). The method of examination and typical findings are summarized in Chapter 3 (section 3.3.2, "Differentiation of Conductive and Sensorineural Hearing Loss"). The diagnosis and treatment of conductive hearing loss and of disorders of the cochlea are the responsibility of the otologist.

Neurologic Disturbances of Hearing
Hearing loss due to a lesion of the inner ear or the vestibulocochlear nerve may be unilateral or bilateral, and its development may be more or less rapid.

Unilateral Hearing Loss
Unilateral hearing loss, if **acute**, is usually due to an infectious process, for example, mumps or another viral infection. If it is **slowly progressive**, a mass lesion compressing the eighth nerve should be suspected, such as an acoustic neuroma (see **Fig. 6.17**) or a meningioma in the cerebellopontine angle (**Fig. 12.26**). Larger masses in the cerebellopontine angle can affect not only the eighth cranial nerve but also the facial and trigeminal nerves.

Bilateral Hearing Loss
Bilateral hearing loss, if acute, is also most commonly due to a viral or other infection; bacterial meningitis is a rare cause. **Progressive** bilateral hearing loss, whether the progression is slow or rapid, should prompt suspicion of chronic basilar meningitis (as in tuberculosis), carcinomatous meningitis, an infectious disease (syphilis, toxoplasmosis), or an intoxication. Very slowly progressive, bilateral hearing loss may be due to a metabolic disorder, for example, Refsum disease, or one of the collagenoses.

Several diseases that can cause hearing loss as their most prominent manifestation are listed in **Table 12.8**.

Tinnitus
Noises in one or both ears are a common complaint. They are usually *subjective*, that is, audible only to the patient. They are termed *objective* when the examiner, too, can hear them with the stethoscope. The more common variety, **subjective tinnitus**, often involves a noise heard continually in both ears. The patient usually finds it most disturbing in quiet surroundings, particularly in bed at night. The cause is unknown and the problem may resolve spontaneously. Various treatments have been proposed, including perfusion-enhancing drugs and oxygen, but are of questionable benefit.

Pulsatile tinnitus is rare in comparison to continual tinnitus. It is caused by a pulsating blood vessel near the petrous bone and must be taken very seriously. The examiner, too, can often hear the pulse-synchronous bruit through a stethoscope (or even without one). The possible causes include the following:
- Carotid dissection.
- Fibromuscular dysplasia.
- High-lying carotid stenosis due to atherosclerosis.
- Arteriovenous malformation.
- Retromastoid dural fistula.
- Carotid–cavernous fistula.
- Glomus tumor (glomus jugulare or glomus tympanicum).
- Tumor in or near petrous bone.
- Infection in or near petrous bone.
- Intracranial hypertension.
- Pseudotumor cerebri.

If the cause of pulsatile tinnitus is not revealed by CT, MRI, CT angiography, or MR angiography, digital

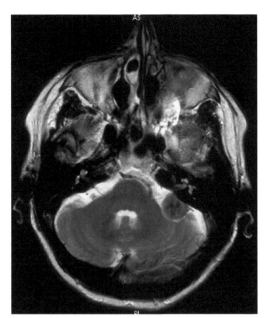

Fig. 12.26 Meningioma of the left cerebellopontine angle seen by MRI. The hazelnut-sized, spherical tumor is based on the pyramid of the petrous bone.

subtraction angiography must be performed. Many of the aforementioned causes are treatable.

12.6.2 Disequilibrium and Vertigo

NOTE

The vestibular organ (semicircular canals and otolith organs) plays a key role in the regulation of balance. Disturbances of the vestibular apparatus (composed of the vestibular organ, the vestibulocochlear nerve, and the vestibular nuclei of the brainstem) cause dysequilibrium, the main symptom of which is vertigo. Unilateral lesions cause directional vertigo accompanied by vegetative symptoms and by spontaneous directional nystagmus; bilateral lesions cause nondirectional vertigo. It should be emphasized that vestibular disturbances are just *one* cause of vertigo, and not even the most common one. Many other causes must always be included in the differential diagnosis.

Regulation of Equilibrium

Equilibrium (balance), that is, the optimal static and dynamic mechanical stability of the human being in three-dimensional space, is maintained by the following neural processes:

- Impulses from the vestibular apparatus concerning the position, movement, and acceleration of the individual in space.
- Impulses from the visual system concerning the body's relation to visual space.

- Impulses from the exteroceptive pathways concerning the body's contact with underlying surfaces (floor, mattress, etc.).
- Impulses from the proprioceptive pathways concerning the positions of the joints and the spatial relations of the parts of the body to each other.
- Impulses concerning movements in the process of being executed, from the pyramidal, extrapyramidal, and cerebellar systems.
- Conscious (cognitive) and unconscious (emotional) influences.
- Finally, the integration of all of these signals in the brainstem, cerebellum, and cortex.

The various components of the regulation of balance are shown schematically in **Fig. 12.27**.

Disturbances of the Regulation of Equilibrium

Vertigo arises if individual informational and/or control components of the regulatory system are lost (see later), if the information coming through different sensory channels seems to be inconsistent (so-called *multisensory mismatch*, e.g., in seasickness), or the sensory input is highly unusual (e.g., uncommon visual input from a great height). So many different structures play a role in the maintenance of equilibrium, and their interactions are so complex, that the causes of vertigo are, understandably, highly varied. Different types of vertigo result from lesions at different sites.

- **Vestibular vertigo** is usually directional; it is characteristic of lesions of the peripheral portion of the vestibular apparatus, that is, the vestibular organ and/or the vestibulocochlear nerve. The patient perceives the environment as if it were in motion when he/she is at rest (= oscillopsia due to spontaneous nystagmus) or during movements of the head (oscillopsia due to absence of the VOR). The vertigo can be either rotatory (like being on a carousel), as in vestibular neuritis, or heaving first in one direction and then in the other (like being on the deck of a boat), as in bilateral vestibulopathy. Vestibular vertigo is often accompanied by autonomic manifestations, such as nausea and vomiting, and by nystagmus. Central vestibular lesions (i.e., lesions of the vestibular nuclei in the brainstem and their connections in the brainstem, thalamus, and cerebellum) also usually cause directional vertigo, albeit less intensely than peripheral lesions. The autonomic manifestations, too, tend to be milder or absent.
- **Nonvestibular vertigo** is nondirectional, unsystematic, and often hard to describe. The patient may report a woozy feeling, emptiness in the head, or darkness in front of the eyes. Oscillopsia is absent and there are usually no autonomic

12

Table 12.8

Diseases that can cause hearing loss as their main clinical manifestation

Category	Disease	Remarks
Hereditary congenital anomalies of the inner ear	— Isolated hereditary deafness — Mondini syndrome — Alport syndrome — Klein–Waardenburg syndrome — Usher syndrome — Laurence–Moon–Biedl syndrome — Mitochondrial encephalomyopathies	— Mostly autosomal recessive inheritance, less commonly dominant or X-chromosomal — Mitochondrial encephalomyopathies are nearly always transmitted in a strictly maternal inheritance pattern (via mitochondrial DNA)
Nonhereditary congenital anomalies of the inner ear	— Thalidomide dysplasia — Measles embryopathy — Hyperbilirubinemia (kernicterus) — Perinatal asphyxia — Cretinism — Congenital syphilis — Toxoplasmosis	— In thalidomide dysplasia and measles embryopathy, the ear anomalies are often accompanied by other anomalies elsewhere in the body — Kernicterus often causes athetosis — Cretinism causes feeblemindedness
Infections	— Viral: herpes, mumps, measles, mononucleosis, HIV, and other neurotropic viruses — Bacterial meningitis — Otitis media and malignant otitis — Chronic otitis media (cholesteatoma) — Syphilis — Borreliosis	— Hearing loss is a common late sequela of bacterial meningitis — Otitis media causes conductive (not sensorineural) hearing loss; otoscopic examination is mandatory
Polyneuropathies	— Refsum disease — Hereditary neuropathy (Charcot–Marie–Tooth)	— Retinitis pigmentosa in Refsum disease
Tumors	— Acoustic neuroma — Glomus tympanicum tumor — Paraneoplastic	— Acoustic neuroma occurs sporadically or as a component of neurofibromatosis, type I or II — The presenting symptom of a glomus tympanicum tumor is often pulsatile tinnitus
Vascular disorders	— Infarct in the territory of the labyrinthine artery — Migraine	
Autoimmune disorders	— Collagen diseases — Susac syndrome — Cogan syndrome	— Various types of autoantibody can be demonstrated in these conditions
Trauma	— Transverse fracture of petrous bone — Labyrinthine contusion — Acoustic trauma — Chronic exposure to noise — Barotrauma	— The history leads to the diagnosis
Toxic/iatrogenic	— Aminoglycosides — Cytostatic agents	— Usually bilateral, often with a bilateral vestibular deficit
Specific ear diseases	— Ménière disease — Lermoyez syndrome — Otosclerosis — Acute hearing loss — Perilymph fistula	— In these conditions, vestibular symptoms are often present in combination (or in alternation) with hearing loss
Miscellaneous	— Superficial hemosiderosis of the CNS	— Progressive hearing loss and ataxia
	— Intracranial hypotension (section 14.2.4)	— Orthostatic headache; MRI reveals pachymeningeal enhancement

Abbreviations: CNS, central nervous system; MRI, magnetic resonance imaging.

manifestations. Central nervous lesions can cause pathologic nystagmus, as listed in **Table 12.2** and **Table 12.3** and shown in **Fig. 12.5**. Nonvestibular vertigo is caused either by a lesion of the nonvestibular parts of the regulatory system for balance or by faulty information processing within the central nervous system (e.g., because of a cerebellar lesion). Pathologic processes outside the central nervous system, such as orthostatic hypotension or aortic stenosis, can also cause nonvestibular vertigo.

The typical features of peripheral and central vestibular vertigo and of nonvestibular vertigo are summarized in **Table 12.9**.

Special Aspects of History-Taking and Diagnostic Evaluation

The clinician should be able to tell whether the patient is suffering from **vestibular** or **nonvestibular vertigo** based on a meticulously elicited clinical history alone. It is also important to determine whether the vertigo is **episodic** or **continuous** and to ask about

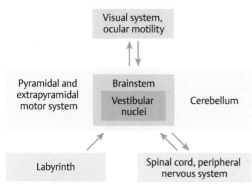

Fig. 12.27   The maintenance of balance by integration of information from multiple channels.

any **precipitating factors** (e.g., changes of position or particular situations that make the vertigo worse). If the vertigo worsens in the dark or when the patient's eyes are closed, the cause is likely to be a disturbance of proprioception (polyneuropathy, posterior column disease) or a bilateral vestibulopathy. The examiner should also always ask about **accompanying symptoms** (in particular, autonomic symptoms, tinnitus, hearing loss, and recent illnesses and infections). The history combined with the physical findings (nystagmus, results of balance tests, any other neurologic abnormalities) usually enables the localization of the functional disturbance. Further testing (e.g., caloric testing of the vestibular organ, ENT consultation, neuroimaging of the head) mainly serves to determine the etiology.

We will now describe the main neurologic causes of vertigo, particularly vestibular disturbances, in greater detail.

Vestibular Vertigo
Acute Loss of Vestibular Function
This condition also called **vestibular neuritis**, **acute vestibulopathy**, or an **acute vestibular crisis**. It can arise by a variety of pathogenetic mechanisms, the most common of which is a viral infection (reactivation of a type 1 herpes simplex virus infection). The patient suddenly experiences acute rotatory vertigo with nausea, vomiting, and falling to the side of the diseased vestibular organ. Every movement of the head makes the vertigo worse; the patient, noting this, tries to lie still. Examination reveals horizontally beating, spontaneous nystagmus away from the side of the lesion, with a rotatory component. The nystagmus is more intense when the patient lies on the affected side, and it can generally be alleviated by visual fixation. The affected vestibular organ is less responsive than normal to caloric stimulation and the head impulse test is abnormal (see "Vestibular Function" in section 3.3.2). Vertigo usually resolves fully within a few days, rarely within a few hours.

Often a so-called "trigger labyrinth" remains as a residual phenomenon, that is, vertigo on acceleration or rapid movements of the head. Recurrences are rare.

> **NOTE**
>
> Acute central vertigo due to a brainstem or cerebellar stroke can be confused with acute dysfunction of the vestibular nerve. The following three clinical signs indicate central vertigo and call for emergency neuroimaging, preferably MRI:
> - A normal head-impulse test.
> - Gaze-evoked nystagmus rather than spontaneous directional nystagmus.
> - Vertical strabismus (=skew deviation), detectable with an alternating cover test (see "Ocular Motility" in section 3.3.2).

Positional and Positioning Vertigo
These types of vertigo arise only with certain positions or positioning movements of the head and manifest themselves as **brief attacks of vertigo** that diminish in intensity if they are provoked multiple times in rapid succession. These conditions have several different causes.

Benign Paroxysmal Positioning Vertigo.
- This is the most common type of positioning vertigo. It is provoked by changes in the position of the head, usually involving lying down rapidly, bending forward, turning in bed, or rapidly sitting up. It manifests itself as very brief (15–30 seconds), very severe **attacks of rotatory vertigo** and nausea.
- As for the **pathogenesis** of this condition, it is thought that small pieces of the otolith membranes of the saccule and utricle can break off and float freely in the endolymph—usually in the posterior semicircular canal, less commonly in the horizontal one. When the head moves, these free particles move together with the endolymph and slide over the hair cells of the cupula, continuing to do so even after the head has stopped moving. The abnormally prolonged activation of the hair cells induces acute rotatory vertigo. The condition is also termed cupulolithiasis or canalolithiasis.
- The **Hallpike positioning maneuver** can be used as a **diagnostic test** (**Fig. 12.28**). The patient is rapidly taken from an upright sitting position into the supine position with the head held down, 30 degrees below the level of the examining table, and turned 60 degrees to the right or left. Within a few seconds, the examiner should be able to observe rotatory nystagmus, which then disappears after 5–30 seconds. This is easiest to see if the patient is wearing Frenzel goggles. If the head is turned to the right, the nystagmus is

counterclockwise; if the head is turned to the left, the nystagmus is clockwise (see also **Fig. 12.5**). In canalolithiasis of the lateral semicircular canal, when the supine patient turns the head, the nystagmus is toward the lower ear; in cupulolithiasis, it is toward the higher ear.

– Certain positioning maneuvers (the Epley and Semont maneuvers for the posterior semicircular canal, and the barbecue or Gufoni maneuver for the horizontal semicircular canal) have been found useful as **treatment** for this condition. These maneuvers work by flushing the floating otoliths out of the affected semicircular canal.

Central positional or positioning vertigo. This is a rarer type of positionally dependent vertigo that arises when the head is tilted into certain positions. The nystagmus usually beats toward the higher ear and does not habituate on repeated provocation. The vertigo is generally not very severe. The cause is a lesion or dysfunction of the cerebellum or its connections with the vestibular nuclei.

Ménière Disease

This disease is a common cause of acute vestibular vertigo. It is due to a pathologic accumulation of endolymph in the inner ear (endolymphatic hydrops) and manifests itself clinically in episodes of acute rotatory vertigo, a tendency to fall to the affected side, and horizontal, directional, spontaneous nystagmus. At the beginning of a so-called Ménière attack, spontaneous nystagmus beats toward the side of the lesion; later on, it beats away from the lesion (as in vestibular dysfunction). Vertigo and nystagmus are accompanied by nausea, vomiting, and tinnitus. There is slowly progressive hearing loss that worsens after each attack.

Bilateral Vestibular Deficits

While unilateral dysfunction of the vestibular apparatus can be compensated for by the intact opposite side within a matter of weeks, bilateral dysfunction deprives the regulatory system for balance of all incoming vestibular information. Consequently, the patient's gait becomes very unsteady in the dark (i.e., when visual input, too, is lost), or when the patient must walk on an uneven or soft surface (i.e., when the incoming proprioceptive information is difficult to interpret). Subjectively, the patient suffers from oscillopsia (apparent movement of the external world) on movement of the head, particularly when walking, because the defective VOR makes visual fixation is unstable. Objectively, the head-impulse test and the caloric irritability of the labyrinth are pathologic on both sides.

Vestibular Migraine

Vestibular migraine is among the more common central vestibular syndromes. It consists of recurrent attacks of vertigo (a sensation of rotatory or back-and-forth movement) that generally last a few minutes to a few hours. More than 60% of the affected patients also have photophobia, phonophobia, and/or headache during their attacks. The obligatory criteria for the diagnosis are: a positive history of migraine as defined by the International Headache Society, the occurrence of at least two attacks of vertigo that are accompanied by at least one typical symptom of migraine (such as a migraine-like headache, phonophobia, a scintillating scotoma, or any other kind of aura), and the exclusion of other causes of recurrent attacks of vestibular vertigo.

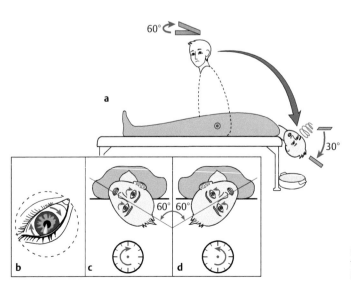

Fig. 12.28   Hallpike positioning test for the demonstration of benign paroxysmal positioning vertigo. See text.

Nonvestibular Vertigo

Dysfunction of the nonvestibular components of the regulatory system for balance can also cause vertigo.

- **Physiologic vertigo** occurs when the incoming proprioceptive information is inconsistent with the incoming visual information (multisensory mismatch). Examples include vertigo induced by looking down from a great height and the vertigo of seasickness.
- **Impaired proprioception**, for example, in polyneuropathy or posterior column disease, can also cause vertigo. The patient's unsteady stance and gait are worse in the dark or with the eyes closed.
- **Cervical vertigo** is thought to be due to faulty proprioceptive information arising in diseased cervical intervertebral joints or the adjacent soft tissues, which is then transmitted to the integrating apparatus for balance in the brainstem. This type of vertigo is also said to increase in the dark. Its existence is debated.
- **Pathologic processes affecting the central motor structures** (e.g., paralysis, cerebellar or extrapyramidal disease, brainstem disorders) impair the patient's motor adaptation to changes in position or cause oculomotor disturbances that can be perceived as dizziness.
- **Partial impairment of consciousness**, for example, in presyncope or certain types of epilepsy (particularly is dyscognitive seizures and absence seizures), is often experienced by the patient as dizziness.
- Another frequent occurrence is **psychogenic vertigo**, particularly due to phobias, in the setting of depression, neurotic conflict situations, anxiety disorders, and panic attacks.
- Finally, all **general medical conditions** that can temporarily diminish blood flow to the brain must be included in the differential diagnosis of dizziness and vertigo, for example, arterial hypotension and heart disease.

12.7 Lesions of the Glossopharyngeal and Vagus Nerves

    Key Point

Lesions of the glossopharyngeal and vagus nerves produce dysphagia, hoarseness, and dysphonia.

Anatomy. The anatomic course and distribution of these nerves is described in section 3.3.2.

Typical deficits. A unilateral lesion of the glossopharyngeal and vagus nerves causes ipsilateral weakness of the soft palate and posterior pharyngeal wall, which is evident as the **curtain sign** (**Fig. 12.29**; see also **Fig. 3.14**). The associated sensory deficit causes dysphagia, and unilateral vocal cord paralysis causes hoarseness. The patient usually does not notice the loss of sensation in the external auditory canal or the loss of taste on the posterior third of the tongue.

Causes. Dysfunction of the 9th and 10th cranial nerves can be caused by **infarction** of the corresponding **brainstem nuclei** (e.g., in Wallenberg syndrome, see **Table 6.17**). **Lesions of the peripheral nerve trunks** of these nerves can be caused by a mass in the posterior fossa or by a bony fracture involving these nerves at their site of exit from the jugular foramen. In the latter case, the injury involves not only these two nerves, but also the accessory nerve (Siebenmann syndrome). Finally, isolated neuritis of 9th and 10th cranial nerves can occur, for example, in the setting of herpes zoster, or as a cryptogenic disturbance.

12.8 Lesions of the Accessory Nerve

    Key Point

Lesions of the accessory nerve, depending on their level, produce weakness of the sternocleidomastoid muscle and trapezius muscle.

Anatomy. The anatomy and method of examination of the accessory nerve are described in section 3.3.2.

Typical deficits. A lesion of the purely motor main trunk of the accessory nerve causes paralysis of the sternocleidomastoid muscle and of the upper portion of the trapezius muscle (**Fig. 12.30**). Lesions of the accessory nerve in the lateral triangle of the neck, however, are much more common. These spare the sternocleidomastoid muscle and weaken only the upper portion of the trapezius muscle, causing a shoulder droop and an externally rotated position of the scapula (i.e., tilting of the caudal angle of the

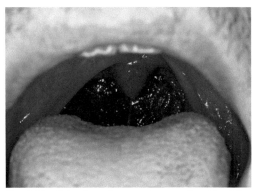

Fig. 12.29 Right glossopharyngeal nerve palsy with a right curtain sign and leftward deviation of the uvula.

12

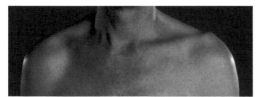

Fig. 12.30 Proximal left accessory nerve palsy with weakness and atrophy of the left sternocleidomastoid and trapezius muscles.

scapula toward the midline). This condition is depicted in **Fig. 12.31**.

Causes. Dysfunction of the main trunk of the accessory nerve is caused by mass lesions in the posterior fossa or at the base of the skull (Siebenmann syndrome, see earlier). Accessory nerve palsy due to interruption of the nerve in the lateral triangle of the neck is practically always iatrogenic, for example, as a complication of lymph node biopsy at the posterior border of the sternocleidomastoid muscle (where such biopsies often used to be taken). Neuritis is a rare cause.

12.9 Lesions of the Hypoglossal Nerve

 Key Point
Lesions of the hypoglossal nerve produce ipsilateral peripheral-type paresis of the tongue, with atrophy of the tongue muscles.

Anatomy. The anatomy and technique of examination of the hypoglossal nerve are described in section 3.3.2.

Typical deficits. The ipsilateral half of the tongue is **paretic** and, in the course of time, becomes **atrophic**. When the tongue is protruded, it deviates to the paretic side. This condition is illustrated in **Fig. 3.17**.

Causes. Unilateral hypoglossal nerve palsy is usually due to a bony fracture or a mass lesion—rarely, a congenital malformation—in the posterior cranial fossa. Carotid dissection is another possible cause. Rarely, isolated hypoglossal nerve palsy arises as a postinfectious or cryptogenic condition.

Differential diagnosis. Unilateral tongue weakness can also be of central origin, that is, due to a lesion of the corticobulbar pathway to the hypoglossal nerve nucleus.

│ NOTE
Central weakness, unlike hypoglossal nerve palsy of nuclear or peripheral origin, is not accompanied by atrophy of the tongue musculature.

— In (true) **bulbar palsy** (section 5.5.5), bilateral tongue weakness and atrophy are due to

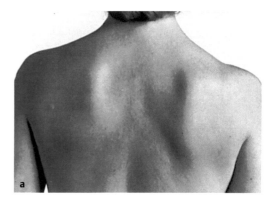

a

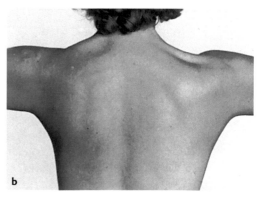

b

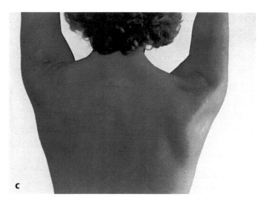

c

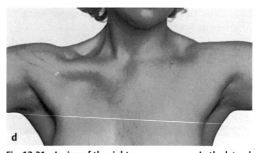

d

Fig. 12.31 Lesion of the right accessory nerve in the lateral triangle of the neck. a At rest, the right shoulder is lower and the right scapula is somewhat farther away from the midline. **b** When the arms are elevated laterally, the contour of the levator scapulae muscle is visible under the atrophic edge of the right trapezius muscle. **c** When the arms are raised, the right scapula tilts and the right shoulder is low. **d** The atrophic edge of the right trapezius muscle is easily seen from the front.

progressive loss of motor neurons in the medullary nucleus of the hypoglossal nerve bilaterally. The condition is slowly progressive and accompanied by fasciculations of the tongue.

— In **pseudobulbar palsy** (section 5.5.5), tongue weakness is due to bilateral, usually ischemic damage of the central corticobulbar pathways. Because the lesion is central, no atrophy or fasciculations are seen. Examination reveals dysarthria, dysphagia, and abnormal prominence of the perioral reflexes.

12.10 Multiple Cranial Nerve Deficits

  Key Point

Lesions affecting more than one cranial nerve at a time can be seen in various combinations.

— Progressive involvement of multiple lower cranial nerves (**Garcin syndrome**) is usually due to a tumor at the base of the skull.

— **Chronic basilar meningitis** (see section 6.7.4), for example, in tuberculosis, or **meningeal carcinomatosis** causes multiple cranial nerve palsies in varying combinations.

— **Cranial polyradiculitis** (see section 11.2.3) affects the cranial nerves symmetrically; the most prominent manifestation is bilateral facial nerve palsy.

— Further causes of multiple cranial nerve palsies include sarcoidosis, paraproteinemia, Wegener granulomatosis, malignant otitis, and others.

12

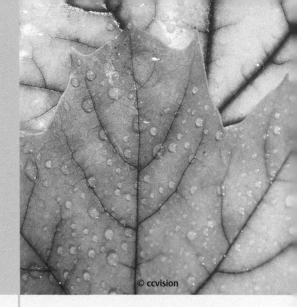
© ccvision

Chapter 13

Diseases of the Spinal Nerve Roots and Peripheral Nerves

Down the Garden Path

The patient, a 52-year-old office worker, had been receiving intramuscular vitamin B_{12} injections every month for the past 3 years because of vitamin B_{12} deficiency. A few days after a physician's assistant in a specialized outpatient clinic gave her such an injection in the right gluteal region, she complained to her family physician of a "fuzzy" feeling over the right shin and dorsum of the foot, as well as occasional pain, "like an electric shock," going down the leg. The doctor suspected an iatrogenic peripheral nerve injury. His physical examination revealed marked dorsiflexor weakness of the right big toe and also, to a lesser extent, of the other toes of the right foot, but foot dorsiflexion was of normal strength. There was diminished sensation to touch, and even more so to noxious stimulation, in the anterolateral quadrant of the right leg below the knee, and on the dorsum of the foot. The knee- and ankle-jerk reflexes were symmetrically elicitable; the tibialis posterior reflex was bilaterally absent. The doctor concluded that the patient had an iatrogenic right sciatic nerve lesion mainly affecting the peroneal nerve fibers.

Lesions of the peripheral nervous system (nerve roots, nerve plexuses, and peripheral nerves) are associated with flaccid weakness, diminution or loss of intrinsic muscle reflexes, and sensory deficits. Autonomic and trophic disturbances may be present as well (but not in nerve root lesions affecting the limbs). Each nerve root and each peripheral nerve have their own highly characteristic pattern of sensory and motor deficits; thus, the clinical findings generally enable the examiner to determine which root or nerve is affected. Sometimes, however, the differential diagnosis is harder. In the case described, the physician was too quick to conclude that the sciatic nerve was damaged in its peroneal component,

on the basis of the history, the pattern of the sensory deficit, and the intact reflexes. All of these findings would, indeed, have been consistent with a peroneal nerve lesion, but not the motor findings. Peroneal nerve lesions markedly impair not just toe dorsiflexion, but foot dorsiflexion as well, because this nerve innervates all the dorsiflexor muscles, including the tibialis anterior muscle—yet this patient could still dorsiflex her foot. Nor did her shock-like pain shooting down the leg conform to the classic picture of a peroneal nerve lesion. The physician should have considered an L5 nerve root lesion in the differential diagnosis.

The family physician sent the patient to a neurologist for a consultation. She told the neurologist that she had, in fact, suffered from severe back pain a few days earlier. The neurologist confirmed the weakness of toe dorsiflexion, also noting weakness of hip abduction and foot inversion. These findings suggested an L5 nerve root lesion. A magnetic resonance imaging (MRI) of the lumbosacral spine revealed a centrolateral intervertebral disk herniation at L4/L5 compressing the right L5 root. Electromyography revealed marked denervation potentials in the right extensor hallucis longus muscle, which is innervated almost exclusively by the L5 root, while there was none in the tibialis anterior muscle (innervated mainly by the L4 root). To confirm the diagnosis, the neurologist studied the gluteus medius muscle, a muscle innervated by the L5 root (via the superior gluteal nerve) but remote from the distribution of the peroneal nerve; here, too, there were typical signs of denervation. The patient's sensory disturbance thus had nothing to do with the intramuscular injection but was, rather, due to the disk herniation.

Key Point
Lesions of the peripheral nervous system cause flaccid weakness, sensory deficits, and auto-nomic disturbances in variable distributions and combinations, depending on their site and extent. They can be classified as follows:
  – Lesions of the anterior horn cells in the spinal cord (see section 7.7).
  – Lesions of the spinal nerve roots (radicular lesions).
  – Plexus lesions.
  – Lesions of individual peripheral nerve trunks or branches.

13.1 Radicular Syndromes

 Key Point
Radicular lesions are usually due to mechanical compression; less commonly, they may be infectious/inflammatory or traumatic. Their main clinical manifestation is pain, usually accompanied by a sensory deficit in the derma-tome of the affected nerve root. Depending on the severity of the lesion, there may also be flaccid weakness and areflexia in the muscle(s) innervated by the nerve root.

13.1.1 Overview

Anatomy
The **spinal nerve roots** constitute the initial segment of the peripheral nervous system. The **anterior (ventral) nerve roots** contain **efferent fibers**, while the **posterior (dorsal) nerve roots** contain **afferent fibers**. The motor roots from T2 to L2 or L3 also contain the efferent fibers of the **sympathetic nervous system**. The anterior and posterior roots at a single level of the spinal cord on one side join to form the **spinal nerve** at that level, which then passes out of the spinal canal through the corresponding **intervertebral foramen**. At this point, the nerve roots are in close proximity to the intervertebral disk and the intervertebral (facet) joint (**Fig. 13.1**).
In their further course, the fibers of the spinal nerve roots of multiple segments form **plexuses**, from which they are then distributed to the peripheral nerves. The areas innervated by the nerve roots thus differ from those innervated by the peripheral nerves.
Dermatomes and myotomes. The sensory component of a spinal nerve root innervates a characteristic segmental area of skin, which is called a **dermatome**. The efferent fibers of a spinal nerve root, after redis-tribution into various peripheral nerves, innervate multiple muscles (the **myotome** of the nerve root at that level). Each muscle, therefore, obtains motor

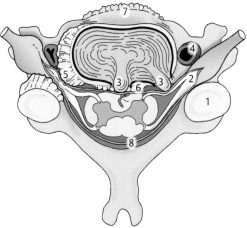

Fig. 13.1   View of a cervical vertebra and intervertebral disk. The normal anatomy of the intervertebral (neural) foramen is shown on the right side of the figure; narrowing of the foramen by uncarthrosis is shown on the left. **1** Facets of the intervertebral joint; **2** root with spinal ganglion; **3** lateral/ medial intervertebral disk herniation; **4** vertebral artery; **5** uncarthrosis; **6** dorsal spondylosis; **7** ventral spondylosis; **8** spinal dura mater. (Reproduced from Mumenthaler M. Der Schulter–Arm-Schmerz. 2nd ed. Bern: Huber; 1982.)

impulses from **more than one** nerve root, even if it is only innervated by a **single** peripheral nerve.
Root segments and root-indicating muscles. Table 13.1 is a list of the muscles that are often affected by radic-ular lesions and are accessible to clinical neurologic examination. The muscles that derive most of their innervation from a single nerve root are called **root-indicating muscles**.
Causes of radicular syndromes. In most patients, the cause is **compression** of the nerve root from outside by a space-occupying lesion, most often a herniated intervertebral disk ("slipped disk"), but sometimes a tumor, abscess, or other type of mass. In the cervical segments, **spondylotic narrowing of the interverte-bral foramina** is a further common cause of radicular pain and brachialgia (**Fig. 13.2**). **Infectious and inflammatory processes** can also cause monoradicu-lar deficits, for example, **herpes zoster** and **borrelio-sis** (Lyme disease; see section 6.7.5 and **Fig. 13.50**). **Diabetes mellitus**, too, can cause monoradiculopathy with pain and weakness. Finally, individual nerve roots can be affected by **traumatic lesions**, for exam-ple, root avulsion (see **Fig. 13.23**) or root compres-sion due to a fracture.

> **NOTE**
>
> Radiculopathy is often due to a mechanical injury or irritation of a nerve root by degenerative disease of the spine, particularly intervertebral disk herniation. A radicular deficit, however, should never simply be assumed to be due to disk herniation. Other causes must always be considered.

Table 13.1

Synopsis of radicular syndromes

Segment	Sensory deficit	Motor deficit	Reflex deficit	Remarks
C3/C4	Pain and hypalgesia in shoulder region	Diaphragmatic paresis or plegia	None detectable	Partial diaphragmatic paresis is more ventral in C3 lesions, more dorsal in C4 lesions
C5	Pain and hypalgesia on lateral aspect of shoulder over deltoid muscle	Deltoid and biceps paresis	Diminished biceps reflex	
C6	Radial side of arm and forearm down to thumb	Biceps and brachio-radialis paresis	Diminished or absent biceps reflex	
C7	Dorsolateral to C6 dermatome down to second, third, and fourth fingers	Triceps, pronator teres, and (occasionally) finger flexor paresis; thenar eminence often visibly atrophic	Diminished or absent triceps reflex	Triceps reflex key to differential diagnosis versus carpal tunnel syndrome
C8	Dorsal to C7 dermatome, i.e., ulnar side of arm and forearm, down to little finger	Intrinsic hand muscles visibly atrophic, particularly on hypothenar eminence	Diminished or absent triceps reflex	Triceps reflex key to differential diagnosis versus ulnar nerve palsy
L3	From greater trochanter crossing over the anterior aspect to the medial aspect of the thigh and knee	Quadriceps paresis	Weakness of quadriceps (knee-jerk) reflex	Differential diagnosis versus femoral nerve palsy: intact sensation in distribution of saphenous nerve
L4	From lateral thigh across patella to upper inner quadrant of calf and down to medial edge of foot	Quadriceps and tibialis anterior paresis	Weakness of quadriceps reflex	Differential diagnosis versus femoral nerve palsy: involvement of tibialis anterior muscle
L5	From lateral condyle above knee across the upper outer quadrant of the calf to the big toe	Paresis and atrophy of extensor hallucis longus muscle, often also of extensor digitorum brevis muscle; paresis of tibialis posterior muscle and of hip abduction	Absent tibialis posterior reflex (of diagnostic value only when clearly elicitable on opposite, unaffected side)	Differential diagnosis versus peroneal nerve palsy: in the latter, tibialis posterior muscle and hip abduction are preserved
S1	From posterior thigh over posterior upper quadrant of calf and lateral malleolus to little toe	Paresis of the peronei muscles, often also of the gastrocnemius and soleus muscles	Absent gastrocnemius reflex (ankle-jerk or Achilles reflex)	
Combined L4, L5	Combination of L4 and L5 dermatomes	Paresis of all foot and toe extensors and of quadriceps muscle	Diminished quadriceps reflex, absent tibialis posterior reflex	Differential diagnosis versus peroneal nerve palsy: peronei muscles spared. Note reflex findings
Combined L5, S1	Combination of L5 and S1 dermatomes	Paresis of toe extensors, peronei muscles, sometimes also gastrocnemius and soleus muscles	Absent tibialis posterior and gastrocnemius reflexes	Differential diagnosis versus peroneal nerve palsy: tibialis anterior muscle spared. Note reflex findings

General Clinical Features and Differential Diagnosis of Radicular Lesions

See also Section 7.1.2.

Regardless of the etiology, a disease process affecting any particular nerve root evokes a **characteristic pattern of symptoms and neurologic findings**:

— **Pain** in the distribution of the affected nerve root.
— A **sensory deficit** and irritative sensory phenomena (paresthesia, dysesthesia) in the dermatome of the affected nerve root.
— **Paresis** of the muscle(s) supplied by the affected nerve root, generally less marked than the paresis

caused by a peripheral nerve lesion (no plegia!), but possibly severe in the root-indicating muscles.

— **Muscle atrophy** is common, but usually less severe than in peripheral nerve lesions. Chronic radicular lesions can, rarely, cause fasciculations.
— **Impaired reflexes** in the segment corresponding to the affected nerve root.

The characteristic syndromes of the individual nerve roots supplying the upper and lower limbs are summarized in **Table 13.1**. The table also provides information on the differential diagnosis of radicular and peripheral nerve lesions in certain common situations.

Radicular syndromes are to be differentiated from **lesions in more distal components of the peripheral nervous system** (plexuses, peripheral nerves), as well as from lesions of the anterior horn of the spinal cord. This can usually be done by careful **clinical examination** alone, but **electromyography** may be required for unambiguous confirmation.

— The **lack of an autonomic deficit** may be a useful clinical criterion in the differential diagnosis of radicular lesions that affect the limbs, because sympathetic fibers travel in the spinal nerve roots only at levels T2 through L2 (see earlier); therefore, an autonomic deficit in a limb always indicates a lesion **distal to the nerve root**.

— When there is a **purely motor deficit**, unaccompanied by a sensory deficit or pain, a **lesion of the spinal motor neurons** (e.g., spinal muscular atrophy or amyotrophic lateral sclerosis [ALS]) should be suspected, rather than a radicular lesion.

— If the patient complains only of pain radiating into the periphery, in the absence of any demonstrable sensory deficit or weakness, the clinician should think of **pseudoradicular pain** (see section 14.7) due to mechanical overuse or another abnormality of the musculoskeletal apparatus.

13.1.2 Radicular Syndromes due to Intervertebral Disk Herniation

 Key Point

The proximity of the spinal nerve root to the intervertebral disk at the level of the intervertebral foramen carries with it the danger of root compression by disk herniation. The nerve root can be compressed either by a merely bulging disk or by a disk herniation in the strict sense, that is, a prolapse of nucleus pulposus material (which is usually soft) through a hole in the annulus fibrosus.

Definitions. In a disk **protrusion** ("bulging disk"), the annulus fibrosus is intact, but bulges outward. This situation is sometimes (misleadingly) called "incomplete disk herniation." Disk **herniation** (alternatively, disk prolapse or "complete" disk herniation) is defined as the emergence of disk tissue through a **hole in the annulus fibrosus**. In a **subligamentous** disk herniation, the herniated disk tissue is still contained beneath the posterior longitudinal ligament; in a **transligamentous** herniation, the ligament, too, has been perforated and there is disk tissue in the spinal canal.

General clinical features. The typical manifestations of acute radiculopathy due to intervertebral disk herniation are the following:

— **Local pain** in the corresponding area of the spine, with painful restriction of movement and a compensatory, abnormal posture of the spine (scoliosis, flattening of lordosis).

— Usually, after a few hours or days, **radiation of pain** into the cutaneous distribution (dermatome) of the affected nerve root.

— **Pain on stretching of the nerve root** (e.g., in the lower limb, a positive Lasègue sign).

— Exacerbation of pain by coughing, abdominal pressing (Valsalva maneuvers), and sneezing.

— Objectifiable **neurologic deficits** (hyporeflexia or areflexia, paresis, sensory deficit, atrophy in the late stage) depending on the severity of the root lesion.

Cervical Disk Herniation

Cervical disk herniation is a common cause of **acute torticollis** and of **(cervico)brachialgia**.

Etiology. Cervical disk herniation may occur as the result of cervical trauma, a twisting injury of the cervical spine, an excessively rapid movement, or mechanical overload.

Clinical features. The most commonly affected segments are **C6, C7, and C8. Subjectively**, patients usually complain of **pain in the neck and upper limb**, and sometimes of a sensory deficit, which does not necessarily cover the entire zone of innervation of the affected root.

Diagnostic evaluation. The **clinical history** and **physical examination** should enable identification of the affected nerve root. The objectively observable

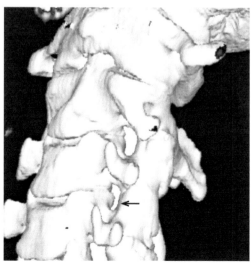

Fig. 13.2 Stenosis of the left C3/C4 intervertebral foramen (arrow); 3D CT reconstruction.

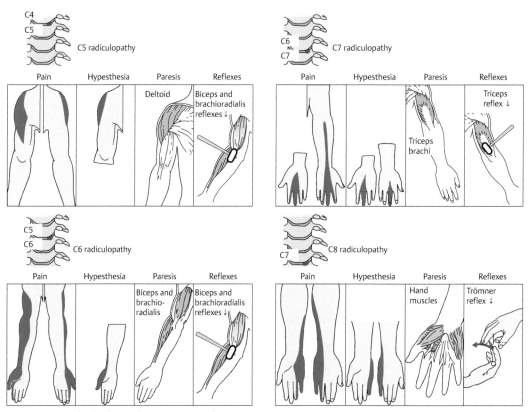

Fig. 13.3 Cervical radicular syndromes. Synopsis of pain radiation, somatomotor deficits, and reflex deficits in the common cervical nerve root compression syndromes. (Adapted from Stöhr M, Riffel B. Nerven- und Nervenwurzelläsionen. Weinheim: Edition Medizin VHC; 1988.)

neurologic deficits are listed in **Table 13.1** and shown schematically (independently of etiology) in **Fig. 13.3**. The **Spurling test** can provide additional evidence of cervical nerve root irritation: the head is leaned backward and the face is turned to the side of the lesion. Carefully titrated axial compression by the examiner's hand may induce pain radiating in a radicular distribution (**Fig. 13.4**).

Imaging studies (CT and/or MRI) are indispensable for the demonstration of nerve root compression by a herniated intervertebral disk. These are sometimes supplemented by **neurography** (i.e., measurement of nerve conduction velocities) and **electromyography**.

NOTES

One should not forget, however, that a mere disk protrusion without any detectable nerve root compression is a common incidental radiologic finding and is of no pathologic significance without clearly correlated symptoms.

Treatment. Temporary rest and **physical therapy**, with the addition of appropriate **exercises** as soon as the patient can tolerate them, usually suffice as treatment. Sufficient **analgesic medication** must also be provided, to prevent the chronification of the pain syndrome through the maintenance of an abnormal, antalgic posture (persistent fixation of the affected spinal segments by muscle spasm) and through nonphysiologic stress on other muscle groups.

Surgical treatment may be needed because of intractable pain, persistent, severe, or progressive paresis, or signs of spinal cord compression. The operation generally involves **fenestration** of the intervertebral space at the appropriate level to expose the affected nerve root and disk, widening of the bony intervertebral foramen (**foraminotomy**), then **discectomy**, and, under some circumstances, **spondylodesis** (fusion) if there is thought to be a risk of spinal instability afterward. Fusion should be performed in such a way as to distract the vertebrae above and below and thereby maintain the patency of the intervertebral foramen. **Disk prostheses** (artificial intervertebral disks) have also become available in recent years.

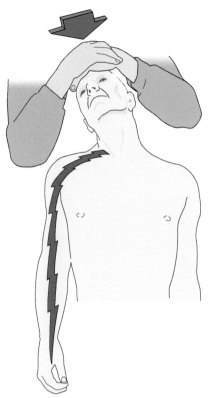

Fig. 13.4   Spurling cervical compression test for the provocation of radicular pain in cervical disk herniation. Pain can often be elicited by reclination and rotation of the head toward the affected side even without axial compression. (Adapted from Mumenthaler M. Der Schulter-Arm-Schmerz. 2nd ed. Bern: Huber; 1982.)

Lumbar Disk Herniation

Lumbar disk herniation is one of the more common causes of **acute low back pain and sciatica**.

The anatomic relationship of the lumbar roots to the intervertebral disks (both normal and herniated) is shown schematically in **Fig. 13.5**.

Pathogenesis and clinical features. A first episode of lumbar disk herniation (and often the first or second recurrence as well) may present with no more than **acute low back pain** (lumbago), a sudden "charley horse." The event may be precipitated by a relatively **banal movement in the wrong direction**; in particular, the lumbar spine may suddenly freeze in a twisted position if the individual incautiously tries to lift a heavy load with the upper body turned to one side. Any further movement of the lumbar spine is blocked by **muscle spasm, a reflex response to the pain**. Even the smallest movement is painful, as are coughing and abdominal pressing (Valsalva maneuvers). The pain usually resolves after a few days of bed rest. It is usually only when the herniation recurs

later that the patient experiences pain radiating into the leg, that is, **sciatica**, possibly in combination with typical **radicular neurologic deficits**.

In our experience, **motor deficits** generally arise only later in the course of this syndrome. The patient must be examined carefully to determine whether a deficit is present. The **L5** root is most commonly affected, usually by an L4–L5 disk herniation, and the **S1** root is the next most commonly affected after that, usually by an L5–S1 disk herniation. The corresponding clinical findings are listed in **Table 13.1** and are depicted schematically, independently of etiology, in **Fig. 13.6**.

For the following special clinical entities that can be caused by lumbar disk herniation, see also section 7.1.2:

- **Epiconus syndrome** (damage to the segment of the spinal cord just above the conus medullaris, at spinal levels T11 and T12).
- **Conus medullaris syndrome** (damage to the conus medullaris at level L1).
- **Cauda equina syndrome** (compression of the nerve roots in the lumbar spinal canal below the L1 level).

Diagnostic evaluation. Often, the **posture** of the standing patient already displays the typical appearance of a lumbar disk herniation (**Fig. 13.7**). As in cervical disk herniation, the level of the affected nerve root can generally be determined from the pattern of referred pain and any motor, sensory, and reflex deficits that may be present. The peripheral nerve trunk containing the axons derived from the affected root is often sensitive to **pressure** (**at the Valleix's pressure points**), and **stretching** of the nerve is often **painful**. The latter can be tested by passive raising of the supine patient's extended leg (the **Lasègue test**). Pain caused by elevation of the leg on the side opposite the sciatica (the **crossed Lasègue sign**) usually indicates a large, sequestrated disk herniation. If a higher lumbar root (L3 or L4) is affected, one should look for the **reverse Lasègue sign**, that is, test for pain on *extension* of the leg in the *prone* patient, which stretches the femoral nerve rather than the sciatic nerve. If the herniation is lateral or extraforaminal, pain may also be inducible by lateral bending of the trunk.

Imaging studies (**CT**, **Fig. 13.8** and **Fig. 13.9**; **MRI**, **Fig. 13.10**) are not absolutely essential if the clinical picture is sufficiently characteristic, but they should be performed if there is any doubt as to the etiology of radiculopathy or if surgery is needed. In evaluating diagnostic images, one should pay attention not only to potentially herniated disks, but also to the foraminal and extraforaminal structures (**Fig. 13.8**).

13

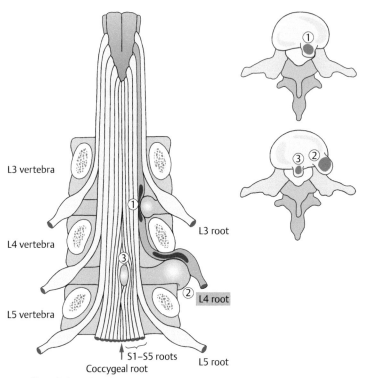

L3 vertebra

L3 root

L4 vertebra

L4 root

L5 vertebra

L5 root

S1–S5 roots
Coccygeal root

① Mediolateral prolapse
② Lateral prolapse
③ Medial prolapse

Fig. 13.5   Anatomic relationships of the lumbar intervertebral disks to the exiting nerve roots.

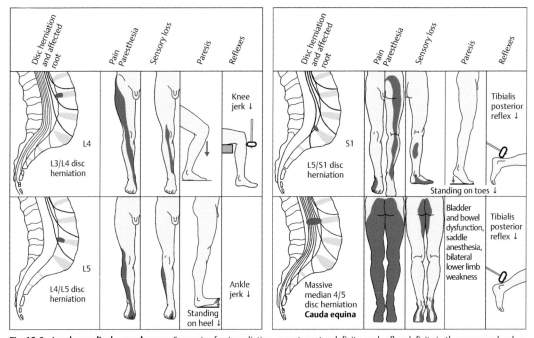

Fig. 13.6   Lumbar radicular syndromes. Synopsis of pain radiation, somatomotor deficits, and reflex deficits in the common lumbar and sacral nerve root compression syndromes. (Adapted from Stöhr M. Riffel B. Nerven- und Nervenwurzelläsionen. Weinheim: Edition Medizin VHC; 1988.)

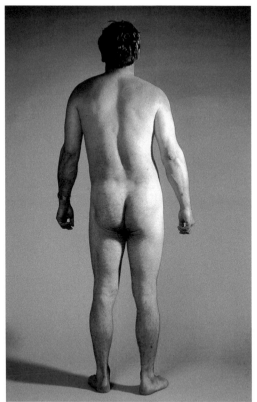

Fig. 13.7   A patient with lumbar disk herniation. The normal lumbar lordosis is no longer present, and scoliosis is seen.

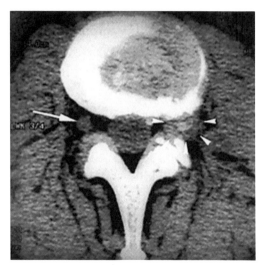

Fig. 13.8   Lateral L3/L4 disk herniation (arrowheads), CT image. The normal spinal ganglion on the right side is visible in the intervertebral foramen (arrow).

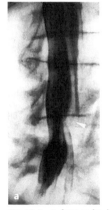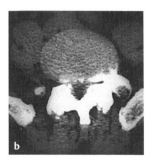

Fig. 13.9   Left S1 radicular compression in a 40-year-old man. **a** Myelography reveals a broadened and shortened left S1 nerve root (arrowhead) and an indentation of the dural sack from the right at this level. **b** CT reveals high-grade spondylarthrosis and bilateral stenosis of the lateral recesses.

| NOTE |

Diagnostic images should always be interpreted critically and in the light of the clinical findings.

Neurography, electromyography, myelography, and postmyelographic CT can sometimes yield additional useful information if the situation is unclear.

Treatment. The initial treatment is almost always **conservative** and follows the same lines as described earlier for cervical disk herniation: **bed rest** with adequate **analgesia** usually suffices. The latter is important to prevent nonphysiologic stress on musculoskeletal structures because of an abnormal, antalgic posture.

Surgery should be considered only if conservative treatment fails. An incipient **cauda equina syndrome** (bladder and bowel dysfunction, saddle hypesthesia, bilateral pareses, and impairment of the anal reflex, cf. section 7.1.2) is an absolute indication for urgent surgery.

| NOTE |

Cauda equina syndrome is an indication for an emergency neurosurgical procedure.

At surgery, the intervertebral space at the appropriate level is opened to expose the affected nerve root and disk (**fenestration**), the bony intervertebral foramen is widened (**foraminotomy**), and the herniated disk tissue is removed (**discectomy**). In rare cases, fusion (**spondylodesis**) is performed as well if there is thought to be a risk of postoperative spinal instability. General rules regarding surgery for intervertebral disk herniation are summarized in the flowchart of **Fig. 13.11**.

| NOTE |

Decompressive surgery is urgently indicated if the radicular pain suddenly disappears while the weakness stays the same or worsens. This is considered to be a sign of the impending **death of the nerve root**.

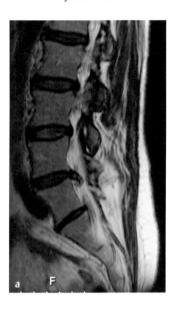

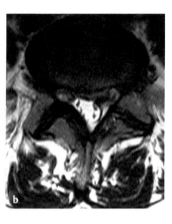

Fig. 13.10   Disk herniation as seen on an MRI scan. Left L4–L5 disk herniation with a caudally displaced free fragment. Clinical examination revealed left L5 and S1 radiculopathy. **a** Sagittal T2-weighted image. **b** Axial T2-weighted image. The free fragment lies behind the L5 vertebral body in the left lateral recess and displaces the dural sac the right.

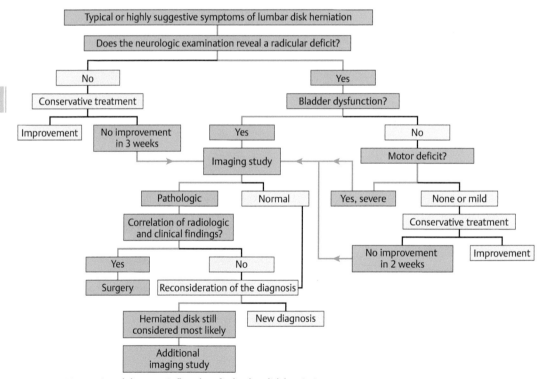

Fig. 13.11   Diagnostic and therapeutic flowchart for lumbar disk herniation.

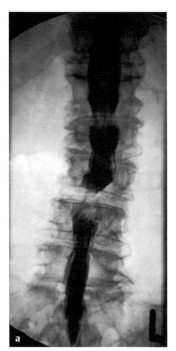
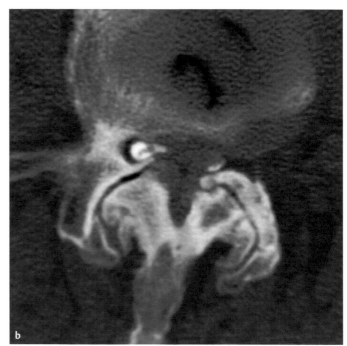

Fig. 13.12   Lumbar spinal stenosis. The myelogram **(a)** and postmyelographic CT **(b)** reveal spinal canal stenosis at the level of the L3–L4 disk. In the myelogram, no contrast medium is seen at this level. In the postmyelographic CT, there is no contrast medium in the dural sac and only a little in the nerve root sleeves. The dural sac is compressed by degenerative changes in the intervertebral disk (note the gas inclusions) and of the facet joints (note the hypertrophic osteophytes).

13.1.3 Radicular Syndromes due to Spinal Stenosis

 Key Point

Slowly progressive mechanical compression of the intraspinal neural structures usually affects elderly patients in whom congenital narrowness of spinal canal has been accentuated by further, progressive, degenerative osteochondrotic and reactive-spondylogenic changes. Lumbar spinal stenosis causes (possibly bilateral) radicular pain and neurologic deficits that arise while the patient is walking (spinal claudication, also called intermittent claudication of the cauda equina). Cervical spinal stenosis causes paresthesiae of the hands and signs of cervical spinal cord compression.

Cervical Spinal Stenosis

A narrow cervical spinal canal can compress not only the cervical nerve roots, but also the spinal cord itself, producing a myelopathy. **Cervical spondylogenic myelopathy** is discussed in detail in section 7.3.2.

Lumbar Spinal Stenosis

For anatomic reasons, a narrow lumbar spinal canal causes an entirely different clinical syndrome than cervical spinal stenosis:

Clinical features. In addition to **low back pain**, which is usually chronic, **intermittent claudication** is the most characteristic symptom: as the patient walks, sciatica-like pain arises on the posterior aspect of one or, usually, both lower limbs and then becomes progressively severe. The pain appears earlier if the patient is walking downhill, because of the additional lumbar lordosis that downhill walking induces. This historical feature differentiates neurogenic from vasogenic intermittent claudication, in which the pain tends to be more severe when the patient walks uphill. A further differentiating feature of neurogenic, as opposed to vasogenic, intermittent claudication is that standing still generally does not, by itself, make the pain go away. The patient must additionally bend forward, sit down, or crouch—these maneuvers induce kyphosis of the lumbar spine and thereby decompress its neural contents.

Diagnostic evaluation. Nowadays, the definitive diagnostic study is **MRI**, though **radiculography** and **myelographic CT** are still sometimes needed (**Fig. 13.12**).

Treatment. Surgery is indicated if the symptoms are very severe and the neurologic deficits are progressive. **Decompression** of the affected segments is performed by opening the narrowed lateral recesses, possibly in combination with a stabilizing spondylodesis (fusion).

13

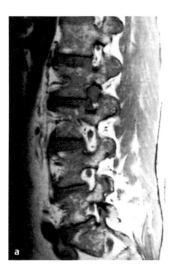
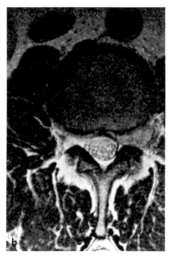

Fig. 13.13   **Neurinoma of the left L2 nerve root** (MRI). The neurinoma completely fills the L2–L3 intervertebral foramen. **a** Normal, nonthickened roots can be seen in the foramina immediately above and below. **b** The transverse image reveals the hourglass-shaped neurinoma on the left side, with both intraspinal and extraspinal extension.

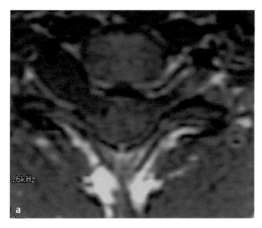

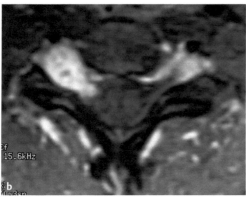

Fig. 13.14   **Neurinoma filling of the right C8 nerve root** in a 26-year-old woman with progressive sensory loss in the C8 dermatome, of one year's duration. **a** T1-weighted spin-echo image: the neurinoma is seen as a thickening of the right C8 nerve root. **b** Neurinomas take up contrast medium. The lesion appears bright in this contrast-enhanced image.

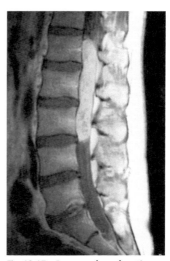

Fig. 13.15   **Sausage-shaped cystic ependymoma** filling the spinal canal from L1 to L3 and compressing the cauda equina (MR image).

13.1.4 Radicular Syndromes due to Space-Occupying Lesions

NOTE

Tumors and other space-occupying lesions can mechanically compress nerve roots and thereby cause radicular deficits and, often, pain.

Etiology.
— Tumors: **neurinoma** in the lumbar (**Fig. 13.13**) or cervical region (**Fig. 13.14**) and **meningioma** are the most common types of primary intraspinal tumor, while **ependymoma** (**Fig. 13.15**), glioma (usually astrocytoma), and vascular tumors are rarer.
— Radiculopathy can also be caused by a **primary destructive process** affecting a spinal vertebra (**Fig. 13.16**), particularly **metastatic carcinoma**.

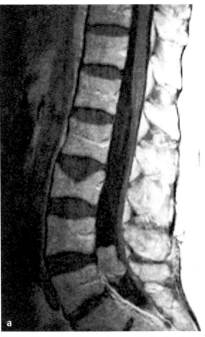
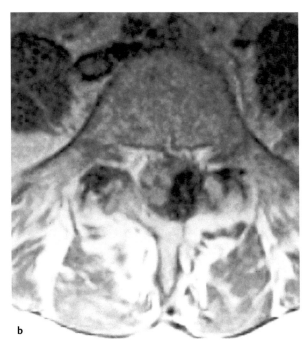

Fig. 13.16   Metastatic melanoma in the lumbosacral spinal canal, 8 years after resection of the primary tumor. The patient presented with cauda equina syndrome. **a** Sagittal MR image. **b** Axial MR image. The nerve roots of the cauda equina are displaced dorsally and to the left by the compressive lesion.

- Finally, **infectious and inflammatory processes** of the vertebrae and intervertebral disks (e.g., spondylodiscitis), as well as **spinal abscesses** and **empyema**, can cause radicular or spinal cord compression.

Clinical features. The patient usually complains of **pain radiating into the periphery**; if the lesion is at a thoracic level, the pain tends to be in a **band-like** distribution around the chest. Motor or sensory deficits may also be clinically detectable, depending on the level of the lesion. A space-occupying lesion within the lower lumbar canal can produce **cauda equina syndrome** of greater or lesser severity (see section 7.1.2).

Diagnostic evaluation. Imaging studies are essential; **MRI** is the study of first choice, though CT can also be informative for bony processes. Plain X-rays are not sensitive enough to be useful in most cases. They can, at most, yield clues to pathologic findings that require further investigation (e.g., a widened intervertebral foramen due to a neurofibroma, or a pedicle that has been destroyed by a metastasis).

Treatment. Surgery (resection of the compressive lesion) is usually needed. Further treatment may also be needed depending on the underlying illness (radiotherapy and/or chemotherapy for neoplastic lesions, antibiotics after the removal of an abscess or empyema).

13.2 Peripheral Nerve Lesions

 Key Point
The typical clinical features of a peripheral nerve lesion are high-grade flaccid paresis, a marked sensory deficit, and diminished sweating in the dermatome of the damaged nerve or nerve segment. Pain may be present, as in radicular lesions. Peripheral nerve lesions are usually due to trauma or nerve compression.

13.2.1 Overview

Anatomy
When we speak here of the "peripheral nerves," we are referring to the **nerve plexuses** formed by the junction and regrouping of fibers derived from the spinal nerve roots, as well as to the more distally lying **peripheral nerve trunks and branches**. The plexuses always contain mixed fiber types and the peripheral nerve trunks nearly always do so, that is, somatic motor, somatosensory, and often also autonomic (particularly sympathetic) fibers. The individual peripheral nerve trunks bear an anatomically invariant relationship to the muscles and cutaneous zones that they innervate. This pattern of innervation differs from that of the spinal nerve roots because of the reassortment of the nerve root fibers in the plexuses. This fact enables the clinician to

13

distinguish a peripheral nerve lesion from a radicular lesion on the basis of the observed pattern of neurologic deficits.

A **peripheral nerve** is a cable-like bundle of **nerve fibers**. The nerve fiber is the smallest "building block" of a peripheral nerve; it consists of an axon and an encasing myelin sheath (if present), which is the membrane of a Schwann cell wrapped around the axon numerous times. Individual nerve fibers are surrounded by a delicate connective tissue called **endoneurium**. The nerve fibers and the endoneurium are bundled together into larger fascicles, each of which is surrounded by a tough **perineurium**. Along the length of the nerve, the individual fascicles make many plexus-like interconnections with one another; they are held together as a single peripheral nerve by an encompassing layer of **epineurium**. This is not a tough husk around the nerve, but rather a loose, lipid-rich layer of connective tissue, reinforced by transversely and longitudinally oriented collagen fibers. It contains not only the nerve fascicles, but also the **vasa nervorum**. The nerve trunks are fixed to the adjacent connective tissue at only a few points, at which they are especially vulnerable to mechanical damage. Larger nerve trunks are often found together with arteries and veins in so-called **neurovascular bundles** surrounded by a common connective tissue sheath. These bundles form an anatomic unit that is clearly demarcated from the surrounding structures.

Causes of Peripheral Nerve Lesions

Most lesions of the nerve plexuses or the peripheral nerve trunks are either **traumatic** (caused by excessive traction, stab wounds, cuts, bony fractures, etc.) or due to **prolonged compression**, that is,

- Compression from outside the body.
- Compression at anatomic bottlenecks.
- Space-occupying lesions within the body in the vicinity of the nerve (especially tumors and hematomas).

Less commonly, plexus and nerve lesions can be caused by **infection and/or inflammation**, for example, neuralgic shoulder amyotrophy, which is probably an autoimmune disorder affecting the brachial plexus (see later in section 13.2.2).

> **NOTE**
>
> Nearly all lesions affecting a single peripheral nerve trunk or branch (**mono**neuropathies) are of mechanical or vascular origin; in contrast, most **poly**neuropathies (see section 11.3) are of toxic, infectious/inflammatory, or metabolic origin.

General Clinical Features of Peripheral Nerve Lesions

Depending on the particular segment of plexus or peripheral nerve trunk/branch that is affected, there may be a motor, sensory, autonomic, or (usually) mixed neurologic deficit:

- **Flaccid paresis** of the muscle(s) innervated by the affected nerve.
- Usually marked **atrophy** of the affected muscle(s).
- The corresponding **reflex deficits**.
- **Diminished sensation** and possibly also **pain and paresthesia** in the cutaneous distribution of the nerve, though the pain is often felt beyond this area as well.
  - All sensory modalities are affected to a comparable extent.
  - In contrast to a radicular lesion, the affected area of skin is more easily demarcated by testing the sense of touch, rather than nociception.
- **Diminished sweating** is often found in the hypesthetic area of skin, because the sudomotor fibers travel together with the somatosensory fibers of the peripheral nerves, and autonomic abnormalities of other kinds may also be present in the distribution of the affected nerve.
  - Radicular lesions affecting the limbs, in contrast, generally leave sweating intact (an important criterion for differential diagnosis).
- **Fasciculations** are only rarely seen; these are much more common in anterior horn disease.

Grades of Severity of Peripheral Nerve Lesions

A peripheral nerve can be damaged more or less severely, with corresponding implications for treatment and prognosis. The traditional, clinically useful threefold distinction is as follows:

- **Neurapraxia**: the nerve is dysfunctional, but its anatomic continuity is preserved (e.g., nerve dysfunction due to pressure on the nerve when the individual has slept for a prolonged period in an unusual posture); the functional deficit is completely reversible.
- **Axonotmesis**: the axons within the nerve are interrupted, but the external structure of the nerve and its internal connective tissue sheaths remain intact; the full clinical picture of a peripheral nerve lesion results; under optimal conditions, full recovery may still be possible.
- **Neurotmesis**: the axons and all surrounding structures are interrupted and the nerve is no longer in continuity (e.g., because of tearing or sharp transection of the nerve); a surgical procedure is needed to restore nerve integrity, and the prognosis for recovery is uncertain.

13

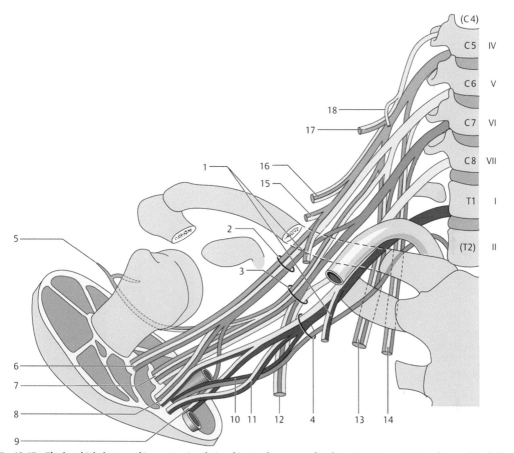

Fig. 13.17   The brachial plexus and its anatomic relationships to the surrounding bony structures. 1 Pectoral nerves (medial/lateral) C5–T1; **2** lateral cord; **3** dorsal (posterior) cord; **4** medial cord; **5** axillary nerve C5, C6; **6** musculocutaneous nerve C5–C7; **7** radial nerve C5–T1; **8** median nerve C5–T1; **9** ulnar nerve (C7) C8–T1; **10** medial brachial cutaneous nerve C8–T1; **11** medial antebrachial cutaneous nerve C8–T1; **12** thoracodorsal nerve C6–C8; **13** subscapular nerves C5–C8; **14** long thoracic nerve C5–C7; **15** nerve to the subclavius muscle C5, C6; **16** suprascapular nerve C4–6; **17** dorsal scapular nerve C3–C5; **18** phrenic nerve C3, C4.

13.2.2 Diseases of the Brachial Plexus

> **NOTE**
>
> In the brachial plexus, axons derived from the **C4 to T1 (or T2)** nerve roots are regrouped and distributed to the various nerves that innervate the upper limb (**Fig. 13.17**). Depending on their localization, lesions of the brachial plexus cause a wide variety of neurologic deficits in the proximal and/or distal portions of the upper limb.

Overview
Anatomy of the Brachial Plexus

The anatomy of the brachial plexus is shown in **Fig. 13.17**. The brachial plexus passes through three **anatomic bottlenecks** on its way to the upper arm; the first two are the **scalene hiatus**, through which it is accompanied by the subclavian artery, and the **costoclavicular space** between the first rib and the

clavicle. At this location, the caudal portion of the plexus is adjacent to the apex of the lung. A bit further distally, the brachial plexus is covered by the pectoralis minor muscle, which originates from the **coracoid process** of the scapula, and it can be compressed here when the arm is elevated. These bottlenecks are illustrated in **Fig. 13.18**.

General Clinical Features of Brachial Plexus Lesions

The complex structure of the brachial plexus and the redistribution of individual radicular elements within it make brachial plexus lesions hard to localize on the basis of the neurologic findings alone. Nonetheless, detailed functional testing of the affected muscles can reveal the root levels that are involved and this, in turn, permits localization of the lesion within the plexus with a fair degree of precision. The information provided in **Fig. 13.19** will be helpful in this regard.

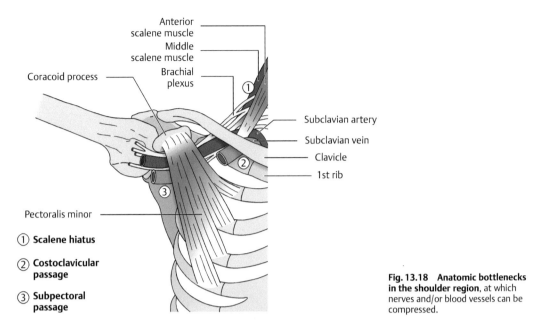

Anterior scalene muscle

Middle scalene muscle

Brachial plexus

Coracoid process

Subclavian artery

Subclavian vein

Clavicle

1st rib

Pectoralis minor

① **Scalene hiatus**

② **Costoclavicular passage**

③ **Subpectoral passage**

Fig. 13.18 Anatomic bottlenecks in the shoulder region, at which nerves and/or blood vessels can be compressed.

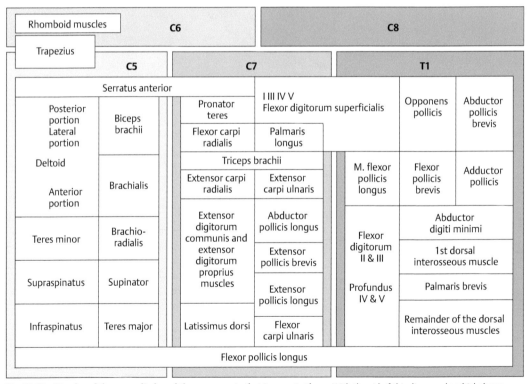

Rhomboid muscles		C6			C8	
Trapezius						
		C5		C7		T1
Serratus anterior						
Posterior portion Lateral portion	Biceps brachii	Pronator teres		I III IV V Flexor digitorum superficialis	Opponens pollicis	Abductor pollicis brevis
		Flexor carpi radialis		Palmaris longus		
Deltoid		Triceps brachii			M. flexor pollicis longus	Flexor pollicis brevis	Adductor pollicis
Anterior portion	Brachialis	Extensor carpi radialis		Extensor carpi ulnaris			
Teres minor	Brachio-radialis	Extensor digitorum communis and extensor digitorum proprius muscles		Abductor pollicis longus	Flexor digitorum II & III	Abductor digiti minimi
				Extensor pollicis brevis		1st dorsal interosseous muscle
Supraspinatus	Supinator			Extensor pollicis longus	Profundus IV & V	Palmaris brevis
Infraspinatus	Teres major	Latissimus dorsi		Flexor carpi ulnaris		Remainder of the dorsal interosseous muscles
Flexor pollicis longus						

Fig. 13.19 Muscles of the upper limb and the nerve roots that innervate them. With the aid of this diagram, brachial plexus lesions can be localized from the pattern of muscle weakness that they cause.

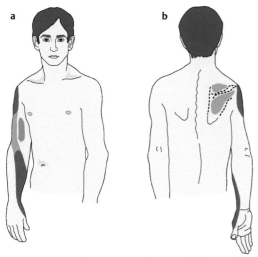

Fig. 13.20   Upper limb posture and sensory deficit in right upper brachial plexus palsy. The deltoid, biceps, and supra- and infraspinatus muscles are atrophic, the arm is internally rotated, and the palm of the hand points posteriorly.

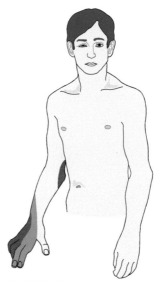

Fig. 13.21   Upper limb posture and sensory deficit in right lower brachial plexus palsy. The intrinsic muscles of the hand are atrophic, there is a sensory deficit in the C7 and C8 dermatomes, and there is an accompanying Horner syndrome.

The Differential Diagnosis of Brachial Plexus Lesions

Meticulous clinical examination, supplemented if necessary by electrophysiologic studies, should always be able to distinguish a brachial plexus lesion from a lesion affecting **multiple nerve roots** or a **peripheral nerve**. In our experience, however, it is not always a simple matter to distinguish a lower brachial plexus lesion (i.e., one affecting the C8 and T1 roots) from a **proximal ulnar nerve lesion** (see section 13.2.3, Ulnar Nerve (C8–T1)). Likewise, an upper brachial plexus lesion (perhaps traumatic) may be hard to distinguish from an **axillary nerve lesion** or an **injury to the rotator cuff**.

Classification of Brachial Plexus Lesions

Topical classification. In addition to total paralysis of the entire upper limb, there are three types of partial lesion in the customary, **topically oriented** classification, namely:
- **Upper** brachial plexus lesion (Erb–Duchenne palsy).
- **Lower** brachial plexus lesion (Déjerine–Klumpke palsy).
- **C7** lesion.

Etiologic classification. Alternatively (or additionally), brachial plexus lesions can be classified by their **cause**—traumatic, compressive, or inflammatory.
In the following sections, the main types of lesion will be presented individually.

Upper Brachial Plexus Lesion (Erb–Duchenne Palsy)

This type of lesion involves the fibers that originate in the **C5 and C6** nerve roots. The affected muscles are:

- The abductors and external rotators of the shoulder joint.
- The flexor muscles of the upper arm.
- The supinator muscle.
- Sometimes the elbow extensors and the extensors of the hand.

A sensory deficit is not necessarily present; if there is one, it is located on the shoulder, the lateral surface of the upper arm, or the radial edge of the forearm (**Fig. 13.20**).

Lower Brachial Plexus Lesion (Déjerine–Klumpke Palsy)

This type of lesion involves the fibers originating in the **C8** and **T1** roots. Its prominent findings include:
- Weakness of the intrinsic muscles of the hand.
- Sometimes also weakness of the long flexors of the fingers.
- Rarely, weakness of the wrist flexors.
- The triceps brachii muscle usually remains intact.

The mechanism of the precipitating injury and the anatomic relationships in this area often lead to an accompanying **cervical sympathetic dysfunction**, resulting in **Horner syndrome** with **impaired sweating**. This finding implies a lesion of the T1 root proximal to the exit of its branch to the sympathetic chain. There is always a **sensory deficit** on the ulnar edge of the forearm, hand, and fingers (**Fig. 13.21**).

C7 Palsy

In the present context, this term does not refer to a lesion of the C7 root itself, but rather to a lesion of the fibers derived from it that make up the C7

13

portion of the brachial plexus. This type of palsy involves deficits in the distribution of the **radial nerve** (see section 13.2.3, Radial Nerve (C5–C8)), while the function of the brachioradialis muscle is preserved.

Traumatic Lesions of the Brachial Plexus

These are usually due to **motor vehicle accidents**; rarer causes include occupational injury and direct stab or gunshot wounds.

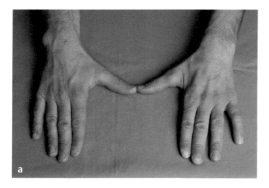

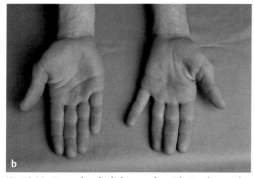

Fig. 13.22 Lower brachial plexus palsy with atrophy mainly affecting the intrinsic hand muscles innervated by the ulnar nerve. **a** On the dorsal aspect of the hand, there is atrophy of the interossei, in particular the first dorsal interosseous muscle. **b** On the volar aspect of the hand, there is atrophy of the adductor pollicis brevis muscle and of the hypothenar muscles.

Clinical features. The initial clinical finding is not uncommonly a **total upper limb paralysis** which may later improve until it resembles one of the types of localized brachial plexus lesion described earlier (**Fig. 13.22**). Upper brachial plexus lesions have a better prognosis.

 Practical Tip
> Bloody cerebrospinal fluid on lumbar puncture and, later, clinical evidence of myelopathy are poor prognostic signs that indicate probable nerve root avulsion. In such patients, MRI may reveal empty nerve root pouches (Fig. 13.23).

Treatment. The treatment consists of an abduction splint and passive exercises to prevent freezing of the shoulder joint. Brachial plexus surgery is highly complex and demanding and is occasionally resorted to in cases of upper brachial plexus injury.

Brachial Plexus Palsy Caused by Birth Trauma

This may result from obstetric complications such as breech delivery. Such cases involve an upper (Erb–Duchenne) brachial plexus palsy in approximately 80% of patients and a lower (Déjerine–Klumpke) brachial plexus palsy in approximately 10%. When the damaged axons regenerate, they may reconnect to the "wrong" muscles and/or muscle groups, leading to pathologic accessory movements and abnormal motor patterns.

Compressive Lesions of the Brachial Plexus

External Compression

External compression can injure the brachial plexus in persons who carry heavy loads on their shoulders or wear heavy backpacks. Lesions of this type usually affect the **upper brachial plexus**, and sometimes only individual branches of it. The **long thoracic nerve** is most frequently involved (see section 13.2.3, Long Thoracic Nerve (C5–C7)).

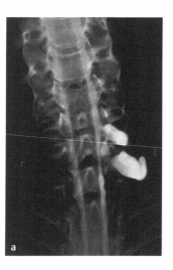

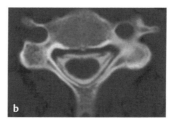

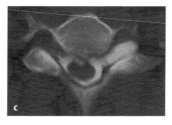

Fig. 13.23 Left C7 and C8 nerve root avulsion. a Myelography: contrast medium flows out via the nerve root sleeves. Root avulsion is usually associated with an injury to the dura mater. **b** Postmyelographic CT: normal findings for comparison. **c** Postmyelographic CT in this case at an affected level: nerve root avulsion.

Compression at Anatomic Bottlenecks

The collective term **"thoracic outlet syndrome"** is commonly used for these conditions, usually nonspecifically and often, unfortunately, as a vague term for brachialgia of undetermined origin, or for other unexplained symptoms relating to the brachial plexus.

Scalene syndrome. This is usually due to the anomalous presence of a **cervical rib**, a fibrous band (which may be visible in a CT scan), or some other structural anomaly in the scalene hiatus (**Fig. 13.18**). Its **typical features** are:

- Clinical evidence of a lower brachial plexus lesion.
- Worsening of symptoms on pulling the arm downward.
- Fixed or motion-induced circulatory insufficiency of the subclavian artery, as revealed by:
  - A vascular bruit.
  - Disappearance of the radial pulse when certain maneuvers are performed, for example, the **Adson maneuver**—turning the chin to the side of the lesion, with simultaneous reclination of the head.

Costoclavicular syndrome. Similar to scalene syndrome, it should be diagnosed only if a causative anatomic anomaly and objectifiable neurologic deficits (usually, a lower brachial plexus palsy) can be found. An arteriogram is occasionally helpful in establishing the diagnosis, as it may demonstrate motion-dependent **compression of the subclavian artery or vein.**

Treatment of compression syndromes. Both the scalene syndrome and costoclavicular syndrome should be treated conservatively at first, once their diagnosis has been definitively established. Special exercises are used to strengthen the shoulder-elevating muscles. Surgical treatment is reserved for the small minority of patients with objectifiable neurologic deficits. A supra- or transclavicular approach gives the surgeon optimal access to the anatomic structures.

Neuralgic Shoulder Amyotrophy

Pathogenesis and epidemiology. This disorder is presumed to be due to an **inflammatory/allergic** affection of the brachial plexus. It affects men more often than women and usually arises **spontaneously**, but is sometimes seen in the aftermath of an infectious disease or, rarely, after vaccination (brachial plexus neuritis).

Clinical features. Neuralgic shoulder amyotrophy affects the right arm more commonly than the left. It typically begins with **intense local pain** in the shoulder, which generally lasts for a few days. Rarely, the pain will persist at a milder intensity for a longer period. Once it subsides, **weakness** of the shoulder girdle and/or arm muscle develops. The weakness

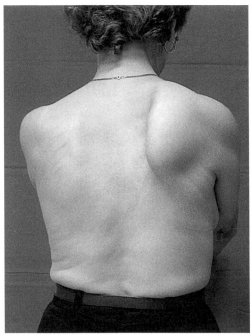

Fig. 13.24   Right serratus anterior palsy in neuralgic shoulder amyotrophy. Marked winging of the scapula is seen on forward elevation of the right arm. (Reproduced from Mumenthaler M, Stöhr M, Müller-Vahl H, et al. Läsionen peripherer Nerven und radikuläre Syndrome. Stuttgart: Thieme; 2007.)

can, in principle, affect any muscle group of the upper limb, but it tends to affect the muscles innervated by the **upper** portion of the brachial plexus. Paresis of the **serratus anterior muscle** is particularly common (**Fig. 13.24**). There may not be any objectifiable sensory deficit.

Treatment and prognosis. No specific treatment is required beyond analgesic medication in the initial, painful phase. The prognosis is generally good, but it may take many months for the weakness to resolve completely.

Radiation-Induced Brachial Plexus Lesions

These usually appear with a **latency** of one or more years after radiotherapy, usually in women who have been treated with surgery and radiotherapy for breast cancer. In 15% of patients, **pain** is the main symptom; it can increase over the course of several years. The **differentiation** of radiation-induced brachial plexopathy from a recurrent malignant tumor is not always easy; very intense pain, or a short interval between the completion of radiotherapy and the onset of pain (except when a very high radiation dose was given), tends to suggest a recurrent tumor rather than radiation injury as the cause. **Imaging studies** are helpful, but even these cannot always reliably distinguish scarring from new tumor tissue.

13

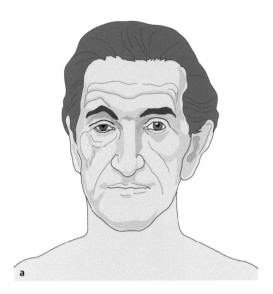

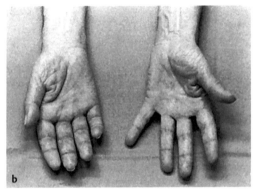

13

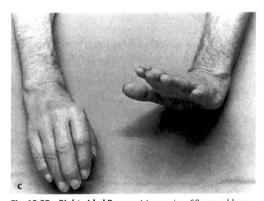

Fig. 13.25 Right-sided Pancoast tumor in a 68-year-old man. There is clinical evidence of compression of the lower brachial plexus and of the sympathetic chain. **a** Right Horner syndrome. **b** Atrophy of the intrinsic muscles of the right hand, especially the thenar muscles. **c** Weakness of the wrist and finger extensors on the right.

Pancoast Tumor

Pancoast tumors of the apex of the lung usually cause a **lower brachial plexus palsy** with severe pain. The sympathetic chain is usually involved as well; thus, **Horner syndrome** and **diminished sweating** in the upper body on the affected side are typical findings (**Fig. 13.25**).

Other Causes

Other, rare causes of brachial plexus palsy include the following:

— Acute palsy due to occlusion of a small artery supplying the plexus.
— Iatrogenic brachial nerve palsy.
— In heroin addicts.
— In familial brachial plexus neuritis.
— Parainfectious and serogenic forms (i.e., brachial plexus palsy mediated by immune complexes, either in the setting of an autoimmune disease or after immune serum administration as a medical treatment).

13.2.3 Diseases of the Peripheral Nerves of the Upper Limbs

> **NOTE**
>
> Lesions of individual peripheral nerves of the upper limbs are very common. Each such disorder has a characteristic clinical picture resulting from the distribution of the affected motor and sensory fibers.

Suprascapular Nerve (C4–C6)

Anatomy. This nerve supplies the **supraspinatus and infraspinatus muscles**. It reaches them after passing through the scapular notch and then running dorsally. It receives sensory tributaries from the shoulder joint, but not from the skin.

Typical deficits. A lesion of the suprascapular nerve produces weakness and atrophy of the two muscles on the dorsal surface of the scapula (**Fig. 13.26**). The first 15 degrees of lateral elevation of the arm are weak (supraspinatus muscle), as is external rotation of the arm at the shoulder joint (infraspinatus muscle) (**Fig. 13.27**).

Causes. Overuse of the arm can lead to mechanical compromise of the nerve in the scapular notch. Other causes include trauma and a ganglion lying in the notch.

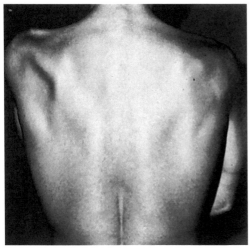

Fig. 13.26   Atrophy of the supra- and infraspinatus muscles due to a lesion of the left suprascapular nerve in a 25-year old man. The etiology remained unclear in this case.

Axillary Nerve (C5–C6)

Anatomy. This nerve (**Fig. 13.28**) provides motor innervation to the **deltoid** and **teres minor muscles** and sensory innervation to a palm-sized patch of skin on the proximal, lateral surface of the upper arm (**superior lateral brachial cutaneous nerve**).

Typical deficits. Axillary nerve palsy manifests itself as marked weakness of lateral abduction and forward elevation of the arm. The normal roundness of the shoulder is flattened. External rotation of the arm at the shoulder joint is lessened at rest because of inactivation of the teres minor muscle, so that the dependent arm is held in mild internal rotation (**Fig. 13.29**).

Causes. The most common cause of axillary nerve palsy is dislocation of the shoulder (forward and downward). The prognosis in such patients is favorable.

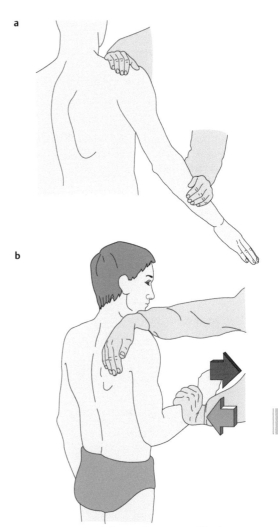

Fig. 13.27   Testing of the muscles innervated by the suprascapular nerve. a Weakness of the supraspinatus muscle is most evident in the first 15 degrees of lateral elevation of the arm. **b** Weakness of the infraspinatus muscle is evident when the arm is externally rotated at the shoulder joint.

13

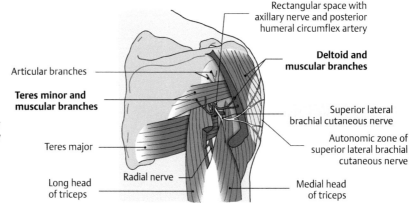

Fig. 13.28   Anatomic course and distribution of the axillary nerve. Sensory (yellow) and motor branches (brown). The autonomous sensory area of the superior lateral brachial cutaneous nerve is shaded in yellow.

Rectangular space with axillary nerve and posterior humeral circumflex artery

Articular branches

Teres minor and muscular branches

Deltoid and muscular branches

Superior lateral brachial cutaneous nerve

Autonomic zone of superior lateral brachial cutaneous nerve

Teres major

Long head of triceps

Radial nerve

Medial head of triceps

Differential diagnosis. A differential diagnosis of axillary nerve palsy includes complex brachial plexus lesions affecting the upper portion of the plexus, rotator cuff lesions, and restriction of movement by pain in humeroscapular periarthropathy (frozen shoulder syndrome).

Long Thoracic Nerve (C5–C7)

Anatomy. This nerve is the longest branch of the brachial plexus. It is a purely motor nerve supplying the **serratus anterior muscle**.

Typical deficits. Long thoracic nerve palsy causes winging of the scapula, which is particularly evident when the arms are held high, or when the patient extends the arms and presses with the palms of the hands against a wall (**Fig. 13.30**). It can also be seen merely on forward elevation of the arms (**Fig. 13.31**).

Causes. Lesions of the long thoracic nerve are usually due to excessive mechanical strain on the shoulder (car-

rying heavy loads) or to neuralgic shoulder amyotrophy (see section 13.2.2). They can also be cryptogenic.

Musculocutaneous Nerve (C5–C7)

Anatomy. This nerve supplies the **biceps brachii** and **coracobrachialis muscles** and a portion of the **brachialis muscle**. Its sensory terminal branch, the **lateral antebrachial cutaneous nerve**, innervates the skin on the radial side of the forearm (**Fig. 13.32**).

Typical deficits. Lesions of the musculocutaneous nerve cause marked weakness of elbow flexion. This

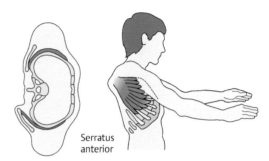

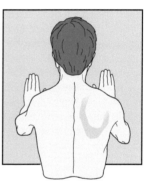

Serratus anterior

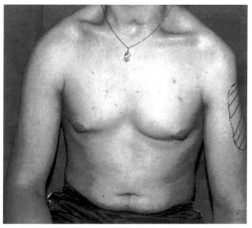

Fig. 13.29   Left axillary nerve lesion in a 26-year-old man. Atrophy of the left deltoid muscle with "pointed" shoulder contour. The sensory deficit in the territory of the superior lateral brachial cutaneous nerve is indicated.

Fig. 13.30   Lesion of the right long thoracic nerve. Weakness of the serratus anterior muscle causes winging of the scapula, which is particularly evident when the patient extends the arms forward and pushes against a wall.

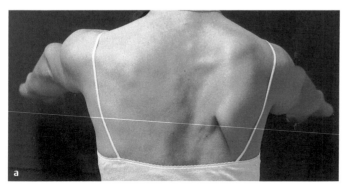

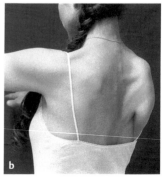

Fig. 13.31   Clinical findings in a lesion of the right long thoracic nerve. Right serratus anterior palsy in a 32-year-old woman with neuralgic shoulder amyotrophy. **a** Winging of the scapula with forward elevation of the arms. **b** Winging of the scapula is especially well seen when viewed obliquely from behind. (Reproduced from Mumenthaler M, Stöhr M, Müller-Vahl H, et al. Läsionen peripherer Nerven und radikuläre Syndrome. Stuttgart: Thieme, 2007.)

must be tested with the forearm in the supinated position (**Fig. 13.33**), because, if the forearm is pronated or in neutral position, the elbow can still be flexed by the powerful brachioradialis muscle, which is innervated by the radial nerve.

Causes. The usual cause is trauma, in which case further signs of an upper brachial plexus lesion may be present. Cryptogenic lesions of the musculocutaneous nerve and palsy of this nerve due to neuralgic shoulder amyotrophy are rarer events.

Differential diagnosis. **Avulsion of the long tendon of the biceps brachialis muscle** only rarely causes weakness of elbow flexion when the forearm is held in the supinated position. This condition is easy to differentiate from musculocutaneous nerve palsy for two further reasons: one is the typical appearance of the belly of the muscle on the volar surface of the forearm (**Fig. 13.34**); the other is the absence of a sensory deficit.

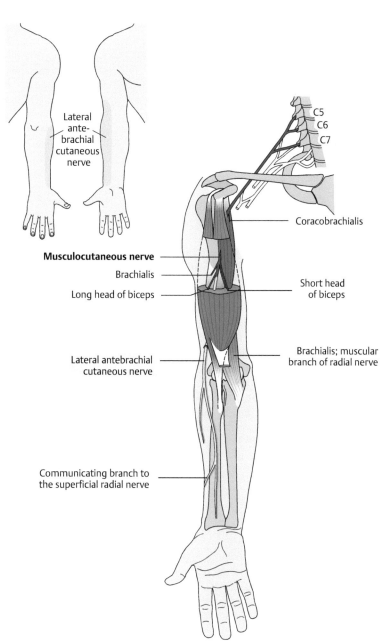

Fig. 13.32   Anatomic course and distribution of the musculo-cutaneous nerve.

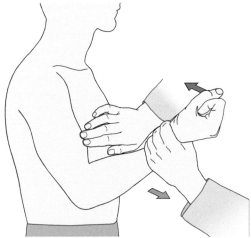

Fig. 13.33 Functional testing of the biceps brachii muscle. The forearm must be held in the supinated position. (Adapted from Mumenthaler M, Stöhr M, Müller-Vahl H, et al. Läsionen peripherer Nerven und radikuläre Syndrome. Stuttgart: Thieme; 2007.)

Radial Nerve (C5–C8)

Anatomy. The anatomy of the radial nerve is depicted in **Fig. 13.34**. It provides motor innervation to the **triceps brachii**, **brachioradialis**, and **supinator muscles**, as well as all the **extensors of the wrist, thumb, and finger joints**. Its sensory innervation is to the dorsal skin of the upper arm and forearm as well as to the dorsum of the hand, with an autonomic zone between the first and second metacarpal bones.

Typical deficits. The clinical features of radial nerve palsy depend on the **level** of the lesion:

- **Lesion in the upper arm**: the radial nerve is particularly vulnerable to injury in the radial nerve canal of the humerus, because it lies directly on the bone at this location. The corresponding, readily apparent neurologic deficit is a **wrist drop** (**Fig. 13.35**), caused by loss of the action of the wrist and finger extensors. In addition, sensation is diminished on the radial portion of the dorsum of the hand. The clinical picture is characteristic (**Fig. 13.36**).
- **"High radial nerve lesion"**: if the nerve is injured more proximally in the upper arm or in the axilla, the triceps brachii muscle is also weak and the elbow can no longer be actively extended against resistance.
- **Supinator canal syndrome**: if the radial nerve is compromised at the site of its passage through the supinator muscle, only its deeply penetrating **motor terminal branch** is affected. The resulting deficit is purely motor. The branch to the extensor carpi radialis muscle and the brachioradialis muscle, which exits the nerve proximal to its passage through the supinator muscle, is unaffected,

but all the other forearm muscles supplied by the radial nerve are weak. Finger extension is impaired, but wrist extension is preserved, particularly on the radial side (**Fig. 13.37**). Typically, there is no sensory deficit.

Causes. Radial nerve lesions can be produced by **trauma** and by **pressure**, for example, by the use of crutches that press in the axilla or by external pressure on the upper arm (humerus; "park-bench palsy"). The supinator canal syndrome is an anatomic bottleneck (**entrapment**) syndrome.

Differential diagnosis. The differential diagnosis of radial nerve palsy must include **mainly distal paresis of central origin**, which can also present with a wrist drop. The flexor weakness and enhanced intrinsic muscle reflexes that are present in central weakness serve to differentiate this condition from radial nerve palsy. **Spinal muscle atrophy** can, in rare cases, initially affect the wrist extensors on one side only. **Curschmann–Steinert myotonic dystrophy** (see section 15.3.2) commonly produces a bilateral wrist drop.

Median Nerve (C5–T1)
Median Nerve Lesions

Anatomy. The anatomy of the median nerve is shown in **Fig. 13.38**. All of the muscles supplied by this nerve are distal to the elbow. In the forearm, these include most of the **long flexors of the fingers** (except the deep flexors of the fourth and fifth fingers, which are innervated by the ulnar nerve), as well as the **flexor carpi radialis**, **pronator teres**, and **pronator quadratus muscles**. After the nerve passes through the carpal tunnel together with the long flexor tendons, it innervates most of the **thenar muscles** (abductor pollicis brevis and opponens pollicis muscle and the superficial head of the flexor pollicis brevis muscle), as well as the **first and second lumbrical muscles**. Its sensory innervation is to the radial side of the palm, the volar surface of the fingers from the thumb to the radial half of the fourth finger, and the dorsal surface of the terminal phalanges of these fingers.

Typical deficits. In median nerve lesions, too, the clinical features depend on the level of the lesion:

- **Median nerve lesion in the upper arm** (i.e., proximal to the origin of its motor branches to the forearm flexors): the typical clinical appearance is that of the "preacher's hand," depicted in **Fig. 13.39**, which is caused by weakness of the radial finger flexors.
- **Median nerve lesion at the wrist**. A lesion of the median nerve in the carpal tunnel causes weakness of the thenar muscles. Clinically, pain and paresthesia are the most prominent symptoms.

Carpal tunnel syndrome (CTS) is discussed separately later, in detail, because of its special clinical importance.

- **Syndrome of the anterior interosseous nerve (Kiloh–Nevin syndrome).** An isolated lesion of the anterior interosseous nerve is a rare occurrence. This nerve is the motor terminal branch of the median nerve; it innervates the flexor pollicis longus muscle, the radial portion of the flexor digitorum profundus muscle (flexion of the terminal phalanges of the second and third fingers), and the pronator quadratus muscle. A lesion of this terminal branch—due to trauma or, sometimes, entrapment—mainly impairs flexion of the terminal phalanges of the thumb and index finger. The patient can no longer form a "0" with these two fingers (**Fig. 13.40**).

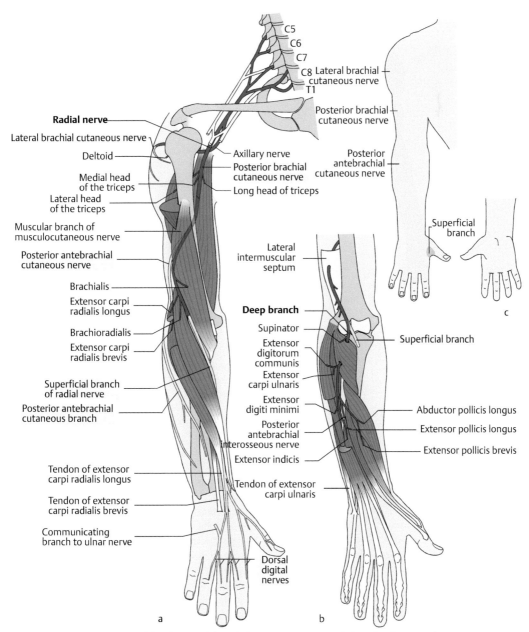

Fig. 13.34   Anatomic course and distribution of the radial nerve. a Proximal muscle branches (brown) and course of the sensory superficial branch (yellow). **b** Course of the motor deep branch. **c** Zones of cutaneous innervation of the branches of the radial nerve and sensory autonomous area of the superficial branch.

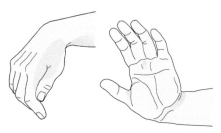

Fig. 13.35   Right wrist drop due to a radial nerve lesion. The yellow color indicates the sensory autonomous area in the distribution of the superficial branch of the radial nerve.

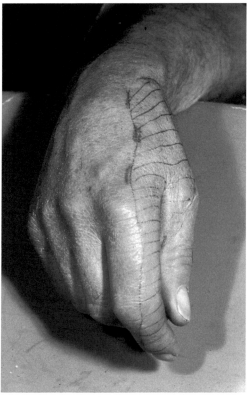

Fig. 13.36   Right wrist drop in radial nerve palsy. The cause is nerve compression in the upper arm. The area of the sensory deficit on the first interosseous space is shaded.

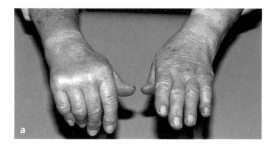

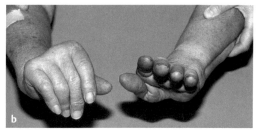

Fig. 13.37   Right supinator tunnel syndrome in a 71-year-old woman. **a** Marked weakness of the finger extensors of the right hand. **b** Preservation of wrist extension on the radial side of the wrist.

Causes. The median nerve is the nerve most frequently injured by **direct trauma**, often by a cut in the wrist. **Pressure palsies** of the median nerve also occur, either in the upper arm (due to prolonged maintenance of an awkward position, or to an Esmarch tourniquet) or in the palm of the hand (e.g., in occupational injuries). Compression at anatomic bottlenecks (**entrapment**) is a further cause of median nerve lesions. In many individuals, a bony spur is present just above the medial epicondyle of the humerus (the **supracondylar process**). A fibrous band (of Struther) may run from this spur to the medial epicondyle, forming a tunnel through which the median nerve passes. The nerve can be compressed either by the supracondylar process or by the fibrous band. Further compression syndromes affecting the median nerve are the **Kiloh–Nevin syndrome** (see earlier) and the **CTS**, discussed later.

Carpal Tunnel Syndrome

CTS, **the most common type of peripheral nerve lesion**, is caused by (mechanical) compression of the median nerve as it passes through the **carpal tunnel**. It is three times as common in women as in men and tends to develop around the time of the menopause; in advanced age, it is equally common in both sexes. Factors that promote or precipitate the development of CTS include hormonal changes (menopause, pregnancy), weight gain, hypothyroidism, diabetes mellitus, and manual activity.

Typical deficits. CTS more commonly affects the **dominant hand**, but it can affect either hand, or both. Its typical features are:

— In the **initial phase**, which lasts **several months or years**, the manifestations are purely subjective: dull pain in the arm at night (**brachialgia paresthetica nocturna**), which is felt not merely in the hand, but in the whole upper limb up to the shoulder, wakes the patient from sleep and can

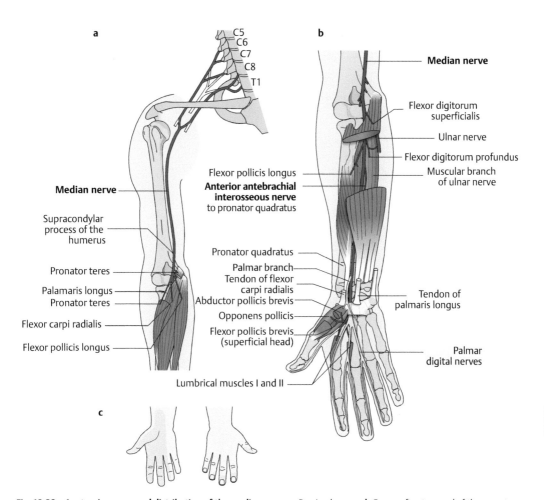

Fig. 13.38   Anatomic course and distribution of the median nerve. a Proximal course. **b** Course after traversal of the pronator teres muscle. **c** Zones of cutaneous innervation in the hand.

be relieved by shaking and massaging the arms. The fingers are stiff and uncoordinated for a short time after the patient wakes up in the morning.
- In the **advanced phase** (**Fig. 13.41**), **abnormal sensations (paresthesiae)** develop and the **sense of touch is impaired**, mainly in the thumb and index finger. Meticulous examination reveals objective sensory and/or motor deficits.

Examination and diagnostic evaluation.
- An occasional objective finding is point tenderness to pressure at the root of the thenar muscles, or a positive **Tinel sign** (paresthesia in the radial portion of the palm and the radial fingers evoked by a tap on the transverse carpal ligament).
- Finger paresthesia can sometimes be evoked by sustained passive hyperflexion or hyperextension of the wrist (**Phalen sign**).

- Only later in the course of CTS is there a mild **impairment of the sense of touch**, particularly in the index finger (e.g., a worsening of two-point discrimination to > 5 mm).
- The major finding, however, is an inability to abduct the thumb fully, particularly when compared with the normal, opposite side, because of weakness of the abductor pollicis brevis muscle. This can be demonstrated by having the patient grasp a cylindrical object; a "**positive bottle sign**" is seen (**Fig. 13.42**).
- Impaired opposition of the thumb is more difficult to observe clinically (**Fig. 13.43**).

Overt CTS is unequivocally demonstrated by a finding of **impaired conduction in the median nerve** across the carpal tunnel, as revealed by **electroneurography** (**Fig. 13.44**).

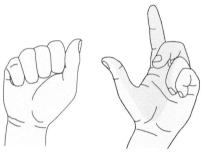

Fig. 13.39 **"Preacher's hand" due to a proximal left median nerve lesion**. The hypesthetic area is shaded yellow.

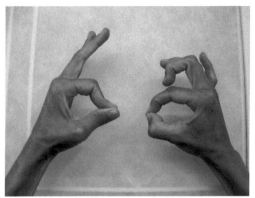

Fig. 13.40 **Kiloh–Nevin syndrome**. The patient cannot flex the distal phalanges of the thumb and index finger. The lesion affects the deep branch of the left median nerve.

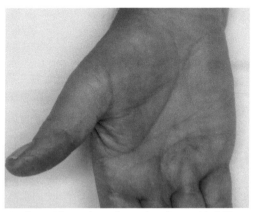

Fig. 13.41 **Advanced carpal tunnel syndrome** with visible atrophy of the abductor pollicis brevis and opponens pollicis muscles.

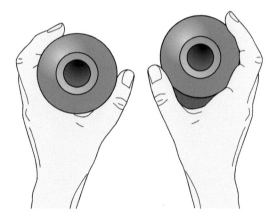

Fig. 13.42 **"Bottle" sign in right median nerve palsy**. The thumb cannot be adequately abducted and opposed.

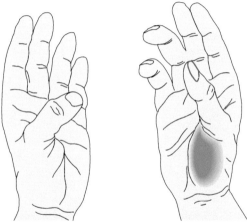

Fig. 13.43 **Inadequate opposition and pronation of the thumb in a patient with a right median nerve lesion**. Because the thumb is insufficiently rotated, the thumbnail is seen tangentially rather than head on (as on the normal left side).

 Practical Tip

Diagnostic electroneurography should always be done before any operation is performed. Diminished conduction velocity alone, in the absence of characteristic symptoms, is not an indication for surgery.

Treatment. Splinting of the hand in the neutral position at night with a well-padded volar splint often brings relief. If it does not, or if objectifiable neurologic deficits are already present, there should be no hesitation in proceeding to surgery. Operative **carpal tunnel release** involves splitting of the flexor retinaculum with an open or endoscopic technique (generally performed either by a neurosurgeon or by a hand surgeon).

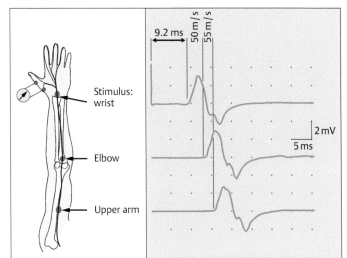

9.2 ms

50 m/s

55 m/s

Stimulus: wrist

2 mV

5 ms

Elbow

Fig. 13.44 Motor median neurography in right carpal tunnel syndrome. The recording is performed over the abductor pollicis muscle. The distal motor latency is prolonged (9.2 ms, compared with normal 3.9 ms). The nerve conduction velocities in the arm and forearm are normal.

Upper arm

Ulnar Nerve (C8–T1)

Anatomy. Among the muscles supplied by this nerve, the ulnar flexors of the wrist and fingers (the flexor carpi ulnaris muscle and the ulnar portion of the flexor digitorum profundus muscle) are functionally much less important than the ulnar-innervated **intrinsic muscles of the hand** (**Fig. 13.45**). The ulnar nerve is, indeed, the most important nerve for finger function: it innervates not only the **hypothenar muscles**, but also all of the **interossei**, the **third and fourth lumbrical muscles**, and, in the thenar region, the **adductor pollicis muscle** and the **deep head of the flexor pollicis brevis muscle**. It provides sensory innervation to the ulnar edge of the hand, the volar surface of the fifth finger, and the ulnar half of the fourth finger. A sensory branch arising from the ulnar nerve in the distal third of the forearm innervates the skin on the ulnar side of the dorsum of the hand, as well as on the dorsal surface of the fifth finger and the ulnar half of the fourth finger.

Typical deficits. The typical clinical picture of ulnar nerve palsy is a **claw hand** (**Fig. 13.46**): because the interossei and lumbrical muscles cannot contract, the ulnar digits are hyperextended at the metacarpophalangeal joints and flexed at the remaining joints. The long fingers can no longer be fully adducted against one another, the fingers cannot be strongly spread apart, and the patient cannot flick the middle finger against the examiner's palm with full, normal strength. A key finding is that, when the patient grasps a flat object (such as a piece of paper) between the thumb and the index finger, weakness

of the adductor pollicis muscle (ulnar nerve) leads to automatic functional substitution by the flexor pollicis longus muscle (median nerve), and therefore to flexion of the thumb at the interphalangeal joint. This finding, called **Froment sign**, is highly characteristic of ulnar nerve palsy (**Fig. 13.47**).

In addition to these general clinical features of ulnar nerve palsy, there are other specific findings that depend on the level of the lesion:

— If the lesion is **proximal** (at the elbow or higher), it will also affect the ulnar portion of the flexor digitorum profundus muscle, thereby impairing flexion of the distal phalanges of the fourth and fifth digits (**Fig. 13.48**).

— If the lesion is **at the wrist**, it can be precisely localized by the involvement or noninvolvement of the palmaris brevis muscle and the configuration of the sensory deficit. The flexor muscles of the forearm that are innervated by the ulnar nerve remain intact.

— **An isolated lesion of the purely motor terminal branch** of the ulnar nerve (its deep branch) causes weakness of the interossei while sparing the hypothenar and lumbrical muscles and the muscles of the forearm innervated by the ulnar nerve. There is typically no sensory deficit (**Fig. 13.49**).

Causes. Ulnar nerve palsy is often of **traumatic** origin. The nerve can be chronically **dislocated** at the elbow, where it can slip out of the ulnar groove on the medial epicondyle of the humerus; it is also vulnerable to **external compression** at this point (the

13

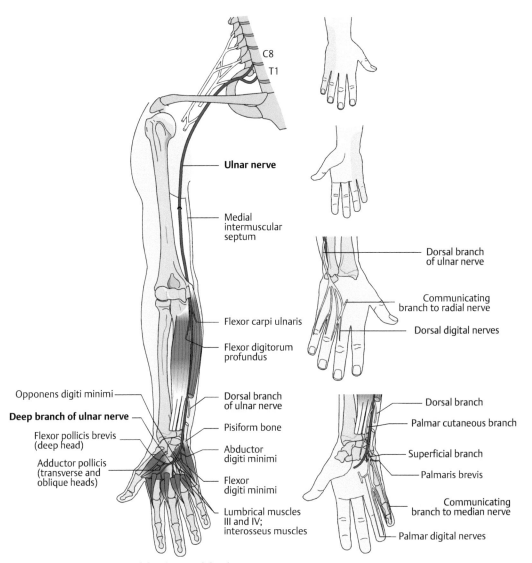

C8
T1

Ulnar nerve

Medial
intermuscular
septum

Dorsal branch
of ulnar nerve

Communicating
branch to radial nerve

Dorsal digital nerves

Flexor carpi ulnaris

Flexor digitorum
profundus

Opponens digiti minimi

Deep branch of ulnar nerve

Flexor pollicis brevis
(deep head)

Adductor pollicis
(transverse and
oblique heads)

Dorsal branch
of ulnar nerve

Pisiform bone

Abductor
digiti minimi

Flexor
digiti minimi

Lumbrical muscles
III and IV;
interosseus muscles

Dorsal branch

Palmar cutaneous branch

Superficial branch

Palmaris brevis

Communicating
branch to median nerve

Palmar digital nerves

Fig. 13.45   Anatomic course and distribution of the ulnar nerve.

13

"funny bone"), as well as to compression due to **anatomic variations** of the ulnar groove (sulcus ulnaris syndrome, **cubital tunnel syndrome**). Similarly, the ulnar nerve can be damaged in the palm of the hand (e.g., by occupational tools), or because of anatomic variations at the wrist (**syndrome of the "loge de Guyon,"** e.g., after a long bicycle ride).

Treatment. The treatment depends on the cause and location of the lesion. Chronic compression of the nerve is treated by removing the source of compression. This may involve splinting or padding of the elbow, or even operative relocation of the nerve from a more dorsal to a more volar position.

13.2.4 Diseases of the Nerves of the Trunk

| NOTE

The nerves of the trunk are in a less vulnerable anatomic position than those of the limbs and are thus much less commonly injured. Lesions of the nerves of the trunk also have less serious functional consequences. On rare occasions, however, such lesions do cause troublesome pain syndromes.

Anatomy. The peripheral nerves supplying the thoracic and abdominal wall are derived from nerve roots T2 through T12. Each peripheral nerve in this region contains fibers that are (nearly) exclusively derived from a single nerve root. We recall that this is not the case in the limbs, where the nerve fibers are reassorted in a plexus interposed between the nerve roots and the peripheral nerves. The clinical features of a peripheral nerve lesion in the trunk are thus very similar to those of a nerve root lesion.

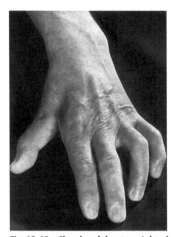

Fig. 13.46   Claw hand due to a right ulnar nerve lesion at the elbow. Typical features include hyperextension at the meta-carpophalangeal joints and hyperflexion at the interphalangeal joints, particularly on the ulnar side of the hand. There is marked atrophy of the interossei and of the hypothenar muscles.

Typical deficits. The most characteristic neurologic syndrome caused by nerve lesions in this area is **intercostal neuralgia**, that is, band-like, usually burning pain radiating around the trunk from back to front, at a single dermatomal level.

Causes. The nerves of the trunk can be damaged by **viral infections** (e.g., herpes zoster), **mass lesions**, or by a diabetic or infectious **mononeuritis** (e.g., in borreliosis). Mononeuritis produces unilateral weakness of the abdominal wall muscles; the corresponding segment of the abdominal wall becomes flaccid and pouches visibly outward (**Fig. 13.50**). Sensation in this area is diminished as well, and the abdominal skin reflex is absent at the corresponding level.

Rarely, painful **entrapment neuropathies** may affect individual sensory terminal branches of the nerves of the trunk:

— **Notalgia paraesthetica** is a neuropathy of this kind causing pain in the back. One of the dorsal rami of the thoracic spinal nerve roots becomes stuck in a small gap in the fascia, producing pain and hypesthesia in a coin-sized, paravertebral area of skin.

— There are similar entrapment syndromes of the ventral rami, causing, for example, the so-called **rectus abdominis syndrome.**

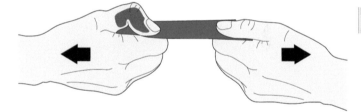

Fig. 13.47   Froment sign in right ulnar nerve palsy. Flexion of the interphalangeal joint of the thumb is seen when the patient pulls on a flat object (piece of paper).

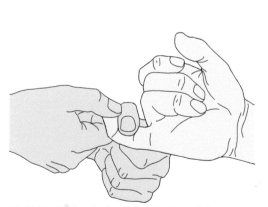

Fig. 13.48   Testing the function of the flexor digitorum profundus muscle of the little finger (ulnar nerve). Flexion of the little finger at the distal interphalangeal joint.

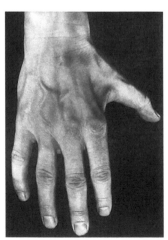

Fig. 13.49   Typical appearance of the hand in a lesion of the deep branch of the ulnar nerve at the wrist. Marked muscle atrophy in the first interosseous space, with preservation of the hypothenar musculature. Sensation was intact in this case.

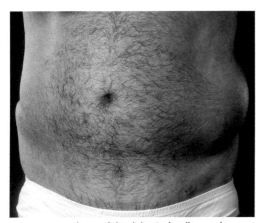

Fig. 13.50 Weakness of the abdominal wall musculature, worse on the left side, caused by neuroborreliosis affecting the caudal thoracic nerve roots.

13.2.5 Diseases of the Lumbosacral Plexus

Anatomy. The structure of the lumbosacral plexus is illustrated in **Fig. 13.51**. It lies in a well-protected location in the posterior wall of the pelvis.

— Its cranial portion (the **lumbar plexus**, L1–L4) gives off, as its main branches, the **ilioinguinal iliohypogastric, femoral**, and **obturator nerves**. These nerves innervate most of the hip flexors and knee extensors.

— Its caudal portion (the **sacral plexus**, L5–S3) gives off the **superior** and **inferior gluteal nerves** to the gluteal muscles, as well as the **sciatic nerve**, which innervates the knee flexors and all muscles of the lower leg and foot.

Typical deficits. The clinical features of a lumbosacral plexus lesion depend on its location; in general, one finds a **combination of the deficits** seen in lesions of the individual peripheral nerve trunks lying distal to the plexus lesion.

Causes. Lumbosacral plexus palsy is usually due to a **local mass**, but it may also be due to prior **radiation**

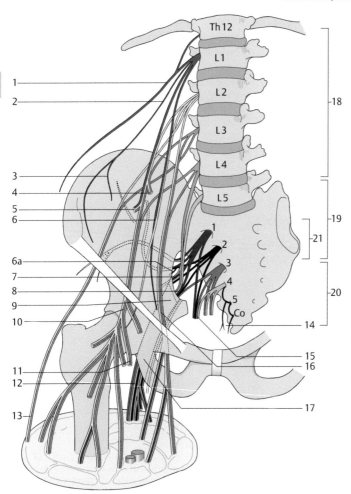

Fig. 13.51 Anatomy of the lumbosacral plexus. 1 Iliohypogastric nerve L1 (T12); **2** ilioinguinal nerve L1; **3** branch to iliacus muscle; **4** branch to psoas muscle; **5** branch to iliacus muscle; **6** genitofemoral nerve L1, L2; **6a** posterior femoral cutaneous nerve S1–S3; **7** superior gluteal nerve L4–S1; **8** inferior gluteal nerve L5–S2; **9** sciatic nerve L4–S3; common peroneal (fibular) nerve L4–S2; tibial nerve L4–S3; **10** femoral nerve L1–L4; **11** saphenous nerve L2–L4; **12** common peroneal (fibular) nerve L2–S2; **13** lateral femoral cutaneous nerve L2–L3; **14** anococcygeal nerves; **15** pudendal nerve S1–S4; **16** obturator nerve L2–L4; **17** tibial nerve L4–S3; **18** lumbar plexus; **19** sacral plexus; **20** coccygeal plexus; **21** "pudendal plexus."

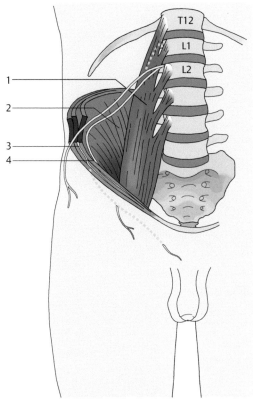

Fig. 13.52 Anatomic course of the iliohypogastric and ilioinguinal nerves. 1 Psoas major muscle, **2** iliacus muscle, **3** iliohypogastric nerve, **4** ilioinguinal nerve.

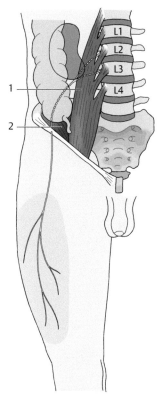

Fig. 13.53 Anatomic course and distribution of the lateral femoral cutaneous nerve. The nerve turns from a nearly horizontal to a nearly vertical course at the point where it traverses the inguinal ligament. **1** Psoas major muscle, **2** iliacus muscle.

therapy or to an **autoimmune disorder** called **chronic, progressive lumbosacral plexopathy.**

Diagnostic evaluation. Ancillary testing, primarily with **MRI** or **CT**, is generally needed to determine the cause of a lumbosacral plexopathy. These imaging studies can, for example, reveal a mass.

13.2.6 Diseases of the Peripheral Nerves of the Lower Limbs

> **NOTE**
>
> Like nerve lesions in the upper limbs, nerve lesions in the lower limbs cause typical clinical syndromes. The sciatic nerve is frequently affected, as is one of its terminal branches, the peroneal nerve. A peroneal nerve palsy causes a foot drop.

Genitofemoral and Ilioinguinal Nerves (L1–L2)

Anatomy. The course of these two (almost) monoradicular, mixed nerves is depicted in **Fig. 13.52.**

Typical deficits. Lesions of these nerves cause local pain in the groin (**ilioinguinal nerve syndrome**), a sensory deficit in the corresponding zone(s) of cutaneous innervation, and sometimes, in men, loss of the cremaster reflex (because the afferent arm of the reflex loop is interrupted). The associated motor deficit only affects oblique muscles of the abdominal wall and is hardly noticeable.

Lateral Femoral Cutaneous Nerve (L2–L3)

Anatomy. This purely sensory nerve passes through the three layers of the abdominal wall and then penetrates the inguinal ligament, usually at a point three finger breadths medial to the anterior superior iliac spine, to emerge onto the anterior fascia of the thigh. It provides sensory innervation to a palm-sized area of skin on the **anterolateral surface of the thigh** (**Fig. 13.53**).

Typical deficits. The lateral femoral cutaneous nerve is vulnerable to injury at the point where it penetrates the inguinal ligament. The resulting clinical disturbance is an entrapment neuropathy called **meralgia paresthetica**, characterized by **burning pain in the cutaneous distribution of the nerve.** The pain is better when the hip is flexed, for example, when the patient raises the ipsilateral foot onto a low stool; it is worse on hyperextension of the leg (**reverse Lasègue sign**). The site where the nerve passes through the inguinal ligament is often tender

13

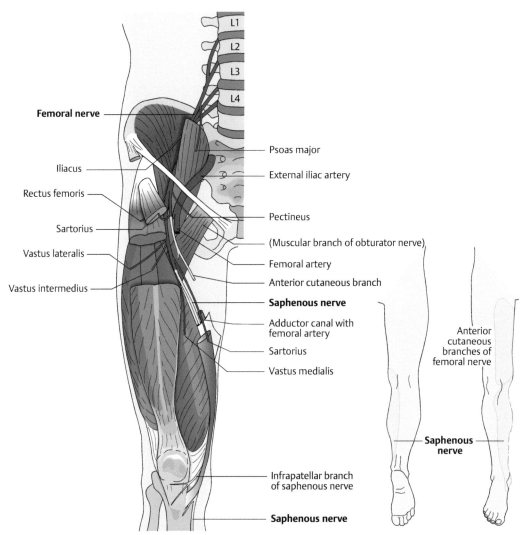

Fig. 13.54 Anatomic course and distribution of the femoral nerve.

to light pressure. Most patients find the symptoms bearable and need only be reassured that the condition is benign. Surgery is only rarely necessary; the goal of the operation is to widen the aperture in the ligament through which the nerve passes, relieving compression.

Causes. Meralgia paresthetica may be due to marked **weight gain** or **pregnancy**. It can also arise after prolonged, sustained extension of the hip joint (supine position). Some cases have no apparent cause.

Differential diagnosis. Meralgia paresthetica must be distinguished from an **L3 nerve root lesion**. L3 root lesions impair the quadriceps reflex; they also produce a more extensive sensory deficit, which, unlike that of meralgia paraesthetica, crosses over the midline of the thigh onto its anteromedial surface.

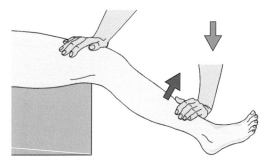

Fig. 13.55 Testing the knee extensors with the patient supine and the lower leg hanging free. In this position, the knee extensors that originate from the pelvis and cross two joints (the rectus femoris and sartorius muscles) can exert their effect optimally.

Femoral Nerve (L1–L4)

Anatomy. The femoral nerve provides motor inner-vation to the **hip flexors** (iliacus and psoas major muscles) and **knee extensors** (quadriceps femoris muscle). It provides sensory innervation through **anterior cutaneous branches** to the anterior surface of the thigh and, through its terminal branch, the **saphenous nerve**, to the medial quadrant of the ante-rior surface of the lower leg. Its anatomic course is shown in **Fig. 13.54**.

Typical deficits. A lesion of the femoral nerve impairs **hip flexion and knee extension**. The hip flexors are tested with the patient sitting up, and the knee extensors with the patient supine (**Fig. 13.55**). In the standing patient, a **low-lying patella** is seen on the side of the lesion. The **quadriceps reflex** (patellar ten-don reflex) **is absent**. The patient cannot climb stairs with the affected leg and keeps it in a hyperextended position while walking (see **Fig. 3.2**). Sensation is

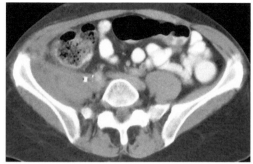

Fig. 13.56   Femoral nerve palsy in a 47-year-old woman with ovarian carcinoma. The CT scan shows a neoplastic process infiltrating the right psoas and iliacus muscles.

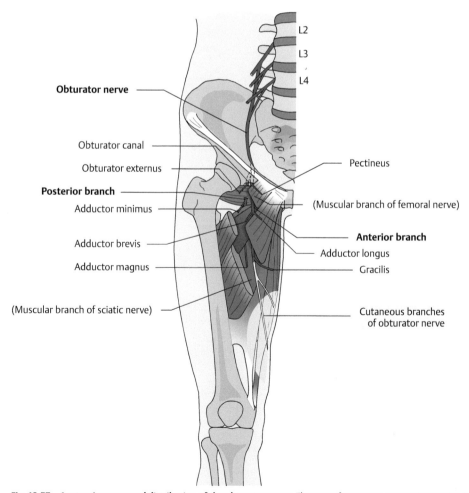

Fig. 13.57   **Anatomic course and distribution of the obturator nerve.** The zone of cutaneous sensory innervation is shaded yellow.

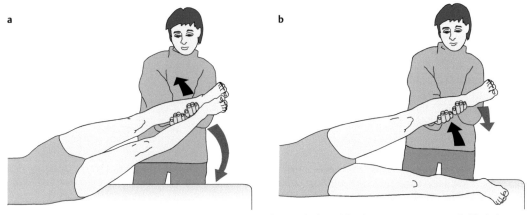

Fig. 13.58 Functional testing of the thigh adductors. a A patient lying in the lateral decubitus position can normally lift the lower leg off the examining table when the examiner lifts the upper leg. **b** A patient with adductor weakness cannot do this.

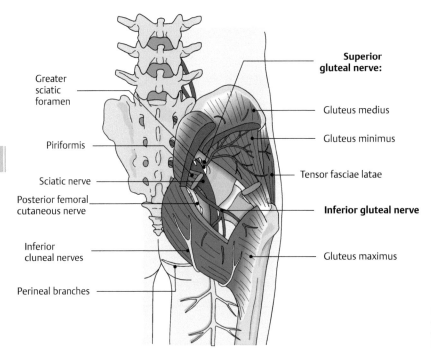

Greater sciatic foramen

Piriformis

Sciatic nerve

Posterior femoral cutaneous nerve

Inferior cluneal nerves

Perineal branches

Superior gluteal nerve:

Gluteus medius

Gluteus minimus

Tensor fasciae latae

Inferior gluteal nerve

Gluteus maximus

Fig. 13.59 Anatomic course and distribution of the superior and inferior gluteal nerves.

diminished in the territory of the sensory terminal branches (anteromedial surface of the thigh and medial surface of the lower leg, **Fig. 13.54**).

Causes. Lesions of the femoral nerve are commonly of **traumatic** or **iatrogenic** (surgical) origin. The nerve can also be involved by a pelvic **tumor** (**Fig. 13.56**) or, acutely, by a **hematoma in the psoas sheath**, for example, in an anticoagulated patient.

Obturator Nerve (L3–L4)

Anatomy. The obturator nerve supplies the **thigh adductors** (**Fig. 13.57**). Its sensory innervation is to a small area of skin just above the medial aspect of the knee.

Typical deficits. A lesion of the obturator nerve impairs thigh adduction. The examining technique needed to demonstrate this is shown in **Fig. 13.58**. The adductor reflex, elicited by a tap on the medial

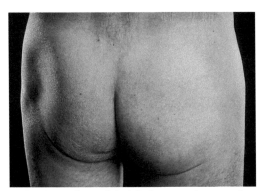

Fig. 13.60   Weakness of the left gluteus maximus muscle. The left buttock, on active contraction, is less voluminous than the right, and the left gluteal fold hangs lower.

condyle of the femur, is diminished and there is a small area of hypesthesia on the medial aspect of the thigh, just above the knee. Sometimes, irritation of the obturator nerve trunk can produce pain in this area as the sole clinical manifestation. This is called the **Howship–Romberg phenomenon**.

Causes. Masses in the pelvis or the obturator foramen are the usual causes; an obturator hernia is rarer.

Gluteal Nerves (L4–S2)

Anatomy. The gluteal nerves are purely motor. They innervate the **hip abductors and extensors**. Their course is shown in **Fig. 13.59**.

- **Lesions of the superior gluteal nerve** produce weakness of the hip abductors (gluteus medius and minimus muscles and tensor fasciae latae muscle). This impairs the stability of the pelvis on the side of the stationary leg when the patient walks; the pelvis tilts to the side of the swinging leg (**Trendelenburg gait**, cf. **Fig. 3.2**). In an incomplete superior gluteal nerve palsy, the patient barely manages to prevent tilting of the pelvis by inclining the trunk to the side of the stationary leg, thus displacing the body's center of gravity laterally (**Duchenne gait**, cf. **Fig. 3.2** and **Fig. 15.3**).
- **Lesions of the inferior gluteal nerve** (L5–S2) produce weakness of the gluteus maximus muscle, impairing hip extension. This makes it difficult for the patient to climb stairs (for example). Atrophy of the gluteus maximus muscle is usually hard to see because of the overlying fatty tissue, but, when the gluteus maximus muscle tones on either side are simultaneously and actively contracted, the

lack of muscle tone on the affected side is easily appreciated by palpation. The natal fold is lower on the affected side.

Causes. The gluteal nerves are often injured by intramuscular **injections** with faulty technique.

Differential diagnosis. Trendelenburg gait can be observed in many diseases of the hip, for example, in **congenital hip dislocation**. Duchenne gait, too, is most often due to hip disease. Weakness of the gluteus maximus muscle is part of the syndrome caused by an **S1 nerve root lesion** (**Fig. 13.60**), while weakness of the gluteus minimus and gluteus medius muscles can be caused by an **L5 nerve root lesion**. Bilateral weakness of the hip abductors is found in myopathies such as **muscular dystrophy**.

Sciatic Nerve (L4–S3)

Anatomy. The sciatic nerve is the common trunk of the peroneal (= fibular) and tibial nerves. It is the longest and thickest nerve in the human body. Its anatomy is shown in **Fig. 13.61**. The portions of the sciatic nerve that are destined to become the peroneal and tibial nerves are already clearly distinct from one another in the sciatic nerve just distal to its exit from the pelvis, but they are usually ensheathed in a common epineurium nearly all the way down to the level of the popliteal fossa. The sciatic nerve trunk, in its proximal portion, gives off cutaneous branches to the buttock and the posterior surface of the thigh (the **inferior cluneal nerves** and the **posterior femoral cutaneous nerve**). Along its further course, it gives off **motor branches to the knee flexors** (the semimembranosus, semitendinosus, and biceps femoris muscles, which are collectively termed the ischiocrural muscles or **hamstrings**).

Typical deficits. The clinical features of a sciatic nerve lesion depend on the level of the lesion and the extent to which it involves the peroneal and tibial portions of the nerve. Proximal lesions (but not distal ones) produce hypesthesia on the buttock and the posterior surface of the thigh and impair knee flexion. The strength and reflexes of the knee flexors are best tested in the prone patient (**Fig. 13.62**). For the clinical features of peroneal and tibial nerve lesions, see below.

Causes. The sciatic nerve trunk can be injured by **fractures** of the pelvic ring or proximal portion of the femur, by **surgical procedures** in the region of the

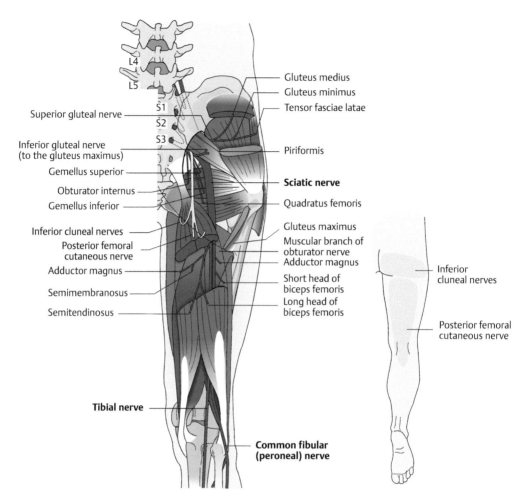

Fig. 13.61   Anatomic course and distribution of the sciatic nerve.

hip, or by faultily delivered **injections. Tumors** are a less common cause of sciatic nerve palsy.

Peroneal (Fibular) Nerve (L4–S2)

Anatomy. The peroneal (fibular) nerve, after it separates from the tibial portion of the sciatic nerve, travels to the lateral margin of the popliteal fossa, winds around the fibular neck, and then enters into the body of the peroneus longus muscle, where it divides into the superficial and deep peroneal (fibular) nerves. The **superficial peroneal nerve** provides motor innervation to the **peroneal muscles** and sensory innervation to the **lateral surface of the lower leg** and the **dorsum of the foot**, except for the space between the first and second toes (the first interosseous space). The latter is supplied by the **deep**

peroneal nerve, which also innervates the **dorsiflexors of the foot and toes** and the **intrinsic muscles of the dorsum of the foot**. The anatomy of the peroneal nerve is shown in **Fig. 13.63**.

Typical deficits. The clinical features of a lesion of the deep peroneal nerve are a **foot drop** and **steppage gait** (cf. **Fig. 3.2**). Sensation is impaired on the dorsum of the foot and completely abolished in the first interosseous space. A lesion of the superficial peroneal nerve causes **weakness of pronation of the foot** (i.e., inability to elevate the lateral edge of the foot); when the patient walks, the lateral edge of the foot hangs downward. Sensation is impaired in the lower leg and on the dorsum of the foot. If the trunk of the peroneal nerve (i.e., the common peroneal nerve) is affected, all of the above deficits are seen.

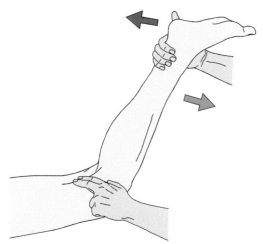

Fig. 13.62   Functional testing of the knee flexors in the prone patient. This is mainly a test of the semimembranosus, semitendinosus, and biceps femoris muscles.

Causes. The common peroneal nerve can be injured by **penetrating** or **blunt trauma**, for example, by knee fractures. **Injection palsies** of the sciatic nerve usually affect its peroneal portion. The most common cause of peroneal nerve palsy, however, is compression of the nerve at the fibular neck by **local external pressure** (faulty surgical positioning, a cast, etc.). The lesion can be precisely localized with electroneurography (cf. **Fig. 4.31**).

Differential diagnosis. A foot drop combined with loss of sensation on the dorsum of the foot can be seen in **combined lesions of the L4 and L5 nerve roots**, but such lesions will additionally impair abduction of the hip and inversion of the foot. Bilateral foot drop caused either by **Steinert myotonic dystrophy** or by peroneal muscle atrophy in **HMSN type I** can mimic a bilateral peroneal nerve palsy. An initially isolated, progressive, unilateral foot drop without any associated sensory deficit may be the first symptom of **spinal muscular atrophy** or **ALS**.

The **tibialis anterior syndrome** often causes difficulties in differential diagnosis. It is caused by **infarction (due to compression) of the muscles in the anterior compartment of the lower leg**, because of overuse, trauma, or a hematoma. Steadily rising local pressure within the anterior compartment, which is tightly encased in fascia, leads first to intense local pain, and then to **muscle swelling**. The pain increases on passive extension of the muscles by plantar flexion of the foot. The muscles become **necrotic** in 12 to 24 hours and are later **replaced by connective tissue**. The resulting contracture prevents the appearance of the flaccid foot drop that would be characteristic of peroneal nerve palsy (**Fig. 13.64**). In the acute

phase of the tibialis anterior syndrome, the deep peroneal nerve can be damaged, because its course passes through the anterior compartment of the lower leg. The resulting sensory deficit may be diagnostically misleading, as it may suggest a peripheral nerve lesion as the primary causative event.

Tibial Nerve (L4–S3)

Anatomy. This nerve, derived from the medial portion of the sciatic nerve, innervates the **plantar flexors of the foot and toes** in the lower leg, as well as all of the **intrinsic muscles of the foot**, except those on the dorsum of the foot. It provides sensory innervation to the heel and sole (**Fig. 13.65**).

Typical deficits. Weakness of plantar flexion makes tiptoe walking impossible, while weakness of the intrinsic muscles of the foot makes the patient unable to fan the toes. If the weakness is mild, the patient may still be able to walk on tiptoe; the weakness can be brought out by having the patient stand on the toes repeatedly while standing on one foot (**Fig. 13.66**). The sensory deficit on the sole of the foot is particularly troublesome because of the important protective function of sensation in this area.

— **Tarsal tunnel syndrome** is an entrapment neuropathy affecting the terminal branch of the tibial nerve as it passes under the medial malleolus. It is seen almost exclusively after **fractures** or **sprains** of the upper ankle joint. Its typical feature is local **pain** behind the medial malleolus or on the sole of the foot, which increases when the patient walks. The nerve trunk is tender to palpation behind the medial malleolus. Sensation is diminished on the sole of the foot and the plantar skin is abnormally smooth and dry. The patient can no longer fan the toes (**Fig. 13.67**).

— **Morton metatarsalgia**. A painful neuroma can develop on a digital nerve (a sensory terminal branch of the tibial nerve) if the nerve is chronically injured by compression between two adjacent metatarsal heads. This condition, called Morton metatarsalgia, causes pain in the forefoot, which is initially felt only on walking, but later also at rest. The pain can be induced by the examiner by laterally compressing the anterior arch of the foot or by squeezing the metatarsal heads against each other. An injection of local anesthetic along the course of the nerve, applied from the dorsal surface of the foot proximal to the site of the neuroma, brings complete, though transient, relief. A specially padded shoe insert with retrocapital support may help. If the pain persists, the neuroma should be surgically excised through a plantar approach (**Fig. 13.68**).

13

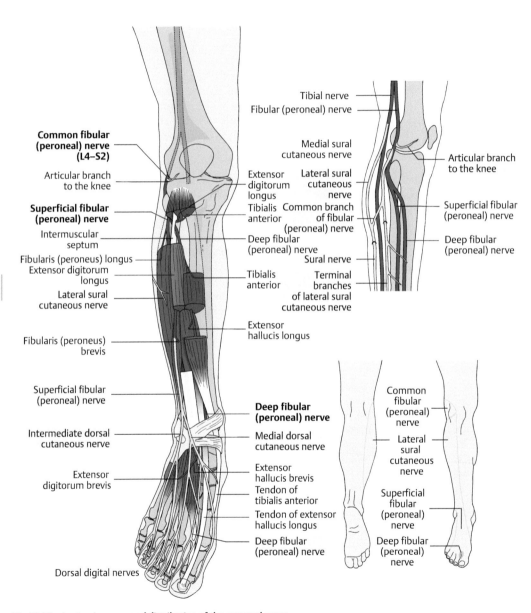

Fig. 13.63   Anatomic course and distribution of the peroneal nerve.

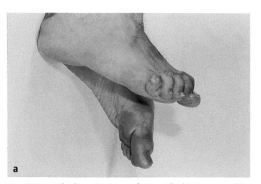
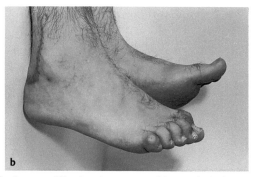

Fig. 13.64 Tibialis anterior syndrome. The big toe resembles a claw because of fibrosis and contracture of the muscles in the anterior compartment of the leg. Plantar flexion of the foot is restricted **(a)**, as is dorsiflexion **(b)**. (Adapted from Mumenthaler M, Stöhr M, Müller-Vahl H, et al. Läsionen peripherer Nerven und radikuläre Syndrome. Stuttgart: Thieme; 2007.)

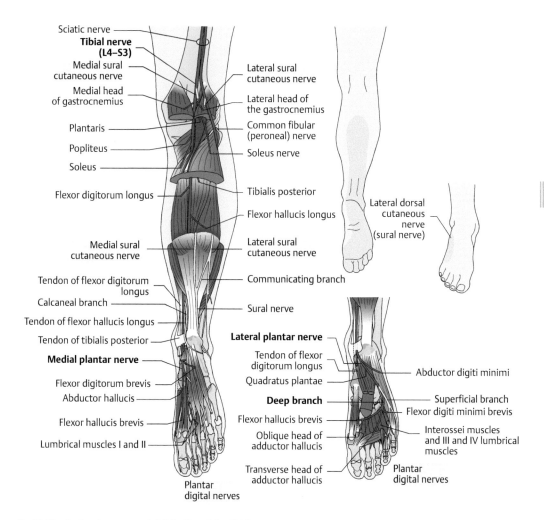

Fig. 13.65 Anatomic course and distribution of the tibial nerve.

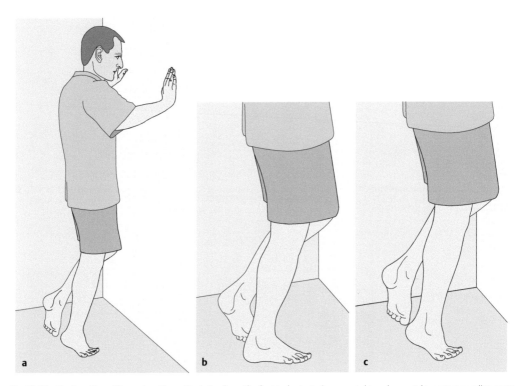

Fig. 13.66 Testing the calf muscles. The patient stands on the foot to be tested, supports his or her weight against a wall to maintain balance, and repeatedly lifts the heel off the floor to stand on his or her toes. This test is particularly useful for the detection of mild gastrocnemius weakness.

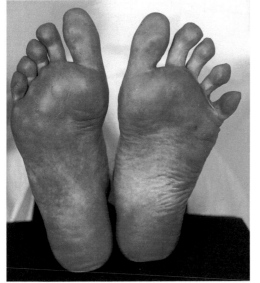

Fig. 13.67 Weakness of the intrinsic muscles of the foot in right tarsal tunnel syndrome (lesion of the tibial nerve behind the medial malleolus). The patient can fan the left toes, but not the right toes.

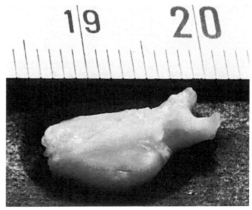

Fig. 13.68 Excised neuroma of an interdigital nerve. The neuroma was found at the branch point of the nerve. The patient suffered from Morton metatarsalgia.

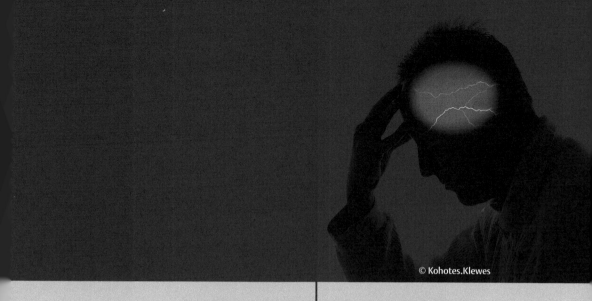

Chapter 14

Painful Syndromes

The Same, Only Different

The patient, a 32-year-old nurse, had suffered from recurrent headaches every few months since childhood. These were generally of a pulsating quality, very intense, and limited to one side of the head, usually the right side. The pain was most intense behind the eye, accompanied by a strong sensation of pressure. Each attack lasted 6 to 8 hours; during the attacks, she was also very sensitive to light and noise. Whenever possible, she withdrew to a quiet, dark room, avoided all activity, and waited for the pain to go away. Her mother had suffered from similar headaches.

She had a severe headache again one Easter Sunday; this surprised her, because the last attack had been only 1 week before. This time, the pain came on not gradually, but suddenly, "out of a clear blue sky," and was much more intense than usual. The pain was "all over my head," and she felt as if her head were about to explode. She went to her room and lay down. Five minutes later, she became nauseated and vomited repeatedly. Over the next half hour, she became progressively confused. Her husband called the emergency medical services.

This patient's prior usual headaches were typical migraine headaches, but the Easter Sunday episode was of another kind entirely. A headache of sudden onset and extreme intensity is characteristic of an intracranial hemorrhage. The most common cause is a ruptured aneurysm of an artery at the base of the brain, causing arterial blood to enter the subarachnoid space (subarachnoid hemorrhage, SAH).

The emergency physician on the scene examined her and found meningismus (a clinical manifestation of leptomeningeal irritation, generally caused either by extravasated blood or by an infectious/inflammatory process). She was somnolent, but responsive and cooperative, and had no other neurologic deficits. Suspecting SAH, the emergency physician had her transported immediately to the emergency room of a tertiary-care hospital for neurosurgical evaluation. A computed tomography (CT) scan confirmed the diagnosis of SAH and revealed a probable ruptured aneurysm of the anterior communicating artery as the cause. This was then confirmed by angiography, whereupon the aneurysm was obliterated with intravascular detachable coils in an interventional neuroradiologic procedure.

Headache is a common symptom in everyday clinical practice and has many causes. Primary diseases of the nervous system often cause intense or unbearable pain as a prominent or even sole manifestation. For this reason, neurologists are often consulted to help in the evaluation of patients with pain. The nervous system plays a key role in the transmission and processing of nociceptive impulses and in the perception of pain.

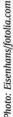

Photo: Eisenhans/fotolia.com

14.1 Fundamentals

Key Point

Many conditions whose most prominent, or sole, symptom is pain lie within the neurologist's field of expertise. In this chapter, we will discuss painful syndromes by location: headache, facial pain, shoulder–arm pain, pain in the trunk, and pain in the lower limb. The differential diagnosis of a painful syndrome cannot be restricted to neurologic conditions and must always include diseases of nonneurologic origin.

14.1.1 The Generation and Perception of Pain

Pain is a type of unpleasant sensation. In terms of **pathophysiology**, it arises when specialized sensory end organs are excited by certain mechanical, thermal, or chemical stimuli of a potentially damaging ("noxious") nature. The pain-related ("nociceptive") impulses are conducted centrally, mainly by way of thin, poorly myelinated fibers, through the posterior root and into the spinal cord. The nociceptive fibers cross the midline in the spinal cord at their level of entry and then ascend in the spinothalamic tract to the thalamus and onward to higher centers in the brain, which enable pain to be consciously felt (see section 5.3 and **Fig. 5.2**). **Biochemical factors** also play an important role in pain perception. In the periphery, the intensity of pain is increased by a variety of biogenic amines, for example, substance P. In the central nervous system, the intensity of pain is modulated by the production of opioid substances in certain areas of the brain. Finally, **psychological factors**—relating to the patient's personality as well as the sociocultural environment—affect the manner in which pain is experienced and processed.

14.1.2 General Aspects of the Clinical History in Patients with Pain

Many painful syndromes have their origin in the nervous system; many others, in which there is no evident neural dysfunction (e.g., most kinds of headache), are nonetheless traditionally evaluated and treated by neurologists. These facts justify the inclusion of painful syndromes in a textbook of neurology. It should be emphasized, however, that the physician confronted by the symptom "pain" should not approach it from the narrow viewpoint of any particular specialty, but must rather apply the full range of general medical knowledge.

This purpose is best served, first, by the taking of a systematic and directed **pain history**. The main elements of the pain history are listed in **Table 14.1**. Further specific questions will need to be asked depending on the nature and location of pain in the particular case, and ancillary diagnostic tests may be needed as well.

14

Table 14.1

Pain history

Aspect	Questions
Where is the pain?	— Precisely localized or diffuse? — Constant or varying localization? — Radiating?
How long has it been present?	— For what length of time and since what precipitating event, if any?
Continuous or intermittent?	— If continuous: of constant or variable intensity? — If intermittent: how long and how frequent are the episodes of pain?
Quality?	— Hammering? — Throbbing? — Stabbing? — Dull? — Burning?
Intensity?	— On a scale of 0 (no pain) to 10 (intolerable pain)
Precipitating and/or aggravating factors?	— None? — Constant factors—which, if any? — Variable factors—which, if any? — Dependence on posture? — Dependence on physical activity—what kind, if any?
Alleviating factors?	— None? — Constant or variable factors—which, if any? — Medications—which ones, in what doses, with what duration of effect?
How severely is the patient impaired by the pain?	— At work? — In personal life?
Current complaints other than pain?	— Other symptoms and complaints? — What is the patient's own explanation for the pain? — Other medical history? — Living situation?

Table 14.2

IHS headache classification

Category	Entities
Primary headaches	— Migraine — Tension-type headache — Cluster headache and other trigeminal autonomic cephalalgias — Other primary headaches
Secondary headaches	— Headache attributed to head and/or neck trauma — Headache attributed to cranial or cervical vascular disorder — Headache attributed to nonvascular intracranial disorder — Headache attributed to a substance or its withdrawal — Medication-overuse headache — Headache attributed to infection — Headache attributed to disorder of homoeostasis — Headache or facial pain attributed to disorder of cranium, neck, eyes, ears, nose, sinuses, teeth, mouth, or other facial or cranial structures — Headache attributed to psychiatric disorder
Cranial neuralgias, central and primary facial pain, and other headaches	— Cranial neuralgias and central causes of facial pain — Other headache, cranial neuralgia, central or primary facial pain

Note: Further subcategories and related information can be found on the Web site of the International Headache Society (http://ihs-classification.org).

In the remainder of this chapter, we will discuss various major painful syndromes, classifying them by location.

14.2 Painful Syndromes of the Head and Neck

Key Point

Headache can be either idiopathic or symptomatic. The most common idiopathic or "primary" types of headache are tension-type headache, migraine, and cluster headache. While migraine and cluster headache are typified by highly characteristic, mostly unilateral attacks of pain, tension-type headache more commonly assumes the form of a diffuse, continuous headache of lesser intensity. Symptomatic ("secondary") headaches are, by definition, a manifestation of some other underlying condition. The possible causes include many neurologic diseases, as well as diseases of the eyes, teeth, jaw, ear, nose, and throat, and many general medical conditions. Spondylogenic headache is caused by pathologic processes in the cervical spine. A third group of conditions characterized by head and neck pain is the neuralgias, the most common of which is trigeminal neuralgia.

Headache can also include a variably significant component of **facial pain**—a typical example is cluster headache, which is felt mainly in the forehead, eye, and temple. Headache and facial pain cannot be cleanly separated from each other and are therefore considered under one heading in the International Headache Society (IHS) classification (see later and also **Table 14.2**). It is nonetheless useful, for clarity, to distinguish syndromes in which the pain is mainly in the head from those in which it is mainly in the face. Headache will accordingly be discussed in this section and facial pain in the next.

14.2.1 IHS Classification of Headache

The classification of headache syndromes proposed by the IHS has won general acceptance. The major categories of headache in this system are listed in **Table 14.2**. The IHS has established obligatory diagnostic criteria for each type of headache. This highly precise approach to headache syndromes is most useful in clinical research, where the findings of different teams of investigators must be compared with each other, but it is also highly practical for routine clinical use.

Practical Tip

The potential benefit of any proposed treatment of a particular type of headache can only be assessed reliably when it is clear that all of the research teams reporting on it are, in fact, treating the same condition. Standardization is the main virtue of the IHS criteria.

For the beginning student of neurology, however, it is more useful to gain a descriptive overview of the more common, "classic" types of headache (**Table 14.3**). In particular, he or she should learn to distinguish the common **primary** types of headache, that is, those not due to any demonstrable structural

Table 14.3

Common types of headache

Headache type	Site of pain	Duration of episodes	Frequency of episodes	Phenomena during episodes	Intensity; other remarks
Tension-type headache	Diffuse, bilateral	Hours to days	Rare to several times per week	No unusual phenomena	— Bearable — Tends to improve with physical activity
Migraine	Two-thirds of attacks are unilateral, one-third bilateral	4–72 h	Rare to several times per week	Occasionally, Horner syndrome	— There may be an aura before the pain begins; photo- and phonophobia, nausea — Sometimes very intense — Worsens with physical activity, improves with rest
Cluster headache	Periorbital, forehead, temple, maxilla	15–180 min	1–8/d	Horner syndrome, periorbital erythema, conjunctival injection, lacrimation, rhinorrhea or stuffed nose	— No prodrome, always on the same side — Intense — The patient is restless, walks around
Trigeminal neuralgia	In the distribution of one of the three divisions of CN V (usually maxillary)	Fraction of a second	1 to 100 per day	Painful contraction of the affected half of the face (*tic douloureux*)	— Generally idiopathic in older patients, generally symptomatic in persons under age 40 y
Secondary headache types	Depends on etiology	Usually continuous or long-lasting	–	Depends on etiology	— Consequence of another underlying disease

Abbreviation: CN, cranial nerve.

lesion in the head, from **secondary** types. The latter are caused by organic disease of the cranial vessels or other structures in the head, or have other organic causes (e.g., infection, disorders of homeostasis). Ninety percent of all cases of headache are of the primary type.

14.2.2 Approach to the Patient with Headache

NOTE

The patient who goes to the doctor because of headache is suffering from pain and, often, anxiety. He or she therefore can rightly expect the following:
- To be taken seriously.
- To be examined carefully.
- To have the cause of the problem identified and clearly explained.
- To be given effective treatment.

The physician must **take the time needed** to meet these expectations fully.

The **clinical history** is a vital step in the evaluation of headache. The systematic interview of the headache patient should address the following points:
- **Family history** of headache?
- **How long** have headaches been present?

- **Nature** of headache:
  • Site?
  • Continuous or episodic?
  • Usual or unusual quality of pain?
  • Timing of onset?
  • Speed of development?
  • Character of pain?
  • Precipitating factors?
  • Duration of episodes?
  • Accompanying signs?
- **Frequency?**
- **Headache-free intervals?**
- **Impairment** of activities at home and at work?
- **Drugs and other measures** against headache:
  • Frequency?
  • Dose?
  • Effect?
- **Other symptoms** besides headache:
  • ENT, ophthalmic, or dental disease?
  • Memory loss?
  • Neurologic/neuropsychological deficits?
  • Epileptic seizures?
  • General symptoms (fatigue, weight loss, circulatory problems, etc.)?
- **Personality** and **external circumstances:**
  • Personality type?
  • Occupation?

14

- Private life?
- Conflict situations?
- Alcohol, tobacco, caffeine, drugs of abuse?
- Current medications?

A carefully elicited history usually leads to a fairly secure diagnosis. Nonetheless, the general physical examination and the **neurologic examination** should never be omitted, not least because they help the physician win the patient's confidence—an important factor for the success of treatment. The examination should include the following:

- **General medical examination:**
  - Cardiovascular system, especially blood pressure.
  - Renal function.
  - Signs of infection.
  - Signs of meningitis.
  - Signs of malignancy.
  - ENT diseases.
  - Eye diseases.
  - Dental diseases, jaw diseases.
  - Cervical spondylosis.
- **Neurologic examination**, with particular attention to:
  - Meningismus.
  - Signs of intracranial hypertension.
  - Focal neurologic signs.
  - Cranial nerve deficits.
- **Mental status**, with particular attention to:
  - Cognitive deficit.
  - Impairment of consciousness.
  - Current psychological conflicts.
  - Depression.
  - Neurotic personality traits.

14.2.3 The Main Types of Primary Headache

Definition and frequency. By definition, primary headache is not a symptom or consequence of any other disease—the pain itself is the disease. About 60 to 70% of people suffer from headache or facial pain at some time in their lives, but only about 15% seek medical attention. Of people with headaches, 90% have one of the two most common types: tension-type headache and migraine.

Pathogenesis. Multiple factors probably play a role in the pathogenesis of tension-type headache and, especially, migraine (see later). Positron emission tomography (PET) studies have revealed activation in the brainstem at the beginning of a migraine attack and in the hypothalamus in cluster headache. In a migraine attack, there is first vasoconstriction, then vasodilation. Dilation of the large arteries of the base of the brain is usually accompanied by unilateral, often throbbing headache. Vasodilation was once thought to cause the headache but is now thought to be an epiphenomenon, that is, a result of

the same **activation of the trigeminovascular system** that separately causes headache. Migraine is presumably initiated when a neural process that is not yet completely understood activates the trigeminovascular system, leading to pain. The dura mater, the large arteries of the base of the brain, and the pial vessels all receive sensory innervation from the trigeminal nerve and the gasserian (trigeminal) ganglion. The main function of the sensory trigeminal system is to protect the head from dangerous external influences and stimuli. The pain that arises in primary headache syndromes is of no use to the organism and is thought to be caused by faulty activation of the system.

These changes in the trigeminovascular system are partly caused, or accompanied, by **changes in humoral mediators**. The neurotransmitter **serotonin** plays an especially important role, and several vasodilator peptides have been discovered in trigeminal neurons, including substance P, neurokinin A, and the calcitonin gene–related peptide. Antagonists of these peptides, and antibodies against them, are now being tested as drugs for the prevention and treatment of migraine attacks.

Tension-Type Headache

Tension-type headache has episodic and chronic forms.

In the IHS classification, sporadic **episodic tension-type headache** (of greater or lesser frequency) is defined as follows:

- **A**: At least 10 previous episodes (once per month or on at least 12 days per year, or else on more than 1 but fewer than 15 days per month) that met criteria B to D and were present on fewer than 180 days per year overall.
- **B**: Each individual headache episode lasts for 30 minutes to 7 days.
- **C**: The pain is characterized by at least two of the following features:
  - Bilateral.
  - Pressing, squeezing, not throbbing.
  - Of mild to moderate intensity.
  - Not exacerbated by physical activity, walking, or climbing steps.
- **D**: Both of the following criteria must be fulfilled:
  - No nausea or vomiting
  - No photophobia or photophobia, or at most one, but not the other.
- **E**: The headache is not due to any other known disease.

Tension-type headache is illustrated schematically in **Fig. 14.1**.

Chronic tension-type headache occurs, by definition, on more than 15 days per month for at least three consecutive months and on at least 180 days per

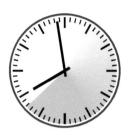

Usually beginning in the morning

Duration: 30 minutes to 7 days
Intensity: mild to moderate
Chronic: ≥ 15 attacks/month
Episodic: < 15 attacks/month

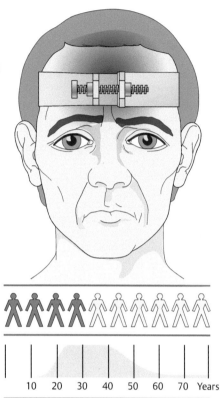

Chronic		June				July				
	S		4	11	18	25	2	9	16	23	30
	M		5	12	19	26	3	10	17	24	31
	T		6	13	20	27	4	11	18	25
	W		7	14	21	28	5	12	19	26
	T	1	8	15	22	29	6	13	20	27
	F	2	9	16	23	30	7	14	21	28
	S	3	10	17	24		1	8	15	22	29

Episodic		June				July				
	S		4	11	18	25	2	9	16	23	30
	M		5	12	19	26	3	10	17	24	31
	T		6	13	20	27	4	11	18	25
	W		7	14	21	28	5	12	19	26
	T	1	8	15	22	29	6	13	20	27
	F	2	9	16	23	30	7	14	21	28
	S	3	10	17	24		1	8	15	22	29

10 20 30 40 50 60 70 Years

Fig. 14.1 Tension-type headache. (These images are provided courtesy of Mumenthaler M, Daetwyler Ch, Kopfschmerz Interaktiv, Instructional Media Department [AUM-IAWF] of the University of Bern Faculty of Medicine, 2001.)

14

year. The pain is usually diffuse, sometimes felt most intensely on the forehead, temples, or vertex, and often of a dull rather than throbbing character. It does not worsen with exercise. It can arise at any time of day, but most often in the morning on awakening or shortly after the patient gets up. There are usually no accompanying symptoms. This type of headache mainly affects young or middle-aged persons, men just as commonly as women, although the subjective suffering of female patients tends to be worse. The headaches are often provoked by weather changes, sleep deprivation, overconsumption of alcohol ("hangover headache"), and emotional tension. The neurologic examination reveals no abnormalities.
Treatment. The main components of treatment are:
— Lifestyle readjustment.
— Dealing with external and internal sources of emotional tension.
— On the pharmacologic level of attack management, acetaminophen 1,000 mg, ibuprofen 200 to 600 mg, or a combination of acetylsalicylic acid 250 mg, acetaminophen 250 mg, and caffeine 50 mg. Excessive intake of drugs to treat chronic tension-type headache can cause medication-

overuse headache (see section 14.2.4, Drug- and Substance-Related Headache).
Important prophylactic measures include **relaxation exercises** (e.g., progressive muscle relaxation by the Jacobson's technique), **endurance training**, and **stress-management training**, ideally in a multidisciplinary treatment program. Acupuncture does not lessen the frequency of attacks of episodic tension-type headache. **Antidepressants** (e.g., amitriptyline) can be considered for patients with the chronic form of the disorder.

Migraine

| **NOTE**

Migraine, a type of primary headache, is the second most common type of headache overall, after tension-type headache (see earlier). It is characterized by intense, often **hemicranial** headaches that last several hours, occur at variable frequency, and are accompanied by **nausea** (and sometimes vomiting), **photophobia**, and **phonophobia**. The pain worsens with physical activity. The first headaches often occur in the patient's teens. Migraine is markedly more common in **women** than in men.

Pathogenesis. The pathogenesis of migraine is discussed more extensively earlier at the beginning of this section.

Epidemiology. The frequency of migraine in schoolchildren is generally estimated at 5%. Among older children, it affects girls more commonly than boys.

In adults, epidemiologic studies have revealed an unexpectedly high prevalence of migraine, roughly **25% in women** and 17% in men. More than half of all "migraineurs" have a **family history** of headache (not necessarily of typical migraine). Women are more commonly affected, or, at least, they more commonly seek medical help.

Simple (Classic) Migraine without Aura

Clinical features. Migraine without aura (also called simple, classic, or common migraine), whose sole neurologic manifestation is **headache**, is distinguished from migraine with aura (also called complicated migraine), in which additional neurologic manifestations are present. The **IHS criteria** for the diagnosis of migraine without aura are as follows:

- **A**: The patient has had at least five attacks fulfilling criteria B to D.
- **B**: The attacks last 4 to 72 hours (if untreated or unsuccessfully treated).
- **C**: The headache has at least two of the following features:
  - Unilaterality.
  - Throbbing character.
  - Moderate or marked intensity.
  - Worsening when the patient walks, climbs stairs, or performs similar everyday physical activities, which are avoided.
- **D**: At least one of the following symptoms is present during the headache:
  - Nausea and/or vomiting.
  - Oversensitivity to light and noise.
- **E**: The headaches are not attributable to any other disease.

Persons with migraine have often had uncharacteristic headache attacks in their childhood. They suffer from episodic abdominal pain and vomiting appreciably more frequently than the general population. Episodic headaches that only arise in adulthood are truly "hemicranial" in only about 65% of cases. The pain is often described as **throbbing**, pulsating, piercing, and deep; it worsens with any kind of **physical exertion**, even as mild as climbing a staircase, and with external stimuli such as **light** and **noise**. It reaches maximum intensity within 1 hour or a few hours, and 60% of patients have **nausea** and/or vomiting. Because of their oversensitivity to light and noise, patients usually withdraw to a dark and quiet room during the attack. They often cannot tolerate odors either. Allodynia, that is, pain felt merely on light touch of certain areas of the skin, has been described as occurring in 70% of patients during attacks. In many patients, the attacks are almost always on the same side of the head, but absolute constancy of the affected side should arouse suspicion of secondary headache. The attacks generally last at least 1 hour and may last for many hours; their frequency varies from a few per year to several per week. The typical features of migraine are shown schematically in **Fig. 14.2**.

Chronic migraine is defined as consisting of attacks that occur on more than 15 days per month for at least three consecutive months. An intense migraine attack that lasts longer than 72 hours is called **status migrainosus**. An **aura without headache** can also last a week or more. (For migraine auras, see the next subsection.)

Precipitating factors. Common triggers are **emotional stress** (responsibilities, worries, excessive demands, tension) or, alternatively, **diminishing stress** and prolonged lying in bed (Sunday or holiday migraine). Further possible precipitating factors are **weather changes** and **photic stimuli** (e.g., bright sunlight). In women, migraine attacks may regularly come just before, or at the same time as, **menstruation**. Certain substances in **food**, such as chocolate or aspartame, can also precipitate migraine in some persons. The pressor substance tyramine, which is found in certain kinds of cheese, is a rare migraine trigger; it can also cause hypertensive crises in patients taking monoamine oxidase inhibitors. Migraine induced by trauma ("footballer's migraine") has been described as well.

Diagnostic evaluation. In persons with classic migraine, the neurologic examination is normal. The electroencephalogram (EEG) may show nonspecific changes, usually slow waves.

Treatment. The treatment of common migraine depends on the frequency and severity of the attacks.

Rare and mild attacks often need no treatment. Moderately severe, not very prolonged attacks that are relatively rare (occurring less than three times per month) can be managed by **treating the individual attacks**. Mild to moderate attacks can be effectively treated early on in each attack with **analgesic drugs** or **nonsteroidal anti-inflammatory drugs (NSAIDs)** in adequate doses, for example, acetylsalicylic acid 1,000 mg, acetaminophen 1,000 mg, ibuprofen 200 to 600 mg, or the fixed combination of acetylsalicylic acid 250 mg, acetaminophen 250 mg, and caffeine 40 mg. For nausea, an **antiemetic drug** should be given as well, for example, metoclopramide 20 mg by mouth or, if necessary, as a suppository. Moderate to severe attacks are often treated with **triptans** (usually by mouth); many patients prefer triptans

Maximum in 1–2 hours

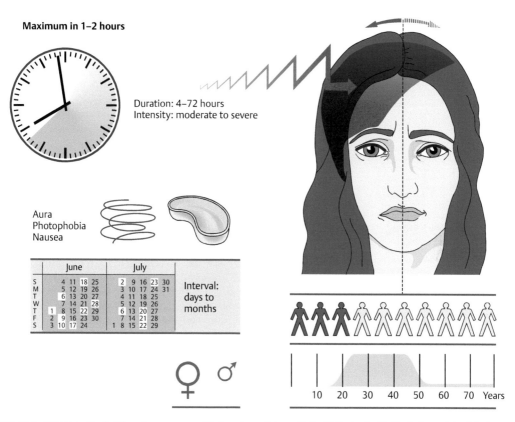

Duration: 4–72 hours
Intensity: moderate to severe

Aura
Photophobia
Nausea

	June				July					Interval: days to months
S		4	11	18	25	2	9	16	23	30
M		5	12	19	26	3	10	17	24	31
T		6	13	20	27	4	11	18	25	
W		7	14	21	28	5	12	19	26	
T	1	8	15	22	29	6	13	20	27	
F	2	9	16	23	30	7	14	21	28	
S	3	10	17	24		1	8	15	22	29

♀ ♂

10   20   30   40   50   60   70   Years

Fig. 14.2   Migraine attack. (These images are provided courtesy of Mumenthaler M, Daetwyler Ch, Kopfschmerz Interaktiv, Instructional Media Department [AUM-IAWF] of the University of Bern Faculty of Medicine, 2001.)

14

because they are more effective than the analgesics and relieve pain faster. They are also more effective than **ergotamines**, which should no longer be given because of their side effects.

 Practical Tip
The available triptan preparations differ in the strength and latency of pain relief and in their side effects. If necessary, a triptan can be given by injection (sumatriptan) or as a nasal spray (sumatriptan, zolmitriptan). The oral triptans that relieve pain fastest are rizatriptan and eletriptan.

If the attacks occur more than three times per month and/or severely hamper the patient's everyday activities because of their duration (>72 hours) or severity, **attack prophylaxis** should be given. Once begun, this must usually be maintained continuously for months (rarely, years) afterward. First-line drugs for attack prophylaxis are the **β-blockers** propranolol and metoprolol, the **anticonvulsants** topiramate and valproate, and the **calcium antagonist** flunarizine. Second-line drugs include antidepressants (amitriptyline,

venlafaxine), gabapentin, naproxen, acetylsalicylic acid, and magnesium. These recommendations also apply to the various types of complicated migraine described later.

Migraine with Aura

NOTE

More than one-third of all persons with migraine suffer from other neurologic manifestations before the headache itself begins, for example, visual or sensory disturbances, difficulty speaking, paralysis, vertigo (see section 12.6.2, Vestibular Migraine), or abdominal symptoms. This condition is called **migraine with aura** or, in the traditional nomenclature, **complicated migraine**.

Migraine auras develop over 5 to 20 minutes and end within 60 minutes at most. They can be very dramatic, sometimes overshadowing the headache to such an extent that the patient's illness is not immediately recognizable as migraine. In pathophysiologic terms, auras have been correlated with the phenomenon of spreading depression (of Leão), a wave of

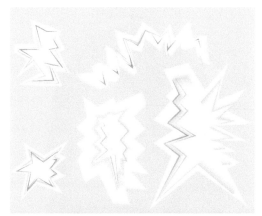

Fig. 14.3   Scintillating scotoma during an attack of ophthalmic migraine: typical fortification figures.

cortical neuronal discharge followed by neuronal silence that begins in the visual cortex and sweeps outward. Regional cerebral blood flow decreases during an aura and increases afterward.

Sometimes, an aura can be the only symptom of a migraine attack. This is called a **typical aura without headache** (or, traditionally, "**migraine sans migraine**").

We will now individually describe the major clinical types of migraine with aura.

Migraine with ophthalmic aura. This is characterized by visual symptoms that precede the headache. About one-third of persons with migraine have ophthalmic auras. The typical kind is a **scintillating scotoma**, that is, a flashing figure bordered by a bright, zigzag line ("**fortification figure**"—think of a crenellated medieval fortress), which is seen in both eyes. It arises in the center of one visual hemifield and then travels outward for 5 to 15 minutes until it falls out of view in the periphery, leaving behind a transient impairment of vision in the hemifield (**Fig. 14.3**). The scintillating scotoma is followed by an attack of hemicranial headache, usually on the opposite side. Occasionally, no headache follows (*migraine sans migraine*); patients with this type of migraine may have a permanent visual field defect. There are also rare cases in which the visual disturbance affects one eye only (**retinal migraine**).

Ophthalmoplegic migraine. This is defined as a migraine-like headache accompanied by ipsilateral weakness of the extraocular muscles, usually due to **oculomotor nerve palsy**. The existence of this type of membrane is questionable. Other causes of ophthalmoplegia must be ruled out.

An aura consisting of a hemisensory deficit or aphasia, previously called **migraine accompagnée**, now appears in the IHS classification under the heading **typical aura with migraine headache**. This variant of

migraine usually begins in childhood or adolescence. In an attack, paresthesia arises in a small area, most often on an arm or the face, spreads within a few minutes to cover a larger area (e.g., from the thumb to the entire arm to the face), and then slowly subsides. Aphasia may follow or may be the sole manifestation of the aura. The typical hemicranial headache usually comes after the neurologic disturbance, on the same or the opposite side, enabling the diagnosis of migraine to be made. Headache may also be absent, in what is called **aura without headache** (traditionally, **migraine accompagnée sans migraine**); this type of migraine is especially common in children and is the initial manifestation of migraine in nearly half of all cases.

An EEG recorded after an aura shows a focal abnormality that may take a few days to resolve. Attacks may also be accompanied by cerebrospinal fluid (CSF) pleocytosis. CSF pleocytosis or auras without headache call for careful diagnostic evaluation to rule out other potential causes of the problem, for example, transient ischemia.

Familial hemiplegic migraine (FHM). This is characterized by recurrent migraine attacks accompanied by a transient hemiparesis, hemiplegia, or hemisensory deficit that resolves within 1 hour. Most patients have, or had, a first- or second-degree relative with the same disorder. There are multiple genetic subtypes. FHM1 is due to a mutation in the CACNA1A gene on chromosome 19, while FHM2 is due to a mutation in the ATP1A2 gene on chromosome 1.

Basilar migraine. In this type of migraine, the symptoms reflect a pathophysiologic process located in both cerebral hemispheres as well as the brainstem. The name of the disorder reflects an earlier belief that the underlying abnormality was limited to the distribution of the basilar artery, which may not be true. The symptoms of the aura include varying combinations of dysarthria, dizziness, tinnitus, hearing loss, double vision, and ataxia, and, typically, simultaneous bilateral paresthesia and visual impairment in both hemifields of both eyes. Consciousness is variably impaired, to an extent ranging from somnolence to coma. The patient may be confused during the attack and amnestic for it afterward. The headache is generally occipital. Basilar migraine mainly affects girls and young women.

Special types of migraine with aura. These include **abdominal migraine**, which is not uncommon, mainly in children, and **cyclic vomiting syndrome**; both of these disorders are often a precursor of migraine (i.e., headache develops later). Adults with migraine may have accompanying psychiatric manifestations such as mood swings (anxiety, depression), cognitive disturbances, confusion, agitation, or even "migraine

Table 14.4

Trigeminal autonomic cephalalgias and other types of paroxysmal headache

Disorder	Site of pain	Duration of attacks	Frequency of attacks	Phenomena during an attack	Remarks
Cluster headache	Periorbital, frontal, temporal, maxillary	15–180 min	1–8/d	Horner syndrome, conjunctival injection, tearing, runny or stuffed nose, periorbital edema	Always on the same side
Paroxysmal hemi-crania	Periorbital, temporal	2–30 min	15/d	Conjunctival injection, tearing, runny or stuffed nose, eyelid edema, sweating, Horner syndrome	Responds to indomethacin
Hypnic headache	Diffuse	At least 15 min	>15 nights per month	None	Headaches awaken patient from sleep, onset after age 50, considered a rare type of primary headache
SUNCT	Periorbital, temporal	5 s to 5 min	≥100 per day	Conjunctival injection, tearing	Must be distinguished from cluster headache and trigeminal neuralgia
Trigeminal neuralgia	Distribution of one branch of the trigeminal nerve (usually maxillary)	Seconds	A few to 100 per day	Painful contraction of the affected side of the face	Usually idiopathic in older patients, often symptomatic in younger ones

Abbreviation: SUNCT, short-lasting unilateral neuralgiform headache with conjunctival injection and tearing.

psychosis" (**dysphrenic migraine**). Recurrent attacks of dizziness, termed vestibular migraine (see section 12.6.2, Vestibular Migraine), have also been described; other syndromes in this class include benign paroxysmal vertigo of childhood and episodic ataxia (**cerebellar migraine**).

Treatment of migraine with aura. Migraine with aura is treated in the same way as simple migraine (see earlier).

Cluster Headache and Other Trigeminal Autonomic Cephalalgias

NOTE

The category called **"trigeminal autonomic cephalalgias"** in the new IHS classification comprises pain syndromes that mainly affect the face and have accompanying autonomic manifestations, for example, conjunctival injection, facial erythema, lacrimation, and altered nasal secretion (**Table 14.4**). All of them are of a more or less paroxysmal nature, with short-lasting individual attacks of pain. They are as follows:

- Cluster headache (see later).
- SUNCT syndrome (see later).
- Trigeminal neuralgia (see section 14.3.1).
- Paroxysmal hemicrania (see later).

Cluster Headache

Epidemiology. Cluster headache (older, alternative name: "Bing–Horton neuralgia") is about 1/10 as common as migraine. Unlike migraine, it is much more common in **men**, particularly **smokers**. It often begins in middle age or old age.

Pathogenesis and etiology. Cluster headache attacks tend to occur in a circadian rhythm. The disorder is attributed to a **functional disturbance of the diencephalon**, as PET studies have shown increased activity in the hypothalamus during the attacks. Individual attacks can be induced by alcohol, histamine, or nitroglycerin. Aside from primary cluster headache, there are also **symptomatic** forms, caused, for example, by mass lesions.

Clinical features. These are highly typical and are illustrated in **Fig. 14.4**.

The headache attacks always occur on the same side of the head. The pain is mainly felt in the temple, eye, and forehead. About one-third of patients are regularly awakened by the attacks at certain times of night. Most patients have one to three attacks per 24-hour period when they are having attacks (i.e., during a "cluster," see later). Photophobia and nausea are occasional accompanying manifestations. During an attack, the patient does not lie down (as in a migraine headache) but sits up or paces around restlessly. Typical physical findings in an attack are

14

Maximum within 20 minutes

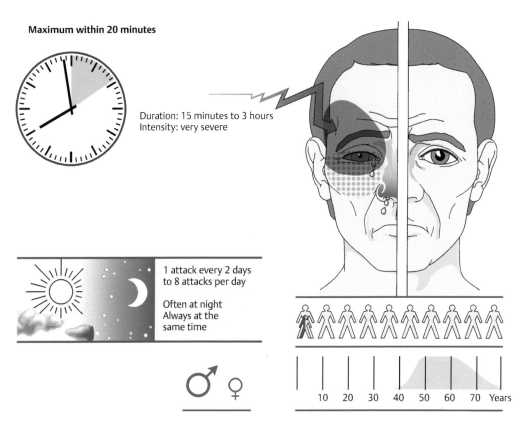

Duration: 15 minutes to 3 hours
Intensity: very severe

1 attack every 2 days
to 8 attacks per day

Often at night
Always at the
same time

10   20   30   40   50   60   70   Years

Fig. 14.4   Cluster headache attack. (These images are provided courtesy of Mumenthaler M, Daetwyler Ch, Kopfschmerz Interaktiv, Instructional Media Department [AUM-IAWF] of the University of Bern Faculty of Medicine, 2001.)

14

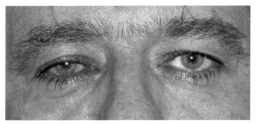

Fig. 14.5   Right-sided cluster headache attack in a 52-year-old patient. Note the narrow palpebral fissure, conjunctival injection, and periorbital erythema.

conjunctival injection, lacrimation, a runny or stuffed nose, and, often, redness of the face, all on the same side as the headache (**Fig. 14.5**).

In **episodic cluster headache**, the attacks occur during periods called "clusters" that may be one to several weeks long, with months or even years of freedom from headache in between. In the rarer, **chronic form** of the disorder, there are no attack-free intervals, and therefore no clusters (despite the name "chronic cluster headache").

Transitional forms. It is not uncommon for typical migraine to be replaced by typical cluster headache (or vice versa) at some point in a patient's life. Some

patients, too, have headaches with some of the features of both.

Diagnostic evaluation. The acute attacks, because they are brief, are only rarely observed by the physician. The diagnosis depends on a **precise clinical history** (as in nearly all types of headache).

Differential diagnosis. This disorder must be carefully differentiated from **facial neuralgias** such as trigeminal neuralgia, nasociliary neuralgia, and Sluder neuralgia (all described in section 14.3.1), as well as from SUNCT syndrome, paroxysmal hemicrania, and hypnic headache (all described later in this section). It must also be borne in mind that **symptomatic headache** may clinically resemble typical cluster headache; the causes include tumors, inflammatory and infectious processes, and multiple sclerosis.

Treatment. The treatment of an **acute attack** is difficult. Triptans can be given by subcutaneous injection, or the patient can be given pure oxygen to breathe (7 L per minute for 15 minutes). Medications for the **reduction of attack frequency** include verapamil and, as a second choice, indomethacin, sometimes in combination with a tricyclic antidepressant. A brief course of cortisone treatment is often effective. The chronic form responds to lithium.

Table 14.5

Some rare types of primary headache

Type	Clinical features	Remarks
Hemicrania continua	Persistent unilateral headache	Responds to indomethacin and sometimes to aspirin
"Ice-cream headache"	Acute headache, usually temporal, lasting 20–30 s, precipitated by a cold stimulus on the palate (such as ice cream)	–
Cough headache	Precipitated by coughing, abdominal straining, or bending over; an intense, diffuse headache lasting a few seconds	Usually innocuous, but sometimes due to a pathologic process in the posterior cranial fossa
Coital headache	Sudden onset, lasts minutes or hours, sometimes accompanied by vomiting	No meningismus (differential diagnosis: subarachnoid hemorrhage)

Paroxysmal Hemicrania

This type of headache usually arises in adulthood and is equally common in men and women. The pain is always **unilateral** and, like cluster headache, located in the **orbit and temple**. The attacks last 2 to 30 minutes and generally occur at least five times per day. They are accompanied by the same **autonomic manifestations** as cluster headache.

The absolutely characteristic feature of paroxysmal hemicrania is that it responds to treatment with **indomethacin**.

SUNCT

This acronym (pronounced "sunked") stands for "short-lasting unilateral neuralgiform headache with conjunctival injection and tearing." The disorder is characterized by brief attacks of pain (lasting 5 seconds to a few minutes each) that always arise on the **same side** of the head, in the **orbital and temporal** area; they are accompanied by ipsilateral **conjunctival injection** and **tearing**, and sometimes by other **autonomic manifestations**. There are 3 to 100 attacks per day. SUNCT with a very high frequency of attacks can easily be mistaken for trigeminal neuralgia. SUNCT occasionally responds to treatment with **antiepileptic drugs**.

The main features and differentiating characteristics of the trigeminal autonomic cephalalgias, and of two other paroxysmal pain syndromes that can resemble them, are listed in **Table 14.4**.

Other Types of Primary (Idiopathic) Headache

Table 14.5 lists a few rarer types of primary headache that will be briefly discussed in this section.

Stabbing ("icepick") headache consists of unprovoked attacks of pain lasting only a few seconds that are felt at variable sites on the skull. The condition is harmless.

Primary **exertional headache** is holocranial and usually of a throbbing type. It can be induced by a variety of physical activities.

Cough headache is induced by heavy coughing. It last a few seconds to a few minutes.

Headache associated with sexual activity (orgasmic or coital headache) is a variety of exertional headache; some patients also have headache induced by other activities. It lasts a few minutes to a few hours. The absence of meningismus generally distinguishes an episode of coital headache from SAH, which can also occur during sexual intercourse.

Primary headache that wakes the patient from sleep is called **hypnic headache** or "alarm-clock headache syndrome." This disorder affects persons over age 65. The headaches are generally not very intense; they generally last 15 minutes to 1 hour and rarely for several hours. This condition, too, is harmless.

Hemicrania continua is always unilateral and always on the same side. The pain is of moderate to severe intensity; it is accompanied by autonomic manifestations like those of paroxysmal hemicrania (see earlier) and, like the latter condition, responds to indomethacin. Acetylsalicylic acid is sometimes effective as well.

New daily persistent headache begins as a diffuse headache in a person who has not suffered from headaches before and then persists. It is felt as a mild to moderately intense pressure in the head. It does not worsen with exercise. This diagnosis should only be made after secondary (symptomatic) headache has been excluded.

14.2.4 The Main Types of Secondary Headache

Secondary headaches are not diseases in themselves but "merely" symptoms of another, underlying disease. **Table 14.6** contains an overview of the major causes of secondary headache. Only a small minority of patients whose chief complaint is headache have secondary headaches. Alarm symptoms indicating the likely presence of secondary headache are listed below under "Dangerous Types of Headache."

14

Table 14.6

The main types of symptomatic headache

Type	Cause	Features, remarks
Subarachnoid hemorrhage (section 6.6.2)	Usually rupture of a saccular aneurysm at the base of the brain	Sudden, extremely severe headache, usually diffuse, accompanied by vomiting, drowsiness, and meningismus
Intracranial mass (section 14.2.4)	Brain tumor, chronic subdural hematoma, brain abscess	Permanent headache of increasing severity; emesis, bradycardia, papilledema, focal neuro-logic deficits; neuroimaging is essential
Occlusive hydrocephalus	Aqueductal stenosis, intraventricular mass, mass in posterior cranial fossa	Manifestations like those of a brain tumor; neuroimaging is essential
Malresorptive hydrocephalus (section 6.12.6)	Prior subarachnoid hemorrhage or meningitis, venous sinus thrombosis	Diffuse, increasingly severe headache, gait ataxia, incontinence; neuroimaging is essential
Intracranial hypotension	Prior LP, (rarely) spontaneous, dural tear	Orthostatic headache that improves or resolves when the patient lies down; normal neurologic examination, CSF not obtainable by LP (or only with aspiration); elevated CSF protein concen-tration; meningeal contrast enhancement
Pseudotumor cerebri	Often seen in overweight young women; may be secondary to prior head trauma, anovulatory drugs, steroid withdrawal, tetracycline, etc.	Chronic headache without any other detectable cause; often papilledema; sometimes, visual loss lasting seconds (amblyopic attacks); CT or MRI reveals slit ventricles; elevated pressure on LP
Meningitis	Bacterial or viral meningitis	Hyperacute in purulent meningitis; very severe headache, meningismus, drowsiness, vomiting
Carcinomatous or leukemic meningitis	Primary tumors of various types, e.g., breast carcinoma	Chronic, diffuse headache, cranial nerve deficits or spinal radicular deficits; LP and CSF cytology are essential; can often be diagnosed by MRI
Postinfectious headache	After recovery from a (viral) infection	Diffuse, often intractable headache without other neurologic abnormalities, resembling tension headache; mild CSF pleocytosis
ENT disease	Chronic sinusitis, neoplasia in the pharynx	Headache or facial pain depending on the site of the disease process; no neurologic deficit
Eye disease	For example, heterophorias (latent strabismus), acute glaucoma, iritis, infectious/inflammatory processes in the orbit	Usually frontal and temporal headache
Dental conditions	Pulpitis, periodontitis, retained teeth, and myo-fascial pain syndrome due to malocclusion	Severe, acute facial pain or chronic facial pain, depending on cause

Abbreviations: CSF, cerebrospinal fluid; CT, computed tomography; LP, lumbar puncture; MRI, magnetic resonance imaging.

Headache due to an Intracranial Tumor

Headache is an early or late major symptom in about half of all patients with brain tumors, particularly those with tumors in the **posterior fossa**.

Headache due to Abnormalities of CSF Circulation

Intermittent obstruction of CSF outflow causes sudden attacks of very intense headache accompanied by nausea, vomiting, and, rarely, brief and transient loss of consciousness. The patient may have opisthotonus as well. The attack may arise gradually over a few seconds or minutes, rarely lasts longer than a few minutes, and generally subsides more slowly than it arose. Any process that obstructs CSF outflow intermittently can produce headaches of this type; a classic example is **colloid cyst of the third ventricle**.

Intracranial Hypotension

Pathophysiology. The intracranial hypotension syndrome has also been called the low CSF volume syndrome, the CSF loss syndrome, and the hypoliquorrhea syndrome. Its symptoms are due to a **reduction of intracranial pressure**. It can arise after traumatic brain injury, because of CSF loss (by lumbar puncture, through a dilated nerve root sleeve, or through a tear in the dura mater, e.g., because of perforation by a bone spur), or without any evident cause.

Intracranial hypotension can be **complicated** by a subdural hematoma or hygroma (**Fig. 14.6b**).

Clinical features. The typical symptom is a very intense orthostatic headache felt whenever the patient stands up, which diminishes on lying down. Persistent, severe intracranial hypotension may be manifested by confusion, nausea/vomiting, tinnitus, hearing loss, and diplopia.

14

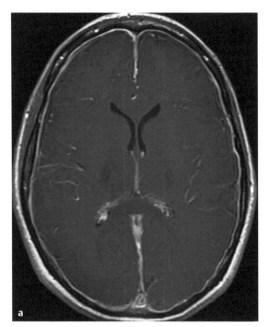

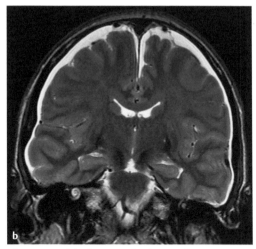

Fig. 14.6   MRI in intracranial hypotension syndrome. a Contrast enhancement of the dura mater (pachymeninx). In meningitis, the leptomeninges take up contrast medium as well. **b** Subdural hygromas over both cerebral convexities.

Diagnostic evaluation. Lumbar puncture in the recumbent patient reveals a CSF pressure below 5 cm H_2O, possibly so low that CSF does not flow spontaneously at all and must be aspirated from the needle. **Magnetic resonance imaging (MRI)** reveals contrast enhancement of the dura mater (pachymeninx) (**Fig. 14.6a**). This differs from the characteristic MRI finding in chronic meningitis, that is, leptomeningeal contrast enhancement (**Fig. 6.44**).

Treatment and prognosis. The prognosis is good: the disorder usually **resolves spontaneously.**

The efficacy of bed rest, fluid administration, and normal saline infusions is debated. **Pharmacotherapy** (e.g., with caffeine) may help. An **epidural blood patch** is an effective treatment. **Surgical closure** of a CSF leak is only rarely necessary.

Pseudotumor cerebri. This syndrome can be considered the opposite of the intracranial hypotension syndrome, so to speak, in that the headaches are due to **intracranial hypertension**. Most patients are overweight young women. The neurologic examination usually reveals **papilledema**, particularly in patients who, when closely questioned, report having had attacks of loss of vision (**Fig. 14.7**). Elevated intracranial pressure is confirmed by **lumbar puncture**. In **imaging studies**, the ventricles are abnormally narrow ("slit ventricles") and the optic nerve sheath is dilated (**Fig. 14.8**). The treatment consists of dehydrating measures, repeated lumbar punctures, and, above all, dedicated and maintained **weight loss**.

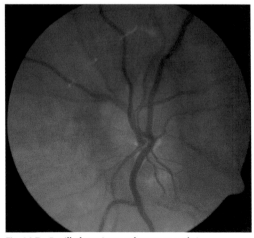

Fig. 14.7   Papilledema in pseudotumor cerebri.

Headache due to Intracranial Infection

Headaches are a prominent symptom of **meningitis** (see section 6.7). In bacterial meningitis, the headache usually begins subacutely or acutely, along with fever and constitutional signs of illness. There is marked meningismus. **Intracranial abscesses** usually cause focal neurologic deficits.

Headache in Vascular Diseases

Ninety percent of patients with acute SAH due to a ruptured aneurysm (see section 6.6.2) complain of headache. Most patients experience an extremely

14

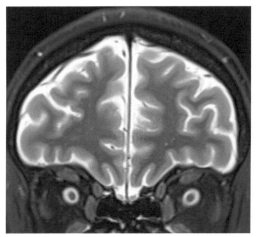

Fig. 14.8　Head MRI in a patient with intracranial hypertension. The coronal images reveal dilatation of the CSF spaces in the optic nerve sheath.

intense headache that begins suddenly ("thunderclap headache") and then persists.

Space-occupying **intracranial hemorrhages** (see section 6.6.1) often cause acute headache, which is frequently initially felt on the side of the hemorrhage. There are always accompanying focal neurologic deficits.

It is not entirely clear whether patients with **arterial hypertension** are more prone to headaches than normotensive persons. An association between blood pressure and headache is well documented only for hypertensive crises.

In **pheochromocytoma**, headaches arise abruptly. The attacks, lasting a few minutes to an hour at most, are usually associated with diaphoresis, palpitations, and pallor.

Headache is only rarely a symptom of intracranial arterial occlusion.

Dissection of the internal carotid artery (Fig. 14.9) can arise spontaneously or after trauma (even mild) to the head or neck. It causes very intense pain on one side of the neck, radiating into the face and temple. It is sometimes accompanied by Horner syndrome (see section 12.3.5). Signs of cerebral ischemia may be absent. Similarly, **vertebral artery dissection** causes pain in the ipsilateral occipital and nuchal region; it can arise spontaneously, after local trauma, or after a whiplash injury of the cervical spine. Clinical manifestations usually arise only if the vertebral artery, the basilar artery, or their branches are narrowed or occluded by an embolus or appositional thrombus.

Cerebral venous thrombosis and venous sinus thrombosis is usually accompanied by headache. For this entity, see the relevant discussion in section 6.5.10. Venous sinus thrombosis can also cause malresorptive hydrocephalus (see section 6.12.6).

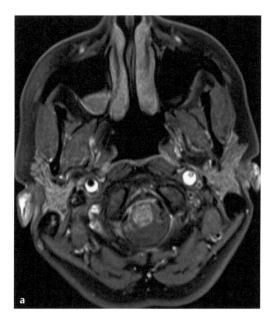

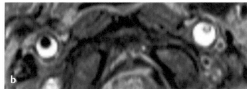

Fig. 14.9　Bilateral carotid dissection of the carotid artery: left, with pseudo-occlusion; right, with high-grade stenosis. **b** is a close-up view of **a**. The typical finding is a sickle-shaped hyperintense mural hematoma eccentrically enclosing the residual lumen, which appears as a low-signal flow void.

Cranial Arteritis

Pathogenesis. Cranial (also called temporal) arteritis is a **giant-cell arteritis**, that is, an autoimmune disease causing typical changes of the tunicae media and elastica interna of large and midsized arteries. It almost exclusively involves the branches of the **external carotid artery**. Large arteries elsewhere in the body can also be affected; involvement of the interior carotid artery is very rare.

Clinical features. This disorder nearly exclusively affects persons over age 50, **women** more often than men. **Headache** is often the initial symptom. It is very intense, usually located in the forehead and temple, and either unilateral or, more commonly, bilateral. The patient may complain of severe, continuous pain, or else of pain on chewing ("claudication" of the tongue and muscles of mastication). The **superficial temporal arteries** are often **thickened** and **tortuous**; they are tender to palpation and cease to pulsate in the advanced stage of the disease (**Fig. 14.10**). In exceptional cases, however, the vessels may appear normal. The headache can also be in an atypical location. If the patient has giant-cell

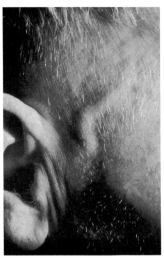

Fig. 14.10 **Temporal arteritis** in a 65-year-old man. Note the thickened, painful, no longer pulsating superficial temporal artery.

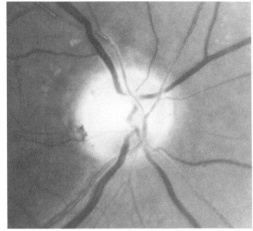

Fig. 14.11 **Ischemia in temporal arteritis**, with disc pallor and thin retinal arteries. (This image is provided courtesy of Prof. Josef Flammer, emeritus head of the Ophthalmological Clinic, University of Basel, Switzerland.)

arteritis as a generalized phenomenon, headache may be absent, but there may be other manifestations such as optic nerve involvement, retinal arterial occlusion, paresis of the extraocular muscles, and polyneuropathy.

Systemic manifestations such as fatigue, anorexia, weight loss, nocturnal diaphoresis, and subfebrile temperature are very common. They are also seen in a further prominent manifestation of giant-cell arteritis—a syndrome called **polymyalgia rheumatica**, characterized by pain in the large proximal joints of the limbs.

> **NOTE**
> The most dreaded complication of giant-cell arteritis is **sudden blindness** due to occlusion of posterior long ciliary arteries (**Fig. 14.11**).

Diagnostic evaluation. The **erythrocyte sedimentation rate (ESR)** and the **C-reactive protein concentration** are markedly elevated in practically all cases; the ESR is generally above 50 mm/h in the first hour.

Color-duplex sonography shows a dark halo around the wall of the superficial temporal artery, which is thickened by arteritis. **MRI** can also reveal inflammation of the arterial wall, but the definitive diagnostic procedure is **biopsy of the superficial temporal artery**.

Treatment. Corticosteroids (e.g., prednisone 1 mg/kg body weight orally once a day in the morning) should be given until the ESR reverts to normal. The dose can then be slowly reduced, but corticosteroid therapy must be continued for many months, often years. A recurrent elevation of the ESR indicates a

new exacerbation of the inflammatory process, which often takes years to "burn out."

> **NOTE**
> If there is a well-grounded **clinical suspicion** of temporal arteritis, **steroids** should be given immediately without waiting for the histologic findings. This is done mainly to prevent serious ocular complications, which can arise rapidly and without warning.

Spondylogenic Headache

Spondylogenic headache, alternatively called cervicogenic headache (or even, inappropriately, "migraine cervicale"), is defined as pain in the head or face caused by a pathologic process in the **bony or soft tissues of the neck**.

Clinical features. Spondylogenic headache is usually, but not always, **unilateral**. It is either nuchal or radiating from the back to the front of the head (in which case patients may accompany their verbal description of the pain with a hat-doffing hand gesture, by way of illustration). It can also be felt in the face. It tends to arise with certain head movements and postures (e.g., prolonged reading) or at night when the head has been kept in an unfavorable position for a long time. The diagnostic criteria are summarized in **Table 14.7**.

Treatment. The treatment is difficult. In acute cases, particularly when torticollis is also present, **traction** can be tried. The immediate success of briefly applied manual traction can also be used as diagnostic evidence for spondylogenic headache.

Persistent or chronic spondylogenic headache can be alleviated by relative immobilization of the cervical spine in a **soft collar** or **hard (Philadelphia) collar** for

14

| Table 14.7 |

Diagnostic criteria for spondylogenic headache

Criteria	Description
Characteristics of the pain	— Radiating from occipital to frontal — Usually unilateral — Episodic pain or permanent pain of variable intensity — Not throbbing — Moderately severe
Cervical spine	— Prior trauma to the head or cervical spine, or prior whiplash injury, or episodes of torticollis (wry neck) — Perhaps accompanied by arm pain — Clinical or radiologic evidence of cervical spine pathology
Precipitating and alleviating factors	— Pain induced by movement or manipulation of the cervical spine, or by keeping the head in a fixed position for a long time, or by local pressure on the nape of the neck or the occiput — Pain temporarily alleviated by infiltration of the greater occipital nerve or the C2 nerve root with local anesthetic
Accompanying symptoms	— Dizziness — Nausea — Blurred vision — Phono- and photophobia — Dysphagia

a few days, as well as by **proper positioning** of the head at night, local **heat application**, **muscle relaxant drugs**, and **NSAIDs**. CT-guided **local anesthetic infiltration** of the cervical intervertebral joints can help in rare cases.

Drug- and Substance-Related Headache
Headache can be an **acute effect of certain drugs and other substances**, among them nitric oxide (NO), nitroglycerin, histamine, carbon monoxide (CO, generated, for example, in a poorly ventilated oven), alcohol, monosodium glutamate ("Chinese restaurant headache"), amyl nitrite ("hot dog headache"), cocaine, and cannabis.

The **withdrawal** of certain drugs and other substances after longstanding use can also cause headaches, for example, caffeine, opioids, and estrogen.

Medication-overuse headache: the longstanding, regular consumption of analgesic drugs by a headache patient can itself cause diffuse, more or less continuous headaches. By definition, medication-overuse headache is present on at least 15 days of each month. It is felt on both sides of the head, usually as a throbbing pain. It is typically of moderate intensity.

| NOTE |

Any analgesic drug—not just ergot derivatives and triptans, but also nonprescription drugs such as acetaminophen—can cause medication-overuse headache if taken to excess.

Chronic **triptan** use, however, causes medication-overuse headache more rapidly than chronic use of other drugs. The diagnosis requires, by definition, that the offending drug has been taken on at least 10 days per month for at least three consecutive months and also that the patient's headache reverts to its original quality once the drug has been discontinued.

The **treatment** is difficult. Analgesic consumption must be markedly reduced; for psychological support, antidepressant drugs may help, but the most important factors are the sustained, direct involvement of the treating physician and the provision of behavior therapy.

Further Kinds of Secondary Headache
The **neck–tongue syndrome** is rare: sudden turning of the head immediately leads to an occipital headache and simultaneous paresthesia of one-half of the tongue.

Ophthalmologic headache can be caused by refractory anomalies but is mainly due to heterophorias (squints) in childhood. The headache arises over the course of the day. The problem resolves after appropriate treatment by an ophthalmologist.

Sinusitis can cause intractable, often sharply localized headache, as can chronic otitis and space-occupying lesions in the nasopharynx.

Goggle headache is a special type of supraorbital neuralgia caused by wearing tight swimming goggles.

Headache due to a systemic disease can be very severe, particularly in some infectious diseases, such as Q fever. The headache can last far longer than the causative acute infection.

Chronic iron deficiency is a further cause of headache.

Emotional factors are said to play an important role in the pathogenesis of so-called **tension headache**. This term has been used with a variety of meanings;

it generally refers to mainly occipital headaches that are attributed to emotional tension and cause more or less persistent contraction of the nuchal muscles. Tension headache is not the same entity as tension-type headache (discussed in section 14.2.3). Headache can also be a heralding symptom of **incipient psychosis**.

Dangerous Types of Headache

All patients who consult a physician because of headache are in pain and therefore deserve our full attention. More than 90% of them, however, will turn out not to have a serious medical problem. An important task facing the physician is to be on guard for the occasional cases of headache that are, in fact, due to a dangerous underlying condition.

The main **alarm signals** are the following:
- Headache of an unusual nature arising **for the first time**, particularly in a patient over age 40.
- **Continuous headache**:
  - that has been continuous from its onset
  - or that has become continuous through the confluence of ever more frequent, previously episodic headaches.
- Progressively severe headache.
- Explosive headache.
- Headache that always occurs on the same side and in exactly the same location (except cluster headache or trigeminal neuralgia, both of which, by definition, always occur in the same place).
- Headache with accompanying features:
  - Vomiting (except in migraine).
  - Progressive personality change.
  - Epileptic seizures.
- Headache with accompanying neurologic abnormalities:
  - Neurologic deficits.
  - Papilledema.
  - neuropsychological abnormalities.
- Headache that does **not** conform to any of the **typical types of headache**.

If any of the above apply, further investigation is needed, usually with an imaging study.

14.3 Painful Syndromes of the Face

  Key Point

Facial pain is often due to a lesion of a sensory nerve in the face, most commonly the trigeminal nerve. It typically presents with very brief, but very intense attacks of pain ("classic" or "genuine" neuralgia). There are also various

kinds of facial pain with other pathogenetic mechanisms, for example, a structural anomaly of the temporomandibular joint. The pain may resemble neuralgia in these conditions as well. Patients with any kind of facial pain always require careful differential diagnostic evaluation.

14.3.1 Neuralgias

Neuralgia is defined as **pain in the distribution of a peripheral nerve**. It is often of a **tearing** or **piercing** quality. The face is a common site of intense, brief (rarely, longer-lasting), lightning-like attacks of pain. Often, these can be induced by touching the faces in certain places (trigger points) or by activities such as speaking, swallowing, or chewing.

Trigeminal Neuralgia

Epidemiology. The prevalence of trigeminal neuralgia is reportedly 100 to 400 per 1 million people.

Etiology and pathogenesis. Excitation of tactile fibers is presumed to cross over abnormally onto nociceptive fibers in what is called "ephaptic transmission." In **idiopathic** trigeminal neuralgia, the underlying cause is thought to be a lesion of the myelin sheath of the trigeminal nerve root at its zone of entry into the pons, brought about either by the **aging** process or else by persistent mechanical irritation from a **pulsating vascular loop** lying on the root. In **symptomatic** trigeminal neuralgia, another underlying disease (e.g., tumor, multiple sclerosis) affects the trigeminal nerve or its brainstem fibers, producing pain.

Clinical features. As mentioned earlier, there is a distinction between idiopathic and symptomatic trigeminal neuralgia:

Idiopathic (essential) trigeminal neuralgia only affects persons over age 50. The pain is always felt in the same area, usually in the distribution of the maxillary and/or mandibular nerve. The pain is always unilateral at first; however, in occasional cases, pain later affects the other side of the face as well. The pain is described as electric or lancinating (lightning-like) and unbearably intense. Each attack lasts only a few seconds, but the attacks can repeat themselves every few minutes and can occur up to a hundred times a day.

  Practical Tip

Patients whose neuralgic attacks occur at very closely spaced intervals may perceive or describe them as continuous. This can cause diagnostic confusion.

The attacks can often be induced by chewing, speaking, or touching particular sites (**trigger points**) on

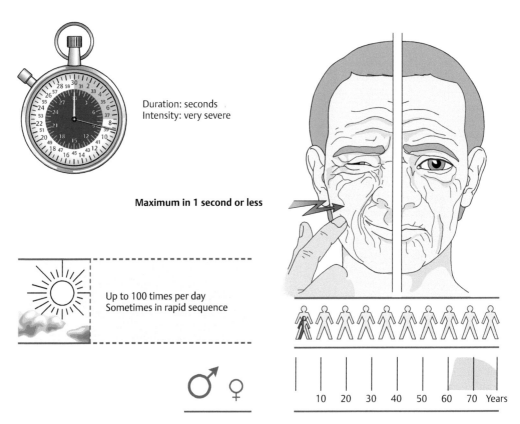

Duration: seconds
Intensity: very severe

Maximum in 1 second or less

Up to 100 times per day
Sometimes in rapid sequence

10 20 30 40 50 60 70 Years

Fig. 14.12   Trigeminal neuralgia. (These images are provided courtesy of Mumenthaler M, Daetwyler Ch, Kopfschmerz Interaktiv, Instructional Media Department [AUM-IAWF] of the University of Bern Faculty of Medicine, 2001.)

14

the face or inside the mouth. Patients with the idiopathic form of the disorder have no abnormalities on neurologic examination. Spontaneous remission is possible, with months or years of freedom from pain. The symptoms of trigeminal neuralgia are illustrated in **Fig. 14.12**.

Symptomatic trigeminal neuralgia can be caused by multiple sclerosis (see the relevant discussion in section 8.2), a pontine infarct, or a tumor of the cerebellopontine angle. Patients with the symptomatic form of the disorder can be of any age; compared with those with idiopathic trigeminal neuralgia, they more commonly suffer from bilateral and/or continuous pain and may have objectifiable neurologic deficits on examination.

Treatment. Symptomatic trigeminal neuralgia is treated by the treatment of its underlying cause. **Idiopathic** trigeminal neuralgia, which is much more common, is initially treated with drugs, usually the anticonvulsant **carbamazepine** (slow dose escalation up to 200 mg three to four times daily) or its structural derivative **oxcarbazepine** (900–1,800 mg/d). If these are poorly tolerated, other anticonvulsants, including gabapentin, lamotrigine, pregabalin, topiramate, and levetiracetam, can be used as second-line drugs.

If pharmacotherapy does not sufficiently relieve the pain, effective **neurosurgical treatments** are available.

Other Neuralgias of the Face

Neuralgias in the face other than trigeminal neuralgia are rare; an overview is provided in **Fig. 14.13**.

In **auriculotemporal neuralgia**, the pain is located in the temple and in front of the ear. It is usually a sequela of ipsilateral parotid gland disease, appearing a few days or months after the parotid condition resolves.

In **nasociliary neuralgia**, either episodic or continuous pain is felt in the nose, on the inner canthus, or in the globe of the eye. It is accompanied by erythema of the forehead, swelling of the nasal mucosa, and sometimes conjunctival injection and lacrimation.

Sluder neuralgia is attributed to a pathologic process affecting the pterygopalatine ganglion. Its clinical features resemble those of nasociliary neuralgia. In many patients, the attacks are accompanied by the urge to sneeze. Sluder neuralgia is occasionally associated with sphenoid, ethmoid, or maxillary sinusitis.

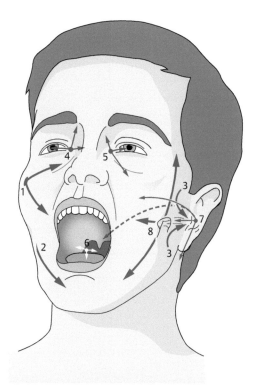

Fig. 14.13   The sites of various types of facial pain and neuralgia. 1 Trigeminal neuralgia in the distribution of the maxillary nerve (V_2). **2** Trigeminal neuralgia in the distribution of the mandibular nerve (V_3). **3** Auriculotemporal neuralgia. **4** Nasociliary neuralgia. **5** Sluder neuralgia. **6** Glossopharyngeal neuralgia. **7** Neuralgia of the geniculate ganglion. **8** Craniomandibular dysfunction (also called temporomandibular joint syndrome or "neuralgia").

Glossopharyngeal neuralgia is characterized by intense, lightning-like attacks of pain in the base of the tongue, the hypopharynx, and the tonsillar fossa, always only on one side of the head. The pain is continuous in some patients.

Neuralgia of the geniculate ganglion was originally described as a sequela of herpes zoster infection, typically associated with a vesicular rash on the tragus and mastoid process and a peripheral facial nerve palsy (**Ramsay Hunt syndrome**). It can, however, arise without any preceding rash or palsy. The pain is felt in front of the ear and in the external auditory canal, and also deep in the roof of the palate, the upper jaw, and the mastoid area. It can be accompanied by abnormal taste perception on the anterior half of the tongue and by hypersalivation.

14.3.2 Pain in the Face Caused by Diseases of the Teeth and Jaws

Acute dental disease can cause severe pain in the face.

Craniomandibular dysfunction, that is, dysfunction of the temporomandibular joint, can cause

neuralgiform pain. This condition has many names, including temporomandibular joint syndrome, temporomandibular "neuralgia," myofascial syndrome, and Costen syndrome. It is usually caused by **malocclusion** and mainly affects young and middle-aged women. Patients typically complain of intermittent or continuous preauricular pain that is brought on, or made worse, by chewing. In about half of all patients, the pain also radiates into the forehead, the lower jaw, and/or the occiput. It is mostly unilateral. Physical examination reveals tenderness of the jaw joint to palpation and, sometimes, restricted opening or closing of the mouth. Dental examination reveals the malocclusion that is the cause of the pain.

14.3.3 Atypical Facial Pain
This term refers to **unilateral, diffusely localized pain in the face**, often of a burning, distressing quality. It may have no apparent cause but can also arise after a dental procedure, often a minor and apparently uncomplicated one. The pain is **always present**, with intermittent exacerbations. Atypical facial pain is most common in middle-aged women.

14.3.4 Further Types of Facial Pain
Several other types of facial pain have been described, most of them rare.

Tolosa–Hunt syndrome consists of intense periorbital pain accompanied by weakness of one or more of the extraocular muscles, probably because of a nonspecific inflammatory process in the cavernous sinus. Treatment with corticosteroids is effective.

Glossodynia ("burning mouth syndrome") is a more or less permanent, dull, burning, distressing pain in the tongue and mouth, accompanied by paresthesia in these areas. It affects women much more often than men, in a 7:1 ratio. It tends to arise in middle age.

14.3.5 Differential Diagnosis of Headache and Facial Pain
The differential diagnosis of headache and facial pain is nearly always based on the patient's detailed description of the pain. The clinical features often provide important clues to the cause. Important aspects of differential diagnosis are summarized in **Table 14.8**.

14.4 Painful Shoulder–Arm Syndromes

   Key Point

Pain in the shoulder and arm is a common complaint. The differential diagnosis includes conditions treated by a wide range of medical specialties: cervical spine pathology (spondylogenic arm pain); degenerative changes of the

14

Table 14.8

Differential diagnosis of headache and facial pain

Clinical features	Syndrome
Recurrent attacks of intense headache with pain-free intervals	— Migraine (unilateral headache) — Cluster headache (unilateral pain in the temple, eye, and face) — Hypertensive crises (diffuse pain)
Recurrent attacks of intense facial pain with pain-free intervals, usually unilateral	— Trigeminal neuralgia (duration, seconds; localization, usually midface) — Auriculotemporal neuralgia (duration, minutes; localization, preauricular) — Nasociliary neuralgia (duration, minutes to hours; localization, inner canthus) — Sluder neuralgia (duration, minutes; localization, inner canthus) — Glossopharyngeal neuralgia (duration, seconds; localization, base of tongue and tonsillar fossa) — Geniculate ganglion neuralgia (duration, seconds; localization, external auditory canal and palatal roof)
Continuous facial pain	— Atypical facial pain (diffuse, usually unilateral pain) — TMJ syndrome (preauricular)
Intense headache of **sudden onset**, which then persists	— Subarachnoid hemorrhage — Intracerebral hemorrhage
Diffuse, usually intense headache of subacute onset, which then persists	— Meningitis — Encephalitis (accompanied by meningismus)
Headache on standing or sitting that improves when the patient lies down	— Intracranial hypotension
Chronic, or chronically relapsing, diffuse headache of insidious onset and mild to moderate severity	— Tension-type headache — Headache due to hypertension — Headache due to intracranial mass — Posttraumatic headache — Headache due to systemic illness (particularly febrile illness); toxic/iatrogenic headache; psychogenic or depressive headache
Chronic, well-circumscribed headache and facial pain	— Spondylogenic headache (pain mainly in the back of the head) — Temporal arteritis (pain mainly temporal) — Eye diseases (pain mainly frontal) — ENT diseases (especially sinusitis, pain mainly frontal, worse on inclination of the head) — Odontogenic headache (jaw and temporal region)

Abbreviation: TMJ, temporomandibular joint.

14

shoulder and elbow joints and the adjacent connective tissues (ligaments, tendons, joint capsules); diseases of the cervical nerve roots, brachial plexus, and peripheral nerves (neurogenic arm pain); and vascular diseases. Finally, there remains "arm pain of overuse," a collection of conditions caused by unusually intense stress on muscles and joints.

An overview of diseases causing pain in the shoulder and arm is provided in **Table 14.9**. The clinical features of the more common conditions in this group are described in the following paragraphs.

14.4.1 Spondylogenic (Cervicogenic) Shoulder and Arm Pain

NOTE

The cause of spondylogenic shoulder and arm pain is usually **degenerative osteochondrosis** with spondylotic narrowing of the intervertebral foramina and, possibly, **cervical disk herniation**. These disease processes compress and mechanically irritate the cervical nerve roots.

Clinical features. Conditions of this type always begin with neck pain and/or a painful restriction of head movement. Later on, the pain radiates into the shoulder and, usually, down the arm (**cervicobrachialgia**). Some patients have diffuse pain, but most have pain in the dermatome of the affected nerve root (i.e., **radicular pain**): C6 lesions cause pain on the lateral aspect of the forearm and the thumb, C7 lesions cause pain in the middle finger, and C8 lesions cause pain on the ulnar side of the hand and in the fourth and fifth fingers. The **objective findings** include painful restriction of head movement and, sometimes, radicular neurologic deficits—weakness, loss of segment-indicating reflexes, and diminished sensation in the dermatome of the affected nerve root (cf. **Table 13.1**). **Treatment.** Physical therapy and analgesic drugs are the mainstays of treatment.

14.4.2 Degenerative and Rheumatic Shoulder and Arm Pain

NOTE

Pain in the shoulder and arm is usually due to degenerative changes of the bones, joints, tendons, and other soft tissues.

Table 14.9

Overview of shoulder–arm pain

Category	Etiology	Remarks
Spondylogenic pain	Spondylosis	Nuchal pain at first; pain often radiates diffusely
	Disk herniation	Acute torticollis at first, only later followed by pain radiation in a radicular pattern; objectifiable neurologic deficits
Nonspondylogenic nerve root lesion	Tumor	Slowly progressive symptoms
	Dissection of the vertebral artery	Acute, unilateral nuchal or occipital pain
Brachial plexus lesion	Tumor	For example, lung apex tumor (Pancoast tumor) with lower brachial plexus involvement and Horner syndrome
	Radiation injury	Pain and progressive neurologic deficits after a latency period
	Neuralgic shoulder amyotrophy	Intense pain for one or more days, followed by weakness of shoulder girdle or arm muscles
	TOS	Overdiagnosed; the diagnosis can be accepted if there is a cervical rib or other anomaly of the thoracic outlet
	Hyperabduction syndrome	The arm "falls asleep" at night in certain positions
	Posttraumatic brachial plexus lesion	Phantom pain, neuroma pain, stump pain, painful and non-suppressible twitching of the stump
Lesion of an individual peripheral nerve (or branch)	Radial nerve	Supinator syndrome
	Median nerve	Pronator syndrome, carpal tunnel syndrome (most common cause of nocturnal arm pain)
	Ulnar nerve	Sulcus ulnaris syndrome
	Cutaneous sensory branches	For example, pain in the elbow pit after paravenous injection
Degenerative and rheumatologic disorders	In the shoulder region	Rotator cuff involvement, impingement syndrome
	In the elbow region	Radial epicondylitis (tennis elbow), ulnar epicondylitis (golfer's elbow)
	In the distal forearm and hand	Radial styloiditis, first metacarpophalangeal joint, e.g., in gout
	Upper or lower limb (often hand)	CRPS
Brachialgia of vascular origin	Arterial	Acute brachial artery occlusion, subclavian steal syndrome
	Venous	Effort thrombosis
Tenomyalgic and pseudo-radicular overuse syndromes	Diffuse brachialgia after non-physiologic overuse of an arm, or secondary to weakness of the shoulder muscles	Various occupations, e.g., bank teller, or in the wake of trapezius weakness
Rarer causes	Glomus tumor	A locally painful blue spot is often visible under the fingernail; the pain increases when the arm is dependent

Abbreviations: CRPS, complex regional pain syndrome; TOS, thoracic outlet syndrome.

14

Rotator cuff dysfunction (formerly called humeroscapular periarthropathy) can arise spontaneously or after shoulder trauma (a blow or sprain) or immobilization. The tendons of the short rotators of the shoulder joint undergo degenerative changes, sometimes with calcification, which lead to irritation of the subdeltoid bursa. The highly typical clinical finding is **local shoulder pain** on **active raising of the arm**, particularly with simultaneous **internal rotation**. It is painful, for example, for the patient to slip the arm into a sleeve while getting dressed. If the abducted arm is then rested on a surface (table, etc.), the pain abates. The diseased tendon(s) is (are) **tender to palpation**, usually ventral to the shoulder joint. Plain radiographs may reveal calcifications. **Rotator cuff tear** makes the patient unable to abduct the arm without pain or at all. Rotator cuff dysfunction can be objectively demonstrated with certain functional tests (the Jobe test, the starter test, and the lag sign).

Impingement syndrome is closely related to degenerative disease of the rotator cuff. In this condition, when the arm is abducted, the sensitive area of the rotator cuff comes into contact with the coracoacromial roof.

Frozen shoulder syndrome sometimes represents the end stage of degenerative disease of the rotator cuff, but more commonly arises as a sequela of hemiparesis or myocardial infarction. It is rarely caused by phenobarbital use, and can also come about spontaneously. It is characterized by **very painful restriction of shoulder movement**, with a slowly progressive course.

Complex regional pain syndrome (CRPS): this often intractable condition was known in the past as reflex sympathetic dystrophy, algodystrophy, or Sudeck dystrophy. The sympathetic nervous system plays an important role in its pathogenesis, particularly as a cause of the characteristic swelling. Faulty information processing in the neurons of the dorsal horn of the spinal cord is thought to be another contributing factor. CRPS can affect any part of the upper or lower limbs but it is particularly common in the hand. It tends to arise after a fracture or other type of trauma, which need not be particularly severe. The clinical findings include the following: **soft tissue swelling**; **smooth, cool, often cyanotic skin**; and a **very painful restriction of joint mobility**. Plain radiographs reveal **patchy osteoporosis** of the bones in the affected area.

Epicondylitis is characterized by pain at the origins of the extensor and flexor muscles of the hand and fingers on the humeral epicondyles. The pain can be felt spontaneously, on contraction of the affected muscles and tendons, or in response to local pressure. The usual cause is muscle overuse. The commonest type is **lateral (radial) epicondylitis**, so-called "tennis elbow." **Medial (ulnar) epicondylitis** ("golfer's elbow") is rarer and is caused by flexor overuse.

Radial styloiditis is characterized by pain at the tendinous origins of the extensor carpi radialis muscles on the styloid process of the radius. **Ulnar styloiditis** is the analogous condition on the styloid process of the ulna. Both are varieties of tendonitis, similar to others occurring elsewhere in the body.

14.4.3 Neurogenic Arm Pain

> **NOTE**
>
> In these conditions, pain in the arm and shoulder is due to a lesion affecting **sensory nerve fibers**, either in the brachial plexus or in the peripheral nerves. The lesion may be either **mechanical** (common) or **infectious/inflammatory** (less common).

Irritation of the Brachial Plexus

Compression of the brachial plexus at the thoracic outlet can occur at any of several anatomic bottlenecks (the scalene hiatus, the costoclavicular passage, or the subacromial space). This generally occurs, however, only when an additional pathogenic factor is present, such as a cervical rib, fibrous band, or anomaly of the scalene attachments, or exogenous pressure. The corresponding clinical syndromes are discussed in Chapter 13.

Brachial plexus tumors sometimes cause progressively worsening arm pain that becomes very severe within a matter of weeks. **Pancoast tumors** of the lung apex (described in section 13.2.1) are a well-known cause.

Neuralgic shoulder amyotrophy (discussed in section 13.2.2) also causes acute, severe pain.

Peripheral Nerve Conditions

Compressive neuropathies can cause severe, intractable pain in the upper limb. These conditions are described in section 13.2.3. The more common types are **sulcus ulnaris syndrome** and **carpal tunnel syndrome**, which causes arm pain, especially at night (brachialgia paraesthetica nocturna).

14.4.4 Vasogenic Arm Pain

> **NOTE**
>
> **Stenosis or occlusion of an artery** supplying the shoulder girdle or the upper limb can cause pain, sometimes only during or after movement of the limb. **Venous occlusion** can cause pain as well.

Arterial Diseases

Stenosis or occlusion of the subclavian artery causes diffuse arm pain on movement, forcing the patient to stop using the limb ("intermittent claudication of the arm"). If the occlusion lies proximal to the origin of the vertebral artery, the arm will be supplied with blood through retrograde flow in the vertebral or basilar artery. Blood can be "stolen" in this way from the cerebral circulation (**subclavian steal syndrome**): movement of the arm diverts blood flow away from the vertebrobasilar territory in the brain, and lightheadedness or sudden falling (drop attacks) may result.

Arterial insufficiency in the upper limb is demonstrated with the **fist-clenching test**: the patient holds the upper limbs high, then rapidly and repeatedly clenches and reopens both hands. Pain arises within a few minutes on the poorly perfused side and the hand turns pale. When the arms are lowered again, the veins on the dorsum of the hand fill slowly on the affected side. The arterial blood pressure is also always lower when measured in the affected arm.

Venous Thrombosis

Occlusion of the axillary or subclavian vein: This condition, also known as **effort syndrome** or **Paget–von Schrötter syndrome**, is seen most commonly in young men, usually on the right side. It is rarely spontaneous; more commonly, it arises after heavy use of the arm, for example, in sports. The venous occlusion manifests itself as a **painful tension** in the arm, often accompanied by **swelling**. The subcutaneous veins of the arm, which provide an alternative path for venous return, are more clearly visible than normal. The thrombosed vein itself can sometimes be palpated in the axilla and is tender. It can often be unequivocally demonstrated with neuroimaging studies and Doppler ultrasonography. The prognosis is generally good; operative thrombectomy is only rarely necessary.

14.4.5 Arm Pain of Overuse

> **NOTE**
>
> The prolonged and repeated performance of specific movements of the upper limb(s), particularly in the workplace (e.g., typing, working at a cash register, or use of other kinds of machines), can produce intractable pain in the upper limb extending well beyond the muscles used in the movement.

Pain of this type leads, in turn, to increased use of other muscle groups, so that these, too, become involved in the pain syndrome. This condition and its pathogenesis are described in greater detail in section 14.7.

14.4.6 Other Types of Arm Pain

Glomus tumors: These are small, benign growths that originate in the glomus organs of the skin. They are composed of **arteriovenous anastomoses** in close association with autonomic fibers. Clinically, they are characterized by a **dull pain** that worsens when the arm hangs down and, particularly, when the arm swings as the patient walks. Local pressure over the tumor also causes pain. Glomus tumors are often found at the **fingertips**, where they may be visible as a bluish spot under the fingernail, but they can also arise practically anywhere else, including on the lower limbs.

Referred pain: Diseases of the internal organs commonly cause referred pain in the shoulder and arm. Pain is felt in the right shoulder in gall bladder disease, for example, and in the left arm in angina pectoris.

Gout: An exacerbation can produce extremely severe, acute pain in a hand (**chiragra**) or foot (**podagra**). The pain is sometimes, but not always, restricted to the first metacarpophalangeal or metatarsophalangeal joint.

14.5 Pain in the Trunk and Back

> **Key Point**
> The back is by far the most common site of pain in the trunk of the body. Back pain is usually due to pathologic abnormalities of the spine that lead to abnormal posture and nonphysiologic muscle activation. Lack of exercise and sedentary occupations are probably the main causes of back pain today. Emotional stress, too, can increase muscle tension and cause muscle spasms and bad posture.

Table 14.10 contains an overview of these painful syndromes, their localization, and the types of pain they produce. A few of them will be described in detail in the following paragraphs.

14.5.1 Thoracic and Abdominal Wall Pain

Diseases of the internal organs are the most common cause of pain in the thoracic and abdominal wall (**referred pain, Table 14.10**). The pain is projected on to the body surface and felt in the corresponding dermatome. **Chest pain** is often due to diseases of the heart and lungs. **Band-like pain** suggests a (possibly intraspinal) process irritating one of the spinal nerve roots or segmental nerves. **Abdominal wall pain** often arises from the internal organs, but may also be caused, for example, by compression of the ventral rami of the spinal nerve roots (e.g., compression of the caudal thoracic nerves in the rectus abdominis syndrome). The rare spigelian hernia is another possibility, as is an abnormally mobile 10th rib.

14.5.2 Back Pain

Back pain is a very common problem that often profoundly affects the sufferer's everyday life at work and at home. The pain cannot always be fully explained on the basis of objectively demonstrable musculoskeletal changes. The visible structural changes are often not commensurate with the intensity of the pain. The major causes of back pain are as follows:

— **Degenerative changes of the spine** cause the vast majority of cases of back pain. Degenerative and osteochondrotic changes affect the vertebral bodies and the intervertebral joints. The damaged cartilaginous surfaces react with osteophyte formation and sclerosis in the adjacent bone. **Spondylosis** and **spondyloarthrosis** ensue and, when under mechanical stress, give rise to inflammation and effusion. These problems lead, in turn, to faulty posture, reflex functional disturbances of the musculature, and more pain. Degenerative changes also cause nerve root irritation, which manifests itself as lumbago, sciatica, or cervicobrachial pain, depending on the segment involved. The pain radiating into the upper or lower limbs can be radicular or pseudoradicular. Other deformations of the spine, for example, Scheuermann disease or scoliosis, can also cause persistent back pain because of nonphysiologic stress on the muscles of the trunk and back. Spondylolisthesis, the sliding of one vertebral body on another (with or without spondylolysis, a defect of the pars interarticularis of the vertebral arch), is often a congenital anomaly that remains clinically silent until later in life. It may not become symptomatic until after an accident.

— **Pathologic changes of the sacroiliac joint** typically produce pain that worsens when the patient stands on or hyperextends the leg on the affected side (Mennell's maneuver).

14

Table 14.10

Overview of pain in the trunk and back

Designation	Mechanism	Localization and clinical features	Remarks
Pain in a band-like distribution	Uni- or bilateral nerve root lesion	Feeling of segmental constriction on one or both sides; continuous pain	For example, spinal tumor, disk herniation, herpes zoster
Abnormally mobile 10th rib ("slipping rib")	Pain on displacement of the free end of the 10th rib	Unilateral pain at the costal margin, on bending over or with local pressure; the pain may be continuous	After thoracic trauma, or spontaneous
Tear and hemorrhage in the abdominal wall musculature	Lesion (rupture) of the rectus abdominis muscle, e.g., after strenuous exercise	Local pain in the abdominal wall	Rarely, compartment syndrome of the rectus abdominis muscle
Spigelian hernia	Hernia next to the rectus sheath, covered by the abdominal oblique muscle and difficult to identify	Pain at a paramedian location on the abdominal wall, local tenderness	–
Rectus abdominis syndrome	Entrapment neuropathy; a medial cutaneous branch of one of the intercostal nerves is caught in a gap in the fascia	Abdominal wall pain on movement; sometimes there is a coin-sized area of cutaneous anesthesia	The pain disappears after the application of local anesthetic
Ilioinguinal nerve syndrome	Compression of the ilioinguinal nerve, or constriction by scar	Groin, external genitalia; dull, continuous pain, worse on hip extension, better on flexion; objective sensory deficit in the distribution of the nerve	Differential diagnosis: inguinal hernia, testicular torsion
Referred pain (zones of Head)	Pain from internal organs projected to the surface of the trunk	Pain localization depends on the affected organ; e.g., chest pain in diseases of the heart and lungs, abdominal pain in GI diseases, lumbar pain in diseases of the retroperitoneal organs; typically a dull, piercing, or acute tearing pain	–
Thoracoabdominal neuropathy	Usually diabetic mononeuropathy	Continuous pain and paresthesia of the thoracic or abdominal wall; diminished sensation, or unilateral weakness of abdominal wall muscles	–
Ankylosing spondylitis (Bekhterev disease)	In 90% of cases, associated with the HLA-B27 histocompatibility antigen	The pain usually begins in the low back, usually at night; progressive thoracic kyphosis and diminishing mobility of the spine; rarely, pain in the chest and heels; typical radiologic findings	Usually affects younger men
Spondylolisthesis and spondylolysis	Prolongation of the pars interarticularis and ventral displacement of the upper vertebral body, ranging to spondyloptosis	Low back pain, worse on exertion and after prolonged standing; palpable "step" in the back; typical radiologic findings	Congenital anomaly; spondylolisthesis can be induced by mechanical stress or can occur spontaneously (in the latter case, usually as a symptom of an underlying condition); differential diagnosis: pseudospondylolisthesis in degenerative osteochondrosis
Sacroiliac strain	Tension on the ligamentous apparatus of the sacroiliac joint	Low back pain, sometimes with pseudoradicular radiation into the lower limbs; worse when the patient stands on one leg, or with the Mennell's maneuver	Relieved by wearing a trochanteric belt
Notalgia paresthetica	Entrapment of the terminal sensory branch of the dorsal ramus of a spinal nerve in a fascial gap in the back	Local, unilateral pain in the back; objective local tenderness and a coin-sized area of paravertebral cutaneous anesthesia	The pain disappears after the application of local anesthetic

Abbreviation: GI, gastrointestinal.

— **Entrapment neuropathies** are a rare, nonosseous cause of back pain. **Notalgia paresthetica**, for example, is an entrapment neuropathy of the sensory dorsal rami of the thoracic spinal nerves as they pass through small apertures in the fascia (see also section 13.2.4).

— **Coccygodynia**, that is, intractable pain in the coccyx, can arise after local trauma (a fall on the buttocks) or spontaneously. In the latter case, the diagnostic evaluation should include a search for tumors or infectious/inflammatory changes in the pelvis, as well as cysts of the lumbosacral nerve root sleeves (= Tarlov's cysts).

14.5.3 Groin Pain

Pain in the groin can be caused not only by urinary tract diseases, gynecologic diseases, and inguinal hernias, but also by peripheral nerve lesions. The **ilioinguinal nerve syndrome**, a type of entrapment neuropathy, is described in **Table 14.10**. The pain of **spermatic neuralgia** is felt in the scrotum.

 Practical Tip
When the cause of groin pain is unclear, a pathologic process should be sought in the pelvis.

14.6 Leg Pain

 Key Point
Pain in the leg, like pain in the arm, has many causes. Common ones are degenerative and traumatic processes affecting the joints and soft tissues, lumbar disk herniation, and other lesions in the lumbar spinal canal. Further ones include polyneuropathies, entrapment neuropathies, and restless legs syndrome. Exercise-induced leg pain can be due to either lumbar spinal stenosis or peripheral arterial occlusive disease (neurogenic vs. vasogenic claudication).

Pain in the hip is usually due to a disease of the hip joint, most often degenerative arthritis (**coxarthrosis**). A diagnosis that is often missed is **periarthropathy of the hip**, in which the joint itself is not diseased, but the soft tissues around it give rise to intractable pain, which frequently lasts for months. In **algodystrophy of the hip**, local pain is followed some time afterward by osteopenia of the femoral head. Both the pain and the osteopenia usually resolve spontaneously.

Thigh pain may be due to a local process such as a **sarcoma**. An upper lumbar disk herniation or other lesion causing **nerve root irritation** can produce referred pain in the thigh. **Meralgia paresthetica** (see

also section 13.2.6, Lateral Femoral Cutaneous Nerve (L2–L3)) is an entrapment neuropathy causing pain in the thigh. Acute thigh pain and femoral nerve palsy can be caused by **diabetic neuropathy** or by a **hematoma in the psoas sheath**.

Knee pain is usually of orthopedic, rheumatologic, or traumatic origin. A proximal lesion of the obturator nerve produces referred pain in the popliteal fossa in **Howship–Romberg syndrome** (see section 13.2.6, Obturator Nerve (L3–L4)). Spontaneous or mechanically induced lesions of the infrapatellar branch of the saphenous nerve are a further cause of pain in the knee.

Calf pain that is present only when the patient walks is typical of **vasogenic intermittent claudication**, a syndrome whose cause usually lies in the arteries, less commonly in the veins. **Neurogenic intermittent claudication** is caused by compression of the cauda equina in lumbar spinal stenosis (see section 13.1.3, Lumbar Spinal Stenosis).

 Practical Tip
Neurogenic intermittent claudication is worse when the patient walks downhill, while vasogenic intermittent claudication of arterial origin is worse when the patient walks uphill. Claudication due to venous stasis is felt when the patient walks and resolves when the legs are elevated.

In the **anterior tibial artery syndrome** (see section 13.2.6, Peroneal [Fibular] Nerve [L4–S2]), pain develops acutely on the anterior aspect of the lower leg, particularly with exercise. The saphenous nerve can be caught in a fascial gap on the medial side of the lower leg or, alternatively, in Hunter's canal in the thigh; pain ensues in the cutaneous zone innervated by this nerve (a type of **entrapment neuropathy**).

Pain in the foot is a common complaint. It is usually **unilateral** and caused by an orthopedic condition or by trauma. **Tarsal tunnel syndrome**, which typically arises after an ankle sprain, causes pain in the sole of the foot when the patient walks; it is described in section 13.2.6, Tibial Nerve (L4–S3). **Morton metatarsalgia** is described in the same section. **Bilateral**, burning pain in the feet characterizes **erythromelalgia**, a condition arising from vasomotor dysfunction otherwise known as **burning feet syndrome**. Similar symptoms may arise in **small-fiber neuropathy** (sometimes with preservation of the ankle-jerk reflexes) or in **polyneuropathy** (loss of ankle-jerk reflexes, distal sensory deficit); see also section 11.3.1, Small-Fiber Neuropathy, and section 11.3, Polyneuropathy.

In **restless legs syndrome**, the restlessness is perceived as painful and forces the sufferer to stand up,

14

walk around, and move the legs time and again, particularly at night. The abnormal sensation tends to arise when the sufferer is lying in bed or sitting on a soft chair. For more on this condition and its treatment, see section 10.2.2.

14.7 Pseudoradicular Pain

 Key Point

This term denotes an etiologically heterogeneous collection of painful syndromes that are attributed to faulty synergy of the muscles and joints, arising either from structural joint changes or from nonphysiologic movements that put excessive stress on the musculoskeletal system.

Pathophysiology. The joints of the body have a continuous, dynamic relationship with the muscles that move them. Afferent nerve impulses arising in the joints are fed back to the muscles to regulate and coordinate the strength and timing of muscle contraction. Pathologic impulses arising from **mechanically damaged or otherwise dysfunctional joints** lead to nonphysiologic patterns of muscle activation. In addition, **monotonously repeated movements** or **movements that put the joints in an unfavorable position** ("nonergonomic" movements) can cause pain of the participating anatomic structures through **overuse**. Different names are used for the resulting pain syndromes, depending on the specialty and school of thought of the physician or other expert consulted: tenomyalgia, tenomyosis, pseudoradicular pain, myofascial syndrome, muscular rheumatism, and so forth.

Clinical features. Pseudoradicular pain can arise in many different regions of the body but is particularly common in the **upper limb**. The pain is chronic and difficult to treat, because it is constantly reactivated by the daily (over)use of the involved joints and muscles.

The general features of pseudoradicular pain are as follows:

— The pain is of greater or lesser intensity.
— It is usually situated in **a single limb**.
— It is exacerbated by the use of this limb.
— It causes an **antalgic restriction of movement**.
— There are **painful trigger points** and painful **tendon insertions**.
— There is no objectifiable sensory deficit, paresis, or reflex abnormality.
— Nonphysiologic, antalgic movement leads to the perpetuation, extension, and chronification of the pain.

Treatment and prognosis. This condition is difficult to treat. The most useful approach consists of good occupational hygiene (using the affected muscles only up to the pain threshold), changing the illness-producing behavior (switching to a different task at work), and symptomatic treatments such as trigger-point therapy, local physiotherapy, and analgesic and anti-inflammatory drugs. Much patience is demanded of both doctor and patient.

14

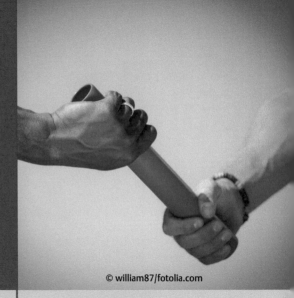

Chapter 15

Diseases of Muscle (Myopathies)

Going Weak

An 81-year-old man with longstanding hypertension and diabetes sustained a myocardial infarction. Coronary angiography revealed stenosis of three coronary vessels, which were recanalized with stents. His clinical condition improved rapidly; after 4 days in the hospital, he was transferred to a rehabilitation center. His doctors in the hospital had optimized his antihypertensive and antidiabetic drug regimen and added a statin (atorvastatin 80 mg orally daily) to treat an elevated cholesterol level.

His condition stabilized in rehabilitation, and he was discharged without symptoms 3 weeks later.

He had barely arrived home when he began to feel diffuse pain in all four limbs, which steadily worsened. He also noted increasing weakness of his entire body, which he interpreted, at first, as fatigue. Ultimately, the pain and weakness bothered him so much that he consulted his family doctor. His urine had also become unusually dark.

The family physician's examination revealed generalized muscle weakness with diminished intrinsic muscle reflexes. The urine was dark brown, and a test strip disclosed high protein content (myoglobin). The serum creatine kinase (CK) concentration was markedly elevated.

These findings clearly indicate rhabdomyolysis, a rapidly progressive loss of striated muscle fibers accompanied by the appearance of myoglobin, creatine, and other muscle enzymes in the blood. This patient's rhabdomyolysis was presumably due to statin treatment: it is known that antilipemic agents (fibrates more often than statins) can, rarely, produce CK elevation, rhabdomyolysis, and toxic myopathy. Elderly patients are at increased risk, as are patients with renal failure or alcoholism. The main symptoms are back pain and muscle pain. If myopathy and rhabdomyolysis are recognized early, the prognosis after discontinuation of the offending drug is good.

A dreaded complication of rhabdomyolysis is acute renal failure: freely circulating myoglobin, a large protein molecule, can obstruct the renal tubules. Forced diuresis is urgently indicated.

The patient was immediately hospitalized and treated with forced diuresis. The statin drug was discontinued. Within a few days, his urine became clear again, and the serum enzymes and renal function tests returned to normal. Acute renal failure was successfully prevented. He was given ezetimibe (a resorption inhibitor) instead of a statin to lower his cholesterol level.

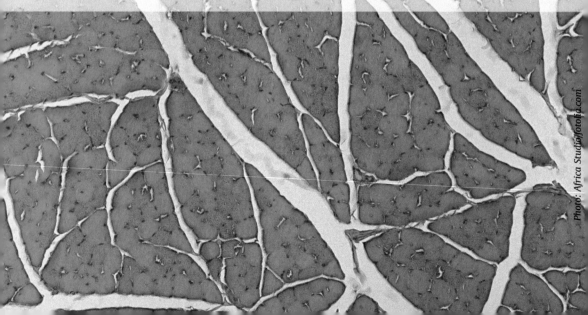

15.1 Structure and Function of Muscle

15.1.1 Microscopic Anatomy of Muscle

The most important structural components of striated skeletal muscle are the muscle fibers (**Fig. 15.1**). The muscle fibers contain contractile elements called myofibrils; these, in turn, are composed of interlacing actin and myosin molecules, which take the shape of filaments. The periodically repeating pattern of molecular structures in skeletal muscle accounts for its characteristic, striped ("striated") microscopic appearance (**Fig. 15.1**). The actin and myosin filaments are connected to each other by intermolecular bridges.

15.1.2 Physiology of Muscle Contraction

When a skeletal muscle contracts, the actin filaments and myosin filaments slide over each other (the sliding filament theory). The connecting bridges between the actin and myosin filaments are disconnected and then reconnected in a ratcheting mechanism, and a net shortening (contraction) of the muscle fiber results. The energy for this process is derived from phosphate compounds: mainly adenosine triphosphate (ATP), but also creatine phosphate when the muscle is under acute stress. The regeneration of creatine phosphate after muscle contraction is catalyzed by CK, the muscle-specific enzyme.

When a muscle is first set in contraction, glycogen within the muscle is anaerobically metabolized, and lactic acid accumulates in the muscle for 5 to 10 minutes. After that, if contraction continues, a switch to aerobic metabolism occurs, with increasing consumption of fatty acids and lactic acid. Enzyme defects that interfere with these energy-liberating processes during muscle contraction can cause clinically manifest abnormalities of muscle function. Much of the aerobic energy metabolism in muscle tissue takes place in mitochondria (**Fig. 15.1**); thus, mitochondrial diseases, too, can impair muscle function.

15.1.3 Impulse Transmission at the Motor End Plate and Impulse Conduction in the Muscle Fiber

Skeletal muscle is set in contraction when a nerve impulse arrives at the so-called **motor end plate** (**Fig. 15.2**) or neuromuscular junction. This "relay station" at the point where a nerve fiber and a muscle fiber meet consists of the following:

— The **presynaptic membrane**, a specialized part of the terminal segment of the motor neuron.
— The **synaptic cleft**.
— The **postsynaptic membrane**, a specialized part of the cell membrane (sarcolemma) of the muscle fiber.

An action potential arriving at the motor end plate induces the release of acetylcholine from the presynaptic membrane. The acetylcholine molecules diffuse across the synaptic cleft and bind to specific receptors on the postsynaptic membrane. This, in turn, leads to depolarization of the sarcolemma.

15

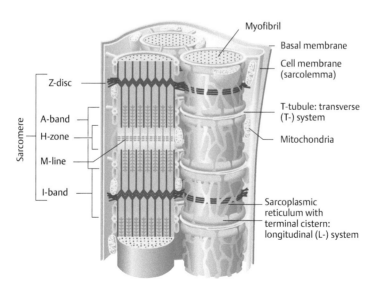

Myofibril
Basal membrane
Cell membrane (sarcolemma)
T-tubule: transverse (T-) system
Mitochondria

Z-disc
A-band
H-zone
M-line
I-band
Sarcomere

Sarcoplasmic reticulum with terminal cistern: longitudinal (L-) system

Fig. 15.1   Microstructure of the sarcomere of a skeletal muscle fiber. (Reproduced from Aumüller G, Engele J, Kirsch J, et al. Duale Reihe Anatomie. Stuttgart: Thieme; 2014.)

Having accomplished their task, the acetylcholine molecules are now rapidly broken down within the synaptic cleft into acetate and choline, a step catalyzed by the enzyme acetylcholinesterase. Meanwhile, the sarcolemmal excitation is carried into the interior of the muscle fiber by way of numerous transverse invaginations of the cell membrane (the tubular system or T-system) and is then transmitted to the longitudinal system, a branched network of cisterns of the endoplasmic (sarcoplasmic) reticulum, which surrounds the individual myofibrils (**Fig. 15.1**). When the depolarizing stimulus arrives here, it induces the secretion of calcium ions from terminal cisterns, and the intracellular calcium concentration rises. This, in turn, activates actomyosin ATPase, leading to muscle contraction.

Functional disturbances of these complex processes and structural changes of one or more elements of muscle or of the motor end plate cause various types of myopathy.

15.2 General Symptomatology

  Key Point

Muscle weakness can be either neurogenic or myogenic. The causes and clinical features of neurogenic muscle weakness have already been discussed in earlier chapters. The present chapter concerns diseases involving a structural or functional defect of the muscle tissue itself, which are called myopathies. These are classified as either primary or symptomatic. Primary myopathies are due to a pathologic process in the muscle itself; symptomatic myopathies are manifestations of muscle involvement by some other underlying disease or condition— for example, an endocrine or toxic disorder.

General etiology. Most primary myopathies are **genetically determined**, for example, the group of muscular dystrophies, which express themselves clinically as progressive weakness, and the channelopathies (functional disorders of individual ion channels of the muscle fiber membrane), which express themselves either as a myotonic syndrome or as episodic paralysis. Most of the diseases caused by enzyme defects are genetically determined (including, among others, the mitochondrial encephalomyopathies). There are also many kinds of **autoimmune myopathy**; prominent among them are polymyositis and dermatomyositis, as well as myasthenia gravis, a disease of the motor end plate.

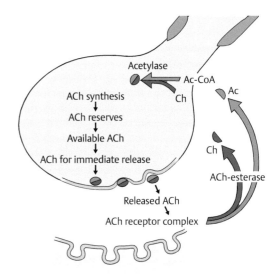

Fig. 15.2 Impulse transmission at the motor end plate. Acetylcholine (ACh), the acetic acid ester of the aminoalcohol choline, is released into the synaptic cleft in response to a depolarizing stimulus and then binds to specific receptors on the postsynaptic membrane. Acetylcholine is inactivated by breakdown into its two components, choline (Ch) and acetate (Ac); this step is catalyzed by the enzyme acetylcholinesterase. Choline is taken back up into the presynaptic nerve terminal with the aid of specific transporters and then reacts again with the activated form of acetic acid (Ac-CoA) to form new acetylcholine molecules.

General clinical features. Myopathies are traditionally considered part of the subject matter of neurology because their most prominent sign is **motor weakness**. The typical manifestations that are common to all myopathies as a class are summarized in **Table 15.1**.

General diagnostic considerations. The evaluation of myopathy comprises the following steps:

— A **complete and precise case history**, including the family history.

— **Physical examination**, with particular attention to the following:
  • Muscle weakness that is already present at rest, or that worsens or is exclusively present on exertion.
  • Muscle atrophy.
  • Fasciculations.
  • Diminished or absent reflexes.
  • Myotonic reactions (see section 15.4) to a tap on a muscle or on muscle contraction.
  • Shortened muscles.

— **Electromyogram (EMG) and electroneurography** (see sections 4.3.4 and 4.3.5).

Table 15.1	

Characteristics of myopathies

Criterion	Typical findings
Onset and progression	— Usually progresses slowly (years); exceptions include myasthenia and inflammatory, toxic, and endocrine myopathies
Appearance of muscles	— Usually atrophic — Sometimes pseudohypertrophic (e.g., calf muscles)
Strength	— Decreased
Localization of atrophy and weakness	— Usually symmetric; exceptions include myasthenia and, sometimes, polymyositis — The weakness is usually proximal; exceptions include myotonic dystrophy and myasthenia (sometimes)
Reflexes	— Diminished or absent
Sensation	— Intact
Contractures	— Usually develop over the course of time (years)
Ancillary testing	— Pathologic EMG — Normal nerve conduction velocity — Elevated serum creatine kinase concentration — Typical biopsy findings
Differential diagnosis	— Mainly spinal muscular atrophy — Muscle weakness of metabolic origin — Functional pseudoparesis

Abbreviation: EMG, electromyogram.

— **Blood tests**, particularly the serum concentration of CK.
— *Further special tests*, as needed in particular clinical situations:
  • Magnetic resonance imaging (MRI) of muscle.
  • Muscle biopsy with conventional light-microscopic histopathologic examination.
  • Special stains for abnormal lipid deposition, dystrophin, mitochondrial anomalies, enzyme defects, etc.
  • Electron microscopy.
  • Quantitative biochemical analysis of biopsy specimens.
  • Stress testing, for example, measurement of the rise in lactate concentration after anaerobic exercise.
  • Genetic analysis.

The classification of muscle diseases. This is based partly on etiology and pathophysiology, partly on clinical manifestations, and increasingly also on genetic criteria:
— Muscular dystrophies.
— Spinal muscular atrophy (see section 7.7.2) and other motor neuron diseases.
— Myotonias and periodic paralyses ("channelopathies").
— Metabolic myopathies.
— Mitochondrial myopathies and encephalomyopathies.
— Congenital myopathies.
— Infectious/inflammatory myopathies.
— Myopathy due to endocrine disorders.
— Muscle involvement by electrolyte disturbances.

— Toxic and drug-induced myopathies.
— Disorders of neuromuscular transmission.
— Tumors.
— Trauma.

The genetic classification of the myopathies changes so rapidly that our listings in **Table 15.2** and **Table 15.3** must be regarded as provisional.

15.3 Muscular Dystrophies

 Key Point
The muscular dystrophies are genetically determined. They typically present with symmetric muscle weakness that is mainly proximal and slowly worsens over the years. (Steinert myotonic dystrophy is the only type with mainly distal weakness.) There is no pain or sensory deficit. The muscles usually become atrophic, though this is masked, in some patients, by intramuscular deposition of fatty tissue (pseudohypertrophy). Connective tissue deposition can lead to muscle shortening and contractures. The reflexes are diminished or absent. Weakness leads to characteristic postural abnormalities and deformities, for example, lumbar hyperlordosis (a common finding), Duchenne or Trendelenburg gait (see Fig. 3.2), winging of the scapula, or scoliosis.

15

Table 15.2 contains an overview of the various types of muscular dystrophy. The major ones are described in detail in the following paragraphs.

Table 15.2

The muscular dystrophies

Type	Inheritance pattern	Chromosomal or genomic defect	Missing or abnormal gene or gene product	Frequency (per 100,000 live births)	Age of onset	Clinical features	Prognosis
Duchenne	X-linked, 30% sporadic	Xp21.2	Dystrophin absent	20–30/ 100,000 boys	Second to third year	Onset in pelvic girdle, pseudo-hypertrophy of calves	Rapidly progressive, most patients die by age 25
Becker	X-linked	Xp21.2	Dystrophin abnormal	3/100,000 boys	First (to fourth) decade	Same as in Duchenne muscular dystrophy, but milder; sometimes cardiomyopathy	Ambulatory till age 15 or later, death in fourth or fifth decade or later
Emery–Dreifuss	X-linked, rarely autosomal dominant	Xp28 or 1q	Emerin (X-linked) Lamin A/C (autosomal)	1/100,000	Childhood, adolescence	Scapuloperoneal dystrophy, contractures, and cardiopathy may be prominent	Ambulatory till third decade or for entire life; cardiac arrhythmia a frequent cause of death
Facioscapulohumeral dystrophy (Duchenne–Landouzy–Déjerine)	Autosomal dominant	4q35 and a second genetic locus	Homeobox gene	5/100,000	Childhood to young adulthood	Weakness of facial, shoulder girdle, and calf muscles	Practically normal life expectancy
Scapuloperoneal dystrophy	Autosomal dominant, autosomal recessive, or sporadic	14q11	? Desmin	Rare	Childhood to adulthood	Weakness of shoulder girdle and dorsiflexors of the feet and toes	Usually normal life expectancy
Limb girdle dystrophy in adults and **severe childhood autosomal recessive muscular dystrophy**	Autosomal recessive, autosomal dominant, or sporadic	17q12–q21.33 4q12 13q12 5q33–q34 15q15.1–q21.1 3q25 20 gene defects are currently known	α-, β-, γ-, and δ-sarcoglycan Calpain 3 Caveolin-3	3–4/100,000	Childhood to adulthood	Mainly proximal weakness of pelvic or shoulder girdle	Depending on type, premature death or only minor disability into old age
Distal myopathies (Welander type, Markesbery–Griggs, Finnish variant)	Autosomal dominant	2p13 (Welander type) 2q31 (Markesbery–Griggs type)	Titin and other unknown gene products	Rare	Middle age	Mainly distal atrophy and weakness	Only minor disability into old age
Distal myopathies (Nonaka and Miyoshi types)	Autosomal recessive	Miyoshi: 2p13.3–p13.1 Nonaka: 9p12-p11	Dysferlin, GNE	Rare	Adolescence to young adulthood	Mainly distal weakness	Progression to inability to walk
Oculopharyngeal dystrophies	Autosomal dominant	14q11.2–q13	Poly-(A-) binding protein 2	Rare	Middle age	Oculofaciobulbar paresis	Often premature death due to dysphagia and aspiration pneumonia

15

| Table 15.2 |

The muscular dystrophies (continued)

Type	Inheritance pattern	Chromosomal or genomic defect	Missing or abnormal gene or gene product	Frequency (per 100,000 live births)	Age of onset	Clinical features	Prognosis
Congenital dystrophies	Autosomal recessive	6q2	Merosin	Rare	At birth	Depending on type: involvement of muscles, eyes, and brain; contractures, arthrogryposis multiplex	Ranging from mild disability to severe intellectual disability
Steinert myotonic dystrophy	Autosomal dominant	19q13.3	Myotonin protein kinase	13.5/100,000, prevalence 5/100,000	Young adulthood, rarely congenital, earlier age of onset in each successive generation ("anticipation")	Mainly distal weakness, faciobulbar paresis, myotonia, cataracts	Age of significant disability depends on age of onset, usually middle age; premature death
PROMM = DM2	Autosomal dominant	3q13.3–q24	Zinc finger protein 9 (ZNF9), an RNA-binding protein	0.5/100,000	Third and fourth decades, sometimes earlier	Mainly proximal weakness, myotonia, and cataracts	Disability in old age

Abbreviations: DM2, type 2 myotonic dystrophy; PROMM, proximal myotonic myopathy.

| Table 15.3 |

Myotonias and periodic paralyses ("channelopathies," channel diseases)

Type	Inheritance pattern	Chromosomal or genomic defect	Missing or abnormal gene product	Incidence (i.e., frequency with respect to live births)	Age of onset	Clinical features	Prognosis
Myotonia congenita, Thomsen type	Autosomal dominant	7q35	Abnormal CLCN1 chloride channels	1/23,000	Early in first decade	Generalized myotonia	Stable, nonprogressive
Myotonia congenita, Becker type	Autosomal recessive	7q35	abnormal CLCN1 chloride channels	1/23,000–1/50,000	End of first decade	Generalized myotonia	Stable, nonprogressive
Myotonia fluctuans, myotonia permanens, acetazolamide-sensitive myotonia	Autosomal dominant	17q23.1–25.3	Abnormal SCN4A sodium channels	Very rare	First decade; myotonia fluctuans in adolescence	Generalized, myotonia fluctuans only episodic, other types severe, potassium loading worsens myotonia, acetazolamide-sensitive myotonia is painful	Nonprogressive
Paramyotonia congenita of Eulenburg	Autosomal dominant	17q23.1–25.3	Abnormal SCN4A sodium channels	Very rare	First decade	Generalized myotonia induced by cold and worsened by exertion, occasionally combined with paramyotonic and hyperkalemic paralyses	Persistent, tendency to improve over time

15

Table 15.3

Myotonias and periodic paralyses ("channelopathies," channel diseases) *(continued)*

Type	Inheritance pattern	Chromosomal or genomic defect	Missing or abnormal gene product	Incidence (i.e., frequency with respect to live births)	Age of onset	Clinical features	Prognosis
Hyperkalemic periodic paralysis	Autosomal dominant	17q23.1–25.3	Abnormal SCN4A sodium channels	Very rare	First decade	Paralysis arises after fasting, or when resting after physical activity	Persistent, often improves over time; permanent myopathy and weakness are less severe than in hypokalemic paralysis
Hypokalemic periodic paralysis	Autosomal dominant	17q23.1– q25.3, 1q32, 11q13-q14	Abnormal CACNL 1A3 calcium channels and SCN4A sodium channels	Very rare	Age 5–30 y, usually in second decade	Paralysis arises after carbohydrate consumption or physical activity	Persistent, often slowly developing permanent myopathy and weakness
Andersen–Tawil syndrome	Autosomal dominant	17q23.1– q24.2	Abnormal KCNJ2 potassium channels	One-tenth as common as hypokalemic paralysis	First or second decade	Clinical triad: periodic paralysis, ventricular extrasystoles and arrhythmias, and skeletal deformities	Permanent, often mild muscle weakness; life-threatening ventricular arrhythmias

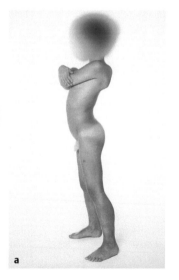

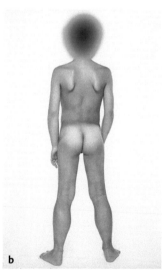

Fig. 15.3 Duchenne muscular dystrophy in a 10-year-old boy. **a** In the lateral view, note the lumbar hyperlordosis; **b** in the posterior view, note the winged scapulae and pseudohypertrophic calves.

15.3.1 Hereditary Muscular Dystrophies of X-chromosomal Inheritance— Dystrophinopathies

The diseases in this group are caused by a genetic defect on chromosome Xp21.2. They are, therefore, almost exclusively seen in boys whose mothers are (healthy) carriers. Dystrophin, a structural protein of the muscle fiber membrane that is also expressed in the brain, is present in reduced amounts or completely absent.

Duchenne Muscular Dystrophy

Clinical features. Boys develop the initial signs of the disease in the first decade of life, usually in the preschool years. The earliest overt abnormalities are **difficulty climbing stairs**, **lumbar hyperlordosis** (**Fig. 15.3a**), and **waddling gait**. Over the next few years, weakness progresses in the proximal muscles of the lower limbs and then of the upper limbs as well. The affected boys can stand up from a squatting position only by climbing up their own legs with their hands and arms (**Gowers sign, Fig. 15.4**). Fat deposition leads to **pseudohypertrophy of the calves**

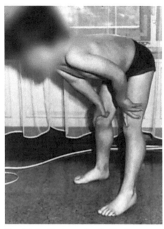

Fig. 15.4   Gowers sign in Duchenne muscular dystrophy.
This 7-year-old boy stands up by climbing up his own thighs.

(**Fig. 15.3b**). The waddling gait is due to bilateral hip adductor weakness (Duchenne or Trendelenburg gait, cf. **Fig. 3.2**). Dystrophin is expressed in the brain as well, and most boys with Duchenne muscular dystrophy are also mentally retarded.

Diagnostic evaluation. The CK is markedly elevated in the initial stages of the disease. The absence of dystrophin can be demonstrated on muscle biopsy specimens with special tissue staining (**Fig. 15.5b**).
Prognosis. The disease progresses relatively rapidly, rendering the affected boys unable to walk in the second decade of life. The scoliosis worsens and causes respiratory difficulty. The myocardium is also affected, though usually not to any clinically evident extent. The affected boys usually die of respiratory insufficiency or secondary complications between the ages of 18 and 25.

Becker Muscular Dystrophy
This type of muscular dystrophy is about one-tenth as common as the Duchenne type. Dystrophin is not

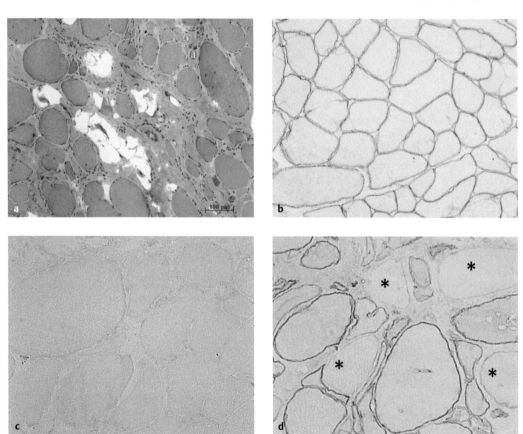

Fig. 15.5   Dystrophinopathy. a Marked myopathic changes with pathologic fiber variation, abundance of centrally located cell nuclei, degenerative and regenerative changes, and replacement of muscle tissue by connective tissue and fat in Duchenne dystrophinopathy (hematoxylin and eosin stain). **b–d** Demonstration of dystrophin with an antibody against the C-terminal end of the molecule. **b** Normal muscle. **c** No dystrophin is seen in a patient with the Duchenne type of progressive muscular dystrophy. **d** Mosaic pattern of dystrophin-positive and dystrophin-negative fibers in a female carrier of the Duchenne muscular dystrophy trait.*, dystrophin-negative fibers. (Reproduced from Zierz S. Muskelerkrankungen. Stuttgart: Thieme; 2014.)

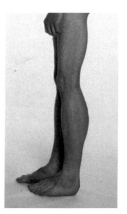
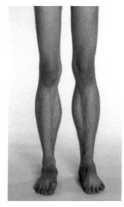

Fig. 15.6   A 19-year-old man with Becker muscular dystrophy. The prominent features are proximal atrophy and pseudohypertrophy of the calves.

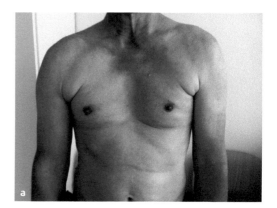

wholly absent but is expressed in reduced amounts. The affected persons show the first signs of the disease in their first or second decade; the progression is much slower than in the Duchenne type (**Fig. 15.6**). Patients typically lose the ability to walk between the ages of 30 and 40, and most die of the disease between 40 and 50. The EMG and laboratory findings resemble those of Duchenne muscular dystrophy.

15.3.2 Hereditary Muscular Dystrophies of Autosomal Inheritance

The genetic localization of the autosomal muscular dystrophies is known in most cases, and many of the gene products are known as well. We will only describe the more common forms here.

Facioscapulohumeral Type

This is a disease of autosomal dominant inheritance due to a genetic defect (deletion) in the 4q35 region of chromosome 4. It begins in the second or third decade of life with **weakness of the facial and shoulder girdle musculature** (eye closure, whistling; elevation of the arms) (**Fig. 15.7**). Sensorineural deafness is often present as well. The muscles of the pelvic girdle and the distal limb muscles are not affected until later decades. The life expectancy is normal.

Limb Girdle Types of Muscular Dystrophy

This is a genetically heterogeneous group of diseases: the inheritance pattern is autosomal dominant for some and autosomal recessive for others. About 20 different causative genetic defects are known at present. The onset of disease can be in

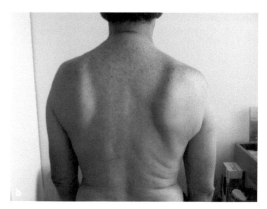
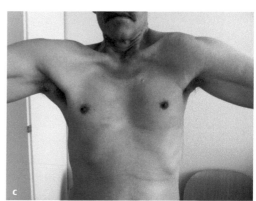

Fig. 15.7   Facioscapulohumeral muscular dystrophy in a 56-year-old man. **a** Atrophy of the trapezii, shoulder girdle, and pectoral muscles. **b** Bilateral winging of the scapula due to shoulder girdle atrophy. **c** The bilateral pectoral muscle atrophy is particularly evident on lateral elevation of the arms.

childhood or in adulthood. The first sign is always mainly proximal **weakness of the muscles of either the shoulder girdle or the pelvic girdle**; over time, the other limb girdle is affected as well (ascending vs. descending type). The prognosis is highly variable: some patients experience rapid progression of the disease within one or two decades, while others live on into old age with hardly any impairment.

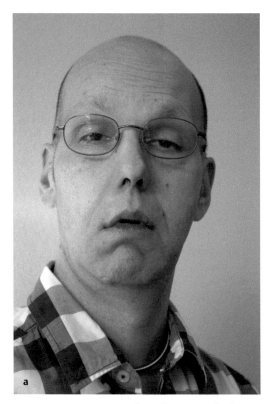 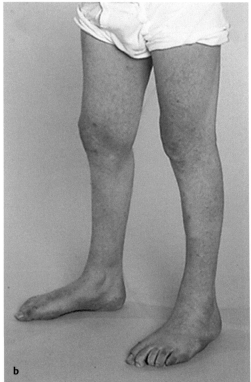

Fig. 15.8   Steinert myotonic dystrophy. a Myopathic facies in a 50-year-old man: flaccid facial features with sunken temples, bilateral ptosis, and frontal baldness. **b** A 41-year-old patient with typical, mainly distal muscle atrophy.

15

Myotonic Dystrophy of Curschmann–Steinert Type

> **NOTE**
>
> Curschmann–Steinert myotonic dystrophy is the most common myopathy of adulthood.

Etiology. This is a disease of autosomal dominant inheritance due to an unstable CTG trinucleotide sequence expansion in a gene on chromosome 19q13.3 that encodes myotonin protein kinase. Clinical manifestations arise when the sequence contains more than the usual 5 to 30 trinucleotide repeats. The expansion lengthens from generation to generation when transmitted in the maternal line; this explains the onset of the disease at an earlier age in each successive generation (**anticipation**).

Clinical features. Muscle involvement is the most prominent sign. **Weakness of the facial and distal limb muscles** usually arises in young adulthood. The face develops a typical "tired" appearance with sunken temples, mild ptosis, and loose folds around the often slightly open mouth (**myopathic facies,** cf. **Fig. 15.8**). Weakness and atrophy of the dorsiflexors of the feet produce a steppage gait. **Myotonia** is a striking phenomenon that may appear in a very early stage of the disease: after the patient firmly grips an object, he or she has difficulty letting it go. Delayed muscle relaxation can also be demonstrated after a sharp blow to a muscle (e.g., tongue, thenar

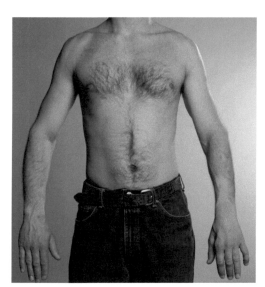

Fig. 15.9 Monomelic amyotrophy. This 32-year-old cabinet maker had slowly progressive muscle atrophy in the left upper limb for more than 10 years. The cause was monomelic amyotrophy, a rare condition. Muscle atrophy is seen mainly in the forearm and hand.

eminence). **Other organs**, too, are affected: early cataracts, dysphagia, sluggish bowel function, cardiomyopathy, pulmonary involvement, diabetes, testicular atrophy, and infertility are all possible manifestations of the disease.

Diagnosis. The diagnosis can be tentatively assigned on the basis of the **typical clinical features** along with myotonic discharges on **EMG**. It is confirmed by genetic testing.

Prognosis. The life expectancy is markedly reduced; most patients die around age 50.

Congenital Myotonic Dystrophy

This disease is due to a genetic defect involving a very large trinucleotide expansion (more than 2,000 copies). It is usually passed on from mothers to their children, particularly when the mother already possesses a long expansion. The affected individuals suffer from birth onward from dysphagia, weakness of drinking, flaccid facial muscles, a high palate, intellectual disability, and other signs like those of Curschmann–Steinert myotonic dystrophy.

15.3.3 Rarer Types of Muscular Dystrophy

Congenital muscular dystrophies are a heterogeneous group of diseases characterized by dystrophic changes in muscle fibers that are present at birth and then either remain constant or slowly progress. Muscular dystrophy that has already exerted its effects in prenatal life presents in the newborn with arthrogryposis multiplex, that is, fixed, abnormal positions of the joints.

Oculopharyngeal dystrophy is a disease of autosomal dominant inheritance that first becomes evident in middle age. The initial signs are progressively severe ptosis and restriction of eye movements, without diplopia. Later, dysphagia develops, which may be life-threatening. Other muscle groups are sometimes paretic as well. This condition must be distinguished from myasthenia gravis (section 15.8.1) and Kearns–Sayre syndrome (KSS; described in section 15.5.2).

Monomelic amyotrophy (muscle atrophy affecting a single limb) is not necessarily a primary disease of muscle; it is sometimes due to a focal lesion of anterior horn cells in the spinal cord. Monomelic amyotrophy of whatever cause is characterized by strictly localized, progressive muscle atrophy (**Fig. 15.9**).

15.4 Myotonic Syndromes and Periodic Paralysis Syndromes

 Key Point

These inherited muscle diseases belong to the group of so-called channelopathies: they involve abnormalities of the chloride, sodium, or calcium channels in the muscle fiber membrane. They are caused by a variety of genetic defects and manifest themselves clinically either with myotonia (delayed relaxation of muscle after active contraction) or with episodic paralysis.

Table 15.3 contains an overview of the main channelopathies. A selection of these will be discussed in the following paragraphs.

15.4.1 Diseases Mainly Causing Myotonia

Congenital Myotonia

Congenital myotonia has both dominant (**Thomsen**) and recessive (**Becker**) forms. Both are due to a genetic defect on chromosome 7q35 that impairs the transporting ability of chloride channels.

Clinical features. The most prominent manifestation is **myotonia**, that is, markedly slowed muscle relaxation after active contraction. A tightly grasped object can be let go again only after a delay. The patient cannot make any sudden movements, but the movements do become more fluid after a few attempts (the warming-up phenomenon). Raw muscle strength may be transiently diminished after a powerful contraction (= myotonic paralysis) but is otherwise normal. There is no atrophy; on the contrary, patients often have a markedly athletic habitus (**Fig. 15.10**). In the Becker form, the myotonic manifestations are more severe and mild distal atrophy may be present in later stages of the disease.

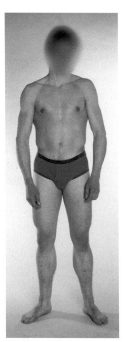 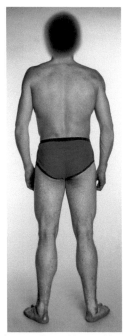

Fig. 15.10   Thomsen congenital myotonia in a 20-year-old man. The patient is of athletic build and has normal muscle strength, but active muscle contraction during the physical examination is followed by marked myotonia.

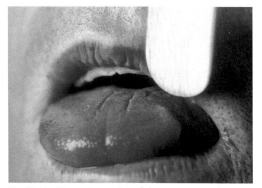

Fig. 15.11   Myotonic reaction of the tongue musculature in Steinert myotonic dystrophy. A forceful blow on the edge of the tongue (here, the left edge) produces a long-lasting indentation.

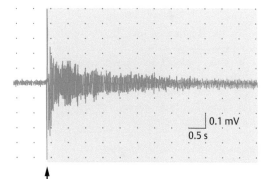

0.1 mV
0.5 s

Muscle percussion

Fig. 15.12   Electromyogram in a 29-year-old woman with Steinert myotonic dystrophy. Tapping on the thenar muscles evokes long-lasting high-frequency electric activity, whose amplitude dies down slowly.

Diagnostic evaluation. A contraction induced by a tap on, or electric stimulation of, a muscle is followed by tonic relaxation and transient indentation of the muscle (**Fig. 15.11**). The diagnosis is confirmed by the **typical EMG findings** (**Fig. 15.12**).

Treatment. Antiarrhythmic drugs such as procainamide and Mexitil, antiepileptic drugs such as phenytoin, and acetazolamide can lessen myotonia by stabilizing the abnormal fluctuations of muscle membrane potential.

Prognosis. The prognosis is favorable, in that the manifestations tend to improve over the years, and the life expectancy is normal.

Other Diseases with Myotonic Manifestations

Other diseases with myotonic manifestations are listed in **Table 15.3**. Curschmann–Steinert myotonic dystrophy is described earlier, in section 15.3.2; a few more rare diseases will be described in the following paragraphs.

— **Proximal myotonic myopathy**, also called type 2 myotonic dystrophy, is characterized by **mainly proximal muscle atrophy** (particularly of the thigh muscles) accompanied by **mild myotonia**. Cardiac arrhythmias and cataracts may also be present. The progression of the disease and the impairment that it causes are mild; walking is impaired only in old age. The disease is due to a CCTG repeat expansion in the zinc finger protein 9 gene on chromosome 3q.1.

— **Neuromyotonia** is a rare condition, also known as the syndrome of continuous muscle fiber activity and as Isaacs syndrome. Its characteristic feature is **continuous generalized muscle stiffness with myokymia**. The patient's movements are correspondingly viscous. The EMG reveals continuous spontaneous muscle activity. This disease can arise at any age and is thought to be due to an autoimmune process. Antiepileptic drugs are an effective form of treatment, as are immunoglobulins or plasmapheresis for some patients.

— **Stiff man syndrome** (recently renamed "**stiff person syndrome**") is also characterized by continuous muscle fiber activity, as revealed by EMG. The muscles are stiff and subject to painful spasms,

15

which worsen in response to external stimuli and emotional stress. The disease manifestations progress slowly over months or years. Here, too, the pathogenesis is thought to be autoimmune. Effective treatments include diazepam, antiepileptic drugs, baclofen, immunoglobulins, and plasmapheresis.

15.4.2 Diseases Causing Periodic Paralysis

The genetically determined periodic paralyses are characterized by suddenly arising abnormalities of the serum potassium concentration, which lead to transient inexcitability of the muscle fiber membrane and thereby to muscle dysfunction. They share the following clinical features:

- **Episodes of paralysis of sudden onset**, of varying severity and duration, which can last for hours to days.
- Usually, sparing of the facial and respiratory muscles.
- In some patients, **permanent muscle weakness** later on in the course of the disease.

There are **normokalemic**, **hyperkalemic**, and **hypokalemic types** (**Fig. 15.3**). We will describe only the last as a paradigmatic example.

Hypokalemic Periodic Paralysis

Pathogenesis. This is a disease of autosomal dominant inheritance caused by dysfunction of the dihydropyridine-sensitive calcium channels in the transverse tubular system of muscle fibers. Various underlying genetic defects are known. The disease has higher penetrance in men.

Clinical features. The initial paralytic attacks occur between the ages of 5 and 30, usually in the second decade of life. Their frequency is highly variable, ranging from daily attacks in some patients to a few attacks per year in others. Each attack lasts from a few hours to an entire day.

Diagnostic evaluation. A positive family history and a low serum potassium concentration during the attacks generally point to the diagnosis. The CK is usually normal. The EMG during an attack reveals only a few motor unit potentials on voluntary contraction, or none at all, and the summed motor potential is small or absent. There are flat T and U waves in the ECG. Rare symptomatic (nonfamilial) cases have been described in persons with thyrotoxicosis.

Treatment. The prognosis of each individual attack is good. The frequency of attacks can be reduced by a low-salt and low-carbohydrate diet and potassium supplementation. The intravenous administration of potassium shortens the duration of an attack.

15.5 Metabolic Myopathies

 Key Point

Normal muscle function depends on an adequate supply and continuous regeneration of the energetic molecule ATP. ATP can be derived from several different sources; glycogen and lipid metabolism, and normal mitochondrial function, play a central role in these processes. Insufficient availability of energy to muscle tissue results in exercise-induced muscle weakness, myalgia, and, ultimately, contractures. The underlying metabolic disorder is usually an inherited enzyme defect. The major clinical entities of this type are the glycogenoses, carnitine deficiency, and the mitochondrial encephalomyopathies.

General clinical features. These metabolic diseases often do not become apparent until adolescence or young adulthood. The following findings suggest the presence of one of these conditions:

- **Muscle exercise** is followed by **muscle weakness, myalgia, and/or contractures**. Rhabdomyolysis sometimes occurs, causing myoglobinuria and an elevated CK concentration.
- **Permanent muscle atrophy and weakness** may develop over time.
- **The serum CK concentration is often elevated**, and sometimes the lactate concentration as well (particularly in mitochondrial diseases).
- The EMG is usually normal; only in rare cases is there any evidence of myopathy.
- Muscle exercise under ischemic conditions normally leads to a fourfold rise of the lactate concentration. This rise does not occur in persons suffering from one of the glycogenoses. On the other hand, an exaggerated rise after only mild exertion suggests the presence of a mitochondrial disease.

The **individual types** of metabolic myopathy are summarized in **Table 15.4**. In the following paragraphs, we will discuss only rhabdomyolysis and the mitochondrial encephalomyopathies in detail.

15.5.1 Acute Rhabdomyolysis

Rhabdomyolysis is the **acute destruction of skeletal muscle tissue**, resulting in the passage of myoglobin into the bloodstream and a marked rise of the serum CK concentration. There are both *idiopathic* forms, with **an autosomal dominant** inheritance pattern, and *symptomatic* forms of rhabdomyolysis, the latter caused either by toxic influences—for example, the consumption of alcohol, heroin, or certain medications, such as statins—or by a disease of muscle metabolism, for example, one of the glycogenoses. Rhabdomyolysis can thus be the symptomatic expression of a wide variety of pathologic processes.

Table 15.4			
Metabolic myopathies with exercise-induced manifestations			
Group of diseases	**Enzyme defect**	**Clinical features**	**Diagnostic evaluation**
Glycogen metabolism	– Phosphorylase – Phosphorylase b kinase – Phosphofructokinase – Phosphoglycerate kinase	Exercise-induced weakness, myalgia, contractures, and sometimes myoglobinuria, even after brief exertion	Lactate ischemia test, electromyogram, muscle biopsy with histochemistry, biochemical analysis of muscle, DNA analysis
Lipid metabolism	– Carnitine deficiency – Carnitine palmitoyltransferase deficiency	Exercise-induced weakness, myalgia, and sometimes myoglobinuria, with prolonged muscle activity	Muscle biopsy with histo-chemistry and perhaps bio-chemical analysis; in systemic carnitine deficiency, the serum carnitine concentra-tion is low
Mitochondrial myopathies	– Decoupling of oxidative phosphor-ylation – Tricarbonic acid cycle defects – Respiratory chain defects	Muscle involvement almost always includes progressive external ophthalmoplegia; the brain is usually involved as well	Serum lactate concentration, muscle biopsy with electron microscopy and biochemical analysis, DNA analysis
Purine nucleotide cycle	– Myoadenylate deaminase	Rarely clinically relevant; exercise intolerance	Absence of rise in ammonia concentration with exercise

Clinical features. The patient develops **rapidly worsening muscle pain and weakness**. Examination reveals loss of reflexes and often muscle swelling; urinalysis reveals myoglobinuria. There is no sensory deficit. The most dreaded complication is acute renal failure.

Treatment. If the patient has myoglobinuria, optimal hydration is given to prevent renal failure. If renal failure nevertheless occurs, dialysis is necessary.

15.5.2 Mitochondrial Encephalomyopathies

Mitochondrial function. Mitochondria are present in every cell of the body; they are the sites of pyruvate, fatty acid, and amino acid metabolism. These processes generate ATP, an essential energy carrier for cellular metabolism and muscle contraction.

The mitochondrial genome. Mitochondria have two copies of the nuclear DNA (nDNA) at their disposal, but also multiple copies of their own mitochondrial DNA (mtDNA). Mitochondrial DNA is transmitted from generation to generation through the oocyte, independently of the nuclear genome. Thus, mito-chondrial diseases caused by mtDNA defects are inherited in a maternal pattern.

General clinical features of mitochondrial disease. Disturbances of mitochondrial metabolism impair the function of nearly all cells in the body. Muscle and brain cells are particularly strongly affected because of their high energy requirements. Thus, mitochondrial diseases often express themselves clinically as an **encephalomyopathy**. The typical clinical features are summarized in **Table 15.5**.

Examples of Mitochondrial Myopathies

Progressive external ophthalmoplegia usually has its onset in adulthood and progresses very slowly. Its

Table 15.5	
Clinical features of mitochondrial diseases	
Organ	**Manifestation**
Muscle	– Myopathy with ragged red fibers – Progressive external ophthalmoplegia – Exercise intolerance
Nervous system	– Myoclonus and generalized seizures – Stroke in younger individuals – Ataxia – Dementia – Polyneuropathy – Deafness – Optic neuropathy – Migraine – Basal ganglionic calcification (Fahr syndrome) – Dystonia – Elevated CSF protein concentration
Eye	– Retinitis pigmentosa – Cataract
Heart	– Cardiomyopathy – Conduction abnormalities
Gastroin-testinal system	– Intestinal pseudo-obstruction – Diarrhea
Endocrine system	– Short stature – Diabetes – Goiter – Hypogonadism
Skin	– Multiple lipomas – Ichthyosis
Abbreviation: CSF, cerebrospinal fluid.	

typical features are progressive ptosis and restriction of ocular motility, so that, in the end, all movements of the eyes are impossible. Skeletal

15

muscle biopsy with Gomori trichrome staining reveals accumulations of mitochondria in so-called ragged red fibers. The condition can appear as a familial disease of maternal inheritance or as a component of KSS.

KSS is characterized by **progressive external ophthalmoplegia** combined with retinal pigment degeneration and an intracardiac conduction defect. There may be further clinical features as well (cf. **Table 15.5**). KSS is usually familial and is due to a single deletion in mitochondrial DNA.

MELAS syndrome consists of mitochondrial **m**yopathy, **e**ncephalopathy, **l**actic **a**cidosis, and **s**troke-like episodes. It presents in childhood with transient cerebral ischemia and episodic vomiting; later on, patients often become demented. The serum lactic acid concentration is elevated.

MERRF syndrome (**m**yoclonus **e**pilepsy with **r**agged **r**ed **f**ibers) is a rare syndrome characterized by myoclonus, generalized epileptic seizures, myopathy, and dementia.

The **MNGIE syndrome** (**m**yo**n**euro**g**astro**i**ntestinal **e**ncephalopathy) involves myopathy, ophthalmoplegia, neuropathy, encephalopathy, and gastrointestinal manifestations (pseudo-obstruction, chronic diarrhea). It is due to a mutation in the thymidine phosphorylase gene. This condition has been alleviated in a few patients by allogeneic stem-cell transplantation to restore the activity of the deficient enzyme.

15.6 Myositis

Key Point

Myositis is an infectious or inflammatory disease of muscle. The various types of myositis include:

– Autoimmune diseases affecting muscle, either as the major disease manifestation (as in polymyositis, which sometimes affects the skin as well = dermatomyositis) or as an accompanying manifestation in a larger syndrome.
– Muscle involvement by a primary, systemic, noninfectious, chronic inflammatory disease.
– Direct infection of muscle (infectious myositis).

The most important types of myositis are listed in **Table 15.6**.

General clinical features. The common features of all types of myositis (infectious/inflammatory myopathies) are:

– Usually symmetric muscle involvement.

Table 15.6

Infectious and inflammatory myopathies (myositides)

Classification	Types
Autoimmune inflammatory disorders mainly affecting muscle	– Dermatomyositis and polymyositis in adults
	– Dermatomyositis and polymyositis in children
	– Dermatomyositis and polymyositis accompanying malignancy
	– Inclusion-body myositis
Autoimmune inflammatory disorders affecting muscle and other organ systems	– Progressive systemic sclerosis
	– Sjögren syndrome
	– Systemic lupus erythematosus
	– Rheumatoid arthritis (=primary chronic polyarthritis)
	– Mixed collagenosis (mixed connective tissue disease, Sharp syndrome)
	– Periarteritis nodosa
	– Behçet disease
Other noninfectious myositides	– Giant-cell myositis
	– Diffuse fasciitis with eosinophilia
	– Eosinophilic polymyositis
	– Polymyalgia rheumatica
	– Sarcoidosis
	– Myositis in Crohn disease
	– Myositis ossificans
	– Myosclerosis
Infectious myositides	– Viral (e.g., influenza virus)
	– Bacterial
	– Borrelial
	– Fungal
	– Protozoal
	– Helminthic

– Usually very rapid progression, with atrophy within a few months.
– Sometimes, local pain.
– No sensory deficit.
– Sometimes, a very high serum CK concentration.
– Negative family history.

In this chapter, we will restrict ourselves to a description of polymyositis and dermatomyositis.

15.6.1 Polymyositis and Dermatomyositis

Epidemiology. These conditions are rare, striking only 5 to 10 per 100,000 persons per year. Women are more commonly affected than men. **Polymyositis** arises almost exclusively from age 35 onward; **dermatomyositis**, on the other hand, tends to arise either before puberty or around age 40.

Pathogenesis. Humoral factors play a role in dermatomyositis, while cellular immune mechanisms are involved in pure polymyositis.

Clinical features. The illness often begins with **constitutional symptoms** such as fatigue, myalgia, joint pain, and sometimes even fever. Thereafter, a **usually symmetric, mainly proximal muscle weakness**

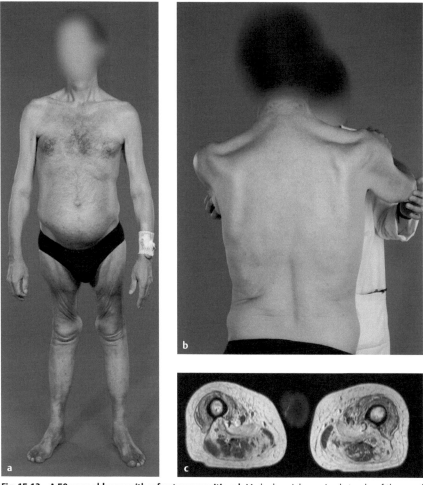

Fig. 15.13   A 50-year-old man with refractory myositis. a,b Marked, mainly proximal atrophy of the muscles of the upper and lower limbs. **c** The thigh muscles are almost entirely destroyed and replaced with fat (MRI).

15

develops, leading to **atrophy** (**Fig. 15.13**). Patients have difficulty rising from a squatting position, getting up from a chair, or raising the arms above the horizontal position. The muscles are often **tender to pressure**. The symptoms and signs progress rapidly over a few weeks or months. About one-third of patients suffer from **dysphagia**, which may lead to **aspiration pneumonia**. If the skin is involved as well (**dermatomyositis**), it is discolored reddish-purple. The discoloration may involve the face in "butterfly" fashion (nose and both cheeks), or it may be visible on the chest, on the dorsum of the hand, or around the fingernails. Subcutaneous calcinosis, joint pain, joint effusions (rare), and Raynaud-like phenomena may also be present. The heart may be involved (extrasystoles, heart failure). When polymyositis arises as a component of a collagenosis (**Table 15.6**) (**overlap syndrome**), other organs are affected as

well. The only other disease affecting both the muscles and the skin is scleroderma.

Diagnostic evaluation. Ancillary testing is usually necessary. The **serum CK concentration** is elevated to 10 times the normal value or more, at least initially. The **EMG** reveals markedly shortened, low, polyphasic potentials, to a highly variable degree in different portions of the same muscle. Pathologic spontaneous activity and denervation potentials are also present. **Muscle biopsy** typically reveals diffusely distributed muscle necrosis and inflammatory infiltrates.

Treatment. Children tend to respond well to treatment with **corticosteroids**. Adults often require treatment with other immunosuppressive drugs, usually **azathioprine. Immunoglobulins** are beneficial in the initial stage of treatment but must always be supplemented with corticosteroids or immune suppressants over the course of time.

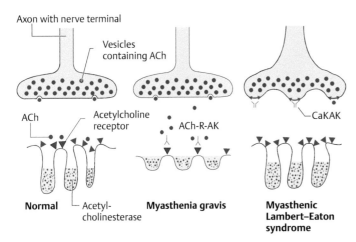

Fig. 15.14 The neuromuscular synapse in normal state, myasthenia gravis, and Lambert–Eaton syndrome. In myasthenia gravis, antibodies against the acetylcholine receptor (Ach-R-Ab) destroy the acetylcholine receptors on the postsynaptic membrane. Acetylcholine (Ach) is still released in normal amounts but has an inadequate effect because of the reduced number of intact receptors. In Lambert–Eaton syndrome, antibodies against calcium channels (CaCAb) on the nerve terminal prevent the release of acetylcholine.

15.7 Other Diseases Affecting Muscle

15.7.1 Myopathies due to Systemic Disease

A variety of general medical conditions cause muscle weakness, among them certain **endocrinopathies** (hypo- and hyperthyroidism, hyper- and hypoparathyroidism, Cushing disease, Addison disease). **Paraneoplastic syndromes** that cause muscle weakness include paraneoplastic poly- and dermatomyositis, as well as Lambert–Eaton syndrome (section 15.8.2), in which neuromuscular transmission is impaired. Among the **electrolyte disorders**, hyper- and hypokalemia (not of genetic origin) can cause muscle weakness, as can **drugs** such as colchicine, chloroquine, fludrocortisone, and antilipemic agents. **Toxic substances** such as gasoline vapor and toluene can produce rhabdomyolysis (be aware of recreational sniffing as a possible cause!), while alcohol can produce an acute alcoholic myopathy. **Malnutrition**, for example, in prison camps, can lead to myastheniform disturbances, and **vitamin E deficiency** can lead to severe myopathy.

15.7.2 Congenital Myopathies

Several types of congenital myopathy have been described, some of which now have a known genetic basis. Their common features are:

- Markedly reduced muscle tone from infancy onward.
- Delayed motor development.
- Later, mainly proximal muscle weakness.
- Often, generally diminished muscle bulk.
- Often, a narrow head with a raised, "Gothic" palate and sometimes further skeletal deformities.
- Slow progression, or none;
- Sometimes, cardiomyopathy and/or intellectual disability.

The following types of congenital myopathy are classified by the histopathologic findings of muscle biopsy:

- Central core myopathy.
- Nemaline (rod) myopathy.
- Centronuclear myopathy.
- Multicore myopathy.
- Fingerprint body myopathy.
- Sarcotubular myopathy.
- Hyaline body myopathy (= myopathy with disintegration of myofibrils in type I fibers).

15.8 Disturbances of Neuromuscular Transmission—Myasthenic Syndromes

 Key Point

The myasthenic syndromes are characterized by abnormal fatigability of muscle. The weakness may affect individual muscle groups in more or less isolated fashion or, alternatively, all of the muscles of the body. Pathophysiologically speaking, these conditions are due to a disturbance of impulse transmission at the motor end plate, usually because of an underlying autoimmune disorder. For example, the most common myasthenic syndrome, myasthenia gravis, is due to the destruction of acetylcholine receptors on the postsynaptic membrane by cross-reacting autoantibodies.

The cellular processes involved in impulse transmission at the motor end plate are discussed in section 15.1.3 and shown pictorially in **Fig. 15.2**. These processes could theoretically be impaired in several different ways:

- Inadequate synthesis of acetylcholine or defective storage of acetylcholine in axon terminals.

- Inadequate release of acetylcholine from axon terminals.
- Impaired transport of acetylcholine in the synaptic cleft.
- Impaired binding of acetylcholine to its specific receptors on the postsynaptic membrane.

The last mechanism in this short list is at work in **myasthenia gravis**, the commonest and clinically most important type of myasthenia. In **Lambert–Eaton syndrome** (section 15.8.2), on the other hand, the underlying problem is inadequate release of acetylcholine from the presynaptic membrane (**Fig. 15.14**).

15.8.1 Myasthenia Gravis

Epidemiology. The incidence of this disorder is 1 to 4 per 100,000 persons per year; its prevalence in the general population is 140 per million. Women are more commonly affected than men, in a ratio of 3:2. The onset of the disease is usually in the second through fourth decade of life in women, but in the sixth decade in men. In principle, however, myasthenia gravis can appear at any age.

It is not uncommon for myasthenia gravis to be accompanied by certain other diseases: thymoma is seen in about 15% of patients with the disease, hyperthyroidism in 5%, hypothyroidism likewise in 5%, and polyarthritis in 4%.

Pathophysiology. Three-quarters of all patients with myasthenia gravis have hyperplasia of the thymus and 15% harbor a thymoma. Antibodies are generated against the myoid cells of the thymus; owing to a misdirection of the immune response, these antibodies also attack the acetylcholine receptors of the motor end plate. **Acetylcholine receptor antibodies are present in the serum in elevated concentration in** nearly all patients with generalized myasthenia. If the serum of an affected patient is injected into an experimental animal, the animal develops a myasthenic syndrome. The antibodies can also be transmitted across the placenta from a myasthenic mother to her child (see later). They are highly heterogeneous and bind to the acetylcholine receptor at several different locations.

About 10 to 20% of patients with clinically diagnosed myasthenia have no antibodies against the acetylcholine receptor—this is called "**seronegative myasthenia.**" About 70% of these patients, however, have antibodies against muscle-specific tyrosine kinase (anti-MuSK antibodies). The affected patients are usually women whose symptoms began before age 40. In the remaining "doubly seronegative" patients, yet another antibody has been found; it is directed against low-density lipoprotein receptor–related protein 4 (LRP4) and interferes with neuromuscular transmission.

Clinical features. The clinical features of myasthenia are summarized in **Table 15.7**. The most prominent feature is **abnormal fatigability of muscle**. Initially, the muscles most obviously affected are those that carry out very fine movements and that accordingly contain unusually small motor units, that is, the extraocular muscles, the levator palpebrae muscle, and the muscles of mastication and deglutition. These are the muscles that react most strongly to a decline in acetylcholine receptor density. Thus, the early manifestations of myasthenia gravis often include **diplopia, ptosis (Fig. 15.15), dysphagia** with frequent aspiration, and **difficulty chewing food**. Nevertheless, practically any other muscle group can be involved, even at the onset of the disease. The disease manifestations worsen over the course of the

15

Table 15.7

Clinical features of myasthenia gravis

	Typical features
Clinical neurologic features	- Progressive weakness of individual muscles
	- The weakness increases on rapid, repeated contraction of the affected muscles
	- Recovery within minutes, or a fraction of an hour, at rest
	- The weakness usually worsens toward evening
	- The eye muscles are often affected first (ptosis, diplopia), or else the pharyngeal muscles (dysphagia, nasal speech)
	- Variably severe weakness of muscles belonging to different motor units
	- Occasionally, crises with sudden deterioration of muscle strength
	- No atrophy or fasciculations
	- More or less complete resolution of disease manifestations after the administration of a cholinesterase inhibitor, e.g., test injection of edrophonium chloride IV (Tensilon test)
Laboratory and EMG features	- Usually, elevated serum titer of antibodies against the acetylcholine receptor (though this not always seen in ocular myasthenia)
	- On EMG, more than 10% decrement (not always seen in ocular myasthenia)

Abbreviation: EMG, electromyogram.

day and are worst in the evening. Repeated activation of an affected muscle group leads to rapidly worsening weakness. This phenomenon forms the basis of several clinical diagnostic tests.

In anti-MuSK-Ab-positive myasthenia gravis, the facial muscles and the muscles of deglutition are most severely affected. Respiratory crises are common.

Diagnostic evaluation. Myasthenic ptosis worsens visibly within 1 minute if the patient rapidly and

repeatedly closes and opens the eyes, or looks upward for a prolonged period (the **Simpson test**, **Fig. 15.16**).

Further diagnostic tests confirm the diagnosis. In the **Tensilon test**, 10 mg of the acetylcholinesterase inhibitor edrophonium chloride are injected intravenously over 10 seconds. This drug inhibits the breakdown of acetylcholine in the synaptic cleft, so that acetylcholine is available to its receptors on the muscle cell membrane for a longer time, compensating for the deleterious effect of diminished receptor density. In myasthenia gravis, an improvement is seen within 30 seconds and lasts for about 3 minutes. A marked ptosis, for example, can transiently disappear. On **EMG**, when a motor nerve is repeatedly stimulated, surface recording from the corresponding muscle reveals a progressive fall-off (**decrement**) in the amplitude of the muscle potentials, by more than 10% (**Fig. 15.17**). In ocular myasthenia that has not yet become generalized, no antibodies may be detectable and the EMG decrement may be normal.

Antibodies against the acetylcholine receptor can be found in the serum of 85% of patients with myasthenia gravis. They are not found, however, in 50% of patients with the purely ocular form, as well as in approximately 15% of patients with generalized myasthenia. In patients without antireceptor antibodies, anti-MuSK and sometimes anti-LRP4 antibodies must be sought as well, as mentioned earlier. A **chest CT or MRI** must be performed to detect or rule out a thymoma. Other diseases that can mimic or accompany myasthenia must be sought and excluded as well (see later).

Classification. Myasthenia can be subdivided into several stages depending on the extent and severity of muscle involvement. The Osserman classification has four main stages and is reproduced in **Table 15.8**.

Spontaneous course. The severity of the disease manifestations fluctuates markedly without treatment,

15

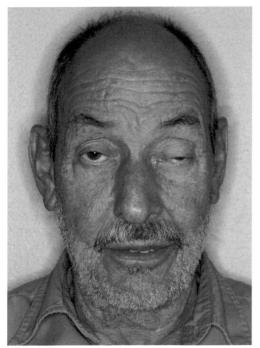

Fig. 15.15   A myasthenia patient with mainly ocular manifestations. There is bilateral ptosis, worse on the left. Note the voluntary contraction of the left frontalis muscle in an attempt to elevate the eyelid and compensate for the ptosis.

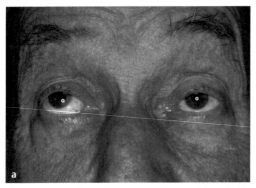
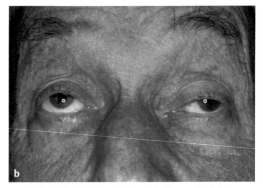

Fig. 15.16   Myasthenia of the extraocular muscles and a Simpson test. The patient's attempt to keep looking up leads to increasing ptosis and abduction of the left eye. **a** The patient looks upward. **b** 20 seconds later, there is a marked ptosis on the left, and the left eye is abducted.

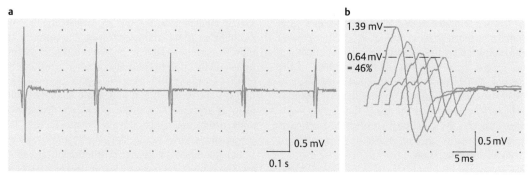

Fig. 15.17   Electromyogram of a 59-year-old man with ocular myasthenia. Electric activity is recorded from the nasalis muscle on repetitive stimulation of the facial nerve in the stylomastoid fossa (stimulation at 3 Hz). **a** The EMG tracing. **b** The same curve is shown on an expanded time scale, and the responses to successive stimuli are superimposed. The summed muscle potential diminishes from one stimulus to the next; the response to the fifth stimulus is 54% smaller than the initial response. Normally there should be no more than a 10% decrement.

Table 15.8

The stages of myasthenia gravis (Osserman classification)

Stage	Features
I	Ocular myasthenia, i.e., limited to the eye muscles
IIa	Mild generalized myasthenia
IIb	Moderately severe generalized myasthenia, not involving muscles of respiration
III	Acute, rapidly progressive myasthenia, beginning abruptly and progressing to involve the muscles of respiration within 6 mo of onset
IV	Chronic, severe myasthenia; may develop from prior stage I or stage II disease after 2 y of a relatively stable course

Note: Patients in stages III and IV are subject to higher mortality and more frequently harbor a thymoma.

---

even over longer periods of time. Spontaneous remissions may be long-lasting, but true spontaneous cures are rare. The eyes are initially affected in 50% of patients; in 16% of these patients, the myasthenic manifestations remain confined to the eyes (ocular myasthenia). The eyes are eventually affected in 90% of all patients. Generalization of manifestations from the eyes to the rest of the body usually occurs, if it does, within 3 years of onset. Transient neonatal myasthenia, caused by placental transmission of antibodies from a myasthenic mother to her child, rarely lasts longer than 2 weeks.

The treatment of myasthenia gravis with antireceptor antibodies. Cholinesterase inhibitors improve the disease manifestations by delaying the breakdown of acetylcholine and thereby prolonging its effect on the remaining functional acetylcholine receptors on the muscle fiber membrane: **pyridostigmine** is given several times a day in individual doses of 10 to 60 mg.

Short-term immune therapies are given for acute exacerbations of myasthenia gravis with impending respiratory failure (**myasthenic crises, Table 15.9**). These include plasmapheresis and intravenous immunoglobulins. Corticosteroids and other immune suppressants,

Table 15.9

Myasthenic crisis versus cholinergic crisis

Myasthenic crisis	Both types of crisis	Cholinergic crisis
– Mydriasis – Ptosis – Tachycardia – Pallor	– Muscle weakness – Dyspnea – Diaphoresis – Urinary and fecal urgency – Anxiety, agitation – Confusion, somnolence	– Miosis – Bradycardia – Bronchial hypersecretion – Fasciculations – Erythematous and warm skin

Source: Grehl H, Reinhardt F. Checkliste Neurologie, 6th ed. Stuttgart: Thieme; 2016.

for example, azathioprine, are given chronically to influence the disease process in the long term. Most patients with myasthenia gravis need these drugs. Steroid treatment can transiently worsen the manifestations of disease and should therefore be initiated very slowly or during a hospitalization. The positive effect generally appears 2 to 4 weeks after the initiation of treatment; the effect of azathioprine usually takes months to appear.

Thymectomy should be considered for every patient with myasthenia. The operation brings about a cure,

15

or at least a substantial improvement, of myasthenia in 80% of operated patients, after a latency of several months or years. There is little controversy regarding the indication for thymectomy in patients under age 60, except those with the mild ocular form of the disease. Good results have also been obtained in older patients. A thymoma, if present, must be surgically removed whatever the age of the patient. Adjuvant radiotherapy must be given if the resection is subtotal, because 25% of these tumors undergo malignant degeneration.

The treatment of myasthenia gravis with anti-MuSK antibodies. Cholinesterase inhibitors often bring inadequate relief or even worsen the manifestations of the disease. Plasmapheresis and long-term immune suppression are helpful; thymectomy is not.

Complications. Patients in the midst of a myasthenic crisis may need such high doses of cholinesterase inhibitors that they develop toxic manifestations such as nausea, diaphoresis, abdominal cramps, excessive tracheobronchial secretions, agitation, and anxiety. This syndrome is referred to, somewhat simplistically, as a **cholinergic crisis**. For the clinical distinction between myasthenic and cholinergic crises, see **Table 15.9**. Long-term immune suppression can also cause complications, including leukopenia, increased susceptibility to infections, hyperkeratoses, and cutaneous tumors.

15.8.2 Lambert–Eaton Syndrome

Etiology and Pathogenesis

This disease is caused by antibodies against voltage-sensitive calcium channels in the motor nerve terminals at the motor end plate. Inactivation of these channels lessens the calcium influx induced by an incoming action potential and therefore results in the release of inadequate amounts of acetylcholine from the nerve terminal. The impairment of neuromuscular transmission in Lambert–Eaton syndrome (unlike myasthenia gravis) is thus **presynaptic**. The underlying etiology in two-thirds of patients is a small-cell carcinoma of the lung: voltage-sensitive calcium channels on the cell membranes of the carcinoma cells initiate a misdirected autoimmune response. Cases of Lambert–Eaton syndrome of nonneoplastic origin are often associated with other autoimmune conditions, such as pernicious anemia, hypo- or hyperthyroidism, myasthenia gravis, Sjögren syndrome, and others. The thymus is not enlarged.

Clinical features. The hallmarks of this condition are muscle **weakness** and, above all, **fatigability**, mainly in the pelvic girdle and lower limbs. The extraocular muscles and the levator palpebrae muscle are sometimes mildly affected. Muscular strength transiently increases, at first, with exercise. The intrinsic muscle reflexes are often absent, and many patients complain of dry mouth or other autonomic manifestations (orthostatic hypotension, impotence).

Diagnostic evaluation. On EMG, the first few muscle action potentials on repeated stimulation are low, and the subsequent ones are larger (increment). This finding is particularly evident with high-frequency stimulation. It contrasts with the decrement typically seen in myasthenia gravis and is thus useful for differential diagnosis.

Treatment. Lambert–Eaton syndrome responds to **immunoglobulins** and **plasmapheresis** and, in the long term, to corticosteroids and azathioprine. Cholinesterase inhibitors are not very effective.

15.8.3 Rare Myasthenia-like Syndromes

Hereditary myasthenic syndromes are usually of autosomal recessive inheritance. These genetic diseases may be due to either pre- or postsynaptic disturbances of neuromuscular transmission. They are clinically characterized by ocular manifestations and generalized muscle weakness. Cholinesterase inhibitors are therapeutically effective, as is 3,4-diaminopyridine in rare cases. These hereditary syndromes include congenital myasthenia gravis (with lifelong manifestations) and familial infantile myasthenia. The latter disease can cause life-threatening episodes of respiratory insufficiency in children but tends to become less severe in later life.

Slow channel syndrome is of autosomal dominant inheritance. It usually becomes clinically evident in young adulthood. The underlying abnormality of neuromuscular transmission is that the cation channels of the acetylcholine receptors open too slowly. In addition to exercise-dependent muscle weakness, patients also develop muscle atrophy. The usual treatments for myasthenia are ineffective against this disease.

Myasthenic phenomena can be caused by various substances, including organophosphates and penicillamine. Other substances can worsen myasthenia that is already present, such as aminoglycosides, quinine, antiarrhythmic drugs, and anticonvulsants.

15

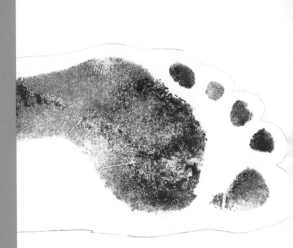

aus Masuhr K. F., Masuhr F., Neumann M.,
Duale Reihe Neurologie, Thieme, 2013

Chapter 16

Diseases of the Autonomic Nervous System

Bad News

The patient, a 54-year-old bank manager, had been feeling "worn out" for months; she was always tired and listless. She also complained of recurrent abdominal pain and a feeling of pressure in the pelvic area. She had gained 3 kg of weight ("mostly belly fat") in recent months, despite a lack of appetite. She had repeatedly formed the intention of seeing her doctor as soon as possible, but then put it off again because her symptoms were so diffuse and because she had too much work to do.

Finally, she developed deep pain in the low back radiating down the back of the right leg down to the sole of the foot, and the sole felt numb. She decided she could not wait any longer and went to see the doctor.

On examination, the doctor found weakness of plantar flexion of the right foot, with an absent ankle-jerk reflex and diminished sensation in dermatomes S1 to S3. On the basis of these findings and the patient's complaint of low back pain radiating down the right leg, the doctor suspected a right L5–S1 intervertebral disk herniation with compression of the S1 nerve root. He ordered a lumbar spinal magnetic resonance imaging scan to confirm the diagnosis and was surprised to find that it was negative.

The doctor had not paid adequate attention to the autonomic nervous system; if he had done so, he would have noted that the sole of the right foot, as opposed to the left, was entirely dry because of the absence of sweating (anhidrosis).

The sympathetic fibers that innervate the sweat glands arise from the intermediolateral cell column of the spinal cord at levels T1 to L2/L3. These spinal segments are the only ones at which sympathetic fibers exit the spinal cord together with the anterior roots; the fibers then join the sympathetic chain and proceed onward to the autonomic nerve plexuses, the viscera, or (in the case of the sudomotor fibers) the skin, by way of the peripheral nerve plexuses and sensory peripheral nerves. The nerve roots above T1 and below L3 contain no autonomic fibers, and thus root lesions below L3 are not associated with autonomic deficits of any kind, including a loss of sweating.

This patient, however, had anhidrosis of the sole of the right foot, which is not consistent with an S1 nerve root lesion. The site of the disturbance had to be further distal. On the other hand, the spatial extent of the sensory disturbance and the sweating abnormality was too large for a lesion of a single peripheral nerve; the hypesthetic skin area corresponded to multiple dermatomes (S1–S3). It follows that the lesion was most likely located in the sacral plexus.

A computed tomography scan of the pelvis revealed a tumor of the right ovary invading the sacral plexus. The patient's more diffuse symptoms, which she had noted long before the neurologic symptoms arose, were also consistent with the diagnosis of ovarian cancer. Her weight gain and increase in girth were probably due to ascites. In retrospect, the physician should have listened more carefully to her full story before formulating his presumptive diagnosis.

16.1 Anatomy

 Key Point

The autonomic nervous system is responsible for the neural control of all of the organs and tissues of the body whose function is involuntary. It thus innervates the internal organs of the throat, thorax, and abdomen, the blood vessels, and the lacrimal, salivary, and sweat glands, among other organs. It can be divided on structural and functional grounds into the sympathetic and parasympathetic nervous systems, which mainly exert mutually antagonistic effects on their target organs. The fundamental structural unit in both systems is a two-neuron chain, in which the first neuron has its cell body within the central nervous system, that is, in the brainstem or spinal cord (the preganglionic neuron), and the second neuron has its cell body in an autonomic ganglion or plexus (the postganglionic neuron). The hypothalamus is the "command center" of the autonomic nervous system.

16.1.1 Sympathetic Nervous System

The cell bodies of the **preganglionic neurons** lie in the lateral horns of the spinal cord at levels T1 to L2/L3 (the intermediolateral cell column or intermediolateral nucleus; the sympathetic nervous system is thus sometimes called the thoracolumbar system). These cell bodies receive neural input from the hypothalamus, whose efferent projection (the central sympathetic pathway) descends through the brainstem and down the spinal cord to the sympathetic nuclei within the cord. The axons of the preganglionic neurons exit the spinal cord in the anterior roots and then travel by way of the rami communicantes into the sympathetic chain, which lies lateral to the spinal cord and consists of a chain of ganglia connected by communicating nerve bundles (interganglionic branches). Some of the preganglionic axons form a synapse onto a postganglionic neuron within the sympathetic chain, while others travel through the entire sympathetic chain without a synapse, only meeting their postganglionic neuron when they have reached the vicinity of the target organ (either in an autonomic plexus or in an intramural ganglion, i.e., a ganglion located within the wall of the organ in question). The **postganglionic neurons** project their axons to the target tissue—for example, the smooth muscle of the internal organs and blood vessels, and various glands. The relationship of the sympathetic fibers exiting the spinal cord to the nerve roots, sympathetic chain, and peripheral nerves is shown in **Fig. 16.1**, while **Fig. 16.2** is an overview of the anatomy of the sympathetic nervous system.

16.1.2 Parasympathetic Nervous System

The **preganglionic neurons** of the parasympathetic nervous system, unlike those of the sympathetic nervous system, are located in two different parts of the central nervous system that lie at a considerable distance from each other: some of them lie in the visceromotor and sensory *brainstem nuclei*, while others lie in the lateral horns of spinal cord segments

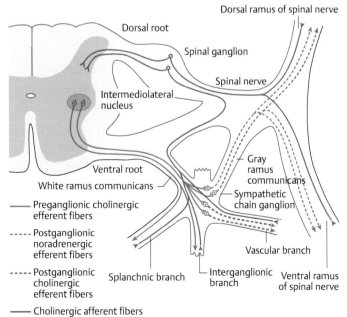

Fig. 16.1 Anatomy of the sympathetic efferent fibers that exit the spinal cord. The sudomotor fibers accompany the spinal nerves (dorsal and ventral rami) to their areas of cutaneous distribution, while the autonomic fibers to the blood vessels and internal organs follow their own paths to their respective targets (vascular ramus, splanchnic ramus).

Dorsal root
Spinal ganglion
Spinal nerve
Dorsal ramus of spinal nerve
Intermediolateral nucleus
Gray ramus communicans
Sympathetic chain ganglion
Ventral root
White ramus communicans
Vascular branch
Interganglioric branch
Ventral ramus of spinal nerve
Splanchnic branch

—— Preganglionic cholinergic efferent fibers
- - - - Postganglionic noradrenergic efferent fibers
- - - - Postganglionic cholinergic efferent fibers
—— Cholinergic afferent fibers

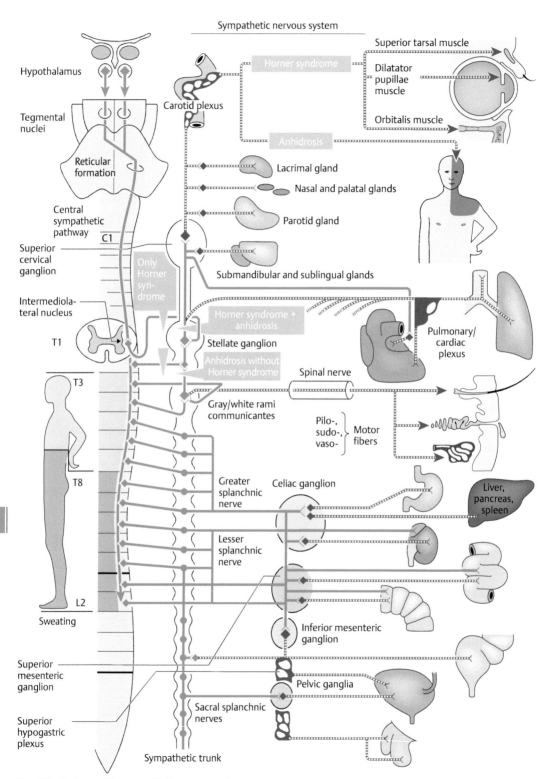

Fig. 16.2 Anatomy of the sympathetic nervous system.

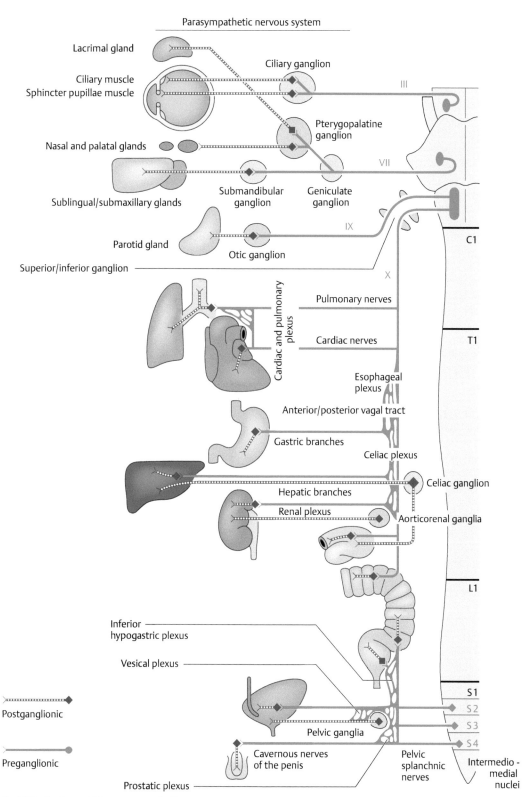

Fig. 16.3   Anatomy of the parasympathetic nervous system.

S2–S4 (the craniosacral system). The axons of the cranial preganglionic neurons exit the brainstem in cranial nerves III, VII, IX, and X and then travel onward to parasympathetic ganglia in the periphery, some of which are intramural, that is, located in the wall of the target organ; inside the parasympathetic ganglia, the preganglionic fibers form synapses onto the postganglionic neurons. The parasympathetic fibers of cranial nerves III, VII, and IX innervate the smooth musculature and glands of the head, while those of the vagus nerve descend in an extensively branched fiber system to innervate the viscera of the throat, thorax, and abdomen, all the way down to the level of the left colic flexure. Beyond this point (the so-called point of Cannon and Böhm), the abdominal and pelvic viscera are innervated by the sacral portion of the parasympathetic nervous system. The axons of the preganglionic neurons whose cell bodies lie in the lateral horns of the sacral spinal cord reach the periphery by way of the anterior roots or the pelvic nerves. They form synapses onto the postganglionic neurons in the pelvic plexus (= inferior hypogastric plexus) or in the intramural ganglia of the abdominal and pelvic viscera. The anatomy of the parasympathetic nervous system is shown in **Fig. 16.3**.

16.2 Normal and Pathologic Function of the Autonomic Nervous System

Key Point
The sympathetic and parasympathetic nervous systems regulate the functions of the internal organs and are responsible for all of the autonomic reflexes of the body. The neurotransmitter used at the synapses of the parasympathetic nervous system is acetylcholine, while the sympathetic nervous system uses acetylcholine at the synapse onto the preganglionic neuron, norepinephrine at the synapse onto the postganglionic neuron, and epinephrine in the adrenal cortex (epinephrine = adrenaline). An overview of the major functions of the two components of the autonomic nervous system is provided in Table 16.1. Diseases of the autonomic nervous system commonly express themselves in disorders of sweating, impairment of bladder, bowel, and sexual function, orthostatic hypotension, and Horner syndrome.

In the following paragraphs, we will describe just a few, clinically relevant functional disturbances and diseases of the autonomic nervous system.

16.2.1 Sweating
The autonomic fibers innervating the sweat glands are exclusively sympathetic. They run in the peripheral nerves together with the somatosensory fibers that innervate the same area of skin. A lesion of a peripheral nerve, therefore, always impairs sweating in the sensory cutaneous distribution of the nerve. The impairment of sweating can be demonstrated with various tests, such as the **ninhydrin test**.

16.2.2 Bladder, Bowel, and Sexual Function

Anatomy
The neural elements that control bladder, bowel, and sexual function are the following:
— **Sympathetic fibers from spinal cord segments T12–L2** and **parasympathetic fibers from spinal cord segments S2–S4** innervate the smooth muscle of the urinary bladder, rectum, and internal genitalia, including the corpora cavernosa. The sympathetic fibers travel to their target organs after a synaptic relay in the superior and inferior hypogastric plexuses, while the parasympathetic fibers do so after a synaptic relay in the inferior hypogastric plexus. There are ganglion cells and synapses not just in the plexuses, but also within the walls of the target organs. Viscerosensory (afferent) fibers return to the spinal cord from the urinary bladder, genitalia, and rectum.
— The spinal center for micturition and defecation receives **supranuclear input from multiple higher cortical areas** (paracentral lobule: voluntary initiation of micturition and defecation) through several different pathways in the spinal cord, and it also sends afferent information back upward to the brain (conscious perception of bladder filling and of noxious and thermal stimuli). These mechanisms are the basis of the voluntary control of micturition and defecation.
— The striated skeletal muscle of the pelvic floor and of the external sphincters of the bladder and rectum, which are under voluntary control, is innervated by the **pudendal nerve**, whose fibers are derived from spinal cord segments S2–S4. This nerve also conveys somatosensory afferent impulses from the urethra, prostate gland, anal canal, and external genitalia.

Disturbances of Bladder, Bowel, and Sexual Function
The clinical manifestations depend on the site of the lesion (peripheral/central, unilateral/bilateral).
Spinal cord transection. Spinal cord transection above the sacral level cuts off the bladder and bowel

from the supraspinally derived (cortical) impulses subserving the voluntary control of micturition and defecation, but the sacral micturition center in the cord and all of the afferent and efferent nerve pathways of the bladder remain intact, including the spinal reflex arc for bladder emptying. The result is a **spastic (automatic) neurogenic bladder**, which empties itself reflexively whenever it is filled to a certain volume (**Fig. 16.4**). In male patients, penile erection remains possible, though there may be retrograde ejaculation into the bladder.

Table 16.1

Functions of the sympathetic and parasympathetic nervous systems

Organ	Effect of the sympathetic nervous system	Effect of the parasympathetic nervous system
Eye	Pupillary dilation	Pupillary constriction
— Dilator pupillae muscle		
— Sphincter pupillae muscle		
Vascular smooth muscle	Vasoconstriction in certain areas of the body, e.g., the skin	Vasodilatation in certain areas of the body, e.g., the GI tract
Salivary glands	Diminished secretion	Increased secretion
Sweat glands	Increased secretion	
Lacrimal glands		Increased secretion
Glands of the GI tract		Increased secretion
Smooth muscle of the GI tract	Diminished motility and peristalsis	Increased motility and peristalsis
Bronchial smooth muscle	Bronchodilation	Bronchoconstriction
Heart	Increased heart rate	Decreased heart rate
Smooth muscle of the vesical wall	Urinary retention	Micturition
Sphincters	Urinary retention	Micturition

Abbreviation: GI, gastrointestinal.

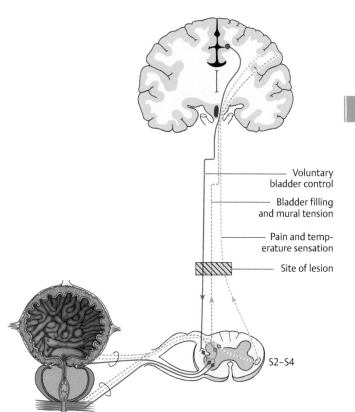

Voluntary bladder control

Bladder filling and mural tension

Pain and temperature sensation

Site of lesion

S2–S4

Fig. 16.4 Spastic neurogenic bladder. The bladder is cut off from the influence of the central nervous system above the level of the lesion, but the spinal reflex arc controlling micturition remains intact and is automatically activated whenever the bladder is filled to a certain volume.

16

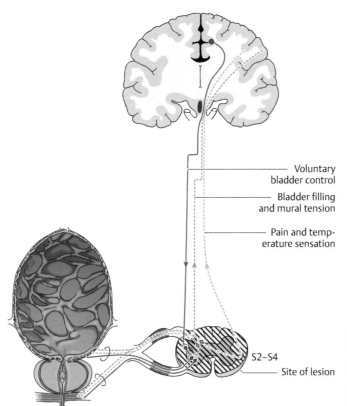

Voluntary bladder control

Bladder filling and mural tension

Pain and temperature sensation

S2–S4

Site of lesion

Fig. 16.5 Flaccid neurogenic bladder. The sacral micturition center is destroyed, and the vesical musculature can therefore no longer be induced to contract. The bladder fills until the intravesical pressure exceeds that of the external vesical sphincter; thereafter, urine is released in small quantities at shorter than normal intervals. The bladder can no longer be completely emptied.

Spinal cord lesions in such disorders as multiple sclerosis can also cause **detrusor-sphincter dyssynergy**. In this condition, the bladder cannot be fully emptied when the detrusor muscle is activated, because the sphincter is simultaneously contracted. Urine often flows back upward into the ureters and renal pelves (vesicoureteral reflux).

Lesions of the conus medullaris, cauda equina, sacral plexus, and pelvic plexus. These lesions inactivate the sacral centers for micturition and defecation. The result is **atony of the bladder and bowel musculature**, leading to severe impairment of emptying. Bladder filling can no longer be perceived. Tone is preserved in the sympathetically innervated internal vesical sphincter; the bladder, therefore, continues to fill until the passive intravesical pressure overcomes the closing force of the sphincter. The continually overfilled bladder lets out small amounts of urine at short intervals (**overflow incontinence, Fig. 16.5**— alternative terms: **hypocontractile detrusor**, **flaccid bladder**, **autonomic bladder**). Defecation, meanwhile, occurs passively and in uncontrolled fashion through a patulous anal sphincter.

Moreover, in the male, lesions of these structures cause erectile impotence. Psychosexually mediated arousal remains possible in rare cases because of the preserved sympathetic efferent innervation through the hypogastric plexus. Thus, a small number of affected men are still able to have an emission of semen, but without ejaculation, and without rhythmic contraction of the pelvic floor muscles.

Lesions of the pudendal nerve. An isolated lesion of the pudendal nerve, which contains parasympathetic fibers from segments S2–S4, causes **erectile dysfunction**: the sacral erection center can no longer be activated because its somatosensory afferent input has been interrupted. Moreover, because the somatic efferent impulses to the bulbocavernosus and ischiocavernosus muscles no longer reach their targets, the maximal tumescence of the corpora cavernosa mediated by these muscles also fails to occur.

Impairment of the sympathetic innervation of the pelvic organs can be caused, for example, by lumbar tumor infiltration or by surgical procedures. Bilateral lesions of the sympathetic chain and lesions of the superior hypogastric plexus abolish seminal emission into the proximal urethra; if ejaculation does occur, then the semen goes into the bladder, in retrograde fashion. As long as the parasympathetic innervation of the genital organs by the pelvic plexus and their somatic sensory and motor innervation by the pudendal nerve remain intact, the affected men are still able to have erections, and affected persons of both sexes can still experience pelvic floor contractions and orgasm. This constellation of symptoms (**preserved ability to experience orgasm, but without seminal emission**) is seen in about half of all men who have undergone bilateral sympathectomy. It does not occur after unilateral lumbar sympathectomy.

16.2.3 The Cervical Sympathetic Pathway and Horner Syndrome

Anatomy
As already discussed at the beginning of this chapter, the spinal cord nuclei in which sympathetic impulses originate are present only from the T2 level downward. Thus, the sympathetic fibers innervating the head must ascend from the thoracic spinal cord and the thoracic segments of the sympathetic chain, by way of the interganglionic branches, to the **cervical sympathetic chain**, where they make a synaptic relay onto the second neuron in one of the three **cervical ganglia** (including the **stellate ganglion**). From these ganglia, the sympathetic fibers continue upward in **periarterial nerve plexuses** until they reach their destinations. Sympathetic fibers in the head innervate the walls of the blood vessels, the sweat glands, and the salivary, lacrimal, nasal, and palatal glands, as well as the dilator pupillae muscle, a smooth muscle. See also **Fig. 16.2**.

Lesions of the Cervical Sympathetic Pathway
Destruction of the stellate ganglion or of the cervical sympathetic chain causes **Horner syndrome**: the pupil is (unilaterally) narrow and, when the patient looks slightly downward, ptosis is evident, or at least a narrowed palpebral fissure. Horner syndrome is usually associated with loss of sweating on the ipsilateral upper quadrant of the body, particularly on the neck and face; depending on the level of the lesion, the arm, hand, and axilla may be affected as well. If the sympathetic chain is interrupted immediately below the stellate ganglion, anhidrosis of the upper quadrant of the body results, but without Horner syndrome. On the other hand, isolated Horner syndrome without anhidrosis can occur as the result of a lesion of the C8–T2 nerve roots between the spinal cord and the sympathetic chain. If the sympathetic pathway is interrupted at the level of the carotid plexus, for example, by carotid dissection, Horner syndrome arises with anhidrosis restricted to the forehead.

16.2.4 Generalized Autonomic Dysfunction
Polyneuropathy often involves autonomic as well as somatic fibers. Affected persons suffer from impaired regulation of blood pressure and sweating, as well as from diarrhea, impaired micturition, and erectile dysfunction. Autonomic manifestations of these kinds are particularly common in **diabetic polyneuropathy**.
Acute pandysautonomia is a type of neuropathy affecting either pre- or postganglionic autonomic nerve fibers. The clinical manifestations include orthostatic hypotension, an invariant heart rate, a lack of sweating and lacrimation, nonreactive midsized pupils, impotence, and an atonic bladder. The cause of this condition is unknown; it gradually resolves spontaneously over the course of a few months.
Familial dysautonomia (Riley) is a hereditary disease with an autosomal recessive inheritance pattern. Its manifestations are probably due to a disturbance of norepinephrine synthesis. They are already evident in infancy and include dysphagia, lack of tears when the infant cries, abnormally intense sweating, diminished ability to feel pain, and impaired temperature regulation. The prognosis is poor.
Certain **other diseases** are accompanied by autonomic dysfunction, including several degenerative diseases of the basal ganglia. Autonomic dysfunction is progressive in multisystem atrophy (earlier term: orthostatic hypotension of Shy–Drager type) and can also result from botulinus intoxication and from congenital sensory neuropathy with anhidrosis.

16

Index